Biology of
the Kinetoplastida

Volume 2

Biology of the Kinetoplastida

Volume 2

Edited by

W. H. R. LUMSDEN

and

D. A. EVANS

Department of Medical Protozoology
London School of Hygiene and Tropical Medicine,
London, England

1979

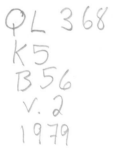Academic Press
London   New York   San Francisco
A Subsidiary of Harcourt Brace Jovanovich, Publishers

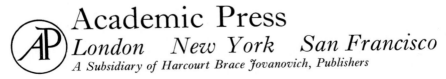

ACADEMIC PRESS INC. (LONDON) LTD.
24/28 Oval Road,
London NW1

United States Edition published by
ACADEMIC PRESS INC:
111 Fifth Avenue
New York, New York 10003

British Library Cataloguing in Publication Data

Biology of the kinetoplastida.

Vol. 2
1. Kinetoplastida
I. Lumsden, William Hepburn Russell
II. Evans, D A
593′.18   QL368.K5   75–19658
ISBN 0–12–460202–9

PRINTED IN GREAT BRITAIN BY
LATIMER TREND & COMPANY LTD PLYMOUTH

List of Contributors

C. J. Bacchi, Haskins Laboratories and Department of Biology, Pace University, New York, N.Y. 10038, U.S.A.

H. Baker, Department of Medicine and Preventive Medicine and Community Health, New Jersey Medical School, East Orange, New Jersey, U.S.A.

W. E. Gutteridge, Biological Laboratory, University of Kent, Canterbury, Kent, England.

W. J. Herbert, University Department of Bacteriology and Immunology, Western Infirmary, Glasgow, Scotland.

S. H. Hutner, Haskins Laboratories and Department of Biology, Pace University, New York, N.Y. 10038, U.S.A.

D. S. Ketteridge, London School of Hygiene and Tropical Medicine, Keppel Street, Gower Street, London WC1, England.

R. Killick-Kendrick, Medical Research Council External Staff, Department of Zoology and Applied Entomology, Imperial College, South Kensington, London SW7, England.

R. Lainson, The Wellcome Parasitology Unit, Instituto Evandro Chagas, Caixa Postal 3, 66000 Belém, Pará, Brazil.

J. Lom, Institute of Parasitology, Czechoslovak Academy of Sciences, Narodni Tr. 3, Prague 1, Czechoslovakia.

W. H. R. Lumsden, London School of Hygiene and Tropical Medicine, Keppel Street, Gower Street, London WC1, England.

M. A. Miles, London School of Hygiene and Tropical Medicine, Keppel Street, Gower Street, London WC1, England.

W. E. Ormerod, London School of Hygiene and Tropical Medicine, Keppel Street, Gower Street, London WC1, England.

D. Parratt, Department of Bacteriology, Ninewells Hospital Dundee, Scotland.

G. W. Rogerson, Wellcome Research Laboratories, Langley Court, Beckenham, Kent, England.

V. P. Sergiev, Department of Epidemiology, Main Board of Sanitation and Epidemiology, Ministry of Health of the USSR, Moscow, U.S.S.R.

J. J. Shaw, The Wellcome Parasitology Unit, Instituto Evandro Chagas, Caixa Postal 3, 66000, Belém, Pará, Brazil.

B. A. Soughgate, London School of Hygiene and Tropical Medicine, Keppel Street, Gower Street, London WC1, England.

W. L. Tafuri, Department of Pathology and Electron Microscopy Centre, School of Medicine, Federal University of Minas Gerais, Belo Horizonte, Brazil.

G. A. T. Targett, London School of Hygiene and Tropical Medicine, Keppel Street, Gower Street, London WC1, England.

P. Viens, Département de Microbiologie et Immunologie, Université de Montréal, P.O. Box 6128, Montreal 101, Province of Quebec, Canada.

F. G. Wallace, 2603 Cohansey Street, Saint Paul, Minnesota 55113, U.S.A.

V. C. L. C. Wilson, London School of Hygiene and Tropical Medicine, Keppel Street, Gower Street, London WC1, England.

Preface

This, the second volume of the *Biology of the Kinetoplastida*, carries out the intention declared in the preface of the first volume, to redress the preponderance of trypanosomes in that volume by paying especial attention to other members of the Order.

We have received many enquiries regarding the content of a third volume. We do not plan another at present. The factors which decide the support of publishers for review volumes such as these cannot be purely scientific: costs have risen to the extent that even essentially interested workers hesitate to purchase such works for their own personal use and so circulations tend to be limited to libraries. But perhaps the continuation of the series may be reconsidered at some time in the future.

We would like to record our appreciation of the unstinted co-operation which we have received from authors and from the editorial staff of Academic Press, which has made the assembly of Volume 2 an enjoyable and rewarding operation to the Editors.

W. H. R. Lumsden
D. A. Evans

Contents

Contributors v

Preface vii

Introduction xxi

1.   The Role of Animals in the Epidemiology of South
American Leishmaniasis
R. Lainson and J. J. Shaw 1

  I. Introduction. 2

  II. Past classification of the neotropical leishmanias. . . 3

  III. Revised classification of the leishmanias 8
      A. Section Hypopylaria 9
      B. Section Peripylaria 9
      C. Section Suprapylaria 9

  IV. Assessment of the importance of phlebotomine sandflies and
mammals as reservoirs of human leishmaniasis . . 14
      A. The human population 14
      B. The phlebotomine sandfly population . . . 15
      C. Mammalian hosts, other than man 22
      D. Detection and isolation of *Leishmania* . . . 27

  V. Neotropical Hypopylaria 34

  VI. Neotropical Peripylaria 35
      A. *Leishmania braziliensis braziliensis* 36
      B. *Leishmania braziliensis guyanensis* 38
      C. *Leishmania braziliensis panamensis* 39
      D. *Leishmania braziliensis*: unidentified subspecies . . 44

  VII. Neotropical Suprapylaria 48
      A. *Leishmania mexicana mexicana* 49
      B. *Leishmania mexicana amazonensis* 55
      C. *Leishmania mexicana pifanoi* 60
      D. *Leishmania mexicana aristedesi* 61
      E. *Leishmania mexicana*: subspecies from Trinidad. . 63
      F. *Leishmania enriettii* 65
      G. *Leishmania hertigi hertigi* 66
      H. *Leishmania hertigi deanei* 67
      I. *Leishmania chagasi*. 68
      J. Unidentified Neotropical Suprapylaria . . . 90

VIII. Neotropical leishmanias of uncertain taxonomic position . 91
      A. *Leishmania peruviana* 91

IX. Concluding remarks 97

X. Acknowledgements 97

XI. References 98

2.   Transmission Cycles and the Heterogeneity of *Trypanosoma cruzi*
      M. A. MILES 117

I. Introduction. 118

II. Morphological and behavioural criteria for the identification of *T. cruzi* 120

III. Diagnosis and survey methods 121

IV. Distribution and transmission cycles 124
      A. Distribution 124
      B. Secondary modes of transmission 125
      C. Transmission cycles 126

V. Circumstantial evidence of the heterogeneity of *T. cruzi* . 137
      A. Biometric comparisons 137
      B. Ultrastructure 138
      C. Virulence and histotropism 138
      D. Enteromegaly 140
      E. Drug sensitivity 141
      F. Infectivity to vectors 142
      G. Immunological differentiation 143

VI. Biochemical characterization—enzyme electrophoresis and DNA studies 144

VII. Prospects of Chagas' disease research 153
      A. Immune response, immunopathogenesis and vaccination 153
      B. Chemotherapy 155
      C. Vector control 156

VIII. Concluding remarks 156

IX. Acknowledgements 157

X. References 157

XI. Appendix 172

      Addendum 184

3.   Epidemiology of Leishmaniasis in the USSR
      V. P. SERGIEV   197

   I.   Zoonotic cutaneous leishmaniases   198

  II.   Anthroponotic cutaneous leishmaniasis   206

 III.   Visceral leishmaniasis   208

  IV.   Conclusion   209

   V.   References   209

4.   Biology of the Kinetoplastida of Arthropods
      F. G. WALLACE   213

   I.   Introduction.   213

  II.   Morphology   215

 III.   Life cycles   216

  IV.   Transmission   218

   V.   Site in host and pathogenicity   219

  VI.   Endosymbionts   219

 VII.   Methods of study   221

VIII.   Systematics   224
         A. Genus *Leptomonas* Kent, 1880   225
         B. Genus *Herpetomonas* Kent, 1880   226
         C. Genus *Crithidia* Léger, 1902   230
         D. Genus *Blastocrithidia* Laird, 1959   233
         E. Genus *Rhynchoidomonas* Patton, 1910   .   .   .   235

  IX.   References   235

5.   Lizard *Leishmania*
      VANESSA C. L. C. WILSON and B. A. SOUTHGATE   .   241

   I.   Historical aspects and evolutionary trends.   .   .   .   242

  II.   Species   243
         A. Lizard parasites   243
         B. Reptilian hosts   243

 III.   Morphology and life cycle   245
         A. Lizard parasite   245
         B. Transmission and vector   247

IV. Relationship of lizard and mammalian leishmaniae . . 248
    A. Susceptibility of lizards to promastigotes of *Leishmania* species 248
    B. Susceptibility of mammals to lizard leishmaniae . 250

V. Leishmaniae of lizards and human leishmaniasis . . 253
    A. Serology 253
    B. Cross immunity between leishmaniae of lizards and man 256
    C. Lizard *Leishmania* and human epidemiology . . 260

VI. Physiology and biochemistry 261

VII. References 263

6.   Biology of the Trypanosomes and Trypanoplasms of Fish
    Jiří Lom 269

I. Introduction 270

II. Cell structure 271
    A. *Trypanosoma* Gruby 271
    B. *Trypanoplasma* Laveran and Mesnil . . . 275

III. Life cycle 279
    A. Transmission 279
    B. Vector phase of the life cycle 280
    C. Vertebrate phase of the life cycle 285
    D. Course of spontaneous infections in nature . . 301

IV. *In vitro* culture 303
    A. *Trypanosoma* 303
    B. *Trypanoplasma* 306

V. Taxonomic considerations 307
    A. *Trypanosoma* 307
    B. *Trypanoplasma* 320

VI. Technique of investigation 325

VII. Conclusions 327

VIII. Acknowledgements 327

IX. References 328

7.   Development of *Trypanosoma brucei* in the Mammalian Host
    W. E. Ormerod 339

I. Introduction 340
    A. Taxonomy of *Trypanosoma brucei* 341

II. The significance of pleomorphic stages in the blood . . 342
    A. Variability of blood trypomastigotes. . . . 342
    B. Methods of examination. 342
    C. Hypotheses to account for the variability of blood forms 345
    D. Filaments of trypomastigotes 352
    E. A view of the significance of pleomorphism . . 353

III. The significance of "Aberrant" forms in the blood . . 354
    A. Spherical forms and "tadpole" forms . . . 354
    B. Filtration of infective blood and tissues . . . 355
    C. Multinucleate forms 356

IV. The significance of culture forms 357

V. Remission, relapse and the relation between parasitaemia and
    pathological lesion 358
    A. Experimental production of remissions . . . 359

VI. Metabolic and fine structural difference between different
    stages and their implications for the life cycle. . . 360
    A. The chondriome 360
    B. Differences in lipid metabolism . . . 361
    C. The autophagosome 362

VII. Tissue stages of *T. brucei* 363
    A. The chancre 363
    B. Lymphatic spread 364
    C. Absence of trypanosomes from the blood . . . 364
    D. Plasmodial and other multinuclear forms . . . 365
    E. Spherical forms and "latent" bodies. . . . 365
    F. The attitude of English-speaking workers . . . 371
    G. The attitude of Italian workers 372
    H. The rediscovery of tissue forms 373

VIII. Hypothetical life cycles of *T. brucei* 375
    A. Sexual dimorphism of blood forms 375
    B. The classical hypothesis 376
    C. The persistence of latent bodies 377
    D. The "two cycle hypothesis" 379
    E. The multinucleate hypothesis 381

IX. Conclusion 383

X. Acknowledgements 384

XI. References 384

8. Biology of *Leishmania* in Phlebotamine Sandflies
    R. Killick-Kendrick 395

I. Introduction. 396

II. Life cycles in the sandfly 398
    A. Mammalian leishmanias 400
    B. Saurian leishmanias 423

III. Pathogenicity of leishmanias to sandflies 428

IV. Factors affecting development in the sandfly . . . 429
    A. Intrinsic insusceptibility of some sandflies. . . 430
    B. Number of parasites ingested 433
    C. Time, temperature and humidity 435
    D. The infecting meal and digestion 437
    E. Sugars 438
    F. Attachment to chitin and invasion of the head . . 441
    G. Concomitant infections 442

V. Physiology and behaviour of sandflies 443

VI. Summary and conclusions 447

VII. Acknowledgements 449

VIII. References 449

9. Immunity to *Trypanosoma* (*Herpetosoma*) Infections
in Rodents
    G. A. T. TARGETT and P. VIENS 461

I. Introduction. 462

II. Course of infection 462

III. Non-immunological factors which determine the pattern of
infection 463

IV. Nature of the immune response 464
    A. Thymus dependency of the immune response . . 464
    B. Immunodepressive treatment 465
    C. Passive transfer of immunity with serum and cells . 466
    D. Trypanocidal antibodies and serological responses to
infection 467
    E. Ablastin 468

V. Antigens, antigenic variation and the cell surface . . 473

VI. Immunization 473

VII. Persistence of infection 474

VIII. Comment 475

IX. References 476

10.   Virulence of Trypanosomes in the Vertebrate Host
       W. J. HERBERT and D. PARRATT   481

   I. Introduction to virulence   482
       A. Definitions   482
       B. Evaluation   482
       C. Pathological basis   485

   II. Evolutionary aspects of virulence   486
       A. Evolutionary adaptation   486
       B. Identification of the natural host   487

  III. Virulence of a single species of trypanosome in different
       vertebrate hosts   491
       A. Range of virulence in different hosts   .   .   .   491
       B. Influence of body-size of the host   493

  IV. Virulence of different stocks of a single species .   .   .   494

   V. Differences in virulence amongst the variable antigen types
       of a trypanosome serodeme   497

  VI. Changes in virulence following passage   500
       A. In laboratory animals or other "unnatural" hosts   .   500
       B. In "natural" hosts.   502

 VII. Changes in virulence induced by drugs   504

VIII. Variation in virulence following exposure to high ambient
       temperatures   504

  IX. General discussion   505
       A. How should the term "virulence" be defined?   .   .   506
       B. Microorganismal multiplication and virulence   .   .   506
       C. Mechanisms of trypanosome pathogenicity in relation
          to virulence   511
       D. Conclusion   514

   X. Acknowledgements   514

  XI. References   515

11.   Heterophile Antibodies in Trypanosome Infections
       D. PARRATT and W. J. HERBERT   523

   I. Introduction.   524

   II. The nature of heterophile antigens   524

  III. The nature of heterophile antibodies   528

IV. Heterophile erythrocyte antibodies in human trypanosomiasis 530
    A. Introduction. 530
    B. Differentiation of the heterophile responses in *Trypanosoma brucei rhodesiense* and *T. b. gambiense* infections 532

V. Antibody specificity of the elevated immunoglobulin levels seen in trypanosomiasis 533

VI. Application of heterophile antibodies for the diagnosis of trypanosomiasis 535

VII. Heterophile antibodies in trypanosomiasis caused by *Trypanosoma* other than *T. brucei* sub-species *gambiense* and *rhodesiense* 537

VIII. Conclusions 539
    A. Diagnostic significance 539
    B. Biological significance 541

IX. Acknowledgements 542

X. References 542

XI. Appendix I 544

XII. Appendix II 544

12. Pathogenesis of *Trypanosoma cruzi* Infections
W. L. TAFURI 547

I. Pathogenetic concept. Parasite- and host-dependent factors playing a role in the pathogenesis of *Trypanosoma cruzi* infections 547
    A. Parasite-dependent factors 548
    B. Host-dependent factors 550

II. Natural history of *T. cruzi* infections 552
    A. The acute phase of *T. cruzi* infections . . . 553
    B. The chronic phase of *T. cruzi* infections . . . 591

III. Lesions of the central nervous system in *T. cruzi* infections. 607

IV. Concluding remarks 609

V. Acknowledgements 609

VI. References 610

13. Biochemical Aspects of the Biology of *Trypanosoma cruzi*
W. E. GUTTERIDGE and G. W. ROGERSON . . . 619

I. Introduction. 620

II. Morphological changes 621

III. Isolation of the various morphological forms . . . 623

IV. Energy metabolism 625
    A. Substrates utilized. 625
    B. End products of metabolism 626
    C. Pathways of metabolism 627
    D. Oxidation of reduced pyridine nucleotides . . 629
    E. Synthesis of ATP 633
    F. Conclusions 634

V. Nucleic acid metabolism 636
    A. Purine metabolism 636
    B. Pyrimidine metabolism 638
    C. Deoxyribonucleotide metabolism 641
    D. Nucleic acid synthesis 642
    E. DNA, especially kinetoplast DNA 643
    F. RNA 644
    G. Nucleic acid catabolism 644
    H. Conclusions 644

VI. Discussion and Conclusions 645

VII. Acknowledgements 647

VIII. References 647

14. Nutrition of the Kinetoplastida
    S. H. HUTNER, C. J. BACCHI and H. BAKER . . 653

I. Introduction. 654

II. Kinetoplastid origins; inferences from nutrition. . . 658

III. *Crithidia fasciculata* as point of departure for nutritional in-
    vestigations; substrates for trypanosomatids . . . 660
    A. Basic requirements 660
    B. Haem and Protoporphyrin 668
    C. Long-chain fatty acids 670
    D. Amino acids; purines and pyramidines; vitaminic
       growth factors 671
    E. Temperature factors 677

IV. Endosymbionts; detection of external contaminants . . 677

V. Lower trypanosomatids, *Leishmania* and *Trypanosoma* com-
    pared . . . . : 678

VI. A perspective 680

VII. Acknowledgements 681

VIII. References 681

15.   Characterization, Nomenclature and Maintenance of
       Salivarian Trypanosomes
       W. H. R. Lumsden and D. S. Ketteridge   .   .   693

I.   Introduction.   694
       A. Current usages in characterization and taxonomy   .   695
       B. Deficiencies of current usages   695
       C. Requirements of a serviceable system   .   .   .   697
       D. Reviews of practice in allied fields   697

II.   Characterization Techniques and their Limitations   .   .   699
       A. Intrinsic characters   699
       B. Extrinsic characters   707
       C. Numerical taxonomy   710
       D. Consideration of usefulness of different characters   .   710

III.   Definitions and Nomenclature.   711
       A. Terms relating to Linnaean taxa   .   .   .   711
       B. Operational terms without implication of characteriza-
           tion   711
       C. Terms implying characterization   .   .   .   712
       D. Nomenclature of variable antigen types (VATs).   .   712

IV.   Relationship of characterized populations to Linnaean taxa .   713
       A. Genus   713
       B. Section   713
       C. Subgenus   713
       D. Species and subspecies   713

V.   Maintenance of reference collections.   .   .   .   714
       A. Living organisms   714
       B. Antigens   714
       C. Antisera   714
       D. Biochemical products   714

VI.   Documentation of reference collections   .   .   .   715
       A. Designation of materials.   .   .   .   715

VII.   References   715

VIII.   Appendix A   719

IX.   Appendix B   720

X.   Appendix C   721

Contents of Volume 1

VICKERMAN, K. The Diversity of the Kinetoplastid Flagellates.

VICKERMAN, K. and PRESTON, T. M. Comparative Cell Biology of the Kinetoplastid Flagellates.

BAKER, J. R. Biology of the Trypanosomes of Birds.

MARINKELLE, C. J. Biology of the Trypanosomes of Bats.

MARINKELLE, C. J. The Biology of the Trypanosomes of Non-Human Primates.

WELLS, E. A. Subgenus *Megatrypanum*.

MOLYNEUX, D. H. Biology of Trypanosomes of the Subgenus *Herpetosoma*.

D'ALESSANDRO, A. Biology of *Trypanosoma* (*Herpetosoma*) *rangeli* Tejera.

NEWTON, B. A. Biochemical approaches to the Taxonomy of Kinetoplastid Flagellates.

BOWMAN, I. B. R. and FLYNN, I. W. Oxidative Metabolism of Trypanosomes.

TERRY, R. J. Innate Resistance to Trypanosome Infections.

GRAY, A. R. and LUCKINS, A. G. Antigenic Variation in Salivarian Trypanosomes.

Dedication

This volume is dedicated to Professor Bronislaw Mark Honigberg who recognized the essential similarity of these organisms by creating the Order Kinetoplastida; and who led the team which revised the classification of the Phylum Protozoa, which revision has greatly aided the systematic advance of protozoology.

Introduction

The days when the Editors of a collection of reviews make Olympian comments upon the contributions which they have marshalled have departed, for what reader will now stop to read these when the real meat of the actual review of his interest is within his grasp? Yet editors may perhaps still be permitted some short survey of what they feel they have accomplished and some remark upon what they consider the significance of their collaboration.

Volume 1 of the *Biology of the Kinetoplastida* was fairly homogeneous: after a definition of the whole scope of the Kinetoplastida, all the other reviews related to one genus of the Order, *Trypanosoma*. The present volume is, by comparison, heterogeneous. Trypanosomes which, because of their pre-eminent importance to man, attract the lion's share of research effort are bound still to figure largely, but they compose only about half the book, the other half dealing with *Leishmania*, other kinetoplastids, or with general aspects.

Two diseases caused by Kinetoplastida, leishmaniasis and trypanosomiasis, have been selected for special attention by the World Health Organization Special Programme for Research and Training in Tropical Diseases. Many of the reviews in this volume will be useful bases for studies of these diseases—those reviews which deal with the development of the organisms in the vertebrate host and in the vector, the immunological response to invasion and mechanisms of pathogenesis, and the patterns of transmission and survival of these organisms in nature. Reviews of the kinetoplastids of lizards, of fish and of insects, and of kinetoplastid nutrition, round out the treatment of the Order, giving attention to some members of it not of immediate economic significance.

For a subject to progress well scientifically it is important that all those working in it should clearly understand one another. It is, however, sometimes the case that people working separated from one another differ in their understanding of the terms used, so that statements may be misinterpreted in discussion. We have, therefore, included one contribution dealing with this problem—the discussions of an international group on the characterization, nomenclature and maintenance of salivarian trypanosomes, which lead up to proposals for internationally acceptable terms, which may also be pertinent to other fields.

We feel that our decision to treat the Kinetoplastida as a whole has been justified, and we think that we have contributed to an interchange of concepts and approaches which will be helpful to all those who work on the Order. A final comment on the probable progress of the subject in the future is that the combined impact of cloning, cryopreservation and biochemical characterization of organisms is opening opportunities for the systematic study of the biology of these organisms (and of other Protozoa) in relation to their pathological effect, epidemiology and prevention, which are analogous to those which have been available for the bacteria since the time of Koch and for the arboviruses since the time of Theiler.

W. H. R. Lumsden
D. A. Evans

1

The Role of Animals in the Epidemiology of South American Leishmaniasis

R. LAINSON

and

J. J. SHAW

Instituto Evandro Chagas,
Fundação Serviços de Saúde Pública,
C. P. 3, Belém, Pará, Brazil

I.	Introduction	2
II.	Past classification of the neotropical leishmanias	3
III.	Revised classification of the leishmanias	8
	A. Section Hypopylaria	9
	B. Section Peripylaria	9
	C. Section Suprapylaria	9
IV.	Assessment of the importance of phlebotomine sandflies and mammals as reservoirs of human leishmaniasis	14
	A. The human population	14
	B. The phlebotomine sandfly population	15
	C. Mammalian hosts, other than man	22
	D. Detection and isolation of *Leishmania*	27
V.	Neotropical Hypopylaria	34
VI.	Neotropical Peripylaria	35
	A. *Leishmania braziliensis braziliensis*	36
	B. *Leishmania braziliensis guyanensis*	38
	C. *Leishmania braziliensis panamensis*	39
	D. *Leishmania braziliensis*: unidentified subspecies	44

VII. Neotropical Suprapylaria 48
    A. *Leishmania mexicana mexicana* 49
    B. *Leishmania mexicana amazonensis* 55
    C. *Leishmania mexicana pifanoi* 60
    D. *Leishmania mexicana aristedesi* nov. subsp. . . . 61
    E. *Leishmania mexicana*: unidentified subspecies . . . 63
    F. *Leishmania enriettii* 65
    G. *Leishmania hertigi hertigi* 66
    H. *Leishmania hertigi deanei* 67
    I. *Leishmania chagasi* 68
    J. Unidentified Suprapylaria 90

VIII. Neotropical leishmanias of uncertain taxonomic position . . 91
    A. *Leishmania peruviana* 91

  IX. Concluding remarks 97

   X. Acknowledgements 97

  XI. References 98

I. Introduction

Our broad usage of the word "animals" in the title of this chapter is deliberate, for the invertebrate and vertebrate hosts are of equal importance to the leishmanial parasite, and the role of each is inseparably linked in the epidemiology of leishmaniasis. Indeed, if we accept the general view of the origin of the genus *Leishmania* from monogenetic flagellates of insects, it is more correct to regard the phlebotomine sandfly vectors (Diptera: Psychodidae) as both primary *and* principal hosts of this parasite.

With the development of the haematophagous habit by the primitive insect hosts, and migration of the flagellates to an anterior station in the gut, the leishmanias have gained entrance into certain mammalian hosts in which they have adapted to survive in the amastigote stage. Parasites located in the skin, or circulating in the blood, thus act as a reservoir of infection for some sandfly species.

As far as is known, all forms of American cutaneous and visceral leishmaniasis of man are zoonotic diseases, with the different leishmanias involved originating from a wide variety of wild or, more rarely, domestic mammals. The great majority of these animals live in the dense neotropical forests, where the parasites are transmitted by an equally wide variety of phlebotomine sandflies (Fig. 1); these insects are adapted to live in shady and highly humid conditions, in which they are active principally at night.

Infection in man is thus dependent on his intrusion into these areas of enzootic leishmaniasis, where he may be bitten by infected sandflies. For this reason, silvatic cutaneous leishmaniasis is very much an occupational hazard, mostly afflicting those engaged in the felling and extraction of timber, collection of rubber or chewing-gum latex and other natural forest products, or the clearance of forest for agricultural purposes, road building, etc. Infection extends, too, to those more specialized professions such as topographers, geologists and naturalists: the nighttime activity of professional and amateur hunters puts them at particularly high risk.

There are two notable exceptions to this general pattern of neotropical leishmaniasis of man, which we will discuss in more detail later. "Uta" (a form of cutaneous leishmaniasis rather resembling "oriental-sore" of the Eastern Hemisphere) is apparently restricted to the barren, mountainous areas of the Western Peruvian Andes, although it probably extends into ecologically similar parts of neighbouring countries: certain peridomestic sandflies are suspected as vectors, but complete proof is lacking. American visceral leishmaniasis is found principally in the drier and more poorly forested areas of Latin America, where the sandfly *Lutzomyia longipalpis* is incriminated as the major vector. In both of these situations the dog is an important reservoir of infection, and the sandfly vectors are much more robust and resistant to dryer conditions than are their silvatic relatives.

It is our intention, in this chapter, to draw together all available information on the sandfly hosts of the recognized species or subspecies of *Leishmania* in the Americas, their source of infection in wild or domestic animals, and the importance of certain leishmanias as pathogens for man and some other animals.

II. Past classification of the neotropical leishmanias

Before we can adequately discuss the role of either invertebrate or vertebrate hosts in the epidemiology of neotropical leishmaniasis it is necessary briefly to define the parasites concerned—a task which is still far from easy.

The resurgence of interest in *Leishmania* and leishmaniasis during the past 15 years resulted in an accumulation of data on which it was possible to lay the foundation of a workable classification of the New World parasites (Lainson and Shaw, 1972a, b, 1973; Zuckerman and Lainson, 1977). Based on a variety of biological, immunological and biochemical criteria, the neotropical cutaneous leishmanias were divided into two major groups as follows:

Leishmania mexicana Complex

L. mexicana mexicana: In the Yucatan, Mexico; Belize; and Guatemala. Proven invertebrate host, *Lutzomyia olmeca olmeca.* Vertebrate hosts, wild rodents and man.

L. mexicana amazonensis: In Brazil, Trinidad. Proven invertebrate host, *Lu. flaviscutellata.** Vertebrate hosts, wild rodents, marsupials, and man.

L. mexicana pifanoi: In Venezuela. Invertebrate host unknown. Vertebrate host, man; wild reservoir hosts unknown.

L. mexicana subsp.: In Panama. Invertebrate host unknown. Vertebrate hosts, wild rodents and marsupials.

L. enriettii: In Paraná State, Brazil. Invertebrate host unknown. Vertebrate host, the guinea pig; wild hosts unknown.

L. braziliensis Complex

L. braziliensis braziliensis: In Brazil, Peru, Ecuador, Bolivia, Venezuela, Paraguay, Colombia. Proven invertebrate hosts, *Psychodopygus† wellcomei, Lu. pessoai, Lu. intermedia.* Vertebrate hosts, wild rodents and man.

L. braziliensis guyanensis: In the Guyanas, and north Brazil. Invertebrate hosts, unknown. Vertebrate hosts, man; wild reservoir hosts unknown.

L. braziliensis panamensis: In Panama. Proven invertebrate hosts, *Lu. trapidoi, Lu. gomezi, Ps. panamensis.‡* Vertebrate hosts; edentates, rodents, procyonids, monkeys and man.

L. peruviana: In west Peruvian Andes. Invertebrate hosts, unknown. Vertebrate hosts; the dog and man. Wild animal reservoirs unknown.

L. hertigi: In Panama. Invertebrate hosts unknown. Vertebrate host, the porcupine (*Coendou rothschildi*).

One important biological character we used in the above scheme was the very different behaviour of the flagellated stages of *braziliensis* and *mexicana* parasites in the gut of the sandfly (Hertig and McConnell, 1963; Johnson *et al.*, 1963; McConnell, 1963; Strangways-Dixon and Lainson, 1966; Coelho *et al.*, 1967a, b; Lainson and Shaw, 1968; Johnson and Hertig, 1970; Lainson *et al.*, 1973, 1976, 1977b; Ward *et al.*, 1973a). *L. b. braziliensis, L. b. guyanensis* and *L. b. panamensis* all undergo prolific development in the pylorus or "hind-gut triangle" (Fig.

* The abbreviation *Lu.* is used, throughout, for *Lutzomyia* to avoid confusion with *L.* for *Leishmania.*

† Some authors (Lewis *et al.*, 1977), prefer to use the name *Psychodopygus* as a subgenus of *Lutzomyia*, e.g. *Lutzomyia* (*Psychodopygus*) *wellcomei.*

‡ The abbreviation *Ps.* is used, throughout, for *Psychodopygus*, to avoid confusion with *P.* for *Phlebotomus.*

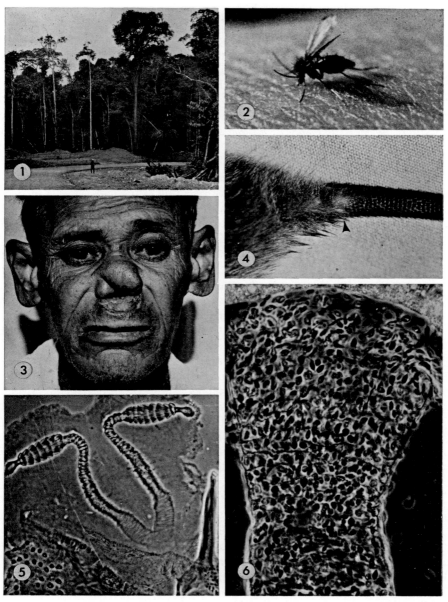

FIG. 1.   Epidemiological aspects of cutaneous and mucocutaneous leishmaniasis in Brazil. 1. Tall, primary forest of the Serra dos Carajás, Pará State, where many men contract cutaneous leishmaniasis due to *Leishmania braziliensis braziliensis*, and where natural infections were found in the sandfly *Psychodopygus wellcomei*. 2. Sandfly biting man. 3. Case of mucocutaneous leishmaniasis caused by *L. b. braziliensis*. 4. Lesion caused by *L. b. braziliensis* on the tail of a naturally infected rodent, *Oryzomys concolor*, from Serra do Roncador, Mato Grosso State. 5. Spermathecae of *Ps. wellcomei*. 6. Pylorus of *Lutzomyia umbratilis* infected with *L. braziliensis guyanensis*. [1 from Ward *et al.*, (1973b); 2 and 4 from Lainson and Shaw (1973).]

1), as well as in the midgut and foregut. In the pylorus the flagellates are predominantly rounded, oval or pear-shaped and firmly attached to the gut wall by their flagellum (for a more detailed account of this attachment, reference should be made to the chapter in this Volume, "Biology of *Leishmania* in the vector", by R. Killick-Kendrick). In striking contrast, this intense hindgut development is not seen in sandflies infected with *L. m. mexicana* and *L. m. amazonensis*, in which growth is limited to the midgut and foregut.

It is very important to remember the morphology and attachment of the hindgut forms of the *L. braziliensis* parasites when one is examining the dissected sandfly. The process of dissection, violent peristalsis of the gut and pressure of the coverslip on the preparation may all contribute to a "backwash" of midgut forms into the hindgut; again, some parasites which are unable to establish themselves well in certain sandfly species will be slowly expelled with the faeces and, at some stage therefore, may be found throughout the hindgut. In either case, such parasites are distinguished by their lack of attachment, elongate form and active swimming movements.

Johnson and Hertig (1970) examined the development of 184 infections of "a strain of *L. mexicana* from Guatemala" in the Panamanian sandflies *Lutzomyia gomezi* and *Lu. sanguinaria*. They noted scanty parasites in the hindgut on rare occasions: "the rarely observed rosettes consisted of oval to spindle-shaped organisms. More usual were single, larger, spindle-shaped to long, thin flagellates attached only by the flagellar tip". The authors nevertheless concluded that *L. mexicana* "typically causes midgut infections alone", and we assume from this that they, too, did not regard the few hindgut forms seen as representing a true development in the pylorus. Hoare (1956) would probably refer to them as the expression of an "atavistic trait" on the part of the Guatemalan parasite. We have seen no evidence of this in 50 specimens of the sandfly *Lu. longipalpis*, experimentally infected with *L. m. mexicana* from Belize (formally British Honduras).

The establishment of closed colonies of *Lu. longipalpis*, a major vector of neotropical visceral leishmaniasis, has enabled observations on the development of a number of *Leishmania* isolates in this insect. Killick-Kendrick *et al.* (1974, 1977b) have found that the pattern of development of *L. m. amazonensis* and *L. b. braziliensis* in this fly is the same as that seen in their natural vectors, and Lainson *et al.* (1977b) have used the presence or absence of pyloric development in *Lu longipalpis* as a means of categorizing recent isolates of *Leishmania* from wild mammals in Brazil. By this method, for example, it was shown that both Brazilian and Panamanian subspecies of *L. hertigi* failed to develop in the pylorus, and for this reason these authors removed the parasite from the *L. braziliensis* complex where they had first placed it.

We have recently discussed the significance of the hindgut development of parasites of the *L. braziliensis* complex in relation to that seen in sandflies infected with a variety of lizard leishmaniae (Lainson *et al.*, 1977b). Many protozoologists support the hypothesis of Léger (1904) that modern Trypanosomatidae evolved from intestinal parasites of arthropods and that the promastigote form was the primitive type (for comprehensive reviews on this subject see Hoare, 1948; Baker, 1963, 1965).

These ancestral flagellates, like their modern counterparts (e.g. *Leptomonas*), presumably occupied the rear part of the arthropod intestine, and spread of infection was by contamination of the environment with cystic, amastigote forms in the faeces.

Arthropods must have formed a prominent part of the diet of certain lizards, and the saurian leishmanias possibly arose when insect flagellates adapted themselves to survival in the gut of the reptilian host. Invasion of the blood and viscera might be regarded as a logical sequence and, in fact, amastigote forms have been demonstrated in some of the lizard leishmanias (Belova, 1971).

With adaptation of the flagellates to life in the peripheral blood of lizards, these reptiles became reservoirs of infections for haematophagous insects (phlebotomine sandflies) in which a major part of the parasite's life-cycle still takes place. The mode of transmission has been poorly studied and remains uncertain: infection of the sandfly must take place after a blood-meal on the infected reptile, but the restriction of the parasites to the posterior part of the insect's intestine in some species of leishmanias such as *L. ceramodactyli* (Adler and Theodor, 1929), suggests that subsequent transmission must take place when the infected sandflies are eaten by another lizard. On the other hand, some other leishmanias of lizards, such as *L. tarentolae* and *L. adleri*, are described as developing in an "anterior station" or the "anterior part of the midgut" (Adler and Theodor, 1929; Heisch, 1958); and Adler (1964) used this feature, with other data, to suggest that "*L. adleri* presents an interesting phase in the evolution of *Leishmania*, i.e. a transition from a purely reptilian to a mammalian parasite". Transmission of *L. tarentolae* and *L. adleri* could, therefore, be by the bite of infected sandflies (although, to our knowledge, final proof of this is still lacking), which has become the mode of dissemination for all those leishmanias now parasitizing mammals.

The primitive hindgut development has disappeared from the life-cycle of most modern leishmanias of mammals, such as those in the *L. mexicana*, *L. tropica* and *L. donovani* groups. In those of the *L. braziliensis* complex, there has also developed a migration to the foregut and mouth-parts, with transmission by the bite of the infected insect: curiously, however, the ancestral hindgut development has persisted, and it still seems to form such an integral part of the life-history of the parasites that it takes place even when sandflies are experimentally infected with promastigotes (Lainson *et al.*, 1977b).

III. Revised classification of the leishmanias

From all the above observations, we have become impressed by the rigidity of developmental pattern of the leishmanias in their sandfly hosts, and feel that this fundamental biological feature should be utilized more strongly than it was in our previous classification of these organisms. This view has to some extent been shared by previous workers on *Leishmania*. Thus, Nicoli (1963) suggested that differentiation on the basis of host-range and host-parasite relationships was artificial and unsatisfactory, and should be replaced by classification based on the vectors and mode of development of the flagellates in the sandfly. He gave as examples the development of the leishmanias of warm-blooded vertebrates in the anterior part of the insect gut, which effectively separates them off from those of cold-blooded animals whose development is restricted to the posterior station. Johnson and Hertig (1970) were clearly impressed by the striking difference in the development of leishmanias of the *L. braziliensis* and *L. mexicana* complexes in their sandfly hosts and suggested that it ". . . may serve as a reliable taxonomic character for the separation of strains or species of *Leishmania*. . . ."

In a modification of Wenyon's classification (1926), Hoare (1964, 1972) divided the mammalian trypanosomes into two Sections: the STER-CORARIA, for those developing in the posterior part of the invertebrate host's gut and with contaminative transmission, and the SALIVARIA, with anterior development and inoculative transmission by bite.

A similar classification of the genus *Leishmania*, based on the mode of development in the gut of the sandfly, seems to us a logical extension of Hoare's scheme. Using the different patterns of development (shown diagrammatically in Fig. I, page 25) we therefore propose to modify our previous grouping of the leishmanias by dividing them into three major Sections, as shown below. These Sections, like those of Hoare, have no taxonomic status.

Classification of the leishmanias

Class ZOOMASTIGOPHOREA Calkins, 1909
Order KINETOPLASTIDA Honigberg, 1963
Suborder TRYPANOSOMATINA Kent, 1880
Family TRYPANOSOMATIDAE Doflein, 1901;
 emend. Grobben, 1905
Genus *Leishmania* Ross, 1903

A. Section HYPOPYLARIA
(from Gk *hypo* = under; Gk *pyl* = gate)

Primitive *Leishmania* species. In the sandfly host the infection moves to a posterior position in the intestine and becomes established in the hindgut (pylorus, ileum and rectum). Reservoir hosts are apparently restricted to lizards, and so far only recorded in Old World species. Parasites in the vertebrate may be in the promastigote and/or the amastigote form, in the blood or viscera. Transmission presumably takes place when the lizard eats infected sandflies.

Leishmania agamae David, 1929
Leishmania ceramodactyli Adler and Theodor, 1929

B. Section PERIPYLARIA
(from Gk *peri* = on all sides; Gk *pyl* = gate)

Leishmanias which still maintain an obligate hindgut development in their sandfly hosts but which, in addition, have now developed an anterior migration to the foregut. The Section includes some lizard parasites of the Old World but is mainly dominated by members of the *L. braziliensis* complex which are limited to mammalian hosts of the Western hemisphere. There is scanty information on the form of the parasite in the lizard hosts, but possibly both promastigote and amastigote stages occur; in mammals the parasites are found only in the amastigote form, in macrophages of the skin, viscera or blood. Transmission of the leishmanias of mammals is inoculative, following the bite of the infected sandfly: that of the lizard parasites may also be by bite, but definite proof is still lacking. All the known species of this Section which infect mammals are accidental and pathogenic parasites in man, causing a variety of cutaneous and/or mucocutaneous leishmaniases.

In lizards: in the Old World.
Leishmania adleri Heisch, 1958
Leishmania tarentolae Wenyon, 1921
In mammals: in the New World.
The *L. braziliensis* Complex
L. braziliensis braziliensis Vianna, 1911
L. braziliensis guyanensis Floch, 1954
L. braziliensis panamensis Lainson and Shaw, 1972

C. Section SUPRAPYLARIA
(from Lat *supra* = above; Gk *pyl* = gate)

Leishmanias which have lost the primitive hindgut development in the sandfly host, with the flagellates now restricted to the midgut and foregut. Vertebrate reservoir hosts in wild and domestic animals of both the Old World and the New World; amastigotes are found in macrophages of the skin, viscera or blood, and transmission is by the bite of the various sandfly vectors. This Section is particularly notable for the two groups of New and Old World parasites, the *L. mexicana* and *L. tropica* complexes: when infecting man, these organisms usually produce a variety of relatively simple and easily curable cutaneous lesions, but they are also capable of causing incurable "diffuse cutaneous leishmaniasis" (DCL) in anergic patients. Also included are Old and New World representatives of the *L. donovani* complex, remarkable for their very exaggerated viscerotropism and resulting high pathogenicity in the human subject.

In mammals: in the New World.

The *L. mexicana* Complex

   Leishmania mexicana mexicana Biagi, 1953
   Leishmania mexicana amazonensis Lainson and Shaw, 1972
   Leishmania mexicana pifanoi Medina and Romero, 1959
   Leishmania mexicana aristedesi nov. subsp.
   Leishmania mexicana subsp., in Trinidad (Tikasingh, 1974)
   Leishmania enriettii Muniz and Medina, 1948

In mammals: in the New World.

The *L. hertigi* Complex

   Leishmania hertigi hertigi Herrer, 1971
   Leishmania hertigi deanei Lainson and Shaw, 1977

The *L. donovani* Complex

In mammals: in the Old World.

   Leishmania donovani (Laveran and Mesnil, 1903)
   Leishmania infantum Nicolle, 1908

In mammals: in the New World.

   Leishmania chagasi Cunha and Chagas, 1937

In mammals: in the Old World.

The *L. tropica* Complex

   Leishmania tropica (Wright, 1903)
   Leishmania major Yakimov and Schockov, 1914
   Leishmania aethiopica Bray, Ashford and Bray, 1973

The lizard parasite *L. adleri* has been shown to produce cryptic, visceral infections in hamsters and transient skin infections in man (Adler, 1964; Manson-Bahr and Heisch, 1961). This and antigenic relationships with mammalian leishmanias (Adler and Adler, 1955) suggests that this parasite represents an evolutionary link between the lizard and mammalian leishmanias.

There remain some species of *Leishmania* which at present are difficult to assign to their correct Section: these include *L. peruviana* Velez, 1913, the cause of "uta" of dogs and man in the western Peruvian Andes, and a number of little studied saurian leishmanias. Among the latter are *L. gymnodactyli* Khodukin and Sofiev, 1947; *L. hemidactyli* Mackie, Gupta and Swaminath, 1923; *L. hoogstraali* McMillan, 1965; *L. zmeevi* Andrushko and Markov, 1955. Experimental infection of sandflies with these parasites, in particular those species suspected as vectors, would be a most rewarding study.

Following observations on the behaviour of *L. hertigi* from Panamanian and Brazilian porcupines (*Coendou* spp.) in sandflies (Lainson *et al.*, 1977b) it has been necessary to remove the parasite from the *L. braziliensis* complex of our previous classification (Lainson and Shaw, 1973). Subspecies of *L. hertigi* are now placed as a separate group within the Suprapylaria (see Part VII, G and H).

Within the *L. mexicana* complex, we propose giving new subspecific rank to the parasite isolated from rodents and an opossum in Panama (Herrer *et al.*, 1971, 1973) and name it *Leishmania mexicana aristedesi* nov. subsp., after Dr. Aristides Herrer who has contributed so much to our knowledge of Panamanian cutaneous leishmaniasis. The parasite is distinguished from other subspecies of *L. mexicana* by biochemical means (Chance *et al.*, 1974; Gardener *et al.*, 1974), using analyses of DNA buoyant densities and electrophoretic variation of malate dehydrogenase. Mammalian hosts include the rodents *Proechimys semispinosus*, *Oryzomys capito* and *Agouti paca*, and the opossum *Marmosa robinsoni*: infection in man has not yet been recorded. The sandfly *Lutzomyia olmeca bicolor* is strongly suspected as the vector on enzootological grounds (Herrer *et al.*, 1971; Christensen *et al.*, 1972). In the hamster, *L. m. aristedesi* produces the large, metastasizing histiocytomata, extremely rich in parasites, which are characteristic of most of the other known members of the *L. mexicana* complex (Fig. 5). The organism will be discussed further in Part VII, D.

There is one other small change in our previous classification: here, we have listed the Trinidadian parasite described as *L. mexicana amazonensis* by Tikasingh (1974) simply as *L. mexicana* subsp. Trinidad is geographically isolated from the type locality of *L. m. amazonensis* in Belém, Brazil, and the parasite may very well be closer to *L. m. pifanoi* from neighbouring Venezuela. It is hoped that continued comparison of the *L. mexicana* subspecies will eventually clarify the situation. Again, this parasite is discussed more fully in Part VII, J.

The old custom of treating the leishmanias from the "Old World" and the "New World" as two separate groups is not, taxonomically, very sound: the proposed use of the three Sections, outlined above, will hopefully offer more freedom for the sub-grouping of any leishmanias, from whatever geographical region, according to their other taxonomic characters. It may also help to dispense with the convenient but misguiding illusion that there is a sharp division between parasites causing "cutaneous" and "visceral" leishmaniasis (see Part IV, C).

Table 1. Natural infections of neotropical sandflies and mammals with parasites which probably were *Leishmania*.

Family	Host species	Localization[b]	Possible identity	Country (State)[a]	Reference
Psychodidae	*Lutzomyia migonei*	int	*L. braziliensis*	Brazil (SP)	Pessôa and Pestana (1940)
		int	?	Venezuela (YC)	Pifano (1943)
	Lutzomyia pessoai	int	*L. braziliensis*	Brazil (SP)	Pessôa and Coutinho (1940)
	Lutzomyia whitmani	int	*L. braziliensis*	Brazil (SP)	Pessôa and Coutinho (1941)
	Lutzomyia whitmani	mh-gut	*Leishmania* sp.?*	Brazil (PA)	Lainson and Shaw (unpub. obs.)
	Lutzomyia permira	int	*L. m. mexicana*	Belize	Disney (1968)
	Lutzomyia intermedia	int	*L. braziliensis*	Brazil (PR)	Forattini and Santos (1952)
	Lutzomyia longipalpis	int	?	Venezuela (YC)	Pifano (1943)
	Lutzomyia longipalpis	fm-gut	*L. chagasi*	Brazil (CE)	Deane and Deane (1954c)
	Lutzomyia longipalpis	fmh-gut	?	Panama	Johnson and Hertig (1970)
	Lutzomyia anduzei	int	?	Venezuela (YC)	Pifano (1956)
	Lutzomyia ovallesi	h-gut	?	Belize	Strangways-Dixon and Lainson (1962)
	Lutzomyia cruciata	?	?	Belize	Strangways-Dixon and Lainson (1962)
	Lutzomyia gomezi	int	*Leishmania* sp.?*	Panama	Johnson et al. (1963)
	Lutzomyia gomezi	h-gut	*Leishmania* sp.?*	Brazil (PA)	Lainson and Shaw (unpub. obs.)
	Lutzomyia shannoni	h and mh-gut	*Leishmania* sp.?*	Panama	Johnson et al. (1963)
	Lutzomyia shannoni	int?	?	Costa Rica	Zeledon and Alfaro (1973)
	Lutzomyia sanguinaria	h and mh-gut	*Leishmania* sp.?*	Panama	Johnson et al. (1963)
	Lutzomyia trapidoi	h and mh-gut	*Leishmania* sp.?*	Panama	Johnson et al. (1963)
	Lutzomyia ylephiletor	h and mh-gut	*Leishmania* sp.?*	Panama	Johnson et al. (1963)
	Lutzomyia yuilli	mh-gut	*Leishmania* sp.?*	Brazil (MT)	Lainson et al. (1977c)
	Lutzomyia anduzei ?	int	*L. b. guyanensis*	Surinam	Wijers and Linger (1966)
	Lutzomyia anduzei	mh-gut	*Leishmania* sp.?	Brazil (PA)	Lainson and Shaw (unpub. obs.)
	Lutzomyia tuberculata	fmh-gut	*L. braziliensis*	Brazil (PA)	Lainson and Shaw (unpub. obs.)
	Lutzomyia dendrophila	mh-gut	*Leishmania* sp.?*	Brazil (PA)	Lainson and Shaw (unpub. obs.)
	Lutzomyia antunesi	mh-gut	*Leishmania* sp.?*	Brazil (PA)	Lainson and Shaw (unpub. obs.)
	Lutzomyia furcata	m-gut	*Leishmania* sp.?*	Brazil (PA)	Lainson and Shaw (unpub. obs.)

Family	Host	Localization[b]	Leishmania sp.[?*]	Country (Region)	Reference
?	Psychodopygus davisi?	int	Leishmania sp.?*	Venezuela (YC)	Pifano (1943)
	Psychodopygus panamensis	h and mh-gut	L. b. braziliensis	Panama	Johnson et al. (1963)
	Psychodopygus amazonensis	h-gut	L. b. braziliensis	Brazil (PA)	Lainson et al. (1973)
	Psychodopygus paraensis	int	L. b. braziliensis	Brazil (PA)	Lainson et al. (1973)
	Psychodopygus wellcomei	fmh-gut	L. b. braziliensis	Brazil (PA)	Lainson et al. (1973)
Bradypodidae	Choloepus didactylus	vis	L. braziliensis	Brazil (PA)	Deane (1948)
Echimyidae	Proechimys semispinosus	bld	L. b. panamensis	Panama	Anon (1957)
	Proechimys guyannensis	sk	L. m. pifanoi	Venezuela (BS)	Convit (1968)
	Hoplomys gymnuras	bld	L. b. panamensis	Panama	Anon (1959)
	Kannabateomys amblyonx	bld and sk	L. mexicana sub sp.	Brazil (SP)	Forattini (1960a)
Cricetidae	Oryzomys eliurus	skls	L. mexicana sub sp.	Brazil (RJ)	Barbosa et al. (1970)
	Zygodontomys microtinus	skls	L. m. pifanoi	Venezuela (BS)	Kerdal-Vegas and Essenfeld-Yahr (1966)
Muridae	Rattus rattus	bld	Leishmania sp.	Brazil (CE)	Alencar et al. (1960)
Dasyproctidae	Dasyprocta azarae	bld	L. mexicana sub sp.	Brazil (SP)	Forattini (1960a)
	Agouti paca	bld	L. mexicana sub sp.	Brazil (SP)	Forattini (1960a)
Canidae	Canis familiaris	skls	Leishmania sp.	Brazil (SP)	Pedrosa (1913)
	Canis familiaris	skls	Leishmania sp.	Argentina (TM)	Romaña et al. (1949)
	Canis familiaris	skls	Leishmania sp.	Argentina (SA)	Mazza (1926a)
	Canis familiaris	skls	L. braziliensis	Venezuela (ZA)	Pons (1968)
	Canis familiaris	skls and vis	Leishmania sp.	Venezuela (YC)	Pifano (1940a)
	Canis familiaris	skls	L. m. amazonensis	Brazil (BA)	Sherlock and Almeida (1970b)
Felidae	Felis catus	skls	Leishmania sp.	Brazil (PA)	Mello (1940)
Phyllostomidae	Phyllostomus hastatus	skls	Leishmania sp.	Venezuela (ZA)	Pons (1968)
Equidae	Equus asinus	skls	Leishmania sp.	Brazil (CE)	Alencar (1959)
	Equus asinus	skls	Leishmania sp.	Venezuela (ZA)	Pons (1968)
	Equus caballus	skls	Leishmania sp.	Argentina (TM)	Mazza (1927)

a Abbreviations of: Argentinian states: SA = Salta; TC = Tucumán; Brazilian states: CE = Ceará; PA = Pará; PR = Paraná; RJ = Rio de Janeiro; SP = São Paulo; MT = Mato Grosso; Venezuelan states: BS = Barinas; YC = Yaracuy; ZA = Zuila. b Localization of parasites: bld = blood; fmh-gut = fore, mid and hind gut; h-gut = hind gut; int = intestine; mh-gut = mid and hind gut; sk = skin; skls = skin lesion; vis = viscera. ?* In these cases the citations refer to a number of infections some of which may have been Leishmania, while others might well have been Endotrypanum or another flagellate.

IV. Assessment of the importance of phlebotomine sandfly and mammalian species as reservoirs of human leishmaniasis

In Table 1 we have listed all the records we can find of natural infections of neotropical sandflies and mammals with parasites which *probably* were *Leishmania*. There are 32 instances of unidentified promastigotes from 25 different sandfly species, and 21 cases of unidentified amastigotes from 15 different wild or domestic mammals. This emphasizes the paramount importance of the isolation of such organisms for future study, for until their true identity is known it is impossible even to guess at the importance of such infections in relation to leishmaniasis of man. To assess the epidemiological situation in any given area, we must consider the following.

A. THE HUMAN POPULATION

If a long-established population is present in an area, these people will clearly give the best indication as to the existence and importance of zoonotic leishmaniasis. We stress this point because although certain leishmanias may be found with remarkable frequency in a wide range of wild mammals and show high incidence in the local sandfly vector, infection in humans may be uncommon or absent if the insect host rarely feeds on man (Lainson and Shaw, 1968). This is the situation with *L. mexicana amazonensis* in Brazil, for example, as discussed in later pages.

If human infection is found, attempts should be made to isolate the parasite from as many cases as possible, by the usual culture of material in blood-agar media or by the inoculation of hamsters. The genus *Leishmania* comprises a very heterogenous group of species and subspecies, particularly in neotropical regions, and their distribution clearly must overlap in certain areas. In our experience it is not uncommon, for example, to isolate parasites of the *L. mexicana* and *L. braziliensis* complexes from men working side by side in the same forest region, or from wild animals in the same trapping area (Lainson and Shaw, 1969a, 1970). In the Serra do Roncador region of Mato Grosso State, Brazil, parasites isolated from skin lesions of man proved always due to a parasite of the *L. braziliensis* complex, and mucocutaneous leishmaniasis was common among the settlers. An examination of the forest rodents and marsupials revealed six different species with cutaneous leishmaniasis—a total of 21 animals out of 107 examined (20%). Our hopes of having discovered a major reservoir of *L. b. braziliensis* for that region were soon dashed, however, for all except one of the isolations from the skin of these animals proved to be *L. m. amazonensis*. The vector of this parasite,

Lutzomyia flaviscutellata, was abundant; but although it was readily trapped with rodent bait, it was rarely taken off man. As far as we could see, human disease due to *L. m. amazonensis* formed no problem. Ironically, only one rodent (*Oryzomys concolor*) (Fig. 1) was found infected with a parasite which was similar to that isolated from man (see Table 2), and only further studies in the Serra do Roncador region may resolve the problem. In the meantime, this experience forms an excellent example of how impossible it is to come to any accurate conclusions regarding the reservoirs of the human disease in a given region unless there is an adequate comparative study of numerous isolates from both man and wild animals.

B. THE PHLEBOTOMINE SANDFLY POPULATION

Table 4 shows the great range of sandflies which can be experimentally infected with neotropical leishmanias. It also shows that sandflies which have no contact with certain parasites in nature (e.g. *Lu. longipalpis* and *L. mexicana*) can nevertheless transmit in the laboratory. Clearly, then, there are biological factors acting as barriers between some sandflies and leishmanias: only careful field studies, therefore, can determine the vector(s) of a given *Leishmania*. It remains to be seen to what extent such barriers depend on the behaviour of the mammalian and/or the insect host; in certain cases, some physiological conditions within the sandfly gut may be important factors.

Incrimination of sandfly species as vectors of *Leishmania* might be regarded as a somewhat academic exercise by many, in particular the public health authorities. If transmission is domiciliary or semi-domiciliary, control measures are possible with insecticide spraying and no one is going to complain if "innocent" species of sandflies are destroyed along with the "guilty" ones. Pin-pointing the major sandfly hosts in the tropical rain-forest again would not appear to help very much in the control of the disease, for extensive insecticide spraying of vast areas of forest such as in the Amazon basin is clearly impracticable for both physical and economical reasons. However, knowledge of certain behaviour characteristics of these vectors may permit some degree of control. Thus, in an area where the vector is strictly nocturnal, a tight control of night-time activities on the part of work-forces will dramatically cut the incidence of leishmaniasis. Some timber and mining companies in north Brazil are now rigorously prohibiting the common pastime of night-time hunting by their workers: in other regions, however, such precautions are useless, for the vectors are known to also be active in the day.

Lutzomyia umbratilis, an important vector of *L. b. guyanensis* in north Brazil, and probably the Guyanas (Lainson *et al.*, 1976; Ward and

Table 2. Hosts of Neotropical Leishmanias

Family	HOST Species	PARASITE Section Species	Localization[b]	Country (State)[a]	Reference
		PERIPYLARIA			
Psychodidae	Lutzomyia pessoai	L. b. brasiliensis	?	Brazil (SP)	Forattini et al. (1972c)
	Lutzomyia intermedia		int	Brazil (SP)	Forattini et al. (1972c)
	Psychodopygus wellcomei		fmh-gut	Brazil (PA)	Lainson et al. (1973)
Cricetidae	Oryzomys capito		skls	Brazil (SP)	Forattini et al. (1973)
	Oryzomys nigripes		nsk	Brazil (SP)	Forattini et al. (1972b)
	Akodon arviculoides		skls	Brazil (SP)	Forattini et al. (1972b)
	Oryzomys concolor		skls	Brazil (MT)	Lainson and Shaw (1969a)
Psychodidae	Lutzomyia umbratilis	L. b. guyanensis	fmh-gut	Brazil (PA)	Lainson et al. (1976)
	Lutzomyia trapidoi	L. b. panamensis	fmh-gut	Panama	Johnson et al. (1963) and Schneider and Hertig (1966)
	Lutzomyia ylephiletor		mh-gut	Panama	Johnson et al. (1963) and Schneider and Hertig (1966)
	Lutzomyia gomezi		mh-gut	Panama	Johnson et al. (1963) and Schneider and Hertig (1966)
	Psychodopygus panamensis		mh-gut	Panama	Christensen et al. (1969)
Bradypodidae	Choloepus hoffmanni		nsk and vis	Panama	Herrer and Telford (1969)
	Bradypus infuscatus		bld, nsk and vis	Panama	Herrer and Telford (1969)
Cebidae	Aotus trivirgatus		sk	Panama	Herrer et al. (1973)
Callithricidae	Saguinus geoffroyi		sk	Panama	Herrer et al. (1973)
Procyonidae	Bassaricyon gabbii		sk	Panama	Herrer et al. (1973)
	Nasua nasua		sk	Panama	Herrer et al. (1973)
	Potos flavus		skls	Panama	Thatcher et al. (1965)
Canidae	Canis familiaris		skls	Panama	Herrer and Christensen

Family	Host	Parasite	Site	Location	Reference
Psychodidae	Lutzomyia ?gomezi				
Didelphidae	Didelphis marsupialis	L. braziliensis sub. sp.	vis	Brazil (PA)	Lainson and Shaw (1973)
Echimyidae	Proechimys guyannensis	L. braziliensis sub sp.	vis	Brazil (PA)	Lainson and Shaw (1973)
Muridae	Rattus rattus	L. braziliensis sub sp.	nsk	Brazil (AM)	Lainson and Shaw (1977a)
Bradypodidae	Choloepus didactylus	L. braziliensis sub sp.	nsk, vis	Brazil (PA)	Shaw and Lainson (1973)
	Choloepus hoffmanni	L. braziliensis sub sp.	bld, liv	Costa Rica	Zeledon et al. (1975)
	Bradypus griseus	L. braziliensis sub sp.	nsk, liv	Costa Rica	Zeledon et al. (1975)
		SUPRAPYLARIA			
Psychodidae	Lutzomyia olmeca olmeca	L. m. mexicana	int	Mexico	Biagi et al. (1965a)
Cricetidae	Nyctomys sumichrasti		fm-gut	Belize	Disney (1968)
			skls	Belize	Lainson and Strangways-Dixon (1962 and 1964)
	Ototylomys phyllotis		skls	Belize	Lainson and Strangways-Dixon (1962 and 1964)
	Sigmodon hispidus		skls	Belize	Disney (1966)
Heteromyidae	Heteromys desmarestianus		skls	Belize	Lainson and Strangways-Dixon (1962 and 1964)
Psychodidae	Lutzomyia flaviscutellata	L. m. amazonensis	fm-gut	Brazil (PA)	Lainson and Shaw (1968)
Didelphidae	Marmosa murina		skls	Brazil (MT)	Lainson and Shaw (1969a)
			skls	Brazil (PA)	Lainson and Shaw (1969b)
	Marmosa sp.		nsk	Brazil (PA)	Lainson and Shaw (1977)
	Metachirus nudicaudatus		nsk	Brazil (PA)	Lainson and Shaw (1973)
Cricetidae	Oryzomys capito		skls	Brazil (PA)	Guimarães and Azevedo (1964)
	Oryzomys concolor		nsk	Brazil (PA)	Lainson and Shaw (1973)
	Oryzomys macconnelli		skls	Brazil (MT)	Lainson and Shaw (1969a)
			skls	Brazil (MT)	Lainson and Shaw (1969a)
			nsk	Brazil (PA)	Lainson and Shaw (1973)
	Neacomys spinosus		skls	Brazil (MT)	Lainson and Shaw (1969a)
	Nectomys squamipes		skls	Brazil (MT)	Lainson and Shaw (1969a)
Dasyproctidae	Dasyprocta sp.		nsk	Brazil (PA)	Lainson and Shaw (1973)

Table 2—cont.

Family	HOST Species	PARASITE Section Species	Localization[b]	Country (State)[a]	Reference
Echimyidae	*Proechimys guyannensis*		skls	Brazil (PA)	Lainson and Shaw (1968)
Canidae	*Cerdocyon thous*		nsk	Brazil (PA)	Lainson and Shaw (1973)
Psychodidae	*Lutzomyia flaviscutellata*	*L. m. pifanoi*	vis	Brazil (PA)	Lainson and Shaw (pres. obs.)
Heteromyidae	*Heteromys anomalus*		fm-gut	Venezuela (AM)	Pifano et al. (1973)
Didelphidae	*Marmosa robinsoni*	*L. m. aristedesi*	skls	Venezuela (CO)	Torrealba et al. (1972)
Cricetidae	*Oryzomys capito*		skls	Panama	Herrer et al. (1971)
Dasyproctidae	*Dasyprocta punctata*		skls	Panama	Herrer et al. (1971)
Heteromyidae	*Proechimys semispinosus*		nsk	Panama	Herrer et al. (1971)
Psychodidae	*Lutzomyia flaviscutellata*	*L. mexicana* s. sp.	nsk	Panama	Herrer et al. (1971)
Didelphidae	*Marmosa mitis*		fm-gut	Trinidad	Tikasingh (1975)
	Marmosa fuscata		skls	Trinidad	Tikasingh (1969)
	Caluromys philander		skls	Trinidad	Tikasingh (1969)
Heteromyidae	*Heteromys anomalus*		skls	Trinidad	Tikasingh (1974)
Cricetidae	*Oryzomys capito*		skls	Trinidad	Tikasingh (1974)
Echimyidae	*Proechimys guyannensis*		skls	Trinidad	Tikasingh (1969)
Caviidae	*Cavia porcellus*	*L. enriettii*	skls	Trinidad	Tikasingh (1974)
Erethizontidae	*Coendou rothschildi*	*L. hertigi hertigi*	nsk, lvr, spl and b.m.	Brazil (PR)	Medina (1946)
				Panama	Herrer et al. (1966)
	Coendou prehensilis	*L. hertigi deanei*	spl and lvr	Brazil (PI)	Deane et al. (1974)
			nsk and vis	Brazil (PA)	Lainson and Shaw (1977b)
	Coendou sp.		nsk and vis	Brazil (PA)	Lainson and Shaw (1977b)
Canidae	*Canis familiaris*	*L. chagasi*	vis	Brazil (PA)	Chagas et al. (1938)
			sk and vis	Brazil (CE)	Deane and Deane (1954b)

Family	Host	Parasite	Localization[b]	Locality	Reference
	Lycalopex vetulus		sk, vis and b.m.	Brazil (SE)	Piva and Barros (1966)
			sk	Brazil (GO)	Coelho et al. (1965)
			b.m., sk and lvr	Brazil (ES)	Martins et al. (1968)
			lvr	Brazil (PB)	Alencar (1962)
			sk, vis and b.m.	Venezuela (GA)	Amaral et al. (1961c)
			b.m. and sk	Venezuela (PG)	Pifano et al. (1962)
			sk, b.m. and spl	Brazil (CE)	Deane and Deane (1954a); Deane (1956)
Felidae	*Cerdocyon thous*				
	Felis catus		ky	Brazil (PA)	Lainson et al. (1969)
			vis	Brazil (PA)	Chagas et al. (1938)

UNCERTAIN TAXONOMIC POSITION

Family	Host	Parasite	Localization[b]	Locality	Reference
Canidae	*Canis familiaris*	*L. peruviana**	skls and nsk	Peru	Herrer (1951c)
Echimyidae	*Proechimys semispinosus*	*Leishmania* sp.	bld	Panama	Anon. (1957)
	Diplomys labilis	*Leishmania* sp.	sk	Panama	Herrer et al. (1971)

[a] Abbreviations of: Brazilian states: AM = Amazonas; BA = Bahia; CE = Ceará; ES = Espírito Santo; GO = Goiás; MT = Mato Grosso; PA = Pará; PB = Paraíba; PI = Piauí; PR = Paraná; SE = Sergipe; SP = São Paulo; Venezuelan states: AM = Federal Territory of Amazonas; CO = Carabobo; GA = Guárico; PG = Portuguesa. [b] Localization of parasites: bld = blood; b.m = bone marrow; fmh-gut = fore, mid and hind gut; fm-gut = fore and mid gut; int = intestine; ky = kidney; lvr = liver; sk = skin (presence or absence of lesions not stated); nsk = normal skin; skls = skin lesion; vis = spleen and liver. *See Addendum.

Fraiha, 1977), rests on the forest tree-trunks during the day (Fig. 2), often in enormous numbers. Although it probably feeds on its natural host(s) during the night-time, it will attack man avidly during the day, particularly when disturbed. Some degree of local control of leishmaniasis among small work-forces would thus seem practical, at least in a limited area, by spraying tree-trunks with insecticides.

Some other vector species are not normally very anthropophilic and only rarely transmit their leishmanias to man. Under certain conditions, however, there may be a population explosion and the numbers attacking man may increase very considerably: this, in turn, will raise the incidence of human leishmaniasis. Knowledge of the habits and population fluctuations of such species of sandflies can enable avoidance of their preferred habitats during the time of year when they are most abundant.

In countries where areas are being colonized for the first time, an assessment of the sandfly population is a useful guide as to whether or not leishmaniasis is likely to be a major health problem for immigrants. An abundance of *Lutzomyia longipalpis* should, for example, alert one to the danger of visceral leishmaniasis: either following the importation of infected dogs by colonists arriving from other regions where the disease is prevalent, or from a local source in the wild animals (e.g. canids). Again, the recognition of sandfly species which are known to be important vectors of cutaneous or mucocutaneous leishmaniasis in other parts of the country would strongly suggest that the newly colonized area is also likely to be enzootic for the same parasites. Alternatively, different anthropophilic species may be found which previously were not associated with the transmission of leishmaniasis: these might prove to be either alternative vectors of known leishmanias, or concerned in unknown enzootics which may, or may not, constitute a potential hazard for the new settlement.

As dissection of the female sandfly is usually prerequisite to rapid identification of the species, dissection of large numbers taken off human bait will simultaneously enable an examination of these flies for promastigotes of *Leishmania*. Needless to say, any flagellates encountered should be isolated for future identification: as discussed above, the position of the parasites in the insect gut provides valuable information on the nature of the parasite, but without isolation it remains impossible to even be certain that the organism is a *Leishmania* (the intra-erythrocytic haemoflagellate of sloths, *Endotrypanum*, produces promastigotes in sandflies which are indistinguishable from those of *Leishmania*) (Shaw, 1964). The importance of certain sandfly species as sources of infection for man will naturally depend on the nature of the parasites they are harbouring.

In this type of investigation, some anthropophilic sandflies may be singled out for particular study; those biting avidly during the day

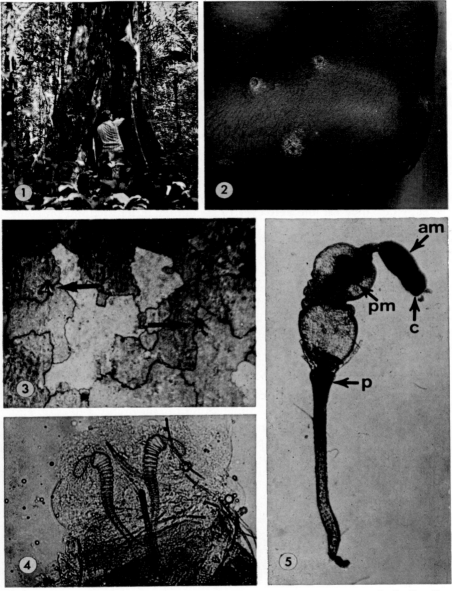

FIG. 2 Epidemiological aspects of *Leishmania braziliensis guyanensis*, in Brazil.
1. Buttressed tree in the Monte Dourado region, Pará State, on which very many
Lutzomyia umbratilis were found. 2. Typical case of "pian-bois". 3. *Lu. umbratilis*
(arrowed) resting on tree-trunk. 4. Spermathecae of *Lu. umbratilis*. 5. Natural
infection of *L. b. guyanensis* in *Lu. umbratilis*. Low-power view showing masses of
parasites in the cardia (c), anterior midgut (am), posterior midgut (pm) and
pylorus (p).

clearly deserve particular attention, for it is during the daytime that man is most active in the forest. The super-abundance of a particular man-biting species of sandfly must, however, be viewed with caution, for it is not always the most ardent man-biter which is the vector. Broadly speaking, there are two quite different epidemiological situations which can result in the same risk of infection for man: one is that in which the fly rarely bites man but has a high infection-rate, and the other is where the fly is highly anthropophilic but is infrequently infected. We will be dealing with such instances when discussing the epidemiology of specific leishmanias in more depth.

Finally, it must again be remembered that a considerable number of sandfly species have been experimentally infected with leishmanial parasites which they are unlikely ever to encounter in nature, and on some occasions have even transmitted them (see Table 4). Finding a *Leishmania* in a single specimen of a given sandfly species and proving it identical with that infecting man in the same region is a great step forward: it is not, however, sufficient for the assumption that this species is the major vector. Infected flies must be found in sufficient numbers, to the exclusion of other species, and wherever possible attempts should be made to correlate behaviour of the fly to its relationship with reservoir hosts and man (see, for example, Part VII, A and B).

C. MAMMALIAN HOSTS, OTHER THAN MAN

Two text-book misconceptions are frequently perpetuated: firstly that leishmanial infection in the mammalian host is inevitably a disease, and secondly that there is a sharp division between "cutaneous" and "visceral" leishmaniasis. Both are principally due to the past emphasis on the clinical aspects of human leishmaniasis, although the severity of canine and vulpine infection due to *L. chagasi* or *L. infantum* must also have contributed.

Where a parasitic association is an ancient one, a well balanced host-parasite relationship is the general rule and infection is usually asymptomatic, with little or no pathology. When their preferred blood-source is scarce, however, many sandflies will turn their attention to unusual hosts, including man, and inoculated *Leishmania* species will find themselves in inhospitable surroundings. In such circumstances the organisms may be quickly destroyed; or they may survive and multiply, producing a violent host reaction and a resulting disease manifested by a variety of skin lesions or severe pathological changes in the internal organs. The latter incidental or accidental hosts cannot be generally regarded as good reservoirs of infection for sandflies, as parasites which are localized in discrete ulcers are not so readily available to the insect as are those scattered through healthy skin. Again, sick animals may die from the disease (e.g. dogs and foxes infected with *L. chagasi*), or fall more ready prey to predators: they will thus be removed as effective, *long-term* reservoirs of infection. The importance of such animals should not be under-estimated, however, in the epidemiology of leishmaniasis: in the presence of abundant *Lu. longipalpis* a single moribund dog, with its skin rich in amastigotes, may initiate a veritable epidemic of visceral leishmaniasis.

As discussed above, there is good reason to regard the leishmanias as an ancient group of parasites, and accumulated evidence does in fact show that these organisms in most cases do not seriously inconvenience the *natural* mammalian hosts. Earlier reports of cutaneous lesions in a variety of wild mammals (Figs 4, 5) do not invalidate this generalization, for at the time these reports were made the authors did not examine the apparently normal skin of other specimens from the same localities (Lainson and Strangways-Dixon, 1962, 1964).

In Panama (Anon., 1957, 1958) *Leishmania* was isolated from the heart-blood of the rodent *Proechimys semispinosus* which showed no skin lesions, and Herrer *et al.* (1966) demonstrated a *Leishmania*, later named *L. hertigi* (Herrer, 1971), in the apparently normal skin of 6 out of 8 porcupines. In Brazil, Lainson and Shaw (1968) isolated *L. mexicana amazonensis* from the ear tissue of *Proechimys guyannensis*: the ears appeared perfectly normal and the authors commented that "it would seem advisable to examine apparently normal skin from wild animals". Later (1973) they concluded that "the most common type of infection is asymptomatic, with parasites scattered through apparently normal dermis". Thus, of 166 *Proechimys* examined, 26 were infected with *L. m. amazonensis* but only 5 showed visible skin lesions: of 64 *Oryzomys capito*, 7 were infected but the skin of all these rodents appeared perfectly normal. Similar cryptic skin infection was noted in another rodent, *Nyctomys squamipes*, and an opossum, *Metachirus nudicaudatus*. Subspecies of *Leishmania braziliensis* were isolated from the apparently normal skin of a specimen of *Rattus rattus*; also from the liver and spleen of *Proechimys*, the opossum *Didelphis marsupialis*, and the sloth *Choloepus didactylus*. All of these animals appeared to be in perfect health. Table 3 brings these observations up to date, with the addition of more recent isolations.

Herrer and Christensen (1975b) also stressed the importance of cryptic infections when they summarized the studies made at the Gorgas Memorial Laboratory, in Panama. Inapparent infections of skin and/or viscera with *L. braziliensis panamensis* were found in 93 of 498 two-toed sloths (*Choloepus hoffmani*), 2 out of 187 three-toed sloths (*Bradypus infuscatus*) and 1 of 8 coatimundis (*Nasua nasua*). Leishmaniotic skin lesions, apparently due to the same parasite, were recorded in single specimens of the monkeys *Aotus trivirgatus* and *Saguinus*

Table 3. Isolates of *Leishmania* from some wild mammals of the Amazon Region of Brazil (Pará State),[a] showing the high frequency of chronic, inapparent infections.

Species	Number examined	Location of parasites as determined by intradermal inoculation of tissues in hamsters and/or culture in blood-agar medium (NNN)				Total infected
		Skin lesions	Normal skin only	Normal skin and viscera	Viscera only	
RODENTIA:						
Proechimys guyannensis (spiny rat)	278	6 (*L. mexicana amazonensis*)	29 (*L. m. amazonensis*)	1	1 (*L. braziliensis* ssp.)	37
Oryzomys spp. (rice rat)	168	0	10 (*L. m. amazonensis*)	0	0	10
Nectomys squamipes (water rat)	35	0	2 (*L. m. amazonensis*)	0	0	2
Dasyprocta sp. (agouti)	8	0	2 (*L. m. amazonensis*)	0	0	2
Rattus rattus (black rat)	4	0	1 (*L. braziliensis* ssp.)	0	0	1
Coendou prehensilis (porcupine)	2	0	1 (*L. hertigi deanei*)	1	0	2
Coendou sp. nov.[b] (porcupine)	16	0	7 (*L. hertigi deanei*)	1	1	9
MARSUPIALIA:						
Didelphis marsupialis (black-eared opossum)	74	0	0	0	1 (*L. braziliensis* ssp.)	1
Marmosa spp. (murine opossums)	30	0	1 (*L. m. amazonensis*)	0	0	1

					(L. braziliensis spp.)		
Choloepus didactylus (two-toed sloth)								2
CARNIVORA:								
Cerdocyon thous (American grey fox)	21	0	6	0	0	3	2[c]	2
Totals	681	56	6	3	8	73		

[a] These figures include some which have already been published (Lainson and Shaw, 1973): In addition the following animals were examined with negative results—RODENTIA: *Neacomys spinosus*, 20; *Agouti paca*, 3; *Zygodontomys* sp., 3; *Oxymycterus hispidus*, 5; *Hydrochoeris hydrochaeris*, 1. EDENTATA: *Bradypus infuscata*, 11. MARSUPIALIA: *Monodelphis* spp., 15; *Philander opossum*, 14; *Caluromys philander*, 29; *Tamandua tetradactyla*, 16; *Dasypus novemcinctus*, 7; *Cyclopes didactylus*, 3. CARNIVORA: *Felis pardalis*, 1; *Nasua nasua*, 1. ARTIODACTYLA: *Mazama americana*, 1; *Tayassu tajacu*, 2. PRIMATA: *Cebus apella*, 2; *Alouatta belzebul*, 3; *Lagothrix* sp., 2. [b] Personal communication, Dr. C. O. Handley, Jr., Smithsonian Institution, Washington, D.C. See also, Pine, R. H. (1973): we understand that a description of the animal is in press. [c] One fox with *L. m. amazonensis* only, in viscera (liver and spleen): one fox with double infection of *L. m. amazonensis* and *L. chagasi* (kidney). Skin not examined in either animal.

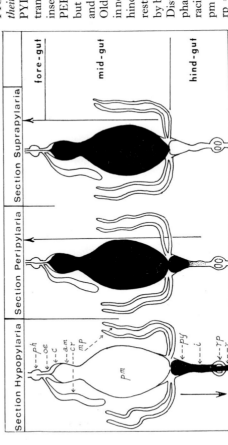

FIG. 1. *Classification of the leishmanias, based on their behaviour in the sandfly host.* Section HYPOPYLARIA: flagellates restricted to hindgut, and transmission presumably after ingestion of infected insect. In reptiles of the Old World. Section PERIPYLARIA: hindgut development retained, but parasites also migrating to midgut and foregut and transmission now by bite. In some reptiles of the Old World, and including the *L. braziliensis* complex in neotropical mammals. Section SUPRAPYLARIA: hindgut development completely lost and parasites restricted to midgut and foregut, with transmission by bite. In mammals of both the Old and New Worlds. Distribution of parasites shown in black: ph = pharynx; oe = oesophagus; c = cardia; am = thoracic midgut; cr = crop; mp = malpighian tubules; pm = abdominal midgut; py = pylorus; i = ileum; rp = rectal ampullae; r = rectum.

Section Hypopylaria | Section Peripylaria | Section Suprapylaria

fore-gut

mid-gut

hind-gut

geoffroyi; and three similar infections were found in procyonid carnivores, 2 in *Potos flavus* (the "kinkajou") and 1 in *Bassaricyon gabbii* (the "olingo").

Subspecies of *Leishmania hertigi* have so far only been found in neotropical porcupines of the genus *Coendou* and are apparently unassociated with any form of human leishmaniasis. It is noteworthy that they are very benign in the natural hosts. Thus, Herrer and Christensen (1975b) record all of 104 animals infected with *L. hertigi hertigi* as showing no visible signs of disease, although parasites were scattered throughout the dermis and sometimes were found in the viscera (Herrer, 1971). In Brazil, all of 11 isolates we have made of *L. hertigi deanei* (Lainson and Shaw, 1977b) have shown a similar lack of virulence in the natural host (Table 3).

The grouping of *L. donovani*, *L. infantum* and *L. chagasi* together as the "visceral" leishmanias has been a convenient clinical method of separating these parasites from *L. tropica*, *L. major*, *L. aethiopica*, and the various other "cutaneous" leishmanias in the *L. mexicana* and *L. braziliensis* complexes, for as long as these parasites have been known to infect man. Many authors in fact still regard all forms of human visceral leishmaniasis as due to the same parasite, *L. donovani*, but this oversimplification is no longer tenable in the light of present knowledge (Lainson and Shaw, 1972a; Bray, 1974; Zuckerman and Lainson, 1977). Leishmanial parasites do not always maintain either a strictly dermotropic or viscerotropic habit (Adler, 1964). Thus, the parasites responsible for human "visceral leishmaniasis" in East Africa and the Sudan may produce primary cutaneous lesions several months before the onset of a visceral disease and sometimes, in fact, the infection does not develop past the cutaneous stage. *L. donovani*, the causative agent of Indian kala azar, may also show a striking invasion of the human skin in the form of the disease known as "post kala azar dermal leishmanoid". In dogs and foxes infected with either *L. infantum* (Mediterranean visceral leishmaniasis) or *L. chagasi* (South American visceral leishmaniasis) there is massive invasion of the skin, which makes these animals very important reservoirs of infection for man.

L. tropica and subspecies of *L. mexicana* and *L. braziliensis* are often regarded as essentially dermotropic parasites. Some "strains" of *L. tropica*, however, give rise to heavy visceral infection in hamsters, while visceral infection by *L. m. mexicana* and subspecies of *L. braziliensis* has been reported in naturally and experimentally infected animals (Disney, 1964; Lainson, 1965; Lainson and Shaw, 1973; and present observations, Table 3). Finally, we have found abundant amastigotes of *L. braziliensis guyanensis* in the spleen and liver of hamsters, only three months after the animals were inoculated by the intradermal route (Lainson and Shaw, unpublished observations). As we have inferred above, it would thus seem time to place less emphasis on location of the parasites in the vertebrate host as an important factor in separating parasites.

There are, nevertheless, at least three leishmanias which do produce a predominantly visceral infection in man—*L. donovani*, *L. infantum* and *L. chagasi*—and it is likely that others will be designated. The East African and Sudanese parasites responsible for visceral leishmaniasis in man are candidates for revised nomenclature, and it is possible that *L. chagasi* is not the only causative agent involved in Latin America (Lainson and Shaw, 1972a, and Part VII, this chapter).

D. DETECTION AND ISOLATION OF *LEISHMANIA*:

1. From man

As man usually presents conspicuous skin lesions when infected with parasites of the *L. braziliensis* and *L. mexicana* complexes (Figs 1, 2 and 5), detection and isolation of the organisms offer few problems, although a considerable degree of practice and patience is needed in finding the very scanty amastigotes typical of many *L. braziliensis* infections. Well stained smears are of the utmost importance, and great care must be taken to avoid the central area of ulcerated lesions, where bacterial and fungal contaminants can cause great confusion in stained smears and can ruin any attempts at sterile culture. If the lesions show an obvious, heavy secondary bacterial contamination, the patient should first be treated with antibiotics and the examination for *Leishmania* postponed till this is completed. Isolation of the parasites depends on the *in vitro* culture of tissue or tissue juices in a suitable medium (usually a variety of blood-agar mixtures), or the inoculation of susceptible laboratory animals, in particular the hamster. These methods simply allow relatively scanty or undetectable parasites to multiply to a readily visible level, either as promastigotes or amastigotes. In our opinion, *both* should always be used.

We have found punch-biopsies of tissue from the borders of skin lesions (Fig. 5) to be much more effective than the method of aspirating material with a syringe. Two or three small biopsies are made, to give pieces for the inoculation of hamsters, for culture and for histology. Impression smears are prepared from the excised tissue and stained by the standard methods: we find that of Giemsa to be the best. The preparations should be air-dried as quickly as possible, fixed at once in absolute methyl alcohol and stained for approximately one hour in double-strength Giemsa (30 drops to 15·0 ml distilled water buffered to pH 7·2–7·4).

In cases of naso-pharyngeal lesions, cultures of snip-biopsies are particularly liable to be contaminated. Care should also be taken to avoid tissue surfaces painted with such antiseptic tinctures as merthiolate or iodine. Introduction of such material into the blood-agar medium will be equally effective in destroying any hope of a positive culture: inoculation of hamsters with triturated material from the biopsies is the most reliable method.

The use of histological sections to detect *Leishmania* is very limited, especially when the amastigotes are very scanty, and the time devoted to their preparation would be better spent in examining several well pre-pared tissue smears in which the amastigotes can be detected much more readily. If sections are required for general histo-pathology, the Giemsa-colophonium method (Bray and Garnham, 1962) is particularly good: for this purpose the tissue must be fixed in Carnoy's fluid.

In those cases suspected to have visceral leishmaniasis, the diagnostic method of choice is usually the culture of bone-marrow, conveniently aspirated by sternal puncture. Some of the material should also be inoculated intraperitoneally into hamsters, and the usual Giemsa-stained smears prepared. Material examined at autopsy should, of course, be extended to spleen and liver tissue, the former organ generally being particularly rich in parasites: in spite of this, spleen-puncture of the living subject does not seem justified in view of the undeniable risks involved.

It is inappropriate here to discuss the variety of media used for the isolation of *Leishmania* and other haemoflagellates. In our laboratory we routinely use both "Difco B45" and "Oxoid CM3" agar base, mixed with 13·0% and 5·0% defibrinated rabbit blood, respectively. The mix-ture is dispensed into 15 × 150 mm test-tubes, which are sealed with rubber stoppers and slanted to give the traditional bacteriological blood-agar slopes. On solidification they are incubated at 37 °C for one or two hours to promote the formation of a few drops of water of condensation, which accumulates in the bottom of the tubes and into which the ma-terial under examination is introduced. As much of the process as possible is carried out in a sterile cabinet: cultures are usually examined after 10 days and rejected as negative if no growth of parasites is seen after one month. Sometimes insufficient condensation is produced in the culture tubes, in which case physiological saline or tissue culture fluids, such as Hanks' solution, may be added to supplement the volume of liquid overlay to about 0·5 ml.

The inoculation of hamsters with material from suspect or proven leishmaniotic lesions is a particularly useful adjunct to *in vitro* culture, for bacteria and fungal spores tend to be eliminated by the animal's bodily defences. The tissue can be triturated with a pestle and mortar, in a small quantity of sterile saline: the addition of a little fine, sterile, sand greatly facilitates the process. It has been found that parasites are more readily isolated when material is inoculated into the skin of the nose or feet of the hamster. The reason for this predilection is generally regarded as due to the slightly lower temperature of the extremities as compared with the rest of the body, a factor considered as more favourable for the growth of the "cutaneous" leishmanias. It remains difficult to reconcile this view, however, with the considerable degree of visceralization shown by such parasites in both wild animals and the hamster, as discussed in earlier pages. Hamsters should not be discarded as negative until at least 9–12 months later, in view of the very slow growth of some of the parasites of the *L. braziliensis* complex in these animals. Material from suspected cases of visceral leishmaniasis is usually inoculated by the intraperitoneal route.

Theoretically, the *in vitro* culture method is the most rapid and sensitive way of isolating *Leishmania*, with the results usually obtained in 1 to 3 weeks. Technically it has its hazards, particularly in the field, due to bacterial or fungal contamination—a problem very prevalent in the humid tropics. The former can to some extent be controlled by incorporating low concentrations of penicillin and streptomycin in the fluid phase of the media (about 200 i.u. and 200 μg per ml, respectively), or by the prior incubation of tissues in saline containing stronger concentrations of these antibiotics (Herrer *et al.*, 1966). Fungal contaminants are the major problem, however, and are virtually impossible to eradicate from cultures. Bacterial and fungal growth are extremely prejudicial to the growth of leishmanial promastigotes.

Members of the *L. mexicana* complex are notable for their luxuriant and easily maintained growth in almost any simple blood-agar medium (e.g. varieties of NNN). On the other hand, difficulties become apparent within the *L. donovani* complex, for *L. chagasi* has, in our experience, proved to be quite selective in the media in which it can be maintained. Its growth is poor in NNN prepared with both the Oxoid and Difco agar bases as formulated by Walton *et al.* (1977), but fairly good in the Yaeger liver-infusion-tryptose (LIT) medium described by Fernandes and Castellani (1966). Subspecies of *L. braziliensis* also tend to be fastidious: some, such as *L. b. panamensis*, do culture relatively easily, but others will either grow only on specialized NNN media or will steadfastly refuse to accept any *in vitro* medium so far tried (Walton *et al.*, 1977). This applies particularly to some of those isolates referred to by us as *L. b. braziliensis* (see Part VI, A). Clearly there is a limit to the number of different media one can use, in practice, during the screening of large numbers of wild animals or persons for different leishmanias, and there remains an urgent need for the perfection of a single, simple medium equally efficient in growing any of these parasites.

The great advantage of hamster inoculation in the isolation of *Leishmania* lies in its application in field conditions which do not permit sterile culture technique. Its disadvantage is the long incubation period before infection of the hamsters becomes apparent, either as a skin lesion or as a visceral involvement (sometimes as long as 6 to 12 months later).

The better known parasites of the *L. mexicana* complex (*L. m. mexicana*, *L. m. amazonensis* and *L. m. aristedesi*) offer the least problems in this respect. Large, tumour-like lesions quickly develop at the site of inoculation, usually within a few months. These have the form of a histiocytoma, with very little host–cell reaction and histiocytes packed with amastigotes. Later in the infection, there is metastatic spread to most of the animal's extremities, where similar histiocytomata occur (Fig. 5). This spread can take place as early as two or three months after the inoculation of the parasites, but on other occasions may require considerably longer. Growth of these lesions continues, unchecked, to the end of the animal's life; which is usually hastened by the large size of the lesions, especially if involving the face.

Among the subspecies of *L. braziliensis*, both *L. b. guyanensis* and *L. b. panamensis* characteristically produce a small, fleshy lesion on the nose of the hamster. Although it may appear relatively quickly, from one to three months after inoculation of the parasites, it *does not take the form of a histiocytoma*, being vascular, with pronounced host–cell response and comparatively few amastigotes. Although we have seen no instances of self-cure, growth of the lesion is arrested and it remains small throughout the animal's life-span. In our experience, metastatic spread does frequently occur in *L. b. guyanensis* infections, but these lesions also remain inconspicuous and histologically similar to the initial lesion. Limited numbers of amastigotes may be encountered in the viscera.

In dealing with infections of man in north Brazil due to the parasite we have referred to as *L. b. braziliensis* (Part VI, A), we have found that in most cases the organism grows even more reluctantly in hamster skin than either *L. b. guyanensis* or *L. b. panamensis*. If lesions develop they may sometimes take as long as 6 to 12 months to become visible. Often appearing as little more than an increased fleshiness and reddening of the nose, they may later develop a slight "crusty" appearance. In other respects the lesions resemble those of the other subspecies of *L. braziliensis*. We have never seen metastasis to elsewhere in the skin, but limited numbers of amastigotes can sometimes be found in the viscera, particularly in those animals with long-term infections.

In studies on the epidemiology of cutaneous leishmaniasis in the Serra do Roncador (Mato Grosso) and Serra dos Carajás (Pará) regions of Brazil, we have on some occasions apparently failed to infect hamsters inoculated with biopsied material from human infections in which amastigotes were seen in stained smears from the lesions (Lainson and Shaw, 1970, 1973). These observations suggest that inapparent *L. b. braziliensis* infections in wild animals may be missed when screening by the inoculation of hamsters, and also that there may well be a variety of *other* leishmania equally reluctant to infect this animal. Thus, we recently cultured liver and spleen suspensions from an opossum, *Didelphis marsupialis*, caught in the forest near Belém; promastigotes appeared in these cultures but could not be maintained *in vitro*, and no infection could be registered in hamsters inoculated both intradermally and intraperitoneally. The area was one in which human infections have been found with a so-far unidentified member of the *L. braziliensis* group, which is difficult to maintain in culture or hamsters.

2. From wild and domestic mammals

If such animals are to be examined in the field, it is best to limit one's technique to the inoculation of tissue-suspensions into hamsters, which we have found to withstand quite arduous conditions, even in tropical rain-forest. If wild animals show skin alterations attention will obviously be focussed on these, and amastigotes may in fact be found in smears from the lesions. Otherwise we inoculate a pooled triturate of apparently normal skin, taken from such points as the ears, nose, tail and feet, intradermally into the skin of one pair of hamsters, and a suspension of liver and spleen tissue intraperitoneally into two other animals. Later, on return to the laboratory, and if a leishmanial infection is established, cultures of skin and/or viscera of the hamsters may be made under more favourable conditions. At the same time, serial passage may be continued in other hamsters and the newly isolated parasite cryopreserved in liquid nitrogen. If wild animals can be transported back to the laboratory, much time may be saved by direct culture from skin and viscera, as already described.

3. From wild-caught sandflies

The method of isolation from sandflies again depends on whether or not the insects can be brought back, alive, to good laboratory facilities. In this respect it is surprising just how well fragile silvatic species will withstand long journeys, if they are kept in suitable conditions of humidity and temperature in a sealed polystyrene container.

Under reasonable laboratory conditions it is possible to dissect sandflies using sterilized instruments, slides and coverslips, after vigorously "washing" the insects by shaking them in sterile saline. If an infected gut is found, it is then carefully transferred from the drop of saline into a tube of blood-agar medium. This method was used at the Gorgas Memorial Laboratory in Panama (Johnson *et al.*, 1963; McConnell, 1963), although even these experienced workers only recorded an over-all success rate of 89 isolations in 218 attempts (40%).

The method is useful in areas where there is a high infection-rate in the sandflies, and it does have the advantage of growing the parasite quickly; there is also the possibility of isolating other interesting haemoflagellates such as *Endotrypanum* and *Trypanosoma* species, which are not infective to hamsters. The high rate of loss due to contamination and the very slow rate of dissection imposed by such a sterile technique are, however, serious drawbacks in other regions where the infection rate is much lower.

When the infection rate is low, or when the sterile technique is impracticable—as in the field, the easiest and most reliable method of isolation is by inoculation of the flagellates into hamster skin. Once more, the nose or feet are the preferable sites for injection. As previously indicated, before this is done careful note must be made of the position of the parasites in the gut, their general morphology and whether or not they are attached to the gut-wall. The spermathecae of the infected fly may give on-the-spot identification of the insect (Figs 1, 2 and 4), but *in all cases* these and other parts should be mounted as a permanent preparation for subsequent confirmation.

As already mentioned, the hamster will usually effectively eliminate the problem of bacterial and fungal contaminants, and if a *Leishmania* is isolated in the animal it can be cultured later under sterile conditions. In view of the very inconspicuous or even inapparent infections produced by some leishmanias in hamster skin, culture should be made from the site of the intradermal inoculation of the flagellates, regardless of the presence or absence of a visible lesion.

The complete failure to infect the hamster does not necessarily mean that the promastigotes seen in the sandfly were not those of a *Leishmania* —even one which commonly produces severe lesions in man. Thus, in an extension of our earlier studies on the parasite we refer to as *L. braziliensis braziliensis*, in Serra dos Carajás, Pará (Lainson et al., 1973), we recently inoculated most of the promastigotes of a naturally infected sandfly, *Psychodopygus wellcomei*, into the nose-skin of a hamster: at the same time we succeeded in obtaining an *in vitro* culture with the few remaining flagellates left in the saline in which the insect was dissected. To our surprise, no infection resulted in the inoculated hamster, but other animals subsequently injected with the culture forms did develop typical lesions containing amastigotes. As previously mentioned, we have several times failed to infect hamsters inoculated with biopsied tissue from lesions of man, in which scanty amastigotes had been seen microscopically: other hamsters *did* become infected, however, when injected with abundant culture forms from blood-agar cultures that had been made from the same lesions.

It is inappropriate to discuss these observations in great depth, here. It seems likely, however, that the number of infective forms inoculated is an important factor in deciding whether or not the parasite will produce an infection in the hamster. This animal is peculiarly susceptible to certain leishmanias, notably subspecies of *L. mexicana*, when very low numbers of either promastigotes or amastigotes will quickly produce rapidly growing lesions in which the parasite proliferates enormously. On the other hand, the same animal is only moderately susceptible to other leishmanias, e.g. certain subspecies of *L. braziliensis*, and much larger inocula of infective stages are necessary to overcome this natural resistance to infection. In this connection it is significant that there is little or no cellular reaction in hamster-lesions due to subspecies of *L. mexicana*, but a very considerable amount in lesions due to those of *L. braziliensis*.

4. Detection of reservoir hosts by the identification of sandfly bloodmeals

The identification of blood from wild-caught, engorged arthropods has been used in epidemiological studies to pin-point the vertebrate reservoir hosts of a number of zoonotic diseases (Weitz, 1956, 1963; Tempelis, 1974; Boreham, 1975). With regard to phlebotomine sandflies, the precipitin test was used as long ago as 1930 by Lloyd and Napier in India, and since that time it has proved a useful tool to establish these insects' preferred vertebrate hosts in many parts of the Old World where sandflies occur. In the Americas such studies seem to have been limited to Panama (Tesh *et al.*, 1971, 1972), and to recent precipitin tests on the bloodmeals of Brazilian sandflies, kindly carried out for us by Dr. P. F. L. Boreham.

The tests in Panama indicated that the feeding habits of different sandfly species not only change from site to site, but also from one time of the year to another. In studies on *Lutzomyia umbratilis*, the vector of *L. b. guyanensis* in north Brazil, we have found it easy to find engorged females resting on tree-trunks and, on some occasions, up to 50% contained fresh blood. One batch of 39 fed flies gave the following results with the precipitin test: primate, 20 (51·3%); rodent, 11 (28%); anteater, 8 (18%): these flies were caught from a number of widely separate trees. On another occasion, however, 36 blood-fed *Lu. umbratilis*, taken from three adjacent trees, showed that 35 had fed on a primate and 1 on a porcupine. Doubtless the primate was a monkey, for the area was uninhabited by man and our own movements precluded ourselves as the blood-source (Lainson, Shaw and Ward, unpublished observations).

Such tests on samples of sandflies from highly localized habitats can be misleading in attempts to pin-point the vertebrate source of their leishmanias, if the species concerned is an opportunistic feeder. Nevertheless, the results of blood-meal tests on a given sandfly species collected from numerous widely dispersed areas, over a long period, must eventually afford some indication of the more likely reservoir(s) of the *Leishmania* of that insect; especially if they are related to the detection of the parasite in dissected sandflies from the same area, at the same time.

V. Neotropical Hypopylaria

In 1918 Leger described leptomonad flagellates in blood smears of 2 out of 30 dead lizards (*Anolis* sp.) from the island of Martinique, West Indies, and gave the organism the name of *Leishmania henrici*. The name stood for many years (Adler, 1964; Johnson and Hertig, 1970) as the only record of a saurian *Leishmania* in the Western Hemisphere, and as such would be included here as the only possible New World representative of the Hypopylaria.

Dollahon and Janovy (1974), however, suggested that "*Leishmania henrici* . . . has not been demonstrated to be a *Leishmania*, since there is the possibility that the leptomonads described (Leger, 1918) from the blood smears . . . were actually contaminants from the guts of the lizards. . . . Recent research (Dollahon and Janovy, 1971) demonstrates that insect flagellates can be found in lizard gut contents and feces. . . . Therefore, it does not appear that any lizard leishmanias of blood and tissues have been adequately demonstrated in New World lizards." It may reasonably be argued, of course, that the evidence for rejecting Leger's name of *L. henrici* is no stronger than that for accepting it, but only a reinvestigation on the parasites of *Anolis* from Martinique will resolve this problem.

Whilst it is not appropriate to devote space here to mere speculation on the future discovery of saurian members of either the Hypopylaria or the Peripylaria in the New World, it may be noted that there are some American phlebotomine sandflies which do feed predominantly on lizards, and which harbour developmental stages of trypanosomes. Thus, Christensen and Telford (1972) described the development of *Trypanosoma thecadactyli* of the Panamanian gecko *Thecadactylus rapicaudus* in naturally and experimentally infected *Lutzomyia trinidadensis*; and we have found what is probably the development of the same parasite in *Lu. rorotaensis* found feeding on *T. rapicaudus* in Pará, Brazil (Lainson, Ward and Shaw, unpublished observations). Sherlock and Pessôa (1966) described flagellates in the alimentary tract of specimens of *Lu. micropyga*, captured on tree-trunks and in animal burrows, in Bahia, Brazil. They suggested that they might represent the development of a lizard *Leishmania*, but from their illustrations the organisms are clearly *not* promastigotes and have much more the appearance of developmental stages of a trypanosome.

To date, too few New World lizards have been examined to suggest that saurian leishmanias do not exist in the Americas, and it is probably only a question of time before they are discovered.

VI. Neotropical Peripylaria

Leishmania braziliensis was the first specific name to be used to differentiate Old World and New World leishmanial parasites but, as Pifano (1960) cautiously concluded, "*L. braziliensis* probably represents an aetiological complex integrated by species, varieties or biologically different races". New evidence has supported this opinion, and to avoid future confusion in talking about reservoir hosts it is necessary to define the parasites as precisely as possible. Some of the organisms recorded in Table 1 were possibly *L. braziliensis*, but unfortunately there was too little information on them to say that they definitely were. Our "possible identities" are, therefore, really nothing more than intuitive guesses.

Vianna (1911) gave the name *L. braziliensis* to the parasite he found in smears made from lesions of a patient with disseminated cutaneous leishmaniasis of the face, arms and legs that was not recognizable clinically as this disease. Subsequently the name was used for the aetiological agent of a variety of clinical forms of cutaneous leishmaniasis, and in particular for the parasite responsible for the mutilating, mucocutaneous form of the disease. Vianna's patient came from a small village called São João de Além Paraíba, Minas Gerais, Brazil which is situated in the valley of the Paraíba river that forms the southern interstate boundary between Minas Gerais and Rio de Janeiro. To date there are, as far as we are aware, no strains of *Leishmania* available from the type area, and the nearest isolates examined have come from Caratinga and the Rio Doce Valley, Minas Gerais: they have, however, been shown to differ greatly from material identified as *L. braziliensis* from South and Central America (Peters, 1975). There is clearly no way of knowing with which parasite Vianna was dealing, and we feel that it is perhaps more prudent, and will cause less confusion, if the name *braziliensis* is used for the neotropical Peripylaria known to infect man, which have a prolific phase of growth in the pyloric region of the sandfly gut, have nuclear and kinetoplast DNA buoyant densities of 1·716 and 1·717 and 1·691 and 1·694 respectively, and have small amastigotes (2·4 × 1·8 μm).

Having defined the use of the specific name *braziliensis* we can now consider the use of subspecific names within the species. Whereas *L. b. guyanensis* and *L. b. panamensis* are relatively easily recognized by a variety of biological and/or biochemical methods, there remains a group of parasites which, although clearly members of the *L. braziliensis* complex, show characters that differ from the above two subspecies. Up to now some of these have, rightly or wrongly, been referred to as *L. b. braziliensis* but, as in the case of Vianna's parasite, some are no longer available for comparative studies. The difficult situation exists, then, in which we are attempting to define new isolations of parasites without an adequate description of the type material. Also biochemical studies have at present been limited to only two isolates referred to as *L. b. braziliensis*, mainly due to the difficulties in producing adequate culture forms. Both of these came from skin and mucosal lesions of men from Pará State, north Brazil, about 2500 km. from Vianna's type locality: all that it is possible to do at this stage is to regard those parasites referred to as "*L. b. braziliensis*" as being the same, until comparative studies on many more isolates prove otherwise. In this respect it would seem essential to examine a collection of these, from man, *in the type locality* of São João de Além Paraiba, for the taxonomic priority for the name *L. b. braziliensis* clearly belongs to a parasite from that area. It is our belief that even more intricacies will appear in the classification of the neotropical leishmanias than already have been found, especially within the *L. braziliensis* complex.

A. *LEISHMANIA BRAZILIENSIS BRAZILIENSIS*

From Table 2 it can be seen that there are only 4 isolations of this parasite from wild mammals, and in each case they are represented by single isolations from a given rodent species. A few other organisms of the *L. braziliensis* complex have been isolated after the examination of numerous animals from endemic areas (Table 3): they were not considered to be *L. braziliensis braziliensis*, however, with the possible exception of a single isolate from the "spiny rat", *Proechimys guyannensis*.

In spite of the small number of animals known as reservoirs of *L. b. braziliensis*, certain important epidemiological features may be linked with their habits and behaviour. In São Paulo, Professor Forattini's group (Forattini *et al.*, 1972a, b, c; 1973) studied an endemic focus associated with small patches of riverine forest in the Moji-Guaçu river valley. They identified the parasite as *L. b. braziliensis* and isolated it from three species of forest rodents and two species of sandflies. Previous studies indicated that one of the sandflies, *Lutzomyia intermedia*, prefers low secondary forest (Barretto, 1943): it also has peridomestic habits and has been found to invade houses (Barretto, 1943) and breed in pig-sties (Forattini, 1953; 1954). The other sandfly, *Lu. pessoai*, is essentially silvatic, but has been found to enter houses that were up to 300 metres away from the forest edge (Forattini, 1954). It would seem that most transmission takes place in the forest, as the infected rodents and sandflies are predominantly silvatic in their habits, but on some occasions it is possible that man could have become infected in or near to houses by stray, infected sandflies.

More recently, in another endemic focus located in the coastal Serra do Mar region of São Paulo State, *Lu. intermedia* was again found to be the major man-biter, and it was captured in and around houses (Forattini *et al.*, 1976).

Guimarães (1955) and Guimarães and Bustamante (1954) studied an "epidemic" of mucocutaneous leishmaniasis in Magé county, Rio de Janeiro State, that occurred in 1947. At this time *Lu. intermedia* was captured both inside and outside the houses: from 1948 onwards the houses were sprayed with DDT, as part of the anti-malaria campaign, and by 1953 only one new case of leishmaniasis had been registered. Sandflies were no longer found in the houses, although many were captured only 20 metres away. It was felt that transmission to man had taken place in or around the houses and that the virtual absence of new cases was due to the insecticide programme. Recently, a similar situation was reported in the Jacarepaguá zone of Rio de Janeiro State, and epidemiological studies (Sabroza *et al.*, 1975) again indicated domiciliary as well as extradomiciliary transmission.

Even though man can acquire cutaneous leishmaniasis in the domestic habitat in such situations, the sandflies presumably become infected from wild animals. If the number of sandflies is sufficiently great inside the houses, however, man-to-man transmission could possibly take place, although we feel that this must be rarely the case. Further studies on the habits and resting sites of fed *Lu. intermedia* would go a long way to resolve the problem.

In the Serra dos Carajás, Pará State, north Brazil, epidemiological studies (Lainson *et al.*, 1973) on a parasite referred to as *L. b. braziliensis* showed that the vector was the sandfly *Psychodopygus wellcomei* (Fig. 1), and that this fly bit man both during the day and the night (Ward *et al.*, 1973b). In this case transmission was confined to virgin tropical rainforest, and the incidence of human cases was exceptionally high due, particularly, to the insect's daytime activities. Although promastigote infections very similar to those of *Ps. wellcomei* were also seen in other man-biting sandfly species, it was impossible to confirm their leishmanial nature (Table 1). It is quite likely, however, that such flies may act as secondary vectors to man and, depending on their relationships with the mammalian reservoir, they may be as important or even more important in the silvan cycle. Such possibilities can only be more fully examined when the mammalian reservoirs are discovered. *L. b. braziliensis* has been isolated from men in other regions of Pará where *Ps. wellcomei* does not occur: in such areas other species must be vectors.

A comparison of the known epidemiological facts from São Paulo and Pará shows that different reservoirs are involved, and even though both groups of workers referred to their parasites as *L. b. braziliensis* it seems unlikely that they were dealing with the same organism.

In the Serra do Roncador, Mato Grosso, *L. b. braziliensis* was isolated from man but the majority of strains from wild rodents were *L. m. amazonensis* (Table 2). A single isolate of *L. b. braziliensis* was obtained from a small, inconspicuous lesion on the base of the tail of a rodent,

Oryzomys concolor (Fig. 1), and it behaved in a similar way, in hamsters, to the strains isolated from man (Lainson and Shaw, 1969). As in the Serra Norte area, however, it was noted that some of the parasites from man apparently failed to infect hamsters, even though amastigotes had been seen in smears of the biopsied material.

B. *LEISHMANIA BRAZILIENSIS GUYANENSIS*

This subspecies occurs in the northern regions of Pará, the Federal Territory of Amapá, in Brazil, and in the Guyanas. In the latter countries the disease caused by this parasite has long been known as "forest yaws", "pian-bois" or "bosch-yaws": in some cases there may be progressive spread of the parasite along the lymphatic system, giving rise to large numbers (Fig. 2) of ulcers all over the body, but to date there is no firm evidence that *L. b. guyanensis* is associated with nasopharyngeal lesions. Unlike *L. b. braziliensis*, initial growth in the hamster is quite rapid, although the resulting skin lesion remains small: visceralization also may occur within a few months of infection, although it does not progress to anything like the extent of that shown by *Leishmania chagasi* (see Part IV, D, 1.). *L. b. guyanensis* is in general much easier to handle in culture than is *L. b. braziliensis*, and may be grown with some degree of success in a number of different diphasic blood-agar media.

To date the only proven reservoir of the parasite is the sandfly *Lutzomyia umbratilis* (Fig. 2), from the Monte Dourado region of northern Pará (Lainson *et al.*, 1976; Ward and Fraiha, 1977). In Surinam, Wijers and Linger (1966) were almost certainly dealing with infections of *L. b. guyanensis* in this same fly, but due to technical difficulties (see Part IV, D, 3.) they were unable to demonstrate the leishmanial nature of the flagellates they found in their dissected sandflies.

The finding of more infected *Lu. umbratilis* in collections from tree-trunks (Fig. 2) than in catches off man (Wijers and Linger, 1966; Lainson *et al.*, 1976) could be due to a higher percentage of parous flies on the tree-trunks. Although *Lu. umbratilis* is not the principal man-biter in endemic "pian-bois" regions (Forattini, 1959; Wijers and Linger, 1966), various catching methods have shown that it rests during the daytime on tree-trunks and, if disturbed, readily bites man. Wijers and Linger (1966) also noted that it attacked man to a greater extent in the early morning and, even though the total number of sandflies caught off man at this time of day was small (an average of only 12 per hour), it was the dominant species. One cannot exclude the possibility that other sandfly species may sometimes be concerned in the transmission of *L. b. guyanensis*, but the very high infection rate of 7·3% encountered by Lainson *et al.* (1976) in Monte Dourado suggests that *Lu. umbratilis* is responsible for the high endemicity of "pian-bois" in that region of Brazil. We feel that the daytime biting habit of *Lu. umbratilis* is the major factor which increases the man/vector contact to an unusual degree—for man normally only works in the forest during the day. This particular situation is an excellent example of how important vector-species may be overlooked merely because they are not the most obvious of the anthropophilic species in an area, and indicates the great importance of determining infection-rates in wild-caught sandflies which are known to feed on man during the night *and* the day.

The high infection rate in *Lu. umbratilis*, as found in Monte Dourado, Brazil, suggests that there is a close relationship of this sandfly species with the mammalian reservoir(s), which are as yet unknown. It is very reminiscent of the high incidence of *Leishmania major* ("oriental sore") found in *Phlebotomus caucasicus* and *P. papatasi* caught in the burrows of infected gerbils, *Rhombomys opimus*, in Iran (Nadim *et al.*, 1968).

C. *LEISHMANIA BRAZILIENSIS PANAMENSIS*

More is known about the reservoirs of this parasite than any other member of the *braziliensis* complex. Table 2 lists the known hosts, which include four species of phlebotomine sandflies and seven species of wild mammals. The only domestic animal so far found infected is the dog (Herrer and Christensen, 1976a), but it would seem that like man, this animal is merely an accidental host which becomes infected in the deeper forest regions, most probably during hunting trips (Herrer and Christensen, 1976b; Herrer *et al.*, 1976). It has been suggested that such dogs may nevertheless serve as an incidental reservoir of infection for sandflies in isolated patches of forest where the wild animal reservoirs no longer exist, and that this might account for sporadic cases of the human disease in areas normally free from infection. The role of the dog as a reservoir surely remains insignificant, however, even in the above-mentioned situations, and the true source of infection is among the wild, forest mammals.

Investigations on flagellate infections found in wild-caught Panamanian sandflies (Johnson *et al.*, 1963) suggested that the source of the parasites was possibly an arboreal animal, or animals, since infection rates were higher in the arboreal sandfly species (e.g. *Lutzomyia trapidoi*) than they were in those which occurred predominantly at ground level (e.g. *Ps. panamensis*).

It remains uncertain exactly what proportion of the promastigote infections observed by Johnson *et al.* (1963) were *Leishmania*. McConnell (1963) studied a number of the isolates made from such infections and concluded that whilst some undoubtedly were developmental stages of *Leishmania*, others were definitely not. During studies on the life cycle of *Endotrypanum schaudinni* of sloths in Panama, Shaw (1964) noted that this parasite developed as promastigotes in the hindgut of sandflies, and suggested that some of the infections recorded by previous workers (Johnson *et al.*, 1963) could have been *E. schaudinni*. Subsequently, an isolate of promastigotes from a naturally infected *Lu. trapidoi*, which had a heavy pyloric infection, proved to be *E. schaudinni* (Shaw, unpublished observations). The workers at the Gorgas Memorial Laboratory, Panama (Anon., 1967), also recorded an isolate from another specimen of *Lu. trapidoi* which appeared to be serologically identical with the porcupine parasite, *Leishmania hertigi*. It seems, then, that the flagellate infections of wild-caught Panamanian sandflies may be either *L. b. panamensis*, *Leishmania* species not normally infecting man, or developmental stages of other haemoflagellates such as *Endotrypanum*.

The link between arboreal animals and some of the natural promastigote infections of sandflies was finally completed by Herrer and Telford (1969) who found a high proportion of sloths to be infected with *L. b. panamensis* and, later, Herrer *et al.* (1973) concluded that the two-toed sloth, *Choloepus hoffmanni* (Fig. 3), is the major host. We have already discussed the importance of inapparent *Leishmania* infections in wild mammalian hosts (Part IV, C): in this respect it may be noted that none of the infected Panamanian sloths showed any outward signs of infection, and amastigotes were scattered throughout apparently normal skin, and in the viscera.

A number of points regarding the epidemiology of *L. b. panamensis* are worthy of further discussion. Of the four species of sandflies that have been incriminated as vectors, *Lu. trapidoi* and *Lu. ylephiletor* bite man readily, have a wide host range (Tesh *et al.*, 1972), and occur in the forest canopy and at ground level. These facts strongly suggest that these two species occupy a position of major importance as vectors of *L. b. panamensis*, especially to man. It is not so easy, however, to assess the importance of *Lu. gomezi* and *Psychodopygus panamensis*, although in the Santa Rita region of Central Panama they are dominant (Johnson *et al.*, 1963): it seems that they are probably secondary vectors that may assume a major role in certain areas. A fifth species, *Ps. pessoana*, was found to be the major man-biter in one endemic area (Herrer and Christensen, 1976a) and has been recorded as preferentially feeding on edentates (Tesh *et al.*, 1972). This circumstantial evidence clearly indicates that *Ps. pessoana* should be considered as a possible vector in some areas of Panama. Flagellates have not been encountered in this fly, but this is probably because insufficient numbers have been dissected (Johnson *et al.*, 1963).

In Panama, Chaniotis *et al.* (1971b) used light traps and the aspiration of resting flies from tree trunks and buttresses to study the distribution and seasonal variation of sandflies. In general they noted that there were more sandflies in the mature forest and that in this habitat the valleys

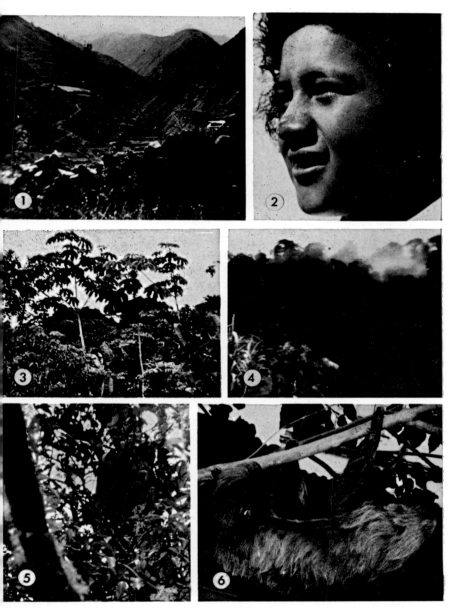

FIG. 3. Some epidemiological and epizootiological aspects of neotropical cutaneous leishmaniasis. 1. Typical endemic area for "uta", due to *Leishmania peruviana*, in the Peruvian Andes. 2. Case of "uta": lesion on external surface of nose. 3. Forest interface in Panama: habitat of *Lutzomyia olmeca bicolor*, suspected vector of *L. mexicana herreri*. 4. Achiote area of Central Panama, endemic for cutaneous leishmaniasis due to *L. braziliensis panamensis*: hilltop forest where the vector *Lutzomyia trapidoi* is particularly abundant. 5. The sloth, *Choloepus hoffmanni* (arrowed), major vertebrate host of *L. b. panamensis*, in natural habitat. 6. The sloth, *Choloepus didactylus*, host of an unidentified subspecies of *L. braziliensis* in Pará State, Brazil. [1 and 2 from Lainson and Shaw (1973).]

(Fig. 3) were less productive than the hill tops. During the dry season, however, when overall populations were low, more sandflies were caught in the valleys. They noted that nearly twice as many anthropophilic species were captured in light traps near the ground than in the canopy. *Lu. trapidoi* and *Lu. ylephilator* populations peaked twice during the year, between July and August and December and January. *Ps. panamensis* was most abundant at the beginning of the wet season while *Lu. gomezi* was most abundant in the period between the end of the dry season and the beginning of the wet season. They noted that dry-season rains were invariably followed by a rapid but temporary increase in adult activity. These authors suggested that the critical factor affecting the sandfly populations is the quantity of ground-water and that seasonal variations in species may reflect varying quantities of ground-water in different breeding sites. In studying the daily and seasonal man-biting activity of Panamanian sandflies, Chaniotis *et al.* (1971a) found no clear relationship between man-biting rates and the respective numbers caught in light traps and from resting sites. They concluded that man-biting activity was, therefore, not only related to the density of the population but also to other undefined factors, such as the physiological state of the flies. In Belize, however, Disney did find a relationship between the number of resting *Lu. o. olmeca* and those found biting rodents, and we have found that there is a correlation between the numbers of *Lu. flaviscutellata* taken in rodent-baited traps and those biting man.

Light-trap catches were made in 11 different localities in the Panama Canal Zone by Rutledge *et al.* (1975) and they concluded that there were two distinct sandfly associations, one dominated by the zoophilic species *Lu. carpenteri* and the other by the anthropophilic species *Lu. gomezi* and *Ps. panamensis*. They also found a third situation in which the *carpenteri* association was dominant in the dry season and the *gomezi/panamensis* association in the wet season. Using the same methods they (Rutledge *et al.*, 1976) studied the sandflies of Empire Range, where American military personnel frequently contract cutaneous leishmaniasis. In this area there were sites where the *carpenteri* association occurred and others where the third type of situation dominated. Where there was little or no evidence of human infection they found the *gomezi/panamensis* association. They concluded that transmission to man occurs in situations or seasons where zoophilic sandfly species are dominant in light-trap catches.

Thatcher and Hertig (1966) investigated sandfly resting sites of Panamanian sandflies in animal burrows, hollow trees, tree buttresses and holes under rocks. The only man-biter that they found was *Lu. ylephiletor*, in rock crevices and buttresses. They concluded that natural cavities were only attractive to sandflies when they concealed a food source or were suitable breeding sites. Chaniotis *et al.* (1972) examined animal burrows, tree holes, tree trunks at different heights, green plants and leaf-litter. Of the anthrophilic species a few, such as *Lu. trapidoi* and *Lu. ylephiletor* were found on tree-trunks at heights up to 5 metres. The majority, however, including *Lu. trapidoi, Lu. gomezi, Ps. pessoana, Lu. olmeca* and *Ps. panamensis*, were found resting on green plants and in forest-floor leaf-litter. Of the sandflies caught off green shrubs and saplings, 96% were *Ps. pessoana* and it was noted that larger numbers were collected after rain or when the forest floor was excessively wet. In order of abundance the following species were found resting in forest-floor leaf-litter: *Lu. trapidoi, Ps. pessoana, Lu. gomezi, Ps. panamensis* and *Lu. olmeca bicolor*. It was noted that very wet leaf-litter gave the poorest catches while the largest were invariably from dry or damp leaf-litter, regardless of the season. In moving around in the forest during the day, man could easily disturb flies resting on green plants or in the leaf-litter which would increase his chances of being bitten. Epidemiologically this could be important since transmission may take place during the night or day.

Hanson (1961) searched for the breeding sites of Panamanian sandflies by collecting immature stages. He obtained 2258 larvae or pupae and of these he reared 600 to the adult stage for identification. Most (2123) of the immature stages were found in soil from the buttresses of trees and, of those that were reared, only one was an anthropophilic species, *Lu. trapidoi*. Immature stages of the anthropophilic species, *Lu. trapidoi, Ps. panamensis, Ps. pessoana*, and *Lu. ylephilator* were found amongst the dead leaves of the forest floor.

Rutledge and Ellenwood (1975a, b) studied the breeding sites of Panamanian sandflies using "soil emergence traps". Their results indicated that drainage and vegetation were important factors: thus, on hilltops (Fig. 3) they found *Ps. pessoana, Lu. gomezi* and *Ps. panamensis* while *Lu. trapidoi* apparently preferred the more unstable leaf-litter found on hillsides and along the edges of streams. The former three species also appeared to prefer the litter under large trees, while *Lu. trapidoi* was more common in soils of areas where there were large lianas. The predominant species captured in the "soil emergence traps" was *Lu. trapidoi* (Rutledge and Ellenwood, 1975a).

The situation in Panama appears to be very complex but this may reflect the kind of epidemiological picture that exists in other *braziliensis* enzootic areas. Generally it would seem that *L. b. panamensis* does not have a uniform enzootic pattern but a mosaic of mammal/sandfly associations which are probably governed by the prevailing ecological conditions. The major mammal/sandfly cycle involves two-toed sloths and *Lu. trapidoi*, but in more limited areas other mammals and sandflies may serve to maintain the cycle. Clearly the risk of infection to man will depend on the infection rate in sandflies and the degree to which they bite man.

D. *LEISHMANIA BRAZILIENSIS:* UNIDENTIFIED SUBSPECIES

PANAMA: We have already dealt with *L. b. panamensis*, but there is some evidence to suggest that other members of the *L. braziliensis* complex occur in Panama. Thus, there is a limited number of case-reports of mucocutaneous leishmaniasis (Jaffé, 1960); since the causative parasites were not isolated, it remains impossible to say if these infections were due to *L. b. panamensis* or another subspecies. Significantly, however, Walton *et al.* (1977) noted a small percentage of cases of cutaneous leishmaniasis from the Caribbean coast of Panama, from which it proved impossible to establish the parasites in a culture medium which was ideal for *L. b. panamensis*. There is also a single isolate (Herrer *et al.*, 1971) from an arboreal "rat", *Diplomys labilis*, which has yet to be characterized (Herrer *et al.*, 1973), and at present it can only be referred to as a *Leishmania* sp.

In Panamanian laboratories the method of choice for isolation of *Leishmania* from man, wild mammals and sandflies has been *in vitro* culture: the more fastidious parasites, such as those encountered by Walton *et al.* (1977), might, therefore, have been missed in the extensive surveys carried out there. It would seem vital to make numerous isolations of parasites *in hamsters*, in particular from the rare cases of mucocutaneous leishmaniasis of man.

COSTA RICA: this is the most northerly point in the Americas from which *braziliensis* parasites have been recorded. They were isolated from two-toed and three-toed sloths (Zeledon *et al.*, 1975) and the sandfly *Lutzomyia ylephiletor* (Zeledon and Alfaro, 1973). From their behaviour in hamsters and in culture, and the geographical proximity to Panama, it seems likely that the parasites belong to the subspecies *panamensis*.

An unusual feature noted by the Costa Rican workers was the isolation of *Leishmania* from the blood of one sloth in the apparent absence of parasites in the viscera. This is atypical of infections in this animal from elsewhere and, even though one might expect parasites at times to enter the peripheral blood from the viscera, the total absence of the organism in the internal organs seems extraordinary.

NICARAGUA, HONDURAS and EL SALVADOR: There seems to be no information on the types of cutaneous leishmaniasis in these countries and, as records from Mexico, Belize and Guatemala only refer to *mexicana* parasites, it would seem that the geographic limit of *L. braziliensis* is somewhere between Costa Rica and Guatemala.

COLOMBIA: There is considerable clinical evidence for the occurrence of *braziliensis* parasites in Colombia; little has been published on the epidemiology of the disease, however, although, as in other Latin

American countries, it appears to be associated with the forested regions. At the time of writing, we are unaware of any studies of Colombian parasites in laboratory animals (including sandflies) or culture. In a country as large as Colombia, which embraces tropical rain-forest on the Pacific and Amazon sides of the Andes, it seems very likely that more than one member of the complex is responsible for the human disease. Barreto (1969) reported that the phlebotomine fauna biting man in the Pacific lowlands, near Buenaventura, was very similar to that of Panama; and it may be that leishmaniasis due to *L. b. panamensis* extends from Costa Rica, down through Panama, and along the Pacific coastal region of Colombia.

VENEZUELA: As in Colombia, there is considerable clinical evidence suggesting the presence of parasites of the *braziliensis* complex. Pifano (1960) discussed the epidemiology of mucocutaneous leishmaniasis (a form of the disease particularly associated with some subspecies of *L. braziliensis*) in members of farming communities which were being established in forested areas. Domestic animals, such as the dog and the donkey, have been found with leishmaniotic skin lesions in such situations (Pons, 1968), but it seems that they, like man, were merely accidental hosts and became infected when they accompanied their owners into the forest. Nothing is known about the wild reservoirs of the parasite(s) in these regions, and although there are records of natural flagellate infections in four species of sandflies (Table 1), the identification of the organisms remains obscure. Infections have been found in some wild mammals (Table 1) but, with the possible exception of the bat parasite, they were probably due to parasites of the *mexicana* complex, which will be discussed later. Until numerous isolates are available for study, from both cutaneous and mucocutaneous cases of Venezuelan leishmaniasis, one can only say that these diseases are most probably caused by members of the *L. braziliensis* complex.

BRAZIL: Isolates, from a "spiny rat" (*Proechimys guyannensis*), an opossum (*Didelphis marsupialis*) and a rat (*Rattus rattus*) (Table 2) have all been shown to be peripylarians from their prolific development in the hindgut of experimentally infected sandflies (Lainson *et al.*, 1977b). These parasites are still being studied, and at the moment we cannot confidently assign them to any of the existing subspecies of *L. braziliensis*. They differ from each other, however, in their behaviour in hamsters and in *in vitro* culture. The *Didelphis* parasite is unique among all other Amazonian Peripylaria we have so far examined in its capacity to grow very well in our simple NN medium made with "Oxoid nutrient agar (CM3)"; biochemically (Chance *et al.*, 1974; Gardener *et al.*, 1974) it appears closest to *L. b. panamensis*, suggesting an extraordinarily wide geographical distribution for this organism. The *Didelphis* parasite appears to differ both morphologically and culturally from strains of *L. b.*

panamensis that we have studied, and it would seem advisable that the biochemical studies should be extended to include isoenzymes other than MDH, upon which its identity was partially based (Gardener *et al.*, 1974).

The *Didelphis* and *Proechimys* parasites were isolated from animals caught at Km 25 of the Itaituba–Altamira sector of the Transamazon highway, Pará, where the major man-biting sandflies were found to be *Ps. complexus*, *Ps. paraensis*, a *Psychodopygus* species close to *squamiventris* and *Ps. tintinnabulus* (Fraiha *et al.*, 1977). The *Rattus* isolate was from an animal captured in a labourers' camp at Km 969 of the Jacaréacanga-Humaita sector of the Transamazon highway, where the major man-biters were found by the same authors to be *Ps. chagasi*, *Ps. paraensis* and *Lu. yuilli*. We see, therefore, a picture slowly emerging in the Amazon region involving different *braziliensis* parasites, and different sandfly and mammalian hosts, even within a relatively restricted area. As yet we have made no isolates of *Leishmania* from man, in the Amazon region, which are comparable with the above mentioned three organisms, but our studies on human infections in the areas from which they came have been few.

The *Leishmania* from *Rattus rattus* is the only one we have so far isolated from a "domestic" animal: although the animal was caught in a camp of the Roads Department, it presumably became infected in the surrounding forest. Examination of 44 small forest mammals from the same area revealed only 3 infections of *Proechimys guyannensis* with *L. m. amazonensis*, and no evidence of any parasite of the *braziliensis* type; it suggests that the source of the *Rattus* parasite was some wild animal not frequently encountered by normal trapping methods.

Rattus rattus is, of course, an introduced species and would be foraging for food among the camp supplies and refuse thrown into the nearby forest. These rats could easily become infected when penetrating the forest edge, but their subsequent rôle as a reservoir of infection for men living in the camps would clearly depend on the anthropophilic tendencies of the sandflies that fed on the rats.

Deane (1948) found amastigotes in the viscera of two-toed sloths captured near Abaetetuba, Pará but he was not certain if they were developmental stages of *Endotrypanum* or *Leishmania*. We have obtained sloths from this same general area and have isolated *Leishmania* from the skin and viscera (Tables 2 and 3). The strains are presently being studied but it is already clear that they differ from *L. b. braziliensis* and *L. chagasi*. From their behaviour in hamsters and culture the sloth parasite appears to be closest to *L. b. guyanensis*.

We have recently studied some cases of cutaneous leishmaniasis from forest near to the Pirelli rubber plantation, some 20 Km from Belém, and the parasite isolated grew very poorly in culture and hamsters. An examination of opossums (*Didelphis marsupialis*) from the Utinga forest,

4 Km from Belém (which is ecologically very similar to the rubber plantation area), led to the isolation of promastigotes in a culture from liver tissue of one animal. Efforts to maintain the isolate *in vitro* failed, however, and the infection did not take in hamsters. Although we cannot even be sure that the parasite was a *Leishmania* species, its behaviour in culture was reminiscent of that of the isolates of *L. braziliensis* we have made from the Pirelli patients, and of those associated with lower Amazonian mucocutaneous leishmaniasis.

In other states, such as Ceará, Minas Gerais, Bahia, Goiás and the Mato Grosso, there is clinical evidence for the existence of *braziliensis* parasites but there have as yet been no detailed studies on the parasites involved and we have been unable to find published records of infections from wild animals and sandflies from these regions. A strain from a case of mucocutaneous leishmaniasis from Ceará has been studied in experimentally infected *Lu. longipalpis* and *Lu. renei* (Coelho *et al.*, 1967a) but the descriptions of the hindgut infections are insufficiently detailed to determine if it behaved as a typical peripylarian. The endemic cutaneous leishmaniasis areas in Ceará are in the cooler mountainous regions where *Lu. whitmani* and *Lu. migonei* predominate over *Lu. longipalpis* in extradomiciliary catches off man (Deane, 1956). There is, therefore, some epidemiological evidence to suggest that the situation in Ceará may be more similar to that found in São Paulo than that in the Amazon region.

We have examined a number of isolates of *Leishmania* from man, sent to us from Goiás and Manaus, Amazonas State, and their behaviour is essentially that of subspecies of *L. braziliensis*. Finally, in the Aripuanã area of Mato Grosso State we have isolated *braziliensis*-like parasites from man; in the same region the predominant anthropophilic species of sandflies were *Ps. complexus*, *Lu. umbratilis*, *Lu. yuilli* and *Ps. davisi*, and the presence of the first two species reminds one of the situation in areas endemic for *L. b. guyanensis*. Dissections of sandflies taken off human bait in Aripuanã revealed attached paramastigotes and free promastigotes in the hindgut of two *Lu. yuilli*, and an epimastigote infection in yet another fly of this species (Lainson *et al.*, 1977c). Flagellates from the first two infections were inoculated into the skin of hamsters, with negative results: possibly they represented developmental stages in the life-cycle of some other haemoflagellate, such as *Endotrypanum*.

ARGENTINA: Cutaneous leishmaniasis occurs throughout the northern states and it seems that more than one aetiological agent is involvedt There are epidemiological situations, such as in the states of Jujuy, Sala. and Catamarca, that resemble that associated with "uta" in Peru (see Part VIII), but there are also descriptions of children with mucocutaneous leishmaniasis (Villalonga, 1963) suggesting the presence of *braziliensis* parasites. There is little information on reservoir hosts but

Mazza (1926a; 1927) described leishmanial infections in dogs and horses. It is not clear, however, if such animals serve as reservoirs or merely represent accidental infections similar to those seen in dogs by Herrer and Christensen (1976a) in Panama. In one area of the Tucumán *Lu. migonei* and *Lu. cortelezzii* have been found (Romaña and Abalos, 1949) which suggests some similarity with endemic areas of São Paulo and Paraná, Brazil.

OTHER COUNTRIES: Cutaneous leishmaniasis has been recorded from Paraguay (Migone, 1935), Bolivia (Barrientos, 1948; Walton *et al.*, 1973) and Ecuador (Escomel, 1922). We have been unable to find any references to reservoir hosts in these countries but the association of the disease with forest suggests the importance of silvatic animals.

VII. Neotropical Suprapylaria

The name *Leishmania tropica mexicana* was originally given by Biagi (1953b) to the parasite causing "chiclero's ulcer" in the Yucatan Peninsula, Mexico, but Garnham (1962) thought it sufficiently distinct from other neotropical leishmanias to raise the name *mexicana* from subspecific to specific rank.

For many years it was considered that this parasite was limited to the northern region of Central America and that the causative agent of cutaneous and mucocutaneous leishmaniasis in man elsewhere in the American continent was *L. braziliensis*. Lainson and Shaw (1972), however, recognized the agent of rodent leishmaniasis in the Lower Amazon region as a new subspecies of *L. mexicana* and named it *L. mexicana amazonensis*. They also noted that this parasite was the causative agent of "diffuse cutaneous leishmaniasis" of man in this general area of Brazil, and that it was also occasionally associated with uncomplicated, single-sore infections. Further studies have now shown *L. mexicana* to be widespread throughout Latin America, and in the future it may well prove that the members of the Suprapylaria have a much greater geographical distribution in the neotropics than do parasites of the Peripylaria.

In the present work we use the name *L. mexicana* in referring to members of the Suprapylaria which readily infect hamsters, grow luxuriantly in a variety of simple blood-agar media, have nuclear and kinetoplast DNA buoyant densities of 1·718 and 1·697–1·700, respectively, and have relatively large amastigotes (3·4 × 2·2 μm). From Table 2 it can be seen that far more reservoir hosts are known for *L. mexicana* than for *L. braziliensis*: this is almost certainly due to the ease with which the former can be cultivated *in vitro* and its virulence for hamsters.

A. *LEISHMANIA MEXICANA MEXICANA*

There are a number of rodent reservoirs of this parasite but, to date, the only sandfly found infected in nature is *Lutzomyia olmeca olmeca*. The first animals to be incriminated were the rodents *Ototylomys phyllotis* (the "big-eared climbing rat") (Fig. 5), *Heteromys desmarestianus* ("Desmarest's spiny pocket-mouse") (Fig. 5) and *Nyctomys sumichrasti* ("Sumichrast's vesper-rat") (Lainson and Strangways-Dixon, 1962). In a more detailed publication (Lainson and Strangways-Dixon, 1964) the highest incidence was found to be in *Ototylomys phyllotis*, with 8 out of 20 of these animals infected (Fig. 5). Disney (1966) added the rodent *Sigmodon hispidus* to the list of reservoirs, although this "cotton-rat" is generally found in grassy savannah and is unlikely to become more than an accidental host, when straying into "fringe" forest. As workers in Belize did not at that time appreciate the importance of inapparent skin infections in wild mammalian reservoir hosts, it remains difficult to assess the individual importance of the first three rodents mentioned. Lainson and Strangways-Dixon (1964) found *Heteromys desmarestianus* to be the most commonly trapped rodent, however, and an examination of apparently normal skin from this animal may show a very much higher infection rate.

During his studies in Belize, between 1964 and 1966, Disney (1966) designed a beautifully simple oil-trap for catching phlebotomine sandflies attracted to a rodent bait. Using this trap, it was soon shown that the predominant sandfly attracted to rats was *Lu. o. olmeca*, whereas the more highly anthropophilic species such as *Lu. cruciata*, *Lu. ovallesi*, *Lu. shannoni* and *Ps. panamensis* were seldom taken in rat-baited traps.

The finding of a sandfly species commonly feeding on known rodent reservoirs was a major breakthrough which ultimately led to the incrimination of *Lu. o. olmeca* as the vector of *L. m. mexicana* (Biagi *et al.*, 1965a; Disney, 1968; Williams, 1970). In October, 1965, Disney (1968) found the first natural infection of *Lu. o. olmeca* with *L. m. mexicana*, in a specimen caught in a rodent-baited trap set in the Central Farm area (Cayo District) of Belize; and in December of the same year Biagi *et al.* (1965a) caught infected *Lu. o. olmeca* off human bait in the Quintana Roo area of Yucatan, Mexico.

The pieces of the jig-saw puzzle had been found, but it remained to organize them to relate the enzootic infection in rodents to the zoonotic disease in man. Basically this is an ecological problem, and in the following text we have attempted to indicate what we feel to be the most plausible explanation.

"Chiclero's ulcer" is a silvatic zoonosis and infected sandflies and wild mammals are restricted to forested areas. Disney (1968) pointed out the difficulties in classifying this habitat and suggested that the "bush" might be subdivided into "low", "medium" or "high" forest, based on the percentage of trees of differing diameter. Williams (1970) also pointed out the problem of using many collecting techniques simultaneously in all study areas, during the same period, in order to determine the relative abundance of the sandfly or mammalian species; with these limitations in mind Disney (1968) and Williams (1970) made the following observations.

Disney found that *Lu. o. olmeca* was a wet-season species, biting in the lower levels of the forest and in particular at a height of up to one metre. There were waves of emergence, detected in rodent-baited traps and catches from natural resting places. He also found *Lu. permira* to be the dominant rodent-biter in the middle zone (4–8 metres): it was most abundant in the dry season and had a restricted distribution. Very significantly, *Lu. o. olmeca* showed a marked preference for the rodent *Ototylomys*—the animal in which most infections had been noted.

In sandfly catches off man *Lu. o. olmeca* usually represented a very small percentage of the total catch (Biagi and Biagi, 1953—0·0%; Garnham and Lewis, 1959—0·8%; Strangways-Dixon and Lainson, 1966 —1·2%; Williams, 1965—0·4%; Williams *et al.*, 1965—0·12%; Biagi *et al.*, 1965a—8·1%), the major man-biting species in this region being *Lu. cruciata*, *Ps. panamensis*, and *Lu. shannoni*. At this point, however, it should be emphasized that data on anthropophilic habits of sandflies is much more meaningful if related to the number of man-hours of capturing.

Dissections of sandflies from Belize and Mexico have revealed promastigote infection-rates in *Lu. o. olmeca* varying from 6·0% (Biagi *et al.*, 1965a) to 0·3% (Disney, 1968). The latter author recorded rates of 0·3% in the Central Farm area and 0·9% in a trapping site on the Chiquibul Road, while Williams (1970) found 1·2% infected at Roaring River, 1·5% at Chiquibul Road (mile 8) and 0·5% at Chiquibul Road (mile 10·5). The variations in infection rates are presumably related to the number of infected mammalian reservoirs; and habitats that support higher populations of rodents are likely to have higher infection rates in *Lu. o. olmeca*. Of the 17 promastigote infections found in this fly by Disney (1968) and Williams (1970), 9 were proven to be *L. m. mexicana*.

Other flagellate infections have been recorded in a variety of sandfly species from Belize, but their true nature remains obscure: the infected flies included *Lu. steatopyga*, *Lu. trinidadensis*, *Lu. shannoni*, *Lu. ovallesi*, *Lu. cruciata*, *Lu. permira* and *Ps. panamensis* (Strangways-Dixon and Lainson, 1966; Disney, 1968; Williams, 1970). Only the parasites of the latter 4 insects appeared to be promastigotes, but none of those inoculated into hamsters produced any leishmanial infection, and those from *Lu. cruciata* and *Ps. panamensis* failed to produce infections when inoculated intradermally into 3 volunteers (Williams, 1970).

Disney (1968) found that the rodents most commonly captured at ground level in "low" and "medium" forest were *Ototylomys*, *Heteromys* and *Sigmodon*, in that order. In a comparison of the numbers caught in paired traps on the ground and in trees, he noted that *Heteromys* was exclusively terrestrial while only 18·0% of the *Ototylomys* captured were taken at ground level. During brief studies in the "high" forest he also captured all three rodents: the presence of *Sigmodon* in such a habitat is unusual as this animal is described by most mammalogists as essentially a grassland species. Lainson and Strangways-Dixon trapped their wild animals in an area in Roaring River, which we feel was comparable with Disney's "high" forest, both before and after a hurricane virtually destroyed the area. They found *Heteromys* to be the most commonly captured rodent, followed by *Ototylomys*, but this was probably because most of their trapping was carried out on the ground: however, they never caught *Sigmodon* in high forest.

The breeding season of *Ototylomys* is mainly during the first half of the year and it has been suggested that it nests on the ground, but moves about on the ground and in the trees during the night: young and pregnant rats seem to be the most commonly associated with the forest floor (Disney, 1968). There is thus an abundant supply of young, non-immune animals during the wet season when *Lu. o. olmeca* populations are at their highest, although the climbing habit during the night would presumably lower the *Ototylomys*–vector contact to some extent. All the ecological evidence available, however, does suggest that the "big-eared climbing rat" is the most likely rodent to become infected with *L. m. mexicana* by virtue of its abundance, behaviour and breeding habits; peak transmission almost certainly takes place during the rains, when the vector is most abundant and there is a large proportion of young, non-immune rats. It is possible that the presence of patent lesions may be related to the age at which the infection takes place, and young animals may develop conspicuous, destructive lesions rather than inapparent skin infection. This aspect will be discussed further when we deal with *L. m. amazonensis*.

From the above data it would seem that the zone below 4 metres is the only one in which the known vector has ample contact with the rodent reservoirs. This also coincides with the zone in which man is most active and it is apparently in the "high" forest that men are most often infected, when collecting chiclé or cutting mahogany trees. Predominance of the disease among such people has led to the name of "chiclero's ulcer" or "chiclero's ear". The chicleros are the most afflicted, as they spend almost all the wet season in the forest (when the chiclé sap is rising), exactly when the sandfly vector population is at its greatest.

Lesions due to *L. m. mexicana* are, as one might expect, usually limited to the exposed parts of the body. Numerous authors, however, have noted that they are much more frequent on the upper part of the body, with up to 40% of the lesions on the ears (Fig. 5): the reasons for this are obscure. Lainson and Strangways-Dixon (1963) felt that it was most probably due to the much greater exposure of the upper body, as the forest workers usually use shirts and long trousers. They also noted that there was a strong tendency for body lesions to cure spontaneously, but for ear lesions to be remarkably persistent: these two factors would influence the incidence on the face and ears considerably. Williams (1970), however, felt that *Lu. o. olmeca* did have a natural tendency to bite the upper body and in particular the ears: he noted that the distribution of bites on man approached that of the lesions, but his observations were based on only eleven bites. This was clearly insufficient evidence, and Williams himself pointed out that ". . . this fly landed too rarely on man for a definite conclusion".

In the Yucatan, Mexico, Biagi (1953a) noted that of 55 chicleros, 31% became infected in their first season of work and about 16% in their second year. Chalmers *et al.* (1968) skin-tested 1442 people from 14 villages in Belize and found only 9·2% to have evidence of present or past infection: of these, 18·1% were men and 3·7% were women, and only 26·8% of those with positive reactions were actually aware of having had the disease.

Compared with the incidence of positive reactions in rural populations in the Amazon region of Brazil, these figures from Belize are low, suggesting that the vector–man contact is poor. There are records of infections acquired during a single daytime visit to the forest (Lainson and Strangways-Dixon, 1963): as some other members of the same group had been working constantly in the same area for nearly two years without becoming infected, however, one might regard such cases as exceptional. Both Lainson and Strangways-Dixon (1963) and Chalmers *et al.* (1968) noted evidence of inconspicuous or inapparent infections with spontaneous cure, which doubtless accounts for the latter authors' high number of persons with positive skin tests in the absence of any remembered infection.

In 1968 Shaw and Lainson discussed evidence indicating that sandflies of the *Lu. flaviscutellata-olmeca* complex rarely bit man, and Williams (1970) agreed that "this is certainly the case in British Honduras" (Belize). The existence of the human disease in the face of such poor contact between the vector among the rodents and man therefore led us to suggest that some other species might possibly act as a vector to man.

Williams (1970) rejected this hypothesis, as he was unable to find *L. m. mexicana* infections in any sandfly other than *Lu. o. olmeca*, and discussed the conditions under which there was some degree of contact between man and this fly. He pointed out (Williams, 1965) that a few specimens of this species were found under dead leaves on the forest floor and, in a more extensive study of this micro-habitat, Disney (1968) had captured 73 female *Lu. o. olmeca* and 147 female *Ps. panamensis*. It was suggested that man, walking through the forest during the daylight hours would disturb such flies and probably be bitten. While working in the forest, Disney (1968) had noted that he and his assistants were in fact bitten in the daytime: while admitting that they missed many of these flies, they did capture 15 *Lu. o. olmeca* during two years.

Williams (1970) went on to compare the catches made between 0500–1000 hours, from stationary men and others who were moving about and intermittently disturbing the forest floor. During 331 hours of catching, they obtained only 1 *Lu. o. olmeca* from the stationary men, but 45 in 71·75 hours from the active men. It is important to stress, however, that these observations were not coincidental; the catches off the stationary men being made during the dry season, when the *Lu. o. olmeca* population is low, and those off the active men during the wet season, when the population is at its highest. Biagi *et al.* (1965a) recorded 376 *Lu. o. olmeca* taken off man between 1630–2200 hours, in the Quintana Roo area of the Yucatan, during December, 1965. There were from 24 to 30 persons engaged in the trapping, however, and this high amount of activity may have been responsible for the unusually large number of this species taken.

From all the above mentioned observations it is clear, then, that small numbers of *Lu. o. olmeca* do bite man, by day and night. In the wet season there are more flies and more risk of being bitten: in addition, there are areas where the infection rate of *L. m. mexicana* in this sandfly is higher than usual and the chances of man becoming infected are still greater. The relatively low incidence of cutaneous leishmaniasis among men of rural populations (Chalmers *et al.*, 1968) reflects the overall poor contact between the vector and man, but all the available evidence does support the view that *Lu. o. olmeca* is responsible for the transmission of *L. m. mexicana* among wild rodents and, under certain conditions, accidentally to man.

Before finally dismissing the role of other sandflies, however, further efforts clearly should be made to elucidate the nature of the promastigote infections seen in other species, in particular *Lu. cruciata*, *Lu. permira* and *Ps. panamensis*. The fact that they did not infect hamsters is particularly interesting in view of the observations of both Disney (1968) and Williams (1970) that some promastigotes in *Lu. o. olmeca* also failed to infect these animals. There remains the possibility, of course that some other species or subspecies of *Leishmania* also exists in the Yucatan and Belize. If so, such flagellate infections, even if not capable of actually infecting man, could produce allergic reactions which would be important both clinically and epidemiologically.

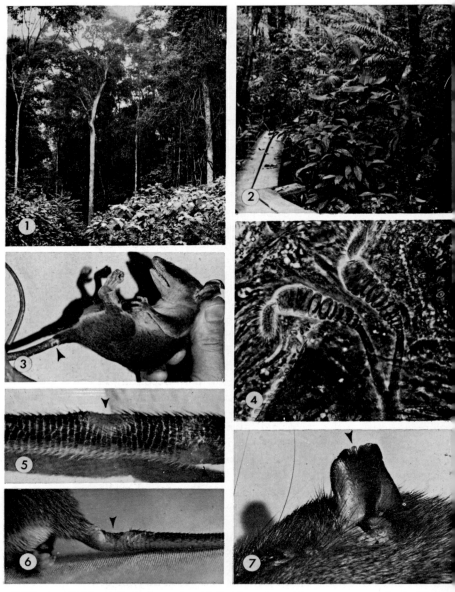

FIG. 4. Epidemiological aspects of *Leishmania mexicana amazonensis*. 1. Tall, secondary forest of Utinga, Belém, Pará State, Brazil, where *L. m. amazonensis* is common in rodents. 2. "Swamp forest" of Catu, Belém, Pará, where large numbers of the vector *Lutzomyia flaviscutellata* are found. 3. Lesion due to *L. m. amazonensis* on tail of opossum, *Marmosa murina*. 4. Spermathecae of *Lu. flaviscutellata*. 5. Tail lesion of naturally infected rodent, *Oryzomys capito*, and 6. *Neacomys spinosus*. 7. Ear lesion of naturally infected rodent, *Proechimys guyannensis*. [3 from Lainson and Shaw (1969b); 6 from Lainson and Shaw (1971).]

B. *LEISHMANIA MEXICANA AMAZONENSIS*

In 1963, one of us (R.L.) had the opportunity to discuss the epidemiology of "chiclero's ulcer" with Dr. Otis Causey, in the arbovirus laboratory of the Instituto Evandro Chagas, in Belém, Brazil. Dr. Causey mentioned having seen skin lesions (Fig. 4) on the tails of some rodents captured during his work in the local forest and he promised to examine them for possible *Leishmania* infections. Within two weeks he had uncovered a remarkably heavy focus of rodent leishmaniasis in the cricetid rodent *Oryzomys capito*. This was studied by Guimarães and Azevedo (1964) who noted tail lesions on 24 out of 111 *O. capito* examined. Guimarães and Costa (1964, 1966) studied the behaviour in hamsters, mice and man of the *Leishmania* isolated from this rodent; they found that in hamsters and mice it behaved very similarly to a strain isolated from a case of diffuse cutaneous leishmaniasis, and that it was infective to man. They concluded that a major reservoir of cutaneous leishmaniasis for man had at last been discovered in the Amazon region, and Giumarães and Costa (1966) in fact referred to the parasite as *L. braziliensis*.

Over a period of some years we compared the behaviour of many isolates of *Leishmania* from man and rodents, and concluded that the parasite found by Causey rarely infected man and was, in fact, distinct from *L. braziliensis*. From its behaviour we considered it to be a new subspecies of *L. mexicana* and (Lainson and Shaw, 1972a) named it *Leishmania m. amazonensis*. Differences were noted between it and *L. m. mexicana* during cross-immunity trials in monkeys (Lainson and Shaw, 1977c); again, its nuclear and kinetoplast DNA buoyant densities are 1·718 and 1·697–1·699, respectively, compared with 1·718 and 1·700 for *L. m. mexicana* (Chance *et al.*, 1974); finally, the malate dehydrogenase (MDH) type of *L. m. amazonensis* is III, while that of *L. m. mexicana* is II (Gardener *et al.*, 1974).

Subsequent investigations in Belém and other foci in Brazil (see Tables 2 and 3), revealed infections in 7 different rodents, 2 genera of marsupials, and foxes (Lainson and Shaw, 1968, 1969a-b, 1970, 1973). It was noted, however, that the most common infections were inapparent, and isolations were made from apparently normal skin (Lainson and Shaw, 1973). Furthermore, appreciation of this fact led to the discovery that the echimyid rodent *Proechimys guyannensis* was clearly the major host of *L. m. amazonensis*, and not *Oryzomys capito* as previously thought (see Table 3). One other interesting finding was that infections in *Oryzomys* captured along the Transamazon highway were all inapparent, unlike those causing destructive skin lesions (Fig. 4), in the same rodent, in the Utinga forest, Belém. Possibly the age of the animal when it acquires the infection may influence the subsequent course of the infection. It is thus noteworthy that adult, laboratory-bred *Oryzomys capito* inoculated with promastigotes of *L. m. amazonensis* all developed inapparent infections. More studies are clearly needed to determine the reasons for the difference between the two types of infection in nature: to date, no biochemical differences have been found between isolates of *L. m. amazonensis* from the Utinga forest, Belém, and those from the Transamazon highway.

Using Disney-traps, we found (Lainson and Shaw, 1968) that the predominant sandfly species biting rodents in the high secondary forest of Utinga was *Lutzomyia flaviscutellata* (Fig. 4), and we felt sure that it must be the vector of *L. m. amazonensis*. No infected flies of this species were found in over 700 specimens dissected from the first trapping site, but a trap 300 metres away caught 8 heavily infected *Lu. flaviscutellata* out of a further 1996 examined, a good indication of focality of the infection, almost certainly due to movements of the reservoir hosts. Since these observations, a further 4802 *Lu. flaviscutellata* have been dissected (Ward *et al.*, 1973a) and a further 37 infections encountered (0·77%). Of the overall total of 45 infections, flagellates from 18 were separately inoculated into hamsters and *L. m. amazonensis* isolated on 15 occasions. In one case the inoculated hamster died one week after the inoculation, and before any detectable infection would have appeared: the final success-rate is therefore more correctly regarded as 15 out of 17 attempted. It is reasonable to suppose, therefore, that the remaining 27 infections seen, but not inoculated, were also due to the same parasite. This, with the failure to find *L. m. amazonensis* in any other species of sandfly dissected from the same area, and the subsequent experimental transmission of the parasite from hamster to hamster with laboratory-bred *Lu. flaviscutellata* on at least four occasions (Ward *et al.*, 1977; Ward, 1977b) leaves us in no doubt as to the importance of this fly as the major and probably the only vector of *L. m. amazonensis* in the Amazon region.

We have studied the feeding habits of *Lu. flaviscutellata* (Shaw and Lainson, 1968) and noted that although it fed avidly on rodents, especially *Proechimys*, it is only rarely taken off man. Based on catching and infection rates, we calculated that an infected fly might bite a rodent once in 23 days, and a man only once in 445 days—an observation reflected in the very high incidence of infection in certain wild rodents and the very low incidence in man. It was noted, however, that some areas of the same forest gave consistently higher catches of *Lu. flaviscutellata* than others and in such micro-areas the rat/fly and man/fly contact must be much greater. The insect has remarkably catholic feeding habits and has been shown to feed readily on most of the known mammalian hosts of *L. m. amazonensis*, including foxes (Ward, 1974).

The most commonly infected wild mammals, *Proechimys* and *Oryzomys* are essentially terrestrial, and, while opossums climb, they do forage

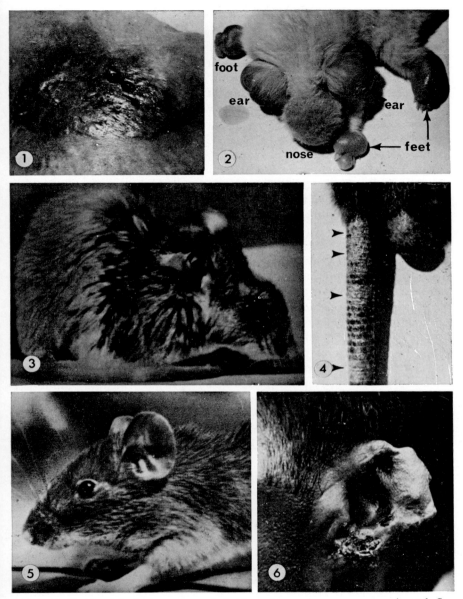

FIG. 5. Epidemiological aspects of *Leishmania mexicana amazonensis* and *L. mexicana mexicana*. 1. Lesion due to *L. m. amazonensis* in man: note marks of punch biopsies. 2. Hamster infected with *L. m. amazonensis*: large histiocytomata following metastatic spread to ears and feet. 3. *Ototylomys phyllotis*, an important rodent host of *L. m. mexicana* in Belize. 4. Multiple lesions on tail of *O. phyllotis*, due to *L. m. mexicana*. 5. *Heteromys desmarestianus*, another rodent host of *L. m. mexicana*. 6. Typical eroded ear-lesion in man due to *L. m. mexicana*: "chiclero's ulcer". [3–5 from Lainson and Strangways-Dixon (1964); 6 from Lainson and Strangways-Dixon (1963).]

around on the forest floor for food. It was not surprising to find, therefore, that the vector *Lu. flaviscutellata* is very much a "low-zone" fly:
approximately 26 times more flies were found attracted to *Proechimys*
bait at 0·2 metres than at 1·2 metres (a difference of only 1 metre!), and
it was noted that a sitting man was bitten by about twice as many *Lu.
flaviscutellata* as a standing man (Shaw *et al.*, 1972). Finally, parasitological examination of 108 cases of human cutaneous leishmaniasis over
the past 8 years (Shaw and Lainson, 1975) showed that only 10 (9·2%)
were caused by *L. m. amazonensis* and, as far as we could ascertain, all
acquired their infections in forests similar to those near to Belém which
have high *Lu. flaviscutellata* populations. All the lesions in adults were
on the lower parts of the body; and 3 cases were in children under 5
years old, whose average height was less than one metre. We have never
seen lesions of the ear (Fig. 5), so typical of "chiclero's ulcer" caused by
L. m. mexicana. These findings support our conclusions of low-level
transmission of *L. mexicana amazonensis*, as does our failure to find any
infections in predominantly arboreal animals such as sloths, kinkajous,
and *Cebus* and *Saimiri* monkeys, although the latter three are susceptible
to experimental infection (Lainson and Shaw, 1968).

Finding cases of infection in very young children is particularly interesting, for they are unlikely to stray far from their homes to play. This
suggests that their infections may have been acquired in the low, secondary forest commonly found very near houses in rural areas.

Long-term studies on the populations of *Lu. flaviscutellata* in different
types of forest (Shaw and Lainson, 1972) showed that there were up to
3 times more flies in the wetter "swamp forest" (Fig. 4) than in the drier
forest, and that this difference may be as high as 5 times at certain times
of the year: the increase in population may augment the fly/man contact
by as much as 25 times, and we feel that it is under such conditions that
transmission to man takes place.

Ward (1974) found that although populations of *Lu. flaviscutellata*
were large in low secondary forest, they were generally much smaller in
the high dry forest. Numbers caught in areas subjected to daily, tidal
flooding were very small indeed. The liking of this sandfly for damp conditions is interesting and Ward and Ready (1975) noted that the exo-
chorion of its eggs have "volcano-like" aeropyles which are undoubtedly
the basis for a well developed plastron, and indicate a successful adaptation to a wet habitat.

Seasonal fluctuations of the *Lu. flaviscutellata* populations have been
extensively studied in the forests around Belém (Shaw and Lainson,
1972; Ward, 1974; Aitken *et al.*, 1975). There is a clear association between numbers of this fly and rainfall, although this appears to vary
according to the type of soil and ground elevation. In the swamp-forest
("igapó") the population builds up during the dry season (June–

December) to reach a peak between October and December; with the onset of the rains (January), it begins to decline and is at its lowest between March and May. In the drier secondary forest ("capoeira") (Fig. 6) the peak is high for a short period, during the beginning of the rains, and then falls sharply. Finally, in the high, dry forest ("terra firme") the population is highest during the earlier part of the dry season (August to September). Ward (1974) suggested that the largest numbers of *Lu. flaviscutellata* are produced when the wet and dry seasons are accentuated, and he noted that fewer flies were caught when the annual rainfall was more evenly spread.

Studies on the *Oryzomys* population by the Belém Virus Laboratory of the Instituto Evandro Chagas (Aitken *et al.*, 1975) showed that the breeding activity of this rodent was mainly during the early months of the year. This, then, would result in an increased number of susceptible, non-immune animals during the middle of the year. During a capture and release programme, however, we noted that there were in fact *fewer* new infections of *L. m. amazonensis* in *Oryzomys* at that time. This suggests that it is the number of sandflies that is the key factor in transmission among this rodent, rather than the presence of non-immune animals. A similar situation was noted by Aitken *et al.* (1975) for the transmission of Pacui virus, which is also transmitted among *Oryzomys* and *Proechimys* by *Lu. flaviscutellata*.

Muirhead-Thompson (1968) discussed the importance of age-grading of insect populations in vector ecology and epidemiology, and notes that extensive work with anophelines has shown physiological changes during the gonotrophic cycle to have a profound influence on behaviour. Such factors could well apply to sandflies, and if one particular method of catching gave more parous flies it would be useful in detecting potential vectors. Studies on the accessory gland secretions of *Lu. flaviscutellata* by Lewis *et al.* (1970) and Ward (1974) have shown that the presence of granules is useful in determining parous rates in this species. Lewis *et al.* (1970) found no evidence that parous flies bit at any particular time of the night. Ward (1974) observed that as *Lu. flaviscutellata* populations decreased, so the proportion of parous flies increased. More work is needed on parous rates in wild *Lu. flaviscutellata* but these preliminary observations do indicate that transmission may take place at any time during the night, and that transmission is likely to lag over into the period when the population is declining. In the Catu forest, Belém, we have found the highest infection rates of *L. m. amazonensis* in *Lu. flaviscutellata* to be in March when the population is falling off.

Recent observations (Ward *et al.*, 1977) on the behaviour of laboratory-reared *Lu. flaviscutellata* showed that infected flies may re-feed up to 3 times: this suggests that the potential of parous flies as vectors is greater than previously suspected. There are no data on how many feeds wild flies take, but the relatively high parous rates recorded (Lewis *et al.*, 1970; Ward, 1974) in wild caught *Lu. flaviscutellata* is perhaps a reflection of its ability to survive oviposition.

In summing up, we conclude that the following factors limit the transmission of *L. m. amazonensis* to man. The swamp-forest is the most likely area where the infection may be acquired, since there are sufficient mammalian reservoirs and a large population of the vector, *Lu. flaviscutellata*. This type of area forms only a relatively small proportion of the Amazon forest, however, and is seldom used by man except for small-scale collection of palm-nuts and palm-hearts: even hunters tend to ignore it, as most of the important game animals are found in the higher, drier forest. The disinclination of *Lu. flaviscutellata* to bite man is perhaps the most important factor limiting the human disease: and even though the population level of this fly may increase to a sufficient degree to enable transmission to man, this is limited to a few months of the year. In the swamp-forest man would seem most likely to become infected during the dry season. The high secondary forest, between the tidally flooded and dry forest, has been shown to be a low risk habitat (Shaw *et al.*, 1972), but in micro-areas of high *Lu. flaviscutellata* density, between November and January, man's chances of being infected become much greater. The low, drier secondary forest is potentially a high risk habitat, but again only for part of the year; it is possible, too, that the *Lu. flaviscutellata* population, here, may be maintained by non-reservoir animals, again reducing the chance of human infection. One can only, therefore, judge the hazards of infection by the dissection of large numbers of *Lu. flaviscutellata* and/or by the finding of infected animals.

C. *LEISHMANIA MEXICANA PIFANOI*

Medina and Romero (1959) originally gave the name of *L. braziliensis pifanoi* to the causative agent of Venezuelan diffuse cutaneous leishmaniasis of man, first seen by Convit (1946) and later described by Convit and Lapenta (1948). To our knowledge, there are no records of the isolation of the parasite from uncomplicated, single-sore infections, although these surely must exist. New isolates of the parasite are badly needed to define accurately *L. mexicana pifanoi*. Thus, Gardener *et al.* (1974) could not distinguish material, sent to them as "*L. mexicana pifanoi*", from *L. mexicana mexicana*: it seems unlikely that the geographic range of *L. m. mexicana* should be interrupted in Panama by the presence of *L. m. aristedesi*, only to commence again in Venezuela.

Material from the lesions of Venezuelan cases of diffuse cutaneous leishmaniasis produce typical *mexicana*-type infections in hamsters (Fig. 5), with metastases to the extremities in older infections (Medina and Romero, 1959). Parasites with a similar behaviour have been isolated from the rodent *Heteromys* by Torrealba *et al.* (1972), and from *Lu. flaviscutellata* by Pifano *et al.* (1973). Cutaneous lesions which were probably due to *L. mexicana* (and possibly *L. m. pifanoi*) were seen in *Proechimys* (Convit, 1968) and *Zygodontomys* (Kerdel-Vegas and Essenfeld-Yahr, 1966). The human infections came from the States of Yaracuy, Lara and Miranda, whereas the infected animals were found in the states of Carabobo and Amazonas.

The wide geographical separation of these areas suggests an extensive distribution of *mexicana*-like parasites in the forested regions of Venezuela. Whether or not they are all the same subspecies can only be determined by the examination of more isolates. The available evidence does suggest, however, that *L. m. pifanoi* is likely to be a parasite of forest rodents that is transmitted by sandflies of the *Lu. flaviscutellata/olmeca* complex. On rare occasions it is transmitted to man, giving rise to diffuse cutaneous leishmaniasis (and presumably single-sore infections). The fact that *L. m. pifanoi* and *L. m. amazonensis* cause diffuse cutaneous leishmaniasis is quite remarkable, suggesting that the *mexicana* subspecies have some inherent property which, in immune-deficient patients, is much more likely to result in this particular clinical form of the disease than infection with other neotropical leishmanias. Cutaneous leishmaniasis caused by *L. braziliensis* subspecies is commoner in man, in the same areas, and yet diffuse cutaneous leishmaniasis has never been attributed to these organisms.

D. *LEISHMANIA MEXICANA ARISTEDESI* NOV. SUBSP.

This subspecies was isolated by Herrer *et al.* (1971) from wild rodents and one marsupial (Table 2), captured in the Sasardi area of the San Blas Territory of Eastern Panama. The parasite has nuclear and kinetoplast DNA buoyant densities of 1·718 and 1·698 respectively, and an MDH Type I (Chance *et al.*, 1974; Gardener *et al.*, 1974).

Of the *Oryzomys capito* examined, 14 (36%) out of 39 were positive, whereas only 8 (4%) of 202 *Proechimys semispinosus* were infected: the remaining infections were in 1 out of 35 murine opossums (*Marmosa robinsoni*), and 1 out of 2 pacas (*Agouti paca*).

In *Oryzomys* and *Marmosa* the parasite characteristically produced destructive lesions, principally on the base of the tail. Of the *Proechimys*, 4 had infections of the skin in the absence of detectable lesions: in the other 4 it was difficult to decide whether ear damage was due to the parasite or was mechanical in origin.

This situation is somewhat at variance with our previous discussion on the importance of benign, inapparent infections of *Leishmania* in natural hosts (Part IV, C). Thus, the low incidence in *Proechimys* does not suggest this animal to be a very important host of *L. m. aristedesi*, even though the infection was of a very mild nature: while the incidence in *Oryzomys* was high, the consistent presence of destructive lesions does not suggest a very well balanced host–parasite relationship.

Studies by Telford *et al.* (1972) showed that both *Oryzomys* and *Proechimys* were only captured in the secondary growth interface (Fig. 3) between the primary forest and deserted agricultural land. From their description of the area it would appear to be relatively low and flat, and subjected to flooding during exceptionally wet years. As in other areas, both *Oryzomys* and *Proechimys* were shown to be essentially terrestrial in habits.

Thatcher (1968) used modified Disney traps in high, primary forest in Central Panama, and found small numbers of *Lu. olmeca bicolor* biting opossums, kinkajous and porcupines at ground level. Chaniotis *et al.* (1971b) studied the distribution of Panamanian sandflies, using light-traps, and caught more *Lu. o. bicolor* in mature, hilltop forest than in the mature lowland or secondary forest. Catches from these three biotopes, during a period of 16 months, indicated *Lu. o. bicolor* to be most abundant during the early wet season.

In the Sasardi region, where the infected wild animals were encountered, Christensen *et al.* (1972) noted that *Lu. o. bicolor* was the third most abundant species taken in light-traps set in secondary forest, but the dominant sandfly on Disney traps baited with *Oryzomys*, *Proechimys* and the opossum *Metachirus*. They also showed it to be the most common species collected from forest-floor leaf litter, and that it was a ground-loving insect.

All the above observations indicate that there is considerable variation in the distribution of *Lu. o. bicolor* in the different types of Panamanian forest, but until more studies are made, preferably using Disney traps, it is still difficult to draw any firm conclusions regarding the relative abundance of this species in the different biotopes. The studies of Chaniotis *et al.* (1971b) and Christensen *et al.* (1972) do suggest, however, that the insect is more common in secondary forest of Eastern Panama, than in that of Central Panama.

Christensen *et al.* (1972) suspected *Lu. o. bicolor* as the most likely vector of *L. m. aristedesi*, on their epizootiological evidence, but failed to isolate the parasite after inoculating pooled triturates of the insects into hamsters; this may have been due to the long storage period before inoculation. No infections were encountered in 449 freshly dissected specimens, but in view of our experiences with the related parasite *L. m. amazonensis* in *Lu. flaviscutellata* this is rather a small number on which to base conclusions (see Part VII, B).

Lu. o. bicolor represented 3·2% of anthropophilic species in Eastern Panama, and only 1·03% in Limbo Field, Central Panama (Christensen *et al.*, 1972; Chaniotis *et al.*, 1971a), which does not suggest that the insect is likely to be of great importance in transmitting *L. m. aristedesi* to man. Although no human cases have been reported to date, it is quite likely that they do occasionally occur: it was not until we routinely isolated *Leishmania* from every available case of cutaneous leishmaniasis, in Belém, that the rare instances of infection with *L. m. amazonensis* were disclosed. It is notable, too, that most isolations of the parasite from man in Panama were carried out in the vicinity of the Canal Zone—a region from which no wild animals have yet been found infected with *L. m. aristedesi*. The apparent absence of the parasite in that area is intriguing, especially as both the mammalian hosts and the suspected vector do occur in the forest bordering the Canal Zone.

E. *LEISHMANIA MEXICANA*: UNIDENTIFIED SUBSPECIES

Worth *et al.* (1968) noted lesions on the tails of rodents and marsupials captured in the Bush Bush forest of Trinidad and remarked on their similarity to those seen in animals infected with *L. m. mexicana*, in Belize. It was Tikasingh (1969), however, who demonstrated amastigotes in material taken from tail lesions of animals captured in the Turure forest. He considered (Tikasingh, 1974) that the parasite was *L. m. amazonensis*, but as Trinidad is over 2000 Km from the type locality of this parasite, and only about 700 Km from that of *L. m. pifanoi* in Venezuela, it is perhaps wiser to refrain from giving a subspecific identification until the parasite's biochemical characters have been fully studied.

Tikasingh (1974) disclosed a variety of rodent and marsupial hosts, but as *Oryzomys* was the most common infected animal and had by far the highest infection rate, he concluded that it was the major host. This can only be confirmed, however, when infections have been looked for in normal skin (see Part VII, B).

Lu. flaviscutellata proved to be the predominant rodent-biting sandfly, both in the drier forest of Vega de Oropouche and the wetter ones of Turure and Aripo-Weller Field (Tikasingh, 1975). Of 1954 dissected, promastigote infections were found in the midgut and foreguts of 20; of these, 3 were shown to be *L. mexicana* subsp., and from Tikasingh's description it seems most likely that the other infections were due to the same parasite. The highest infection rates were found in flies from the drier forest of Vega de Oropouche, where most of the infected animals were found; strangely enough, however, the density of *Lu. flaviscutellata* here was *less* than in the wetter forest of Turure and Aripo-Weller Field, where fewer infected mammals had been trapped. This suggests that population dynamics of the mammalian hosts controls the infection rate in the sandfly host, rather than variation in populations of the vector.

Studies on the habits of *Lu. flaviscutellata* once more confirmed that this species is very much restricted to the forest floor. Highest densities were found in the better drained forest of Vega de Oropouche during the rainy season, while in the wetter forests the peak occurred at the beginning of the wet season and then declined as the rainy season progressed.

Human infections with *Leishmania* are rare in Trinidad, and none has been recorded since 1930 (Tikasingh, 1974): it is impossible to say, however, if these early cases were due to *L. mexicana* or *L. braziliensis* subspecies. Clearing of forest for sugar and citrus plantations at the beginning of the century greatly reduced the areas of natural forest, and almost certainly this resulted in the apparent disappearance of human cases. The continued existence of enzootic leishmaniasis in the wild mammals, in the absence of human infection, is doubtless a reflection of the very limited man-biting habits of *Lu. flaviscutellata*.

In conclusion, it appears that subspecies of *L. mexicana* are principally parasites of silvatic rodents belonging to the genera *Ototylomys*, *Proechimys* and *Oryzomys*, among which they are transmitted by sandflies of the *Lu. flaviscutellata/olmeca* complex. Other rodents and marsupials act as secondary mammalian reservoirs, but no secondary vector species have yet been incriminated. Our knowledge of the biology of the mammalian and insect hosts indicates that transmission occurs at ground level, where man also becomes infected.

Infections of *L. mexicana* in man are commoner in the Yucatan region of Central America than in the rest of the South American continent, where they are mostly known as relatively rare cases of "diffuse cutaneous leishmaniasis". In no part of the Americas does the incidence of *L. mexicana* infection reach that recorded for *L. braziliensis*, and this is principally due to the limited man-biting habits of the vectors *Lu. flaviscutellata* and *Lu. olmeca*.

Judged on the incidence in man (which may be misleading, due to excessive occupational contact with the forest in particular areas) it would seem that infection in the Yucatan is found principally in the high, primary forest (*L. m. mexicana*). In South America, enzootics are most frequent in the swamp-forest and high secondary forest (*L. m. amazonensis* and *L. m. aristedesi*), although natural and man-inspired felling of large trees in areas of primary, high forest may create pockets of secondary growth suitable for the establishment of small foci of *L. mexicana*.

Man is most likely to become infected in those forests with unusually high vector populations, and where the infection is circulating efficiently among the mammalian reservoirs. In those habitats where the vector is in more normal proportions, we tend to find the enzootic but not the zoonotic form of the disease.

F. *LEISHMANIA ENRIETTII*

This is perhaps the best known of all the *Leishmania* parasites, simply because it readily infects guinea-pigs and, therefore, is an ideal immunological tool. In contrast, little is known of the organism's epizootiology or its possible epidemiological importance.

In March 1945, Medina (1946) planned to inoculate some laboratory reared guinea-pigs (*Cavia porcellus*) with cultures of pathogenic fungi causing blastomycosis. He noted, however, that one of the animals had a tumour-like lesion on one ear and the skin near the testicles. He made stained smears from these lesions and found a few large amastigotes: material was then inoculated by various routes into further guinea-pigs, and Medina noted that there was metastatic spread of the infection to extremities such as the feet, ears and nose. The spleen became enlarged, and he isolated the organism from this organ as well as from the liver, bone-marrow and blood.

Muniz and Medina (1948) continued to study the parasite and noted that it would apparently not infect rhesus monkeys, wild guinea-pigs (*Cavia aperea*), dogs or white mice. Six weeks after inoculation, a small lesion was seen in the skin of one out of eight hamsters, and histological sections showed scanty amastigotes in the macrophages. Two volunteers were also inoculated intradermally with culture forms, and after three months neither showed any evidence of infection. Muniz and Medina noted that the amastigotes of the guinea-pig parasite were very much larger than those of other leishmanias, such as *L. donovani* and *L. braziliensis*, and this plus their inability to infect man and most laboratory animals led them to give a new name to the organism, *Leishmania enriettii*.

Later, Luz et al. (1967) found new foci of domestic guinea-pig leishmaniasis in the outskirts of Curitiba, Paraná State. They captured sandflies in the Paraná pine woods (*Araucaria angustifolia*) near the foci, and caught the species *Lu. monticola* off man and on the tree-trunks. The catches were made during the warmer months of the summer at about two o'clock in the afternoon: ten *Lu. monticola* were fed on an infected guinea-pig and six became infected. The infections were described as heavy, with parasites distributed throughout the whole gut, and on one occasion they were inoculated into a "clean" guinea-pig. No infection resulted, though the reasons for this are not clear: Luz and his colleagues concluded that *Lu. monticola* could possibly be the natural vector of *L. enriettii* in the Curitiba region.

More studies are needed to substantiate this suggestion, but this interesting paper raises a number of points to be considered. The fact that spontaneous outbreaks of guinea-pig leishmaniasis were found to occur in domestic guinea-pigs some 20 years after its discovery does suggest some source in wild animals. Although experimental infection could not be produced in *wild* guinea-pigs (*Cavia aperea*), no attention seems to have been paid to the possibility that such animals may have developed a disseminated, inapparent infection of the skin, as occurs in porcupines infected with *L. hertigi* and as we found to result in *Oryzomys* inoculated with *L. m. amazonensis*. Such infections could be the rule, in nature, among the wild guinea-pig (the "preá").

The finding on tree-trunks of a suspected vector which attacks man in the day, is reminiscent of the situation in enzootic areas of *L. braziliensis guyanensis* in north Brazil. In the highlands of southern Brazil there is a timber industry based on the exploitation of the Paraná pine, and possibly men involved in logging might be repeatedly bitten by *Lu. monticola*, or other sandflies. If there is a vector of *L. enriettii* among these, man would stand a good chance of periodic inoculation with this parasite; in this respect it would be most interesting to have figures on the incidence of positive leishmanin tests among those persons closely associated with the Paraná pine forests. Human leishmaniasis has been reported in this State, but seems to be concentrated in the lowland areas of the Paraná valley, and the region of the Paranapanema river valley between Londrina and Jaguariaíva (Pessôa, 1967).

G. *LEISHMANIA HERTIGI HERTIGI*

There is no evidence, till now, that either of the two known subspecies of *L. hertigi* are capable of infecting man but, as stressed in our discussion on *L. enriettii*, man may be occasionally bitten by their sandfly vectors, with subsequent serological or immunological responses.

L. hertigi hertigi was described from the Panamanian porcupine, *Coendou rothschildi* Thomas, and appears only to infect that animal in nature. The host–parasite relationship is clearly an ancient and well adjusted one, for the infection is completely asymptomatic, with small numbers of amastigotes scattered throughout the dermis and viscera, in the absence of any apparent host-cell response. Usually the infection is only detected following culture of tissues in blood-agar medium, in which the parasite grows abundantly. Infections can be induced in the hamster after the intradermal inoculation of either promastigotes or amastigotes, but it is of very low grade, and eventually dies out; the parasites appear to be restricted to the site of inoculation in the skin, and the viscera are uninvolved. The incidence of *L. h. hertigi* in Panamanian porcupines is astonishingly high (up to 88%), and the infection is of long duration, probably for life.

Herrer (1971) gave the new specific name on the grounds of the parasite's apparent host specificity, its failure to immunize hamsters against subsequent challenge with *L. b. panamensis* and the peculiar elongate amastigotes, which measured from 3·5 to 4·8 × 1·2 to 2·5 μm; biochemical studies (Chance *et al.*, 1974; Gardener *et al.*, 1974) have since confirmed this specific identity.

Lainson and Shaw (1973) provisionally placed *L. h. hertigi* in the *L. braziliensis* complex, but subsequently removed it to a group of its own (here, tentatively within the Suprapylaria) because of its failure to undergo any development in the pylorus of sandflies (Lainson *et al.*, 1977b), and its distinct biological and biochemical characters. The subspecific name became necessary when Lainson and Shaw (1977b) described *Leishmania hertigi deanei*, from Brazilian porcupines.

H. *LEISHMANIA HERTIGI DEANEI*

Deane *et al.* (1974) examined spleen smears from a porcupine which was shot in the Mato do Cafundó forest, Município of José de Freitas, State of Piauí, Brazil. They found scanty amastigotes but the organism was unfortunately not isolated and no other tissues were examined. Later, they found similar parasites in the liver of another porcupine, apparently of the same species, and from the same locality: none were detected in the skin, spleen, kidney, lung or peripheral blood. Again, the organism was not isolated, but Deane *et al.* regarded it as "a *Leishmania* proper to the porcupines". The host was not identified with certainty, but suspected to be *Coendou prehensilis prehensilis* (L.). The amastigotes of the Brazilian parasite differed considerably from those of Panamanian *L. hertigi* in their larger size, highly vacuolated cytoplasm and rod-shaped kinetoplast. In view of the scanty material, however, it remained unnamed.

Lainson and Shaw (1977b) examined 18 porcupines from the State of Pará, Brazil, and isolated a *Leishmania*, in blood agar cultures of skin and viscera, from 11 (61.1%). Two of the infected animals were identified as *Coendou prehensilis*, but the others were all considered to be a previously undescribed species of *Coendou*.*

Scanty amastigotes were seen in stained smears of the liver and spleen of one of the porcupines (*Coendou* n.sp.) and were remarkably similar to those described by Deane *et al.*: they were also seen in histological sections of skin from the same animal. In view of the very different morphology, and other criteria of serology and biochemistry,† the authors gave a new subspecific name to the organism, *Leishmania hertigi deanei*.

* Personal communication, Dr. C. O. Handley, Smithsonian Institution, Washington, D.C. See, also, Pine, R. H. (1973): we understand that a description of this porcupine is in press.

† Electrophoretic mobility patterns of glucose phosphate isomerase and glucose-6-phosphate dehydrogenase (personal communication from Mr. S. L. Croft, and Drs. M. L. Chance and L. F. Schnur, Liverpool School of Tropical Medicine).

The amastigotes of *L. h. deanei* are large compared with most other leishmanias: they range from 5·1 × 3·1 to 6·8 × 4·5 μm (average 6·1 × 3·7 μm), approximately the same size as those of *L. enriettii* and very much larger than *L. h. hertigi*. The cytoplasm is highly vacuolated and the kinetoplast appears as a small curved rod: in these features the parasite again differs from *L. h. hertigi*, in which the amastigotes were figured as non-vacuolated and with a small rounded kinetoplast.

Like the Panamanian parasite, *L. h. deanei* is scattered throughout the upper dermis of the porcupine and is also found in the liver and spleen. Infections are asymptomatic and the parasites evoke no host-cell reaction in the surrounding tissues. *L. h. deanei* has not yet been found in any animal other than the two porcupine species referred to above and it is probably highly host-specific: our attempts to produce infections in hamsters and the guinea-pig have failed.

The vectors of both subspecies of *L. hertigi* remain unknown, but it is reasonable to suppose that they are phlebotomine sandflies. Porcupines are common rodents in Brazilian forests and, considering their high incidence of infection, it is surprising that we have not yet found sandflies with promastigote infection which might be considered as *L. h. deanei*. This suggests that transmission is by a very host-specific fly which lives in close association with the porcupine, possibly in its home in hollow tree-trunks. Workers in the Gorgas Memorial Laboratory in Panama found *L. h. hertigi* to develop very poorly in the local sandfly species, *Lutzomyia sanguinaria* and *Lu. gomezi* (Anon., 1967), and Lainson *et al* (1977b) had no greater success with *L. h. hertigi* and *L. h. deanei* in *Lutzomyia longipalpis*.

I. *LEISHMANIA CHAGASI*

1. Distribution and incidence of infection in man

In 1913 Migone described the first autochthonous case of visceral leishmaniasis of man in the Americas, in Paraguay. The patient, however, had spent some time in Porto Esperança, Mato Grosso State, Brazil, and most probably contracted the disease there.

Mazza and Cornejo (1926) registered further Latin-American cases, when they found amastigotes in spleen smears from two Argentinian children who had never left that country. It was not until the viscerotomy studies of Penna (1934), however, that some real idea of the importance of the disease was gained, when he demonstrated 41 parasitologically proven cases of visceral leishmaniasis in various States of Brazil. They included Ceará (15 cases), Bahia (9), Sergipe (5), Alagoas (4), Pará (3), Piauí (3), Rio Grande do Norte (1) and Pernambuco (1). Later Brazilian workers registered further infections elsewhere in the country: in the

States of Mato Grosso (Oliveira, 1938; Chagas and Chagas, 1938), Paraíba (Almeida, 1945), Minas Gerais (Maciel and Rosenfeld, 1947), Goiás (Barbosa, 1966), and Espírito Santo (Martins et al., 1968).

Sporadic cases also appeared in other South and Central American countries: in Venezuela (Martinez and Pons, 1941), Bolivia (Barros and Rosenfeld, 1942; Alencar, 1955), Colombia (Gast Galvis and Rengifo, 1944), Paraguay (Boggino and Haas, 1945), Guatemala (Cabrera and Léon, 1949), El Salvador (Bloch and Guillon, 1950), Mexico (Villaseñor et al., 1953; Biagi and Tay, 1963), Surinam (Winckel and Aalstein, 1953), Ecuador (see Deane and Deane, 1964), Honduras (Nuernberger et al., 1975) and even the tiny West Indian island of Guadeloupe (Courmes et al., 1966).

Although visceral leishmaniasis is widespread in the neotropics, from Mexico to Argentina, by far the majority of cases have been recorded in Brazil. Even the next highest incidence, that of Venezuela, pales into insignificance in comparison. Thus, in a review of the existing literature, Deane and Deane (1964) gave the total figure of 3200 cases from all of Latin America up to that date; with 3120 from Brazil (97·5%), 48 from Venezuela (1·5%) and 32 (1%) from other countries. From 1964 until 1976 there have been 501 more cases reported from Brazil, 50 from Venezuela and 11 from other Latin American countries (Ward, 1977a).

While these figures suggest a decrease in the number of human cases, they may only be a reflection of the fact that there has been little intensive epidemiological study of the disease during the last 10 years or so: some recent records of outbreaks of the disease in various parts of Brazil and, less dramatically, in other countries, however, leaves no doubt as to the continued problem of visceral leishmaniasis in Latin America (Baruffa and Cury, 1973; Guedes et al., 1974; Fernandes et al., 1976 and Chaddad et al., 1976 in the States of Mato Grosso, Paraíba, Rio Grande do Norte and Bahia, Brazil; Pifano and Romero, 1973, in Isla de Margarita, Venezuela; Nuernberger et al., 1975, in Honduras).

2. Identification of the parasite

Both L. donovani and L. infantum had been shown to infect a variety of laboratory animals, and when Cunha and Chagas (1937) failed to establish infections in similar hosts with the organism isolated from cases of visceral leishmaniasis from Pará and Sergipe States, they concluded that this warranted the new name of Leishmania chagasi for the parasite. In later experiments, however, Cunha (1938a) succeeded in infecting hamsters, monkeys and dogs, and concluded that their previous failures had been due to the inoculation of non-viable flagellates from old cultures. He extended his studies (Cunha, 1938b, 1942) to serology, and suggested that absorption/agglutination tests showed the causative agent of American visceral leishmaniasis to be identical with L. infantum Nicolle of the

Mediterranean region. Although Wenyon (1946) questioned the value of these tests, Cunha's altered opinion did find some support from Senekjie (1944) who, however, synonymized *L. chagasi* with *L. donovani* on the basis of biochemical and cultural characteristics, thermal death-points, and the lytic effect of bile on the two organisms.

Differences of opinion exist to this day on the identity of the *Leishmania* responsible for American visceral leishmaniasis, and the following points of view may be considered.

(a) That all visceral leishmaniasis is due to the same parasite, *Leishmania donovani*. This extreme view is largely founded on the *overall* clinical similarity of the disease, whether in Asia, Europe or the Americas. On such grounds alone, one might equally argue that all cutaneous leishmaniasis is due to *Leishmania tropica*.

(b) That there are two forms of visceral leishmaniasis. One caused by *L. donovani*, in Asia, and the other due to *L. infantum* or closely allied parasites in the Mediterranean countries, parts of Asia, the Middle East and Africa, and virtually all the South American continent. The parasite of American visceral leishmaniasis is regarded as most probably imported into Latin America as recently as post-Columbian times by European or African immigrants (presumably slaves, in the latter case).

While it remains impossible to refute this theory completely, there are some arguments against it. It does suggest, for example, that there was either an unusually rapid spread of the disease throughout all 14 of the affected neotropical countries, or a virtually coincidental introduction of the parasite(s) at various points, from Mexico to Argentina. Again, as far as we are aware, the source of slaves for both the Portuguese and Spanish colonists of South and Central America was the notorious "Slave Coast" of West Africa (in particular Guinea), and visceral leishmaniasis is absent from this region. Even if some infected slaves had originated from East Africa, where the disease *is* endemic, it remains to explain the different clinical and epidemiological features between Kenyan and Sudanese "kala-azar" (not infantile, and no canid reservoirs) and American visceral leishmaniasis (very much infantile, and much more common in canids than in man).

What of the colonists themselves? One of the interesting features of Mediterranean visceral leishmaniasis is the extremely poor infection rate obtained when the sandfly vectors feed on man: so poor, in fact, that Adler (1940) and Adler and Theodor (1957) did not consider that man serves as a source of infection. In the dog and other canids, however, parasites are extremely abundant in the unbroken skin of the animals and give a very high infection rate in sandflies. It would seem, then, that man himself is most unlikely to have introduced *L. infantum* into the Americas, and the real question to resolve is whether or not the disease was imported in dogs. Canids (e.g. foxes) were, of course, well distributed throughout the Latin American continent before the European invasion, and there is no reason why they should not already have had their own leishmanial parasites.

As Adler and Adler and Theodor pointed out, Mediterranean visceral leishmaniasis appears to have a very stable epidemiology and has not been known to establish itself in any new foci in recent times. Vectors of *L. infantum* are limited to sandflies of the *Phlebotomus major* group and the parasite has not adapted to other species in the endemic areas, in spite of ample opportunity to do so. It would seem unlikely, therefore, that this should suddenly happen following the introduction of infected man or dog into Latin America, where the phlebotomine fauna is so different that the sandflies have actually been removed from the genus *Phlebotomus*.

It might be argued that Adler and Theodor's reasoning has been somewhat shaken by recent laboratory transmissions of some leishmanial parasites, other than *L. chagasi*, by *Lutzomyia longipalpis* (see Table 4): the following points should be noted, however. Firstly, the natural vectors of those parasites (*L. m. mexicana* and *L. m. amazonensis*) are of the same genus (*Lu. o. olmeca* and *Lu. flaviscutellata*) and one might expect, therefore, some degree of development in *Lu. longipalpis*. Secondly, development of *L. m. amazonensis* in *Lu. longipalpis* clearly did *not* follow a normal pattern in many instances; thus Killick-Kendrick *et al.* (1977a) stated that "Transmission was exceptional" and "parasites degenerated in the foregut of some flies . . .", finally, "The common failure of leishmanias to become established in the foregut of many experimentally infected sandflies may be because parasites die after migration. . . ." These authors' observations contrasted with the consistently massive foregut establishment and relatively easy transmission achieved with *L. m. amazonensis* in the natural vector, *Lu. flaviscutellata* (Ward *et al.*, 1977).

We have already discussed the rôle(s) of environmental and physiological barriers which may limit the natural sandfly vectors of different leishmanias, and there is increasing evidence that this is so. Thus, in many years of study, we have been unable to find evidence that *L. m. amazonensis* is transmitted by any sandfly other than *Lu. flaviscutellata* in nature; *L. b. guyanensis* seems restricted to *Lu. umbratilis*, and *L. m. mexicana* to *Lu. o. olmeca*. This is quite remarkable when one considers that there may be 20 or more other sandfly species present in the forests where these parasites occur. All this would indicate a very ancient insect–mammal–parasite relationship, which is possibly the case, too, with *L. chagasi* and *Lu. longipalpis*. It is likely to have been established long before post-Columbian times.

(c) That there is a multiplicity of parasites responsible for American visceral leishmaniasis, including imported *L. infantum* and one or more indigenous leishmanias.

Table 4. Experimental infection of New World sandflies with neotropical *Leishmania* species and recorded transmissions by bite of the infected insect.

Sandfly species	Source of fly	*Leishmania* species	Source of infection	Location of infection	Transmission	Reference
Lu. intermedia	wild	*Leishmania* sp.	Man	al-tract	NAT	Aragão (1922)
Ps. panamensis	wild	*Leishmania* sp.	Man	al-tract	NAT	Pifano (1940b)
Lu. fischeri	wild	*Leishmania* sp.	Mnk	al-tract	NAT	Pessôa and Coutinho (1941)
Lu. whitmani	wild	*Leishmania* sp.	Mnk	al-tract	NAT	Pessôa and Coutinho (1941)
Lu. longipalpis	lab.	*L. b. braziliensis*	Ham	mh-gut	NAT	Lainson et al. (1977b)
Lu. longipalpis	lab.	*L. b. guyanensis*	Ham	mh-gut	NAT	Lainson et al. (1977b)
Lu. gomezi	lab.	*L. b. panamensis*	Mcpt[a]	fmh-gut	NEG	Hertig and McConnell (1963)
Lu. sanguinaria	lab.	*L. b. panamensis*	Mcpt[a]	fmh-gut	NEG	Hertig and McConnell (1963)
Lu. ylephilator	lab.	*L. b. panamensis*	Mcpt[a]	h-gut	NAT	Hertig and McConnell (1963)
Lu. trapidoi	lab.	*L. b. panamensis*	Mcpt[a]	mh-gut	NAT	Hertig and McConnell (1963)
Ps. paraensis	lab.	*L. b. panamensis*	Mcpt[a]	mh-gut	NAT	Hertig and McConnell (1963)
Lu. sanguinaria	lab.	*L. b. panamensis*	Ham	fmh-gut	NAT	Johnson and Hertig (1970)
Lu. gomezi	lab.	*L. b. panamensis*	Ham	fmh-gut	NAT	Johnson and Hertig (1970)
Lu. longipalpis	lab.	*L. b. panamensis*	Ham	mh-gut	NAT	Lainson et al. (1977b)
Lu. longipalpis	wild	*L. braziliensis* ssp.	Ham	fmh-gut	NEG	Coelho et al. (1967a, d)
Lu. renei	wild	*L. braziliensis* ssp.	Ham	fmh-gut	NAT	Coelho et al. (1967a)
Lu. sanguinaria	lab.	*L. braziliensis* ssp.	Ham	fmh-gut	NAT	Johnson and Hertig (1970)
Lu. gomezi	lab.	*L. braziliensis* ssp.	Ham	fmh-gut	NAT	Johnson and Hertig (1970)
Lu. longipalpis	lab.	*L. braziliensis* (M1580)	Ham	mh-gut	NAT	Lainson et al. (1977b)
Lu. longipalpis	lab.	*L. braziliensis* (M1597)	Memb[a]	mh-gut	NAT	Lainson et al. (1977b)
Lu. longipalpis	lab.	*L. braziliensis* (M2737)	Memb[a]	mh-gut	NAT	Lainson et al. (1977b)
Ps. geniculata	wild	*L. m. mexicana*	Ham	m-gut	NEG	Strangways-Dixon and Lainson (1962)
Ps. pessoana	wild	*L. m. mexicana*	Ham	al-tract	POS	Strangways-Dixon and Lainson (1962)

Species	Source	Leishmania	Membrane	Site	Result	Reference
Lu. ylephilator	wild	*L. m. mexicana*	Ham	fm-gut	NEG	Strangways-Dixon and Lainson (1962)
Lu. longipalpis	wild	*L. m. mexicana*	Ham	fm-gut	POS	Coelho and Falcão (1962)
Lu. renei	wild	*L. m. mexicana*	Ham	fm-gut	POS	Coelho and Falcão (1962)
Lu. cruciata	wild	*L. m. mexicana*	Ham	?	POS	Williams (1966)
Lu. cruciata	wild	*L. m. mexicana*	Ham	m-gut	NEG	Strangways-Dixon and Lainson (1966)
Ps. bispinosa	wild	*L. m. mexicana*	Ham	m-gut	NEG	Strangways-Dixon and Lainson (1966)
Lu. shannoni	wild	*L. m. mexicana*	Ham	m-gut	NEG	Strangways-Dixon and Lainson (1966)
Lu. ovallesi	wild	*L. m. mexicana*	Ham	m-gut	NEG	Strangways-Dixon and Lainson (1966)
Lu. olmeca olmeca	wild	*L. m. mexicana*	Ham	m-gut	NEG	Strangways-Dixon and Lainson (1966)
Lu. longipalpis	wild	*L. m. mexicana*	Ham	fm^c-gut	POS	Coelho et al. (1967b, d)
Lu. renei	wild	*L. m. mexicana*	Ham	fm^c-gut	POS	Coelho et al. (1967b, d)
Lu. sanguinaria	lab.	*L. m. mexicana*	Ham	fm^d-gut	NAT	Johnson and Hertig (1970)
Lu. gomezi	lab.	*L. m. mexicana*	Ham	fm^d-gut	NAT	Johnson and Hertig (1970)
Lu. longipalpis	lab.	*L. m. amazonensis*	Ham	fm-gut	POS	Killick-Kendrick et al. (1977a)
Lu. longipalpis	lab.	*L. m. amazonensis*	Memb[b]	fm-gut	NAT	Lainson et al. (1977b)
Lu. flaviscutellata	lab.	*L. m. amazonensis*	Ham	fm-gut	POS	Ward et al. (1977)
Lu. longipalpis	wild	*L. mexicana* ssp.	Ham	fm^c-gut	NEG	Coelho et al. (1967a, d)
Lu. renei	wild	*L. mexicana* ssp.	Ham	fm^c-gut	NEG	Coelho et al. (1967a, d)
Lu. intermedia	wild	*L. mexicana* ssp.	Ham	m-gut	NAT	Coelho et al. (1967a)
Lu. whitmani	wild	*L. mexicana* ssp.	Ham	m-gut	NAT	Coelho et al. (1967a)
Lu. sallesi	wild	*L. mexicana* ssp.	Ham	m-gut	NAT	Coelho et al. (1967a)
Lu. shannoni	wild	*L. mexicana* ssp.	Ham	m-gut	NAT	Coelho et al. (1967a)
Lu. monticola	wild	*L. mexicana* ssp.	Ham	m^c-gut	NAT	Coelho et al. (1967a)
Lu. coelhoi	wild	*L. mexicana* ssp.	Ham	m-gut	NAT	Coelho et al. (1967a)

Table 4—cont.

Sandfly species	Source of fly	Leishmania species	Source of infection	Location of infection	Transmission	Reference
Lu. cavernicola	wild	L. mexicana ssp.	Ham	m[c]-gut	NAT	Coelho et al. (1967a)
Ps. arthuri	wild	L. mexicana ssp.	Ham	m-gut	NAT	Coelho et al. (1967a)
Lu. gomezi	lab.	L. enriettii	Mcpt[a]	m-gut	NAT	Hertig and McConnell (1963)
Lu. monticola	wild	L. enriettii	G-pig	m-gut	NAT	Luz et al. (1967)
Lu. longipalpis	lab.	L. enriettii	Memb[a]	m-gut	NAT	Lainson et al. (1977b)
Lu. sanguinaria	lab.	L. hertigi hertigi	Porc.	m-gut	NAT	Anon. (1967)
Lu. gomezi	lab.	L. hertigi hertigi	Porc.	m-gut	NAT	Anon. (1967)
Lu. longipalpis	lab.	L. hertigi hertigi	Memb[a]	m-gut	NAT	Lainson et al. (1977b)
Lu. longipalpis	lab.	L. hertigi deanei	Memb[a]	m-gut	NAT	Lainson et al. (1977b)
Lu. longipalpis	wild	L. chagasi	Dog	al-tract	NAT	Ferreira et al. (1938)
Lu. longipalpis	lab.	L. chagasi	Dog	al-tract	NAT	Chagas (1939)
Lu. intermedia	lab.	L. chagasi	Dog	al-tract	NAT	Chagas (1939)
Lu. longipalpis	wild	L. chagasi	Man	fm-gut	NAT	Deane and Deane (1954d)
Lu. longipalpis	wild	L. chagasi	Fox	fm-gut	NAT	Deane and Deane (1954e)
Lu. longipalpis	wild	L. chagasi	Ham	fm[c]-gut	NEG	Coelho et al. (1967c, d)
Lu. longipalpis	lab.	L. chagasi	Dog	fm-gut	NEG	Sherlock and Sherlock (1972)
Lu. longipalpis	lab.	L. chagasi	Memb[b]	fm-gut	POS	Lainson et al. (1977a)
Lu. renei	wild	L. chagasi	Ham	fm[c]-gut	NAT	Coelho et al. (1967c, d)

[a] Promastigotes from culture. [b] Amastigotes from hamsters; al-tract = alimentary tract; h-gut = hind gut; mh-gut = mid and hind gut; fmh = fore, mid and hind gut; fm = fore and mid gut; Ham = hamster; Mcpt = Micropipette; Memb = membrane; Mnk = Macacus rhesus; G-pig = guinea pig; Porc. = porcupine; NAT = transmission not attempted; NEG = transmission attempted but negative; POS = transmission successful; Lu = Lutzomyia; Ps = Psychodopygus; b. = braziliensis; m = mexicana. [c] No mention is made of the presence of attached forms in the hind gut and the mere presence of active flagellates is not considered as hind gut development; free flagellates may be carried back during the early phase of the infection with the remains of the digested blood meal or, in dissections of heavily infected flies, flagellates are often washed backwards from the mid gut. [d] A very small percentage of flies had light hind gut infections most of which were single, long thin flagellates attached by the tip of their flagellum; rosettes were rarely observed. The authors concluded that L. mexicana "typically caused midgut infections alone".

In spite of the above arguments, this compromise is probably the best attitude to take, at least until really large numbers of isolates have been adequately compared from cases of the human disease throughout the entire geographical range of visceral leishmaniasis in South and Central America.

There is little doubt that the genus *Leishmania* is of great antiquity (Lainson *et al.*, 1977b) and that leishmaniasis is one of man's oldest protozoal diseases (Adler, 1940). Although there has been considerable speciation within the genus, this has principally been studied in the group of leishmanias characterized by their pronounced dermotropic tendencies in the mammalian host: a total of 14 species or subspecies are now recognized, and more will certainly be discovered. Phylogenetically distinct parasites may also have independently evolved the common feature of exaggerated viscerotropism, and it remains to be seen if there is not a multiplicity of organisms which, we strongly suspect, are at present "lumped" under the names of *L. donovani* and *L. infantum* in both the Old and the New Worlds. In the meantime we at least accept the additional name of *L. chagasi*.

3. The epidemiology of visceral leishmaniasis in Brazil

Penna's viscerotome studies quickly aroused the interest of the eminent Brazilian parasitologist, Evandro Chagas, who soon recorded his observations on the first living case of American visceral leishmaniasis to be studied (Chagas, 1936). The patient was a boy of 16, from Aracaju, Sergipe State: his sister was confirmed to have died from the disease, and his mother had also recently died with identical symptoms. Chagas noted the abundance of the sandfly *Lutzomyia longipalpis* (Fig. 6) in the house— to the exclusion of all other haematophagous arthropods.

(*a*) *Amazonian visceral leishmaniasis:* Heading a commission of enquiry, Chagas was anxious to extend his studies to other endemic areas, in particular those indicated as the most seriously affected by the disease in Penna's viscerotome examinations. He was offered little more than excuses of administrative and financial problems, however, and the only State prepared to offer the facilities and technical help he needed was that of Pará, in the north. In many ways this was unfortunate: his subsequent investigation was to show that this was an area with only sporadic cases of visceral leishmaniasis, associated with an ecology which was utterly different from that of the major endemic areas of the northeast (Fig. 6).

Nevertheless, between the years 1936–1940, the various members of the commission were able to publish very detailed accounts of a meticulous study made in the hot, humid and heavily forested districts of Abaeté and Moju, in the mouth of the Amazon and where Penna had registered the first three cases of visceral leishmaniasis in Pará. A total of

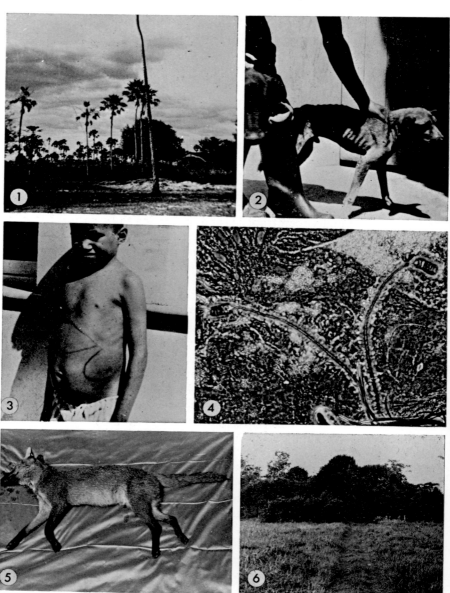

FIG. 6.   Epidemiological aspects of *Leishmania chagasi* in Brazil. 1. Endemic area for visceral leishmaniasis in Ceará State. 2. Naturally infected dog. 3. American visceral leishmaniasis in a boy, showing enlarged liver and spleen. 4. Spermathecae of the vector, *Lutzomyia longipalpis*. 5. The fox, *Cerdocyon thous*, which has been found naturally infected in Belém, Pará. 6. Low, secondary forest in the area in which the infected fox was captured. [1 and 2 from Lainson and Shaw (1971); 5 from Lainson *et al.*, (1969).]

539 people were examined, mostly by spleen puncture, and infections found in 7 more children and one adult. In addition, they detected amastigotes in the viscera of 7 dogs and one cat: most of these animals were showing severe symptoms, and their owners gave instances of other dogs which had died in the past under similar circumstances.

Captures of haematophagous insects were made, with and without bait (man, horse, cow, dog and chicken), both inside and outside houses, and by day and by night. By far the most common insects caught were phlebotomine sandflies, and of 909 specimens 904 were identified as *Lu. longipalpis* (Fig. 6). All were captured at night, almost entirely in rural houses situated in or very near to the forest. Very few were encountered in or near houses in the urban area or suburbs of the nearest major town of Abaeté.

Unfortunately, the method of capture of the sandflies (not stated, but probably with baited and lighted "Shannon" traps) gave an overwhelming proportion of male flies: it would seem unlikely, therefore, that many female *Lu. longipalpis* were dissected in attempts to find infected insects. Again, although the commission captured 737 wild mammals, the last reports on this aspect of the work (Chagas *et al.*, 1938; Deane, 1956) do not make it clear as to the method of examination. Mention was made, however, of suspicious bodies seen in a spleen smear from a specimen of the forest rodent *Proechimys oris*, suggesting that it was limited to a search for amastigotes in stained smears of the viscera—a truly monumental task and one which, in our opinion, would stand little chance of revealing the parasite in what would almost certainly be chronic, inapparent infections. No mention is made of blood-agar culture of tissues, or the inoculation of such material into hamsters.

From their observations, Chagas and his colleagues came to the following conclusions regarding visceral leishmaniasis in the State of Pará. The disease was sporadic, and with no evidence of any cyclical appearance. Its distribution was essentially rural, far from urban centres and only in the proximity of high, or medium–high forest. It was restricted to the drier areas ("terra firme") and was not to be found in the lower, wetter "varzea" or riverine forest which was subjected to frequent flooding. Phlebotomine sandflies were the most likely vectors, being commonly found in the primitive thatched huts in or near the forest of the "terra firme"; these insects were rarely found in urban areas or the suburbs. Dogs, and more rarely man, occasionally became infected but played no vital role in the maintenance of the disease in nature. The silvatic association strongly suggested a reservoir of infection in some wild animal, probably a canid or a rodent: dogs, having acquired the disease, served as a secondary source of infection for man.

According to Costa (1966) 6 further cases of visceral leishmaniasis were diagnosed in villages near Abaeté, Pará, all post-mortem, by a Dr. Madureira Pará, but no details are given. He himself described what appears to be the last recorded case from this general area (Costa, 1966), in Cachoeira do Ararí in the southern part of the Island of Marajó. The patient, like all those previously examined, lived in "terra firme" forest; none of 9 dogs associated with this isolated case was found to be infected, and no sandflies were captured.

The only other focus of infection reported in the Brazilian Amazonian region appears to have been in villages near the small town of Santarém, Pará, about 700 kilometres from Abaeté (Alencar et al., 1962). Three children were found infected, out of 500 persons examined, and 19 dogs —11 parasitologically, after the examination of liver smears, and 8 serologically by the complement fixation test. Sandfly captures, inside and outside houses, produced mainly tree-trunk dwelling species not known to be associated with any form of human leishmaniasis, but two flies identified as Lu. longipalpis were taken from trees in two villages. An important feature, not apparently encountered by Chagas et al. in Abaeté, was the finding of 2 other infected children who had undoubtedly acquired their infections in the State of Ceará, where they had lived before immigrating to Pará. Could they have been the source of infection for local sandflies, thus establishing a focus of infection in an hitherto unaffected region?

In spite of this alternative suggestion for the origin of Amazonian cases of visceral leishmaniasis, most evidence points to the existence of a wild mammalian reservoir, with a wide distribution. Deane (1948, 1956) examined tissue smears from 29 two-toed sloths, Choloepus didactylus, some of which were captured in forest near the Abaeté focus of visceral leishmaniasis. He found amastigotes in the spleen and liver of 7, but thought they were more likely to be developmental stages of Endotrypanum schaudinni. Lainson and Shaw (1971) discussed the possibility that they may in fact have been L. chagasi but, as the parasites had not been inoculated into hamsters, it remained impossible to be sure of their true nature. Subsequently, however, we have found what is probably the same organism in the viscera and skin of a number of C. didactylus from various parts of Pará State and shown it to be a Leishmania of the L. braziliensis complex (Shaw and Lainson, 1973).

The possibility of a wild mammalian host of L. chagasi in the Amazon region remained completely speculative until 1969, when what we believe to be this parasite was isolated from a fox (Cerdocyon thous) which was shot in the grounds of the Agricultural Institute, Belém, Pará (Fig. 6). The isolation was made following the intraperitoneal inoculation of two hamsters with a suspension of kidney tissue during studies on Leptospira (Lainson et al., 1969). Both animals developed fulminating and fatal visceral leishmaniasis, with very large numbers of amastigotes throughout the viscera, principally the spleen: the infection was indistinguishable from that seen in hamsters inoculated with *L. chagasi* from man. At first the parasite grew moderately well in NNN culture but growth diminished with each sub-culture and the *in vitro* line was eventually lost. In our experience this is a common feature of *L. chagasi*.

In a recent publication on the biochemical taxonomy of *Leishmania*, Gardener *et al.* (1974) referred to an isolate of ". . . *L. chagasi*" (acquired from our laboratory) ". . . which would appear to be *L. mexicana amazonensis*". They suggested that "certain anomalous results which are unsupported by other methods of taxonomy" may be accounted for by ". . . misleading information accompanying isolates, due to mixing of strains during long periods of laboratory sub-culture, to errors in cryo-banks, or to the occurrence at the time of isolation of a mixed infection".

In view of the considerable epidemiological importance of isolating *L. chagasi* from a wild animal in the Amazon region, we wish to take this opportunity of removing any doubt that these authors' remarks may have cast on the validity of the *L. chagasi* isolate made from the fox, *C. thous*. Some time after the isolation was made, splenic material from infected hamsters was inoculated intradermally into other hamsters and, to our surprise, gave rise to large, tumour-like lesions at the site of the injection. The lesions were identical to those produced by local strains of *L. mexicana amazonensis* (Lainson and Shaw, 1972), and they contained enormous numbers of amastigotes with the characteristic morphology of that parasite (Shaw and Lainson, 1976). In our opinion the fox was infected with two parasites. During intraperitoneal passage of spleen and liver suspensions in hamsters, these animals showed the typical visceral infection of *L. chagasi* and died before any skin-lesions due to *L. mexicana amazonensis* could become apparent; the latter parasite appeared only when spleen suspension was actually inoculated *intradermally* into the hamster, rather than by the customary intraperitoneal route used for the maintenance of *L. chagasi*. Unhappily, further passage in hamsters was made only with material from the skin-lesions, and the isolate of *L. chagasi* was thus lost. NNN culture of *L. m. amazonensis* from the skin gave the usual luxuriant growth of promastigotes (quite unlike the poor growth of *L. chagasi*) and samples were sent to Liverpool for confirmation of our above-mentioned conclusions. Unfortunately, although the situation was made quite clear at the time, it would appear that this information was not passed on to those actually conducting the biochemical study of the parasite and it erroneously became designated as "*L. chagasi*".

During our studies on the reservoir hosts of cutaneous leishmaniasis in the Amazon region of Brazil we have examined 681 wild mammals by the inoculation of spleen, liver and skin suspensions into hamsters and the culture of such material in blood-agar media (Table 3). Promastigote flagellates appeared in cultures of the liver and spleen of one opossum (*Didelphis marsupialis*) captured near Belém: we were unable to maintain the parasite *in vitro*, however, and neither cutaneous nor visceral infection resulted in hamsters inoculated with tissue suspensions from the opossum. Otherwise there was no other isolate suggestive of *L. chagasi*, although *L. m. amazonensis* was isolated from the skin of a considerable number of animals and, more rarely, subspecies of *L. braziliensis* were obtained from skin and/or viscera.

As we will discuss later, a different species of fox had been previously incriminated as a host of *L. chagasi* in other parts of Brazil (Deane and Deane, 1954a; Deane, 1956), and it remains possible, therefore, that *Cerdocyon thous* could be the natural host in the Amazon forests, or wherever it is abundant. It is notable that the infected animal from Belém was in excellent condition and, apart from pathological changes seen in the infected kidney, showed no visible signs of disease. In Venezuela, Torrealba (1964) inoculated a specimen of *C. thous* with cultural forms of *L. chagasi* originating from a naturally infected dog: seven months later numerous amastigotes were found in bone-marrow smears, although the animal appeared quite healthy. The development of such a chronic, inapparent infection in this fox is strong supportive evidence for suspecting *C. thous* as a reservoir of *L. chagasi* in nature.

It is a sad fact, then, that in spite of the enormous amount of work undertaken by the Chagas commission and later workers, there is no existing isolate of *L. chagasi* from man or dogs in the Amazon region, and no illustration or adequate description of the suspected sandfly vector which was identified as "*Phlebotomus longipalpis*". Are we in fact dealing with the same epidemiological situation as that seen in the more highly endemic areas of Ceará, Bahia, Sergipe and Minas Gerais? Is the causative agent of Amazonian visceral leishmaniasis identical with that elsewhere in Latin America, and is the vector really *Lutzomyia longipalpis*? Until Amazonian isolates of the parasite are available for study we cannot answer the first question: with regards the latter, no specimens of the sandflies collected by the Chagas commission would appear to have been preserved and we have been unable to re-encounter *Lu. longipalpis* during 12 years of study in Pará. Mangabeira (1969) clearly had grave doubts as to the identity of the "*Phlebotomus longipalpis*" of Chagas *et al.* (1938), and he may be justly regarded as one of the greatest experts ever on the taxonomy of South American sandflies. He drew attention to slight morphological differences between the male insects from Pará and those from northeast Brazil (e.g. Ceará): even greater differences were noted between the females. This, and the contrasting ecology of the tropical rain-forest of the Amazon and the semi-desert conditions of the endemic areas of Ceará, led Mangabeira to conclude that one must seriously consider the likelihood of (at least) two species of sandflies which have till now been confused under the same name of *Lutzomyia longipalpis*. The paucity of human cases of visceral leishmaniasis in the Amazon region is probably due to the relatively poor contact between man and the sandfly vector, which is not particularly anthropophilic and much more inclined to feed on dogs. In this respect it may be noted that the dog is much more frequently infected than is man: Chagas and colleagues recorded no capture of *"Phlebotomus longipalpis"* off man, even at times when considerable numbers were being taken off dogs or other animals; infected dogs were found in houses which were free of human infection.

Only another intensive study such as that carried out by the Chagas commission will indicate the true situation regarding Amazonian visceral leishmaniasis, with more isolates from man, dogs (and possibly wild animals) which can be directly compared biologically and biochemically with the parasite from other endemic areas *throughout* the Latin American continent. No further cases of the disease in Pará have come to our notice since that reported by Costa (1966), but we feel that this is merely a reflection of declining interest and lack of surveillance in this area.

(b) *Visceral leishmaniasis elsewhere in Brazil:* Much of the interest in American visceral leishmaniasis undoubtedly died with Evandro Chagas in 1940 and, apart from occasional case reports, no new epidemiological features were forthcoming until 1953. In that year an outbreak of epidemic proportions was estimated to have been responsible for a hundred or more deaths in the vicinity of the small town of Sobral, in northwest Ceará (Aragão, 1953; Deane, 1956; Silva, 1957). Again, most of the cases were in young children (Fig. 6), principally in the rural areas, and the presence of *Lu. longipalpis* was noted in and near the houses. Startled into renewed activity, the authorities set up another inquiry into the problem (the "Campanha Contra a Leishmaniose Visceral"), with the express intention of elucidating the epidemiology of the disease so that some form of prophylactic measures could be taken.

Between 1953–1955 these investigators registered nearly 1000 new cases of visceral leishmaniasis in Ceará and other States, and defined the basic epidemiology of the disease as we know it today in the major endemic areas of the Americas. Much of the credit for this success belonged to three prominent personalities in the field of tropical medicine in Brazil, J. E. Alencar, L. M. Deane and M. P. Deane.

Leonidas and Maria Deane had been members of the Evandro Chagas commission in Pará, and they must have been very impressed with the different ecological features facing them in northwest Ceará, when they selected their four areas of study in Boqueirão (District of Sobral), Pé da Serra das Contendas (Massapê), Ubari (Viçosa do Ceará) and Trapiá (Tianguá). These localities shared three main-biotopes: (i) the lower plains ("sertãos"), with little rain, periodic and lengthy droughts and a sparse, xerophytic vegetation: (ii) the hill-tops or "serras", with more rain and generally thickly covered with low forest: (iii) the foothills or "boqueirãos", in the narrow valleys; usually humid, sheltered from strong winds, partially cultivated but with considerable areas of low shrubbery.

The Deanes found that of 170 cases of visceral leishmaniasis, 63·5% were in the "boqueirãos", 21·7% in the "sertãos" and only 14·0% in the "serras". Fewer people lived in the "boqueirãos" than in the other two regions, and evidently the conditions in the foothills were most favourable for transmission. Deane (1956), for example, referred to one unfortunate couple who had lost seven of their children and were bringing in the eighth for treatment! In contrast, cases were only sporadic in the "sertãos" and "serras", where extreme dryness and strong winds were unfavourable for the sandflies.

From their previous experience in Pará, it was logical that the Deanes should suspect dogs as reservoirs of infection for man, and 49 out of 936 examined (5·2%) proved to be infected. Deane (1956) considered that the true figure was probably very much higher, as field conditions only permitted the direct examination of smears made from liver-biopsies and skin. Interestingly, no infections were found in 142 cats.

Foxes (*Lycalopex vetulus*) were numerous in the study areas and of 33 examined, 4 (12·1%) were infected; 3 came from a single locality ("boqueirão") where the incidence was as high as 3 out of 9 (33·3%). Deane rightly concluded that foxes must be important wild reservoirs, but wisely considered that other animals might be involved. Direct examination of smears was made from the following animals, with negative results: primates: 4 monkeys (*Callithrix jacchus*); carnivores: 1 racoon (*Procyon cancrivorus*); edentates: 2 anteaters (*Tamandua tetradactyla*); marsupials: 6 opossums (*Didelphis paraguayensis*); rodents: 19 domestic rats (*Rattus rattus*), 5 rice-rats (*Oryzomys* spp), 3 *Rhipidomys cearanus*, 9 *Zygodontomys pixuna*, 3 *Echimys spp* (all small rat-like rodents), 1 wild "guinea-pig" (*Galea spixii*) and 4 *Kerodon rupestris* (a large, rabbit-like rodent); 5 bats of various species.

In discussing the results, Deane mentioned a similar examination of 127 wild animals by Pondé et al (1942) in other foci of visceral leishmaniasis in Ceará and the neighbouring State of Pernambuco. No parasites were seen in stained smears of the viscera, including those from 3 foxes (*Cerdocyon thous*). We have already discussed the great importance of NNN culture and hamster inoculation in the detection of chronic, inapparent infections with *Leishmania*, and the small chances of ever finding amastigotes in tissue smears from most of these animals. From experience under similar conditions, we appreciate the impractability of sterile culture in the field and the problems and expense that would have been involved in inoculating hamsters with material from all the above-mentioned animals. The sad conclusion is inescapable, however, that none of these studies in the Amazon region or northeast Brazil has eliminated the likelihood of animal reservoirs other than the fox and the dog.

The disease in the dog is usually fatal: in the final phase of infection there is extreme wasting, weakness of the legs, oedema of the feet, exaggerated elongation of the claws, ulceration and depilation of the skin, various eye conditions leading to blindness, and diarrhoea (Fig. 6). With such a poor host–parasite relationship the dog is clearly not the normal host of *L. chagasi*, important though it may be as a reservoir of infection for man.

Deane considered the number of foxes he examined as too small to say whether or not these animals have chronic, symptomless infections in nature. Only 1 of the 4 foxes appeared healthy, however, and this was probably in an early phase of the infection because amastigotes were found in the viscera but not in the skin: the other 3 animals showed severe symptoms, like the dogs, and 1 was virtually moribund. This does not suggest *Lycalopex vetulus* to be the proper host of the parasite, either, and we feel that it is most likely that this animal is an accidental host following the bite of some sandfly species (possibly not *Lu. longipalpis*) which normally maintains a cryptic infection in some other wild animal (a silvatic species?). Sherlock and Almeida (1970a) made the interesting and significant observation that there was a marked drop in the incidence of visceral leishmaniasis following an outbreak of rodent plague which, with attendant anti-rodent campaigns, had practically eliminated these animals in an area of study near Jacobina, Bahia State.

Neotropical foxes spend much of their time in the safety of wooded areas but, like their European relatives, they frequently invade man's habitations for easy prey in the chicken-house, or for other food. Infected foxes, their skin laden with parasites, would provide a rich source of *L. chagasi* for peridomestic *Lu. longipalpis* (which are particularly abundant in chicken-houses) and these, in turn, could feed on and infect the local dogs. As we have seen, this sandfly is much more attracted to dogs than it is to man, and canine infection is thus much more common than the human one; Deane (1958) gives an example of one locality in which the proportion of canine/human infections was 39/2. Nevertheless, when a sufficiently dense population of *Lu. longipalpis* coincides with the continued presence of numerous infected dogs, the increased number of infective sandflies results in a proportional increase in the human disease, such as occurred in the Sobral outbreak.

Deane and Deane (1954d) were able to demonstrate very scanty parasites in the apparently normal skin in some human infections, and succeeded in infecting up to 15% of *Lu. longipalpis* fed on some patients.

Adler and Theodor (1957) considered this an important difference between *L. chagasi* and *L. infantum* infections in man, the latter rarely providing sufficient parasites in the skin to infect any of the *Phlebotomus perniciosus* fed on patients. Deane nevertheless concluded that man probably could only rarely serve as a source of infection for *Lu. longipalpis*; in contrast, parasites were so abundant in the skin of the fox and the dog that they often provided a 100% infection-rate in sandflies fed on them.

Since the Deanes' pioneer work, there have been numerous studies confirming the role of the dog as an intermediary reservoir of *L. chagasi* in Ceará and other States of Brazil (Alencar *et al.*, 1956, Nussenzweig, *et al.*, 1957, Alencar, 1961, in Ceará; Oliveira *et al.*, 1959, in Minas Gerais; Alencar, 1962, Guedes *et al.*, 1974, in Paraíba; Sherlock and Santos, 1964, Sherlock and Almeida, 1970b, in Bahia; Coelho *et al.*, 1965, in Goiás; Martins *et al.*, 1968, in Espírito Santo). As far as we are aware, no further infected foxes have been found other than the single *Cerdocyon thous* we have discussed above, from Belém, Pará, and no further light has been shed on the existence of other wild mammalian hosts.

4. The vector—*Lutzomyia longipalpis*

In most areas where this insect occurs, engorged females may be aspirated in large numbers, particularly from the more gloomy corners of internal walls in houses and animal shelters. Other resting-sites include holes in tree-trunks, caves, the cracks and spaces in piles of stones, and fissures in rocks. Whilst making collections in Ceará, one of us (R. L.) found them to be particularly abundant in between stacked roofing tiles which are commonly stored in the back-yards of rural houses. *Lu. longipalpis* is very abundant during or shortly after the rainy season, but it is a robust insect (unlike its silvatic relatives) and survives, albeit in reduced numbers, through long periods of severe drought. It has a wide range of hosts, including dogs, horses, cattle, chicken and man (Deane, 1956).

The major breeding places of *Lu. longipalpis* have yet to be discovered, and Deane (1956) thought that the extreme difficulty he had in finding immature stages suggested a large variety of widely dispersed sites. Using cone emergence-traps, he obtained 9 females from the soil in a donkey shed, and 3 more emerged in samples of this soil taken to the laboratory. One male emerged from another sample of soil taken from on and between rocks.

There has long been strong epidemiological evidence suggesting that *Lu. longipalpis* is the major vector of *L. chagasi* in almost all the principal endemic foci in Brazil, for it has been found to be by far the most common haematophagous arthropod associated with both canine and human visceral leishmaniasis (Chagas, 1936; Deane and Deane, 1937; Mangabeira, 1942; Pondé *et al.*, 1942; Deane, 1956, 1958; Martins *et al.*, 1956; Oliveira *et al.*, 1959; Alencar, 1962; Coelho *et al.*, 1965).

This, early on, prompted a series of studies on the development of the parasite in wild-caught and/or laboratory-bred *Lu. longipalpis* and *Lu. intermedia* which had been fed on naturally infected dogs. Promastigotes were found to develop in the gut of both insects (Ferreira *et al.*, 1938b; Chagas, 1939, 1940; Paraense and Chagas, 1940), and suspensions of crushed, infected flies produced visceral leishmaniasis in inoculated hamsters. No transmission was made by the bite of the sandflies, although the titles of the latter two papers rather misleadingly implied so.

Deane and Deane (1954e) fed *Lu. longipalpis* on an infected fox and obtained development of *L. chagasi* in 10 flies. On the 4th and 5th days the flagellates had moved forward to the oesophagus and packed the oesophageal valve: small, thin and very active promastigotes were seen in the distal part of the epipharynx on the 8th day of the infection. No attempts were made to transmit infection by the bite of the sandflies.

The same authors (1954c) found natural promastigote infections in 2 out of 141 *Lu. longipalpis* caught in a focus of visceral leishmaniasis in Ceará, and where two infected foxes were captured. A third infection was noted in a subsequent dissection of 876 more flies, giving the total of 3 positives in 1017 (0·3%) insects examined. One of the infected flies was taken inside a house, another in a stable, and the third off a donkey which was being used as bait. Although it is likely that these flagellates were *L. chagasi*, they were not inoculated into any experimental animal and the chance of obtaining final proof of the role of *Lu. longipalpis* as a vector was lost. Apart from the Deanes' monumental efforts, no other really intensive dissection programme appears to have been carried out in spite of the large number of endemic areas studied, the abundance of *Lu. longipalpis* in most of them, and the relatively good facilities that go with domestic or peri-domestic situations. Pifano (1943), in Venezuela, mentioned one infected *Lu. longipalpis* taken in a house in which there were cases of cutaneous leishmaniasis, but once again the parasite was not identified. Johnson *et al.* (1963) found promastigotes in the only example of *Lu. longipalpis* they ever captured, in Panama, but the infection included attached forms in the hindgut—effectively eliminating the possibility of an infection with *L. chagasi* (see Parts II and III).

It is a surprising fact that although *Lu. longipalpis* was reared in the laboratory by Chagas, as long ago as 1938, no serious attempt to transmit *L. chagasi* experimentally by the bite of *Lu. longipalpis* appears to have been made until that of Sherlock and Sherlock (1972). These authors fed 31 laboratory-reared flies on infected dogs and, later, re-fed them on two young, uninfected dogs. No transmission was achieved, although 9 of the flies proved to be heavily infected when dissected at the end of the experiment.

It was not until 1977, exactly 64 years after the first record of visceral leishmaniasis in the Americas, that the chain of evidence against *Lu.*

longipalpis was finally completed, with five separate transmissions of *L. chagasi* from hamster to hamster by the bite of infected, laboratory-bred insects (Lainson *et al.*, 1977a).

5. Other possible vectors of *L. chagasi*

Despite the coincidental distribution of *Lu. longipalpis* and visceral leishmaniasis in most localities, there are instances when observers have found difficulty in finding this sandfly or when it has appeared to be altogether absent.

Thus, Potenza and Anduze (1942) were unable to find any evidence of this species in two districts of the State of Bolivar, Venezuela, where two cases of infantile visceral leishmaniasis had been diagnosed. Oliveira *et al.* (1959) discussed the epidemiological features of the disease in Minas Gerais, Brazil, and pointed out that in addition to the specimens of *Lu. longipalpis* taken in and near houses, there was also a "wild form" commonly found in limestone caves. In one village which had a high incidence of human infection, however, it proved impossible to find *Lu. longipalpis*, and suspicion fell on *Lu. cortelezzii, Lu. intermedia* and *Lu. whitmani*. Their presence might well be regarded as incidental, however, for Forattini (1960b) recorded the latter two species in large numbers in houses in São Paulo State, where visceral leishmaniasis appears to be absent (Forattini *et al.*, 1970). Other workers (Coelho *et al.*, 1965) were also unable to find evidence of *Lu. longipalpis* in a focus of infection in the southwest of Goiás State, Brazil, where the disease had been confirmed in 3 out of 29 dogs. The sandflies they did encounter included *Lu. intermedia, Lu. whitmani, Lu. shannoni, Ps. davisi* and *Lu. anduzei* (?).

Observations on the apparent absence of *Lu. longipalpis* in foci of visceral leishmaniasis should be viewed with caution, for on numerous occasions the fly has been found in the same localities by other workers. These conflicting results are probably due to seasonal variations in the sandfly population or changing climatic conditions. Thus, *Lu. evansi* became suspected as a vector, in the absence of *Lu. longipalpis*, in a focus of infection in the Turmiquire hills, Sucre State, Venezuela (Pifano and Romero, 1964b): the latter sandfly was found there, however, by later workers (Henríquez *et al.*, 1970). Again, *Lu. atroclavata* (= *Lu. guadeloupensis*) was suspected as a possible vector on the island of Guadeloupe, with no really good reasons other than the apparent absence of *Lu. longipalpis*. It enjoyed a further brief spell of notoriety when a similar situation occurred on the Venezuelan island of Margarita, during the investigation of a single case of visceral leishmaniasis (Pifano and Romero, 1964a): but Pifano and Romero (1973) did find *Lu. longipalpis* there when they studied a further 3 cases of the disease, nine years later.

Perhaps the most likely candidate as a secondary vector is *Lu. intermedia*. This sandfly shares a similar habitat and is known to feed on dogs and man: furthermore it has been infected experimentally with *L. chagasi* (Chagas, 1940; Paraense and Chagas, 1940). Forattini (1953) found this insect to breed commonly in pigsties in rural districts in São Paulo State.

Sherlock (1964), in Brazil, drew attention to the presence of canine visceral leishmaniasis where *Lu. longipalpis* appeared to be rare or absent; he suggested that there may possibly exist some other cycle of development which does not involve sandflies, such as transmission *in coitus* or by the ingestion of infected tissues. Promastigotes were seen in the alimentary tract of the common dog tick which had fed on an infected dog, and these produced visceral leishmaniasis when inoculated into hamsters. No infections could be induced in the flea species *Ceratophyllus canis*, *C. felix* and *Pulex irritans*.

One might easily dismiss this apparent recapitulation of the old theories of the early workers on Indian kala-azar, were it not for the great deal of experience that this author has had in the field of American visceral leishmaniasis, in particular its epidemiology. Could there be a passive transfer of the infection from dog to dog, perhaps by entry of the flagellates *via* the mucous membranes of the mouth when dogs bite at the ticks during their cleaning operations? It would seem to be a well worth-while field of further study.

6. The Control of American Visceral Leishmaniasis

The periodic spraying of houses with insecticides in the malaria control programmes has probably acted as an indirect check on the incidence of visceral leishmaniasis in many parts of Latin America; possibly this is the reason for the apparent disappearance of both the suspected vector and the human infection in the Amazonian foci.

Specific control measures have been carried out in Brazil, largely in the major endemic regions of Ceará and Bahia States (Deane *et al.*, 1955; Alencar, 1961, 1963; Sherlock and Almeida, 1970a, b). Usually these have taken the form of a three-pronged attack—the treatment of diagnosed human infection, the wholesale slaughter of infected dogs, and regular spraying of houses with DDT. Unsprayed areas have in some cases shown an increase of up to 12% of cases during a period of 4 years, whereas those sprayed showed up to a 58% reduction.

In general, then, these campaigns have greatly reduced the incidence of human infection and clearly indicated the importance of both the dog and *Lu. longipalpis* in the epidemiology. Sherlock and Almeida (1970b) emphasized, however, that there still remained some inexplicable fluctuations in the incidence of the disease and that these could be the result of a hidden source in some wild animal, which is unaffected by the eradication programmes, or the existence of asymptomatic human infections.

7. Visceral Leishmaniasis in other Latin American Countries

Next to Brazil, the highest incidence of visceral leishmaniasis appears to be in Venezuela, although this may only be a reflection of insufficient interest and means of diagnosis in the other affected countries. In all of these the geographical and ecological features associated with the disease are very similar to those described for Brazil: the cases have been sporadic and principally confined to children. Where epidemiological studies have been made, there once more emerges the picture of a probable wild mammalian host, secondary infection of dogs, and transmission to man by sandflies identified as *Lu. longipalpis*.

In Venezuela, only 21 cases were recorded between 1941 and 1960, but a further 30 were disclosed by Amaral *et al.* (1961a), and Torrealba (1964) concluded that the true importance of visceral leishmaniasis in Venezuela had yet to be assessed. The human disease has been reported in 8 States but appears to have its highest incidence in Guárico, an important agricultural area in the "llanos" or plains of central Venezuela.

The reservoir of infection for man remained undetected until 1960, when Medina *et al.* recorded the first canine infection in that country: this prompted a series of epidemiological studies, principally in the States of Guárico, Cojedos, Portuguesa and Sucre in the western and central plains (Amaral *et al.*, 1961a, b, c; Torrealba *et al.*, 1961; Pifano *et al.*, 1962; Torrealba *et al.*, 1963; Torrealba, 1964; Pifano and Romero, 1964a, b; Diaz-Ungría, 1969; Henríquez *et al.*, 1970).

Torrealba (1964) summarized most of these authors' findings as follows. Dogs are the most important reservoir for man, and of a total of 1561 examined, in various areas, 38 were found infected: in one focus in Guárico State the incidence was as high as 7 out of 24. No infections were detected in 50 specimens of the fox, *Cerdocyon thous*. Sandflies identified as *Lu. longipalpis* were common in and near houses: the insect has a wide range of hosts, including dogs, pigs and cows, but only feeds on man when the sandfly population increases markedly. Some evidence has been obtained that pigsties are an important breeding site. Pifano *et al.* (1962) mentioned the finding of *Lu. longipalpis* adults in animal-burrows and hollow trees, together with other species: this is a particularly interesting observation which could throw some light on the vexed question of wild mammalian hosts other than the fox. Mention is made of the examination of wild animals, with negative results, including wild rabbits (*Sylvilagos* sp), opossums, armadillos, monkeys and forest rodents, but these have been far too few in number for any conclusions to be drawn.

In Guatemala (León and Figueroa, 1959) *Lu. longipalpis* has been recorded in one of the rare foci of the human disease, but no infections have been found in dogs or any other animal; a similar situation was found in Mexico (Biagi and Tay, 1963; Biagi *et al.*, 1965b; López *et al.*, 1966). The latter authors used a *Mycobacterium butyricum*-derived antigen for complement fixation tests on 468 dogs and 329 wild mammals, and recorded positive reactions in 3·5% of the dogs. Positive tests were also found among some wild rodents, including *Mus musculus, Liomys irroratus, Neotoma mexicana* and *Baiomys musculus*. No parasites were isolated from any of these animals, or the dogs, and one can only speculate as to the specificity of this test in animals and the significance of these findings.

In El Salvador, Trejos *et al.* (1966) recorded the presence of the sandflies *Lu. longipalpis, Lu. evansi, Lu. cayennensis, Lu. cruciata, Lu. barretoi, Lu. deleoni, Lu. gomezi* and *Lu. chiapanensis*, associated with an area in which 4 cases of the human disease had been reported: no other information appears to be available in this country.

These, then, are the major features in the epidemiology of American visceral leishmaniasis. Inevitably some literature will have escaped our attention, but we feel that this would not be likely to cause a modification of the following conclusions, which may or may not be acceptable to all students of leishmaniasis.

1. Although American visceral leishmaniasis could possibly have originated after the importation of *L. infantum* from Europe, in post-Columbian times, it is likely that one or more indigenous leishmanias are also involved.

2. There is probably some hitherto undetected mammalian host which is the *primary* reservoir of infection for foxes and the dog; as is mostly the case in ancient host–parasite relationships, this animal is likely to be relatively unaffected by the infection. It is most likely to be silvatic, and its infection maintained by silvatic sandflies.

3. Foxes spend much of their time under the cover of wooded areas and occasionally become infected, when they usually develop a serious disease in which unusually large numbers of parasites are found in the skin.

4. During their frequent excursions to forage for food around human habitation, infected foxes are fed on by the peridomestic sandfly *Lutzomyia longipalpis*, in which the parasite can undergo complete development as in the silvatic vector.

5. *Lu. longipalpis* has catholic feeding habits; it is particularly attracted to dogs, however, to which it periodically transmits the infection. Canine visceral leishmaniasis is thus much more prevalent than the human disease.

6. If the number of infected dogs and the *Lu. longipalpis* population reach high levels, explosive epidemics may occur. Normally this does not happen and cases are sporadic.

7. It remains likely that there is: (a) a *Lu. longipalpis* complex of very

similar sandflies, which may account for certain anomalous situations such as that occurring in areas of tropical rain-forest in the Amazon region; and (b) different leishmanias associated with visceral leishmaniasis in such areas.

Until more information is forthcoming in this respect, it seems best to retain the name *Leishmania chagasi*. Comparative studies need to be made on isolates from cases of visceral leishmaniasis in man, dogs, foxes or other wild animals throughout Latin America. A taxonomic revision is needed of the sandflies referred to as "*Lutzomyia longipalpis*" from the same areas.

J. UNIDENTIFIED SUPRAPYLARIA

These are parasites which have been only partially characterized, but do seem to have features which are similar to those of other, better known, members of this Section.

Rassi *et al.* (1972) described an outbreak of cutaneous leishmaniasis in the Barra de Garças region of Mato Grosso State. Infections were acquired by men clearing areas of forest for cattle ranches in the wettish lowlands of the Serra do Roncador foothills bordering the Amazon basin. The notable features of the disease were the predominance of lesions on the head, arms and trunk, and frequent involvement of the lymphatics, similar to the clinical picture of "pian-bois", due to *L. braziliensis guyanensis*.

A single isolate from one of these patients was found to have buoyant densities of 1·718 and 1·702 for nuclear and kinetoplastic DNA, and type XII MDH (Chance *et al.*, 1974; Gardener *et al.*, 1974). The DNA buoyant densities are closest to those of *Leishmania major* (Old World "oriental-sore"); while the MDH type, although different, is very close to that of *L. major* and *L. m. mexicana*.

Barbosa *et al.* (1976) studied the biology of the same strain, and found that it would not infect hamsters. We (Lainson, Shaw and Ward, unpublished observations) have attempted to obtain infections in laboratory-bred *Lu. longipalpis*, fed on culture forms of the parasite through membranes—a method highly successful with other leishmanias: no development occurred in the pylorus, and that in the midgut was extremely poor. This failure to develop in a sandfly which supports excellent growth of most parasites of the *mexicana* and *braziliensis* complexes is puzzling, although it may have been influenced by the fact that the isolate had been in culture for over six years. Failure of the organism to infect hamsters is less easy to explain, for the parasite was apparently inoculated into these animals very shortly after its isolation from man, and before it was likely to have lost its infectivity (Barbosa *et al.*, 1976).

The finding of cutaneous leishmaniasis of the dog in the Caratinga and

Rio Doce valleys, Minas Gerais, led Dias (1975) to suspect this animal as the reservoir of the human disease in the same areas. Unless large numbers of dogs can be shown to be infected, however, there seems no reason to regard canine infection as any more than accidental, just as it is in man, after the bite of sandflies which normally feed on some wild animal host. The situation is perhaps comparable with that we have discussed in Panama (see Part VI, C).

In Minas Gerais State, an isolate from man in the Rio Doce valley had buoyant densities of 1·718 and 1·704 for nuclear and kinetoplastic DNA, and type I MDH (Peters, 1975), while one from the Caratinga area had type III MDH (Brazil, 1976).

Biochemically, it would seem that the Mato Grosso and Minas Gerais strains mentioned here are similar, but not identical. Epidemiologically there are apparent differences, too, in that the former has a wild, silvatic reservoir while the latter may have a domestic one in the dog. It is clear that the epidemiology of cutaneous leishmaniasis in the two areas will only be resolved following the biological and biochemical study of many more strains from man, dogs, wild animals and sandflies.

VIII. Neotropical leishmanias of uncertain taxonomic position

A. LEISHMANIA PERUVIANA

Peru is sharply divided into three major natural regions: the coastal desert of the Pacific Ocean, the Andes mountains, and the eastern forest which slopes gently down to merge with the Amazonian region of Brazil.

Peru and Brazil share the problem of mucocutaneous leishmaniasis due to *L. braziliensis* on the Amazonian side of the Andes: the disease is essentially silvatic in origin, with a vast reservoir of infection in wild forest animals. The cooler, barren mountain slopes (Fig. 3), on the western side of the Andes, are in such complete contrast that it comes as no surprise to find another *Leishmania* with an entirely different epidemiology, and associated with a different form of cutaneous leishmaniasis known as "uta".

1. The early history of "uta"

"A written account implicating *Phlebotomus* sandflies as vectors of Carrion's disease and cutaneous leishmaniasis in Peru was published by Cosme Bueno in 1764. Buenos' report precedes other publications implicating sandflies in the transmission of human pathogens by nearly a century and a half" (Herrer and Christensen, 1975a). As Carrion's disease is limited to the western side of the Peruvian Andes, it is fairly safe to say that Bueno's observations referred to "uta" rather than mucocutaneous leishmaniasis. Another interesting historical observation was made by Matta (1918) who recalled that a certain Dr. L. Villar had written in 1859 that "the disease ("uta") is very like the Aleppo button": exactly 39 years before Borovsky (1898) established the protozoal nature of the parasite causing oriental sore.

According to Townsend (1915) credit for the first recognition of "uta", "tiacc-araña" or "llaga" as a form of dermal leishmaniasis goes to a Dr. A. L. Barton, of Lima, who said that he had seen the parasite in smears from a skin lesion in 1910. He concluded, however, that the disease was simply "oriental sore" due to *L. tropica* and had not bothered to publish his observation. In this respect it is significant that Lindenberg (1909) had discovered the existence of cutaneous leishmaniasis in Brazil, only one year earlier, which doubtless inspired all clinicians to a greater interest in human skin lesions.

It remained for Velez (1913) to publish a similar observation, and he proposed the name of *Leishmania peruviana* for the parasite. This name has been accepted by most, although some authorities cling to Dr. Barton's belief that the organism is *L. tropica*, presumably imported into Peru by European settlers. Up till now there is no evidence to support this view other than a clinical resemblance between "uta" and "oriental sore". So few isolates have been available for study other than in Peru, however, that the true nature of *L. peruviana* is still not settled and, in the absence of any observations on natural or experimental infections in phlebotomine sandflies, one cannot even place the organism in either of the Sections Peripylaria or Suprapylaria.

2. Experimental infections of animals with *L. peruviana*

Strong *et al.* (1913, 1915) were apparently the first to infect an experimental animal, when they inoculated material from the lesion of a case of "uta" into the skin of the nose and ears of a dog. Fifty-three days later the animal showed a number of small nodules on the internal surface of the ears, in which amastigotes could be demonstrated microscopically: no signs of infection were seen in the skin of the nose. Similar experiments by Geiman (1940) produced positive lesions of the nose and ears of a dog and the infection was successfully transferred to another. The parasite was also isolated in culture from the spleens of mice which had been inoculated by the intraperitoneal route, one month previously.

Herrer and Battistini (1951) experimentally infected dogs by the intra-dermal inoculation of promastigotes from NNN cultures, and amastigotes in material taken from lesions, but it was noted that *L. peruviana* lost its capacity to infect these animals if kept in culture for a number of years. Lesions were most readily produced in the skin of the nose, less frequently in that of the ear, and usually showed as inconspicuous plaques or nodules with some depigmentation. Parasites were very scanty in smears made from these lesions, and no isolations were made from blood, spleen and liver tissues cultured in NNN medium.

Herrer (1951a) made similar inoculations of *L. peruviana* into the skin of the nose and ear of a number of foxes captured in endemic areas. Only three survived captivity long enough to enable any observations to be made, and two of these showed scanty amastigotes in smears made from apparently normal skin at the site of the injection: the third developed a small lesion similar to that produced in dogs. Two months after the animal was infected, no parasites could be isolated, in NNN medium, from the blood, liver, or spleen. Herrer concluded that the fox (species not stated) could possibly act as a reservoir of infection under certain circumstances, although he was later unable to find natural infections in seven he examined.

3. The epidemiology of "uta"

(*a*) *The human disease.* Herrer and Battistini (1951) and Herrer (1951a-d, 1957) have made the only detailed epidemiological studies of "uta" that we are aware of. The endemic areas were found to be restricted to regions between 900 to 3000 metres above sea level, with maximum endemicity located from 1800 to 2700 metres. Cases occurred mostly in rural communities completely devoid of any wooded areas. At the time of these studies, mainly in the Province of Huarochiri, the incidence was remarkably high in some villages, affecting up to 94% of school children, as judged by the presence of old scars and active lesions. Infection took place at an early age and, as there was usually spontaneous cure and firm protection to reinfection, the disease in adults was infrequent. Although rare cases were recorded of multiple lesions, the infection was usually limited to a single or few ulcers, mostly located on the head or upper parts of the body (Fig. 3). The disease was of a relatively mild nature, unless accompanied by severe, secondary, bacterial contamination: there was no evidence of naso-pharyngeal involvement. Herrer concluded that acquisition of "uta" was peridomestic.

(*b*) *Reservoirs of infection for man:* In 1945 Herrer (1951c) searched for reservoir hosts of *L. peruviana* in various endemic areas in the Province of Huarochiri, principally in the Rimac, Lurin, Canchacalla and Santa Eulalia valleys. He concentrated on domestic animals and examined a total of 513 dogs, 78 cats, 22 donkeys, 7 pigs and 1 horse by means of stained smears of skin, usually taken from the nose. Amastigotes were found in 46 of the dogs and an NNN culture was achieved on one occasion.

From the behaviour of the isolated parasite in culture and in inoculated dogs, Herrer concluded that it was identical to *L. peruviana* of man. He remarked on the parallel distribution of the canine and human disease, found both under the same roof on some occasions, and verified acquisition of infection by dogs which had recently been imported from non-endemic regions. The natural canine infection closely resembled that described for the experimentally infected animal and, in addition, Herrer noted some dogs with parasites in apparently normal skin; continued observations on these animals showed no subsequent development of a visible lesion.

"Considerable numbers" of wild rodents (mostly *Phyllotis* and *Oryzomys* spp.) and opossums (the "muca", species not stated) were trapped in the endemic areas. At that time, however, Herrer was unaware of the inconspicuous nature of the cutaneous infection in the dog, and smears of skin from the wild animals were only examined "in exceptional cases". No mention is made of any examination of the viscera, and it appears that no tissues were inoculated into laboratory animals.

(*c*) *The vector.* Townsend (1915) suspected ceratopogonid "gnats" (*Forcipomyia* species) as vectors of *L. peruviana* and claimed to have produced a lesion containing amastigotes after the intradermal inoculation of a suspension of these insects into a guinea-pig. Other workers, however, soon drew attention to the coincidental distribution of mucocutaneous leishmaniasis and phlebotomine sandflies in other parts of South America (Neiva and Barbará, 1917) and, with the later incrimination of these insects in the transmission of Old World leishmaniasis, Townsend's suggestion was soon discarded.

Attempts to incriminate any of the species of sandflies known to occur in areas endemic for "uta" have almost entirely been based on previous studies of "Carrion's disease" (Bartonellosis due to *Bartonella bacilliformis*), which has an almost coincidental distribution in the Peruvian Andes (Townsend, 1914; Battistini, 1929; Noguchi *et al.*, 1929; Hertig, 1937, 1939, 1942). Between them these authors have: (a) subjected monkeys (*Macacus rhesus*) to the bites of 683 wild-caught sandflies (*Lutzomyia verrucarum*); (b) cultured either whole insects, or the dissected guts, of another 682 (mostly *Lu. verrucarum*, some *Lu. noguchii*); (c) inoculated dogs and monkeys with suspensions of 1290 sandflies (mostly *Lu. verrucarum*, some *Lu. peruensis* and *Lu. noguchii*) and (d) examined histological sections of 434 more (mostly *Lu. verrucarum*, some *Lu. peruensis*). While the results of these studies led to the incrimination of *Lu. verrucarum* as the vector of *Bartonella bacilliformis*, it shed no light on the role of local sandfly species in the transmission of "uta". As Herrer pointed out, however, even though the dog and the rhesus monkey are susceptible to infection, they were almost certainly not observed over a long enough period to allow any leishmanial lesion to appear. Also, experimentally produced lesions due to *L. peruviana* are so inconspicuous that they would probably have escaped attention, anyway.

Lu. verrucarum nevertheless remains the most highly suspect vector of "uta" and, in Herrer's experience, was to be found throughout the entire endemic area. It frequented both houses and animal-sheds and seemed equally attracted to man, dogs and a wide variety of domestic animals; it would feed readily on guinea-pigs and rabbits and presumably, therefore, on wild rodents. The insect was frequently found in fox-holes and other resting-sites far removed from human habitation.

Lu. peruensis was found to be less abundant and more restricted in its distribution in the endemic areas of "uta". Its habits are much less well known than those of *Lu. verrucarum*, but Herrer gained the impression that it was less domesticated and probably fed principally on wild animals. It was nevertheless shown to readily feed on man, as well as domestic birds; in some localities it even outnumbered *Lu. verrucarum*.

Lu. noguchii seems to be an unlikely candidate as a vector to man or the dog, as it is disinclined to bite them and apparently devotes its attention to the wild animal inhabitants of rocky and arid habitats. The fly was frequently found infected with *Trypanosoma phyllotis*, a parasite of a small rodent, *Phyllotis*, which appears to be the principal host of *Lu. noguchii* (Herrer, 1942).

Lu. battistinii and *Lu. pescei* were described by Hertig (1943) from specimens captured in an endemic zone in the Province of Andahuaylas. Both have been captured in houses and animal-sheds, and the latter is known to feed on man. The scarcity of both species in the majority of the foci of "uta", however, rather precludes them as important vectors. The same may be said of *Lu. imperatrix*, described from the outskirts of Huancayo, at about 2850 metres, and believed by Dampf (1950) to be a synonym for *Lu. pescei*: nothing is known of its distribution or its feeding habits. Finally, Herrer (1943) captured one specimen of an undescribed sandfly, biting man, in the endemic area of Molino in the Department of Cajamarca; again, its rarity excludes any important role in the transmission of *L. peruviana* to man.

Whichever species is the major vector remains obscure, but DDT spraying campaigns made it fairly obvious that one or more of these sandflies is involved. Thus, in 1945, Herrer's epidemiological studies in the Rimac valley were effectively halted by a spraying programme for the control of Carrion's disease (Hertig and Fairchild, 1948). Sandflies virtually disappeared from the houses and animal sheds, and control of these insects in two large construction camps was followed by an almost complete cessation of new cases of cutaneous leishmaniasis and bartonellosis. Herrer (1956a) recorded similar results in other parts of the same valley, when sandflies were reduced to an insignificant level in houses and schools and the incidence of cutaneous leishmaniasis in the dogs dropped from 22% to 1·6%: the incidence of the disease in schoolchildren decreased so greatly that transmission was believed to have completely stopped. Continued fall in the number of cases up to 1956, in the absence of renewed spraying programmes, was considered due to private, domestic use of modern insecticides (Herrer, 1956b).

In spite of Herrer's great efforts there are still many questions unanswered on the epidemiology of "uta". Possibly the dog *is* the sole reservoir of infection for man. In the light of modern knowledge on the vital role of wild animals in all other forms of American cutaneous leishmaniasis, however, we feel sure that Dr. Herrer would be the first to agree that further investigations of this possibility are needed in the endemic areas of "uta". It is particularly interesting that species of the rodent *Oryzomys* were found in considerable numbers, for these are commonly infected with *Leishmania* in many other parts of Latin America.

With regards to the vector, it seems that the small number of species of sandflies involved makes it only a question of time before either *Lu. verrucarum* or *Lu. peruensis* (or both) is incriminated by the isolation of *L. peruviana* from wild-caught insects. In the meantime, the behaviour of the parasite in these or other species of *Lutzomyia* (e.g. *Lu. longipalpis*) would enable us to place it in either the Peripylaria or the Suprapylaria. If in the former, this would immediately eliminate the possibility of *L. peruviana* being synonymous with *L. tropica*.

Whether or not the geographical range of "uta" extends into the highlands of other countries within the Andes is not clear, but there seems no reason why *L. peruviana* should not be found in the mountainous parts of Argentina, Bolivia, Ecuador and Colombia.

Mazza (1926a, b, c, and 1927) discussed the coincidental distribution of human and canine cutaneous leishmaniasis in the Argentinian highlands, principally in the provinces of Tucumán, Salta and Jujuy. The disease appeared to be peridomestic and remarkably similar to that later described by Herrer in Peru. It was associated with a sandfly which they indentified as *Lu. verrucarum*, and one instance was cited in which large numbers of this species were caught in a house in which there occurred 1 canine and 5 human cases of cutaneous leishmaniasis. Mazza saw amastigotes in smears from skin lesions, found principally on the ears of the dogs, and was unable to find parasites in the internal organs or bone-marrow of autopsied animals.

Romaña *et al.* (1949) and Romaña and Abalos (1949) discussed similar foci of cutaneous leishmaniasis, principally in the Department of Burruyacú, Tucumán, in relation to the various species of sandflies encountered in Argentina. Of 21 cases examined, most were in children from 7 to 14 years old; the lesions were ulcerous, but with no nasopharyngeal involvement and a great tendency to heal spontaneously; infected dogs were encountered and amastigotes demonstrated in skin lesions; the disease appeared to be domestic or peridomestic, and associated sandflies included *Lu. migonei* and *Lu. cortelezzii*.

It is clear that only further epidemiological studies throughout the Andean countries will establish the geographic range of *L. peruviana*: isolates from man, dog and sandflies are badly needed for direct biological and biochemical comparison.

IX. Concluding remarks

From a deceptively simple beginning the subject of *Leishmania* and leishmaniasis has assumed an astonishing complexity, capturing the interest of the protozoologist, epidemiologist, entomologist, immunologist, biochemist and taxonomist alike. Great advances have been made in our knowledge of the leishmanias over the last 15 years, giving workers a new awareness that these important organisms are not the small group of dubious species, with monotonously identical morphology and uninspiring life-histories, that we once thought them to be.

It is abundantly clear that whatever case may be made for purely anthroponotic leishmaniasis in certain regions of the Old World, there is no doubt whatever of the consistent and dominant role of wild and/or domestic mammals in the epidemiology of the New World disease. It is equally obvious, however, that in spite of the rapidly growing list of species and subspecies of *Leishmania*, we have no more than scraped the surface in our efforts to determine just how extensive is the range of parasites in this actively speciating complex, their individual importance in diseases of man, and the complexities of their natural history. Thus, although *Leishmania b. braziliensis* and *L. b. guyanensis* have long been recognized as responsible for the two most important forms of cutaneous and mucocutaneous leishmaniasis in the Amazon region of Brazil, the recent discovery of two major vectors of these parasites has also necessitated description of these insects as two new species of sandflies!

Probably no-one is more aware of the enormity of the subject of neotropical leishmaniasis than the epidemiologist, in the field. His chance isolation of *Leishmania* from a sandfly or wild mammal gives him a glimpse of the bare materials. Establishing its common identity with a parasite in man, in the same area, lays the foundations. Only many years of arduous field-work in correlating the behaviour of parasite, sandfly, wild mammalian hosts and man will allow him to build his final and accurate epidemiological picture.

X. Acknowledgements

Our thanks are due to the Wellcome Trust, London, whose support over the past twelve years has enabled a continuity of study which is rarely available and yet so essential in any programme on the epidemiology of leishmaniasis; also to the Superintendência de Desenvolvimento da

Amazônia (SUDAM) and the Pan American Health Organization, for their collaboration. Thanks, too, are due to our Brazilian colleagues who have given us every available facility at the Instituto Evandro Chagas; in particular to the late Dr. Orlando Costa, Dr. Miguel Azevedo, and Dra. Gilberta Bensabath. Dr. Habib Fraiha collaborated in identification of much of the sandfly material collected during our studies in Brazil. We are particularly indebted to our staff for their devoted and efficient service: Srs. Roberto Naiff, Sebastião Oliveira, Henrique Buna, Manoel de Souza and José Almeida, and Srtas. Graça Soares, Maricleide Farias, Cristina Loureiro, and Cesarina Arcanjo. Srta. Graça Soares typed the manuscript; and Dr. Richard Ward devoted much time checking it, and offered many useful suggestions. Permission to use certain illustrations was kindly given by the editors of the *Transactions of the Royal Society of Tropical Medicine and Hygiene*, Fig. 1 (1); Fig. 4 (3); Fig. 5 (3–6); Fig. 6 (5): *The Bulletin of the Pan American Health Organization*, for Fig. 1 (2 and 4) and the University of Toronto Press, for Fig. 3 (1 and 2); Fig. 4 (6) and Fig. 6 (1 and 2).

XI. References

Adler, S. (1940). Notas sôbre a *Leishmania chagasi*. *Memórias do Instituto Oswaldo Cruz*, **35**, 173–175.

Adler, S. (1964). *Leishmania*. *In*: "Advances in Parasitology" (Ed. B. Dawes), **2**, 35–96, Academic Press, New York and London.

Adler, S. and Adler, J. (1955). The agglutinogenic properties of various stages of the Leishmanias. *Bulletin of the Research Council of Israel (Section B)*, **4**, 396–397.

Adler, S. and Theodor, O. (1929). Observations on *Leishmania ceramodactyli* n. sp. *Transactions of the Royal Society of Tropical Medicine and Hygiene*, **22**, 343–356.

Adler, S. and Theodor, O. (1957). Transmission of disease agents by phlebotomine sand flies. *Annual Review of Entomology*, **2**, 203–226.

Aitken, T. H. G., Woodall, J. P., Andrade, A. H. P., Bensabath, G. and Shope, E. S. (1975). Pacui virus, Phlebotomine flies, and small mammals in Brazil; an epidemiological study. *American Journal of Tropical Medicine and Hygiene*, **24**, 358–368.

Alencar, J. E. (1955). Leishmaniose visceral no Novo Mundo. *XII Congresso Brasileiro de Higiene, Belém, Pará*, 9–15th January 1955.

Alencar, J. E. (1959). [cited by Forattini (1960): *q.v.*]

Alencar, J. E. (1961). Profilaxia do calazar no Ceará, Brasil. *Revista do Instituto de Medicina Tropical de São Paulo*, **3**, 175–180.

Alencar, J. E. (1962). Investigações em tôrno de foco de calazar na Paraíba. *Revista Brasileira de Melariologia e Doenças Tropicais*, **14**, 367–370.

Alencar, J. E. (1963). Influência da dedetização sôbre a incidência do calazar humano no Ceará—novos dados. *Revista Brasileira de Malariologia e Doenças Tropicais*, **15**, 417–424.

Alencar, J. E., Holanda, D. and Cavalcante, J. D. N. (1956). Calazar no Vale do Jaguaribe, Ceará. *Revista Brasileira de Malariologia e Doenças Tropicais*, **8**, 33–47.

Alencar, J. E., Pessôa, E. P. and Fontenele, Z. F. (1960). Infecção natural de *Rattus rattus alexandrinus* por *Leishmania* (provavelmente *L. braziliensis*) em zona endêmica de leishmaniose tegumentar do estado do Ceará, Brasil. *Revista do Instituto de Medicina Tropical de São Paulo*, 2, 347–348.

Alencar, J. E., Pessôa, E. P. and Costa, O. R. (1962). Calazar em Santarem, Estado do Pará. *Revista Brasileira de Malariologia e Doenças Tropicais*, 14, 371–377.

Almeida, E. (1945). Um caso de leishmaniose visceral na Paraíba. *Brasil-Médico*, 59, 82–83.

Amaral, A. D. F., Torrealba, J. W., Henríquez, C. E., Kowalenko, W. and Barrios, P. A. (1961a). *Phlebotomus longipalpis* Lutz y Neiva, probable transmissor de la leishmaniasis visceral em Venezuela. *Gaceta Médica de Caracas*, 70, 389–408.

Amaral, A. D. F., Torrealba, J. W., Henríquez, C. E., Kowalenko, W. and Barrios, P. A. (1961b). Revisión sobre el kala-azar en Venezuela. *Folia Clinica et Biologica (São Paulo)*, 30, 14–24.

Amaral, A. D. F., Torrealba, J. W., Henríquez, C. E., Kowalenko, W. and Barrios, P. A. (1961c). Studies on visceral leishmaniasis in Venezuela. *Revista do Instituto de Medicina Tropical de São Paulo*, 3, 91–98.

Anon. (1957). The twenty-ninth annual report of the work and operation of the Gorgas Memorial Laboratory, covering the fiscal year ended June 30, 1956. United States Government Printing Office, Washington.

Anon. (1958). The thirtieth annual report of the work and operation of the Gorgas Memorial Laboratory, covering the fiscal year ended June 30, 1957. United States Government Printing Office, Washington.

Anon. (1959). Thirty-first annual report of the work and operation of the Gorgas Memorial Laboratory, covering the fiscal year ended June 30, 1958. United States Government Printing Office, Washington.

Anon. (1967). Thirty-eighth annual report of the work and operations of the Gorgas Memorial Laboratory, fiscal year 1966. United States Government Printing Office, Washington.

Aragão, H. B. (1922). Transmissão de leishmaniose no Brasil pelo *Phlebotomus intermedius*. *Brasil Médico*, 36, 129–130.

Aragão, T. C. (1953). Surto de leishmaniose visceral na zona Norte do Ceará. Communication made at the *III Reunião de Saúde Publica do Estado do Ceará*, September 1953.

Baker, J. R. (1963). Speculations on the Evolution of the Family Trypanosomatidae Doflein, 1901. *Experimental Parasitology*, 13, 219–233.

Baker, J. R. (1965). The evolution of parasitic protozoa. *Symposium of the British Society of Parasitology*, 3, 1–27.

Barbosa, F. S., Mello, D. A. and Coura, J. R. (1970). Nota sôbre a infecção natural de roedores por *Leishmania* sp. nos limites dos municipios Teresopolis-Nova Friburgo, estado do Rio de Janeiro. *Revista da Sociedade Brasileira de Medicina Tropical*, 4, 113–115.

Barbosa, W. (1966). Subsídios ao estudo do calazar em Goiás. *Revista Goiana de Medicina*, 12, 5–30.

Barbosa, W., Souza, M. C. M., Souza, J. M., Rassi, D. M., Gerais, B. B. and Oliveira, R. L. (1976). Note on the classification of the *Leishmania* sp. responsible for cutaneous leishmaniasis in the East Central Region of Brazil. *Annals of Tropical Medicine and Parasitology*, 70, 389–399.

Barreto, P. (1969). Artropodos hematofagos del Rio Raposo, Valle, Colombia. *Caldasia*, 10, 459–472.

Barretto, M. P. (1943). "Observações sôbre a biologia, em condições naturais, dos flebótomus do Estado de São Paulo". Thesis. 162 pp. Tipografia Rossolillo, São Paulo.

Barrientos, L. P. (1948). Um caso atipico de leishmaniose cutâneo-mucosa (Espundia). *Memorias do Instituto Oswaldo Cruz*, **46**, 415–418.

Barros, O. M. and Rosenfeld, G. (1942). Leishmaniose visceral americana. Um caso da Bolivia. *Revista Clínica de São Paulo*, **11**, 91–99.

Baruffa, G. and Cury, P. (1973). Contribuição ao estudo do calazar em Mato Grosso. *Revista de Patologia Tropical*, **2**, 345–361.

Battistini, T. (1929). Estudios sobre la verruga peruana. *La Acción Médica (Lima)*, January 1929.

Belova, E. M. (1971). Reptiles and their importance in the epidemiology of leishmaniasis. *Bulletin of the World Health Organization*, **44** (4), 553–560.

Biagi, F. F. (1953a). Sintesis de 70 historias clinicas de Leishmaniasis Tegumentaria de México (ulcera de los chicleros). *Medicina (México)*, **33**, 385–396.

Biagi, F. F. (1953b). Algunos comentarios sobre las leishmaniasis y sus agentes etiológicos, *Leishmania trópica mexicana*, nueva subespecie. *Medicina (México)*, **33**, 401–406.

Biagi, F. F. and Biagi, B. A. M. (1953). Algunos *Flebotomus* del área endémica de leishmaniasis tegumentaria americana del Estado de Campeche (Méx.). *Medicina (México)*, **33**, 315–319.

Biagi, F. F. and Tay, J. (1963). Observaciones sobre un nuevo foco endemico de kala-azar en México. *Revista de la Facultad de Medicina (México)*, **5**, 7–11.

Biagi, F. F., Biagi, B. A. M. and Beltran, H. F. (1965a). *Phlebotomus flaviscutellata*, transmissor natural de *Leishmania mexicana*. *Prensa Médica Mexicana*, **30**, 267–272.

Biagi, F. F., López, M. R. and Biagi, B. A. M. (1965b). El kala-azar en México: problema ecológico por estudar. *Revista del Instituto de Salubridad y Enfermedades Tropicales (México)*, **25**, 3–12.

Bloch, M. and Guillen, G. (1950). Kala-azar en E. Salvador. *Archivos del Colegio Médico de El Salvador*, **3**, 90–96.

Boggino, J. and Haas, L. C. (1945). Primer caso ciertamente autoctono de leishmaniasis visceral. *Anales de la Facultad de Ciencias Médicas Universidad Nacional del Paraguay*, **5**, 319–324.

Boreham, P. F. L. (1975). Some applications of bloodmeal identifications in relation to the epidemiology of vector-borne tropical diseases. *Journal of Tropical Medicine and Hygiene*, **4**, 83–91.

Borovsky, P. F. (1898). [On Sart Sore]. Voenno-Medicinskij Zurnal [Military-Medical Journal], *Part cxcv*, No. 11 (76th year), 925. [In Russian].

Bray, R. S. (1974). Leishmania. *Annual Review of Microbiology*, **28**, 189–217.

Bray, R. S. and Garnham, P. C. C. (1962). The Giemsa-Colophonium method for staining protozoa in tissue sections. *Indian Journal of Malariology*, **16**, 153–155.

Brazil, R. P. (1976). "Comparative studies on the culture forms of four isolates of *Leishmania* from Brazil". Thesis for degree of M.Sc., pp. 49. University of Liverpool.

Cabrera, M. A. and León, R. (1949). Historia del primer caso clinico de leishmaniasis visceral descubierto en Guatemala. *Publicaciones, Instituto de Investigaciónes Científicas (Guatemala)*, **2**, 1–36.

Chagas, A. W. (1939). Infecção de *Phlebotomus intermedius* pela *Leishmania chagasi*. *Brasil-Médico*, **53**, 1–2.

Chagas, A. W. (1940). Criação de Flebótomus e transmissão experimental da leishmaniose visceral americana. *Memórias do Instituto Oswaldo Cruz*, **35**, 327–333.

Chagas, E. (1936). Primeira verificação em individuo vivo, da leishmaniose visceral no Brasil. *Brasil-Médico*, **50**, 221–222.

Chagas, E. and Chagas, A. W. (1938). Notas sobre a epidemiologia da leishmaniose visceral americana em Mato Grosso. *Hospital (Rio de Janeiro)*, **13**, 471–480.

Chagas, E., Cunha, A. M., Ferreira, L. C., Deane, L., Deane, G., Guimarães, F. N., Paumgartten, M. J. and Sá, B. (1938). Leishmaniose visceral americana. (Relatório dos trabalhos realizados pela Commissão Encarregada do Estudo da Leishmaniose Visceral Americana em 1937.) *Memórias do Instituto Oswaldo Cruz*, **33**, 89–229.

Chaddad, M. S. A., Ferreira, J. M., Shiroma, M. and Meira, J. A. (1976). Calazar: análise de 60 casos. *Tema Livre No. 43, XII Congresso da Sociedade Brasileira de Medicina tropical*, 15th–19th February 1976. Belém, Pará, Brasil.

Chalmers, A. H., Harris, J. C., Swanton, R. H. and Thorley, A. P. (1968). A survey of the distribution of dermal leishmaniasis in British Honduras. *Transactions of the Royal Society of Tropical Medicine and Hygiene*, **62**, 213–220.

Chance, M. L., Peters, W. and Shchory, L. (1974). Biochemical taxonomy of *Leishmania*. I. Observations on DNA. *Annals of Tropical Medicine and Parasitology*, **68**, 307–325.

Chaniotis, B. N., Correa, M. A., Tesh, R. B. and Johnson, K. M. (1971a). Daily and seasonal man-biting activity of phlebotomine sandflies in Panama. *Journal of Medical Entomology*, **8**, 415–420.

Chaniotis, B. N., Neely, J. M., Correa, M. A., Tesh, R. B. and Johnson, K. M. (1971b). Natural population dynamics of phlebotomine sandflies in Panama, *Journal of Medical Entomology*, **8**, 339–352.

Chaniotis, B. N., Tesh, R. B., Correa, M. A. and Johnson, K. M. (1972). Diurnal resting sites of phlebotomine sandflies in a Panamanian tropical forest. *Journal of Medical Entomology*, **9**, 91–98.

Christensen, H. A. and Telford, S. R. (1972). *Trypanosoma thecadactyli* sp. n. from forest geckoes in Panama, and its development in the sandfly *Lutzomyia trinidadensis* (Newstead) (Diptera, Psychodidae). *Journal of Protozoology*, **19**, 403–406.

Christensen, H. A., Herrer, A. and Telford, S. R. (1969). *Leishmania braziliensis* from *Lutzomyia panamensis* in Panama. *Journal of Parasitology*, **55**, 1090–1091.

Christensen, H. A., Herrer, A. and Telford, S. R. (1972). Enzootic cutaneous leishmaniasis in eastern Panama. II. Entomological investigations. *Annals of tropical Medicine and Parasitology*, **66**, 55–66.

Coelho, M. V. and Falcão, A. R. (1962). Transmissão experimental de *Leishmania braziliensis*, II. Transmissão de amostra mexicana por picada de *Phlebotomus longipalpis* e de *Phlebotomus renei*. *Revista do Instituto de Medicina Tropical de São Paulo*, **4**, 220–224.

Coelho, M. V., Cunha, A. S. and Falcão, A. R. (1965). Notas sôbre um foco de calazar no sudoeste do Estado de Goiás. *Revista Brasileira de Malariologia e Doenças Tropicais*, **17**, 143–148.

Coelho, M. V., Falcão, A. R. and Falcão, A. L. (1967a). Desenvolvimento de espécies do gênero *Leishmania* em espécies brasileiras de flebótomos do gênero *Lutzomyia* França, 1924. I. Evolução de *L. braziliensis* em flebótomos. *Revista do Instituto de Medicina Tropical de São Paulo*, **9**, 177–191.

Coelho, M. V., Falcão, A. R. and Falcão, A. L. (1967b). Desenvolvimento de espécies do gênero *Leishmania* em espécies brasileiras de flebótomos do género *Lutzomyia* França, 1924. III. Ciclo vital de *L. mexicana* em *L. longipalpis* e *L. renei*. *Revista do Instituto de Medicina Tropical de São Paulo*, **9**, 299–303.

Coelho, M. V., Falcão, A. R. and Falcão, A. L. (1967c). Desenvolvimento de espécies do gênero *Leishmania* em flebótomus brasileiras do gênero *Lutzomyia* França, 1924. IV. Ciclo vital de *L. donovani* em *L. longipalpis* e *L. renei*. *Revista do Instituto de Medicina Tropical de São Paulo*, **9**, 361–366.

Coelho, M. V., Falcão, A. R. and Falcão, A. L. (1967d). Desenvolvimento de espécies do gênero *Leishmania* em espécies brasileiras de flebótomus do gênero *Lutzomyia* França, 1924. V. Infetividade de leptomonas evoluindo no flebótomo e experiências de transmissão de leishmanioses. *Revista do instituto de Medicina Tropical de São Paulo*, **9**, 367–373.

Convit, J. (1946). [cited by Pifano, C. F. (1949): *q.v.*]

Convit, J. (1968). [cited in Pifano *et al.* (1968): *q.v.*]

Convit, J. and Lapenta, P. (1948). Sobre un caso de leishmaniasis tegumentaria de forma diseminada. *Revista de la Policlinica (Caracas)*, **18**, 153–158.

Costa, O. R. (1966). Calazar no Município de Cachoeira do Ararí, Pará. *Revista do Serviço Especial de Saúde Pública (Rio de Janeiro)*, **12**, 91–98.

Courmes, E., Escudie, A., Fauran, P. and Monnerville, A. (1966). Premier cas autochtone de leishmaniose viscérale humaine a la Guadeloupe. *Bulletin de la Société de Pathologie Exotique*, **59**, 217–226.

Cunha, A. M. (1938a). Infections expérimentales obtenues en partant de la leishmaniose viscérale amèricaine. *Comptes Rendus des Séances de la Société de Biologie et de ses Filiales (Paris)*, **129**, 428–430.

Cunha, A. M. (1938b). A agglutinação e o diagnostico differencial das leishmanias. *Brasil-Médico*, **52**, 849–855.

Cunha, A. M. (1942). A sôro-aglutinação das leishmanias. *Memórias do Instituto Oswaldo Cruz*, **37**, 35–76.

Cunha, A. M. and Chagas, E. (1937). Nova espécie de protozoário do gênero *Leishmania* pathogenico para o homem. *Leishmania chagasi*, n. sp. Nota Prévia. *Hospital (Rio de Janeiro)*, **11**, 3–9.

Dampf, A. (1950). Notas sobre flebótomos americanos (Dipt. Psych.). *Review of Applied Entomology*, **38** (B), 137.

Deane, L. M. (1948). Abstract of discussion on C. A. Hoare's paper "The relationship of the haemoflagellates". *In Proceedings of the 4th International Congress of Tropical Medicine and Malaria*, Washington, D.C., 10th–18th May 1948.

Deane, L. M. (1956). "Leishmaniose Visceral no Brasil". Serviço Nacional de Educação Sanitária, Rio de Janeiro, Brasil.

Deane, L. M. (1958). Epidemiología e profilaxía do calazar americano. *Revista Brasileira de Malariologia e Doenças Tropicais*, **10**, 431–450.

Deane, L. M. and Deane, G. (1937). Estudos sôbre a leishmaniose visceral americana. Nota no. 1. Aspectos clínicos da doença. *Hospital (Rio de Janeiro)*, **12**, 189–199.

Deane, L. M. and Deane, M. P. (1954a). Encontro de leishmânias nas visceras e na pele de uma raposa, em zona endêmica de calazar, nos arredores de Sobral, Ceará. *Hospital (Rio de Janeiro)*, **45**, 419–421.

Deane, L. M. and Deane, M. P. (1954b). Encontro de cães naturalmente infectados por *Leishmania donovani* no Ceará. *Hospital (Rio de Janeiro)*, **45**, 703–707.

Deane, M. P. and Deane, L. M. (1954c). Infecção natural do *Phlebotomus longipalpis* por leptomonas, provàvelmente de *Leishmania donovani*, em foco de calazar, no Ceará. *Hospital (Rio de Janeiro)*, **45**, 697–702.

Deane, M. P. and Deane, L. M. (1954d). Infecção experimental do *Phlebotomus longipalpis* em caso humano de leishmaniose visceral. *Hospital (Rio de Janeiro)*, **46**, 487–489.

Deane, M. P. and Deane, L. M. (1954e). Infecção experimental do *Phlebotomus longipalpis* em rapôsa (*Lycalopex vetulus*) naturalmente parasitada pela *Leishmania donovani*. *Hospital (Rio de Janeiro)*, **46**, 651–653.

Deane, L. M. and Deane, M. P. (1964). Leishmaniose visceral nas Américas do Sul e Central. *Arquivos de Higiene e Saúde Pública (São Paulo)*, **29**, 89–94.

Deane, L. M., Deane, M. P. and Alencar, J. E. (1955). Observações sôbre o combate ao *Phlebotomus longipalps* pela dedetização domiciliária em focos endêmicos de calazar no Ceará. *Revista Brasileira de Malariologia e Doenças Tropicais*, **7**, 131–141.

Deane, L. M., Silva, J. E. and Figueiredo, P. Z. (1974). Leishmaniae in the viscera of porcupines from the State of Piauí, Brazil. *Revista do Instituto de Medicina Tropical de São Paulo*, **16**, 68–69.

Dias, M. (1975). "Contribuição Ao Estudo Da Leishmaniose Tegumentar No Municipio De Caratinga, M. Gerais, Brasil". Thesis for degree of M.Sc. Universidade Federal de Minas Gerais.

Diaz-Ungría, C. (1969). Las leishmaniasis en Venezuela. *Ciencias Veterinarias*, **1**, 151–163.

Disney, R. H. L. (1964). Visceral involvement with dermal leishmaniasis in a wild-caught rodent in British Honduras. *Transactions of the Royal Society of Tropical Medicine and Hygiene*, **58**, 581.

Disney, R. H. L. (1966). A trap for phlebotomine sandflies attracted to rats. *Bulletin of Entomological Research*, **56**, 445–451.

Disney, R. H. L. (1968). Observations on a zoonosis: leishmaniasis in British Honduras. *Journal of Applied Ecology*, **5**, 1–59.

Dollahon, N. R. and Janovy, J. (1971). Insect flagellates from feces and gut contents of four genera of lizards. *Journal of Parasitology*, **57**, 1130–1132.

Dollahon, N. R. and Janovy, J. (1974). Experimental infection of New World lizards with Old World *Leishmania* species. *Experimental Parasitology*, **36**. 253–260.

Escomel, E. (1922). "Leishmaniosis y blastomicosis en America", Arequipa, Lima.

Fernandes, J. F. and Castellani, O. (1966). Growth characteristics and chemical composition of *Trypanosoma cruzi*. *Experimental Parasitology*, **18**, 195–202.

Fernandes, P., Gouveia, F. and Cunha Lima, D. P. (1976). Calazar na Microregião da Borborema Potiguar—RN. *Tema Livre No. 44*, *XII Congresso da Sociedade Brasileira de Medicina Tropical*, 15th–19th February 1976, Belém, Pará, Brasil.

Ferreira, L. C., Deane, L. and Mangabeira, O. (1938a). Infecção de *"Flebotomus longipalpis"* pela *"Leishmania chagasi"*. *Hospital (Rio de Janeiro)*, **14**, 2–3.

Ferreira, L. C., Mangabeira, O., Deane, L. M. and Chagas, A. W. (1938b). Notas sôbre a transmissão da leishmaniose visceral americana. *Hospital (Rio de Janeiro)*, **14**, 1077–1087.

Forattini, O. P. (1953). Nota sôbre criadouros naturais de flebótomos em dependências peri-domiciliares no Estado de São Paulo. *Arquivos da Faculdade de Higiene e Saúde Pública da Universidade de São Paulo*, **7**, 157–167.

Forattini, O. P. (1954). Algumas observações sôbre biologia de flebótomus (Diptera: Psychodidae) em região da Bacia do Rio Paraná (Brasil). *Arquivos da Faculdade de Higiene e Saúde Pública da Universidade de São Paulo*, **8**, 15–136.

Forattini, O. P. (1959). Sôbre os flebótomus do território do Amapá, Brasil. *Arquivos da Faculdade de Higiene e Saúde Pública da Universidade de São Paulo*, **13**, 159–164.

Forattini, O. P. (1960a). Sôbre os reservatórios naturais da leishmaniose tegumentar americana. *Revista do Instituto de Medicina Tropical de São Paulo*, **2**, 195–203.

Forattini, O. P. (1960b). Novas observações sobre a biologia de flebótomos em condições naturais (Diptera: Psychodidae). *Arquivos da Faculdade de Higiene e Saúde Pública da Universidade de São Paulo*, **25**, 209–215.

Forattini, O. P. and Santos, M. R. (1952). Nota sôbre infecção natural de *Phlebotomus intermedius* Lutz e Neiva 1912, por formas em leptomonas, em um foco de leishmaniose tegumentar americana. *Arquivos de Higiene e Saúde Pública*, **17**, 171–174.

Forattini, O. P., Rabello, E. X. and Pattoli, D. G. B. (1970). Sobre o encontro de

Lutzomyia longipalpis (Lutz e Neiva, 1912) no Estado de São Paulo, Brasil. *Revista de Saúde Pública (São Paulo)*, **4**, 99–100.

Forattini, O. P., Pattoli, D. B. G., Rabello, E. X. and Ferreira, O. A. (1972a). Nota sôbre um foco de Leishmaniose tegumentar na região nordeste do Estado de São Paulo, Brasil. *Revista de Saúde Pública*, **6**, 103–105.

Forattini, O. P., Pattoli, D. B. G., Rabello, E. X. and Ferreira, O. A. (1972b). Infecções naturais de mamíferos silvestres em área endêmica de Leishmaniose tegumentar do estado de São Paulo, Brasil. *Revista de Saúde Pública*, **6**, 255–261.

Forattini, O. P., Pattoli, D. B. G., Rabello, E. X. and Ferreira, O. A. (1972c). Infecção natural de flebotomíneos em foco enzoótico de leishmaniose tegumentar no estado de São Paulo, Brasil. *Revista de Saúde Pública*, **6**, 431–433.

Forattini, O. P., Pattoli, D. B. G., Rabello, E. X. and Ferreira, O. A. (1973). Nota sôbre infecção natural de *Oryzomys capito laticeps* em foco enzoótico de leishmaniose tegumentar no estado de São Paulo, Brasil. *Revista de Saúde Pública*, **7**, 181–184.

Forattini, O. P., Rabello, E. X., Serra, O. P., Cotrim, M. D., Galati, E. A. B. and Barata, J. M. S. (1976). Observações sobre a transmissão da leishmaniose tegumentar no Estado de São Paulo, Brasil. *Revista de Saúde Pública*, **10**, 31–43.

Fraiha, H., Ward, R. D., Shaw, J. J. and Lainson, R. (1977). Fauna antropófila de flebótomos da Rodovia Transamazônica, Brasil. *Boletin de la Oficina Sanitaria Panamericana*, **84**, (2), 134–139.

Gardener, P. J., Chance, M. L. and Peters, W. (1974). Biochemical taxonomy of *Leishmania*. II. Electrophoretic variation of malate dehydrogenase. *Annals of Tropical Medicine and Parasitology*, **68**, 317–325.

Garnham, P. C. C. (1962), Cutaneous leishmaniasis in the New World with special reference to *Leishmania mexicana*. *Scientific Reports of Instituto Superiore di Sanita*, **2**, 76–82.

Garnham, P. C. C. and Lewis, D. J. (1959). Parasites of British Honduras with special reference to leishmaniasis. *Transactions of the Royal Society of Tropical Medicine and Hygiene*, **53**, 12–40.

Gast Galvis, A. and Rengifo, S. (1944). Leishmaniasis visceral. Estudo epidemiológico del primer caso diagnosticado en Colombia. *Anales de la Sociedad de Biología de Bogotá*, **1**, 1–8.

Geiman, Q. M. (1940). A study of four Peruvian strains of *Leishmania braziliensis*. *Journal of Parasitology* (Suppl.), **26**, 22–23.

Guedes, G. E., Maroja, A., Chaves, E., Estélio, J., Cunha, M. J. and Arcoverde, S. (1974). Calazar no litoral do Estado da Paraíba, Brasil. Encontro de 70 casos humanos e 16 caninos. *Revista do Instituto de Medicina Tropical de São Paulo*, **16**, 265–269.

Guimarães, F. N. (1955). Estudo de um foco de leishmaniose muco-cutânea na Baixa Fluminense (Estado do Rio de Janeiro). *Memórias do Instituto Oswaldo Cruz*, **53**, 1–11.

Guimarães, F. N. and Azevedo, M. (1964). Roedores silvestres ("*Oryzomys goeldi*") da Amazônia com infecção natural por "*Leishmania*". (Primeira nota.) *Hospital (Rio de Janeiro)*, **66**, 279–285.

Guimarães, F. N. and Bustamante, F. M. (1954). A aplicação domiciliária de DDT como base da profilaxia das leishmanioses. Estudo de um foco de leishmaniose muco-cutânea cinco anos depois da aspersão periódica com aquêle inseticida. *Revista Brasileira de Malariologia e Doenças Tropicais*, **6**, 127–130.

Guimarães, F. N. and Costa, O. (1964). Observações sôbre o comportamento da "*Leishmania*" produtora de infecção natural em "*Oryzomys goeldi*", na Amazônia. (Segunda nota.) *Hospital (Rio de Janeiro)*, **66**, 287–292.

Guimarães, F. N. and Costa, O. (1966). Novas observações sobre a Leishmania isolada de "*Oryzomys goeldi*", na Amazônia. (4a. nota.) *Hospital (Rio de Janeiro)*, **69**, 161–168.

Hanson, W. J. (1961). The breeding places of *Phlebotomus* in Panama (Diptera, Psychodidae). *Annals of the Entomological Society of America*, **54**, 317–322.

Heisch, R. B. (1958). On *Leishmania adleri* sp. nov., from lacertid lizards (*Latastia* sp.) in Kenya. *Annals of Tropical Medicine and Parasitology*, **52**, 68–71.

Henríquez, L. C. E., Rasi, E. and Garcia, L. (1970). *Phlebotomus (Lutzomyia) longipalpis* Lutz and Neiva, 1912 (Diptera: Psychodidae) en foco de kala-azar del oriente medio Venezolano. *Revista Venezolana de Sanidad y Asistencia Social*, **35**, 761–768.

Herrer, A. (1942). *Trypanosoma phyllotis* n. sp. e infecciones associadas en una titira, el *Phlebotomus noguchii*. *Revista de Medicina Experimental (Lima)*, **1**, 40–55.

Herrer, A. (1943). Observaciones sobre la verruga en el departamento de Cajamarca. II. Observaciones entomológicas. *Revista de Medicina Experimental (Lima)*, **2**, 354–361.

Herrer, A. (1951a). Estudios sobre leishmaniasis tegumentaria en el Perú. II. Infección experimental de zorros con cultivos de leishmanias aisladas de casos de uta. *Revista de Medicina Experimental (Lima)*, **8**, 29–37.

Herrer, A. (1951b). Estudios sobre leishmaniasis tegumentaria en el Perú. IV. Observaciones epidemiológicas sobre la uta. *Revista de Medicina Experimental (Lima)*, **8**, 45–86.

Herrer, A. (1951c). Estudios sobre leishmaniasis tegumentaria en el Perú. V. Leishmaniasis natural en perros procedentes de localidades utógenas. *Revista de Medicina Experimental (Lima)*, **8**, 87–117.

Herrer, A. (1951d). Estudios sobre leishmaniasis tegumentaria en el Perú. VI. Relación entre *Phlebotomus* y leishmaniasis tegumentaria. *Revista de Medicina Experimental (Lima)*, **8**, 119–137.

Herrer, A. (1956a). *Phlebotomus* y DDT en el Perú. Experimentos sobre control de la verruga y la uta. *Revista de Medicina Experimental (Lima)*, **10**, 99–137.

Herrer, A. (1956b). Repercusión del uso casero de los insecticidas en la incidencia de la leishmaniasis tegumentaria del perro. *Revista de Medicina Experimental (Lima)*, **10**, 139–145.

Herrer, A. (1957). Verruga y uta en el valle de Huaillacayán (Dpto. de Ancash). I. Determinación de los límites altitudinales de la zona endêmica y de la incidencia de ambas enfermadades. *Revista de Medicina Experimental (Lima)*, **11**, 40–49.

Herrer, A. (1971). *Leishmania hertigi* sp. n., from the tropical porcupine, *Coendou rothschildi* Thomas. *Journal of Parasitology*, **57**, 626–629.

Herrer, A. and Battistini, G. M. (1951). Estudios sobre leishmaniasis tegumentaria en el Perú. I. Infección experimental del perro con cepas de leishmanias procedentes de casos de uta. *Revista de Medicina Experimental (Lima)*, **8**, 12–27.

Herrer, A. and Christensen, H. A. (1975a). Implication of *Phlebotomus* sandflies as vectors of bartonellosis and leishmaniasis as early as 1764. *Science, Washington*, **190**, 154–155.

Herrer, A. and Christensen, H. A. (1975b). Infrequency of gross skin lesions among Panamanian forest mammals with cutaneous leishmaniasis. *Parasitology*, **71**, 87–92.

Herrer, A. and Christensen, H. A. (1976a). Epidemiological patterns of cutaneous leishmaniasis in Panama. I. Epidemics among small groups of settlers. *Annals of Tropical Medicine and Parasitology*, **70**, 59–65.

Herrer, A. and Christensen, H. A. (1976b). Epidemiological patterns of cutaneous leishmaniasis in Panama. III. Endemic persistence of disease. *American Journal of Tropical Medicine and Hygiene*, **25**, 54–58.

Herrer, A. and Telford, S. R. (1969). *Leishmania braziliensis* isolated from sloths in Panama. *Science, Washington*, **164**, 1419–1420.

Herrer, A., Thatcher, V. E. and Johnson, C. M. (1966). Natural infections of *Leishmania* and trypanosomes demonstrated by skin culture. *Journal of Parasitology*, **52**, 954–957.

Herrer, A., Telford, S. R. and Christensen, H. A. (1971). Enzootic cutaneous leishmaniasis in eastern Panama. I. Investigation of the infection among forest mammals. *Annals of Tropical Medicine and Parasitology*, **65**, 349–358.

Herrer, A., Christensen, H. A. and Beumer, R. J. (1973). Reservoir hosts of cutaneous leishmaniasis among Panamanian forest mammals. *American Journal of Tropical Medicine and Hygiene*, **22**, 585–591.

Herrer, A., Christensen, H. A. and Beumer, R. J. (1976). Epidemiological patterns of cutaneous leishmaniasis in Panama. II. Incidental occurrence of cases in non-endemic settlements. *Annals of Tropical Medicine and Parasitology*, **70**, 67–71.

Hertig, M. (1937). Carrion's disease. V. Studies on *Phlebotomus* as the possible vector. *Proceedings of the Society for Experimental Biology and Medicine*, **37**, 598–600.

Hertig, M. (1939). *Phlebotomus* and Carrion's disease. *Proceedings of the VIth Pacific Scientific Congress*. **5**, 775–779.

Hertig, M. (1942). *Phlebotomus* and Carrion's disease. *American Journal of Tropical Medicine* (Suppl.), **22**, 1–81.

Hertig, M. (1943). Notes on Peruvian sandflies with descriptions of *Phlebotomus battistinii*, n. sp., and *P. pescei*, n. sp. *American Journal of Hygiene*, **37**, 246–254.

Hertig, M. and Fairchild, G. B. (1948). The control of *Phlebotomus* in Peru with DDT. *American Journal of Tropical Medicine*, **2**, 207–230.

Hertig, M. and McConnell, E. (1963). Experimental infection of Panamanian *Phlebotomus* sandflies with *Leishmania*. *Experimental Parasitology*, **14**, 92–106.

Hoare, C. A. (1948). The relationship of the haemoflagellates. *Proceedings of the IVth International Congresses on Tropical Medicine and Malaria*, **2**, 1110–1116. Department of State, Washington.

Hoare, C. A. (1956). Morphological and taxonomic studies on mammalian trypanosomes. VIII. Revision of *Trypanosoma evansi*. *Parasitology*, **46**, 130–172.

Hoare, C. A. (1964). Morphological and taxonomic studies on mammalian trypanosomes. X. Revision of the systematics. *Journal of Protozoology*, **11**, 200–207.

Hoare, C. A. (1972). "The Trypanosomes of Mammals. A Zoological Monograph". Blackwell, Oxford and Edinburgh.

Jaffé, L. (1960). Further observations on leishmaniasis Americana of the upper respiratory passages in Panama. *Archives of Otolaryngology (Chicago)*, **72**, 464–470.

Johnson, P. T. and Hertig, M. (1970). Behavior of *Leishmania* in Panamanian phlebotomine sandflies fed on infected animals. *Experimental Parasitology*, **27**, 281–300.

Johnson, P. T., McConnell, E. and Hertig, M. (1963). Natural infections of leptomonad flagellates in Panamanian *Phlebotomus* sandflies. *Experimental Parasitology*, **14**, 107–122.

Kerdel-Vegas, F. and Essenfeld-Yahr, E. (1966). American leishmaniasis in a field rodent. *Transactions of the Royal Society of Tropical Medicine and Hygiene*, **60**, 563.

Killick-Kendrick, R., Molyneux, D. H. and Ashford, R. W. (1974). *Leishmania* in phlebotomid sandflies. I. Modifications of the flagellum associated with attachment to the mid-gut and oesophageal valve of the sandfly. *Proceedings of the Royal Society, London (B)*, **187**, 409–419.

Killick-Kendrick, R., Leaney, A. J., Ready, P. D. and Molyneux, D. H. (1977a). *Leishmania* in phlebotomid sandflies. IV. The transmission of *Leishmania mexicana amazonensis* to hamsters by the bite of experimentally infected *Lutzomyia longipalpis*. *Proceedings of the Royal Society, London (B)*, **196**, 105–115.

Killick-Kendrick, R., Molyneux, D. H., Hommel, M., Leaney, A. J. and Robertson, E. (1977b). *Leishmania* in phlebotomid sandflies. V. The nature and significance of infections of pylorus and ileum of the sandfly by leishmaniae of the *braziliensis* complex. *Proceedings of the Royal Society, London (B)*, **198**, 191–199.

Lainson, R. (1965). Visceral involvement in rodents naturally and experimentally infected with *Leishmania mexicana*. *Transactions of the Royal Society of Tropical Medicine and Hygiene*, **59**, 103–104.

Lainson, R. and Shaw, J. J. (1968). Leishmaniasis in Brazil. I. Observations on enzootic rodent leishmaniasis—incrimination of *Lutzomyia flaviscutellata* (Mangabeira) as the vector in the lower Amazonian basin. *Transactions of the Royal Society of Tropical Medicine and Hygiene*, **62**, 385–395.

Lainson, R. and Shaw, J. J. (1969a). Some reservoir-hosts of *Leishmania* in wild animals of Mato Grosso State, Brazil. Two distinct strains of parasites isolated from man and rodents. *Transactions of the Royal Society of Tropical Medicine and Hygiene*, **63**, 408–409.

Lainson, R. and Shaw, J. J. (1969b). Leishmaniasis in Brazil. III. Cutaneous leishmaniasis in an opossum, *Marmosa murina* (Marsupialia, Didelphidae) from the lower Amazon region. *Transactions of the Royal Society of Tropical Medicine and Hygiene*, **63**, 738–740.

Lainson, R. and Shaw, J. J. (1970). Leishmaniasis in Brazil. V. Studies on the epidemiology of cutaneous leishmaniasis in Mato Grosso State, and observations on two distinct strains of *Leishmania* isolated from man and forest animals. *Transactions of the Royal Society of Tropical Medicine and Hygiene*, **64**, 654–667.

Lainson, R. and Shaw, J. J. (1971). Epidemiological considerations of the leishmanias with particular reference to the New World. *In*: "Ecology and Physiology of Parasites" (Ed. A. M. Fallis), pp. 21–57.

Lainson, R. and Shaw, J. J. (1972a). Leishmaniasis of the New World: Taxonomic problems. *British Medical Bulletin*, **28**, 44–48.

Lainson, R. and Shaw, J. J. (1972b). Taxonomy of the New World *Leishmania* species. *Transaction of the Royal Society of Tropical Medicine and Hygiene*, **66**, 943–944.

Lainson, R. and Shaw, J. J. (1973). Leishmanias and leishmaniasis of the New World, with particular reference to Brazil. *Bulletin of the Pan American Health Organization*, **7** (4), 1–19.

Lainson, R. and Shaw, J. J. (1977a). [cited in Lainson *et al.* (1977): *q.v.*]

Lainson, R. and Shaw, J. J. (1977b). Leishmanias of neotropical porcupines: *Leishmania hertigi deanei* nov. subsp. *Acta Amazônica*, **7** (1), 51–57.

Lainson, R. and Shaw, J. J. (1977c). Leishmaniasis in Brazil. XII. Observations on cross-immunity in monkeys and man infected with *Leishmania mexicana mexicana*, *L. m. amazonensis*, *L. braziliensis braziliensis*, *L. b. guyanensis*, and *L. b. panamensis*. *Journal of Tropical Medicine and Hygiene*, **80**, 29–35.

Lainson, R. and Strangways-Dixon, J. (1962). Dermal leishmaniasis in British Honduras: some host-reservoirs of *L. braziliensis mexicana*. A preliminary note. *British Medical Journal*, **1**, 1596–1598.

Lainson, R. and Strangways-Dixon, J. (1963). *Leishmania mexicana*: the epidemiology of dermal leishmaniasis in British Honduras. *Transactions of the Royal Society of Tropical Medicine and Hygiene*, **57**, 242–265.

Lainson, R. and Strangways-Dixon, J. (1964). The epidemiology of dermal leishmaniasis in British Honduras. Part II. Reservoir-hosts of *Leishmania mexicana* among the forest rodents. *Transactions of the Royal Society of Tropical Medicine and Hygiene*, **58**, 136–153.

Lainson, R., Shaw, J. J. and Lins, Z. C. (1969). Leishmaniasis in Brazil. IV. The fox, *Cerdocyon thous* (L) as a reservoir of *Leishmania donovani* in Pará State, Brazil. *Transactions of the Royal Society of Tropical Medicine and Hygiene*, **63**, 741–745.

Lainson, R., Shaw, J. J., Ward, R. D. and Fraiha, H. (1973). Leishmaniasis in Brazil. IX. Considerations on the *Leishmania braziliensis* complex: importance of sandflies of the genus *Psychodopygus* (Mangabeira) in the transmission of *L. braziliensis* in north Brazil. *Transactions of the Royal Society of Tropical Medicine and Hygiene*, **67**, 184–196.

Lainson, R., Ward, R. D. and Shaw, J. J. (1976). Cutaneous leishmaniasis in north Brazil: *Lutzomyia anduzei* as a major vector. *Transactions of the Royal Society of Tropical Medicine and Hygiene*, **70**, 171–172.

Lainson, R., Ward, R. D. and Shaw, J. J. (1977a). Experimental transmission of *Leishmania chagasi*, causative agent of neotropical visceral leishmaniasis, by the sandfly *Lutzomyia longipalpis*. *Nature (London)*, **266**, 628–630.

Lainson, R., Ward, R. D. and Shaw, J. J. (1977b). *Leishmania* in phlebotomid sandflies. VI. Importance of hindgut development in distinguishing parasites of the *Leishmania mexicana* and *L. braziliensis* complexes. *Proceedings of the Royal Society (B)*, **199**, 309–320.

Lainson, R., Ward, R. D., Young, D. G., Shaw, J. J. and Fraiha, H. (1977c). Preliminary entomological and parasitological studies in Humbolt, Aripuanã, Mato Grosso State, Brazil. *Acta Amazônica*, **6** (4) Suplemento, 55–60.

Léger, L. (1904). Sur les affinités de l'*Herpetomonas subulata* et la phylogène des trypanosomes. *Compte Rendu Hebdomonadaires des Séances et Mémoires de la Société de Biologie*, **56**, 615–617.

Leger, M. (1918). Infection sanguine par *Leptomonas* chez un saurien. *Comptes Rendus des Seances de la Société de Biologie et de ses Filiales*, **81**, 772–774.

León, J. R. and Figueroa, L. N. (1959). Descubrimiento de la primera zona endémica de kala-azar Guatemalense y sus condiciones epidemiológicas. *Revista del Colegio Médico (Guatemala)*, **10**, 240–245.

Lewis, D. J., Lainson, R. and Shaw, J. J. (1970). Determination of parous rates in phlebotomine sandflies with special reference to Amazonian species. *Bulletin of Entomological Research*, **60**, 209–219.

Lewis, D. J., Young, D. G., Fairchild, G. B. and Minter, D. M. (1977). Proposals for a stable classification of the Phlebotomine sandflies (Diptera: Psychodidae). *Systematic Entomology*, **2**, 319–332.

Lindenberg, A. (1909). A úlcera de Baurú e seu micróbio. *Revista de Medicina, Universidade de São Paulo*, **12**, 116–120.

Lloyd, R. B. and Napier, L. E. (1930). The blood-meal of sandflies investigated by means of precipitin antisera. *Indian Journal of Medical Research*, **18**, 347–359.

López, M. R., Martínez, G. A., Molinari, J. L. and Biagi, F. F. (1966). Kala-azar en México. Primeras observaciones sobre posibles reservorios. *Revista de la Facultad de medicina (México)*, **8**, 533–539.

Luz, E., Giovannoni, M. and Borba, A. M. (1967). Infecção de *Lutzomyia monticula* por *Leishmania enrietii*. *Anais da Faculdade de Medicina da Universidade Federal do Paraná*, **9–10**, 121–128.

Maciel, P. and Rosenfeld, G. (1947). Leishmaniose visceral americana. Um caso de um novo foco. *Revista Clínica de São Paulo*, 21, 51–61.

Mangabeira, O. (1942). 11ª Contribuição ao estudo dos *Flebotomus*. *Flebotomus oswaldoi* Mangabeira, 1942. *Memórias do Instituto Oswaldo Cruz*, 37, 287–295.

Mangabeira, O. (1969). Sôbre a sistemática e biologia dos *Phlebotomus* do Ceará. *Revista Brasileira de Malariologia e Doenças Tropicais*, 21, 3–26.

Manson-Bahr, P. E. C. and Heisch, R. B. (1961). Transient infection of man with a *Leishmania* (*L. adleri*) of lizards. *Annals of Tropical Medicine and Parasitology*, 55, 381–382.

Martinez, N. A. and Pons, A. R. (1941). Primer caso de kala-azar en Venezuela. *Gaceta Médica de Caracas*, 48, 329–332.

Martins, J., Souza, J. C. and Silva, E. (1968). Primeiros casos autóctonous de calazar no Espírito Santo. *Hospital* (*Rio de Janeiro*), 73, 745–774.

Martins, V. A., Brener, Z., Mourão, O. G., Lima, M. M., Souza, M. A. and Silva, J. E. (1956). Calazar autóctone em Minas Gerais. *Revista Brasileira de Malariologia e Doenças Tropicais*, 8, 555–563.

Matta, A. (1918). Notas para a historia das leishmanioses da pelle e das mucosas. *Amazonas Médico*, 1, 11–17.

Mazza, S. (1926a). Existencia de la leishmaniosis cutánea en el perro en la República Argentina. *Boletín del Instituto de Clínica Quirúrigica* (*Buenos Aires*), 2, 147–149.

Mazza, S. (1926b). Leishmaniosis tegumentaria y visceral. *Boletín del Instituto de Clinica Quirúrgica* (*Buenos Aires*), 2, 209–216.

Mazza, S. (1926c). Consideraciones sobre flebótomus encontrados en Tabacal y el papel de estos dipteros en la transmission de las leishmaniosis. *Boletín del Instituto de Clinica Quirúrigica* (*Buenos Aires*), 2, 310–317.

Mazza, S. (1927). Leishmaniose cutánea en el caballo y nueva observacion de la misma en el perro. *Boletín del Instituto de Clínica Quirúrigica* (*Buenos Aires*), 3, 462–464.

Mazza, S. and Cornejo, A. J. (1926). Primeros casos autóctonos de kala-azar infantil comprobados en el norte de la República (Tabacal y Orán, Salta). *Boletín del Instituto de Clínica Quirúrigica* (*Buenos Aires*), 2, 140–144.

McConnell, E. (1963). Leptomonads of wild-caught Panamanian *Phlebotomus*: culture and animal inoculation. *Experimental Parasitology*, 51, 336–339.

Medina, H. (1946). Estudos sôbre leishmaniose. I. Primeiros casos de leishmaniose espontânea observados em cobaias. *Arquivos de Biologia e Tecnologia* (*Curitiba*), 1, 39–74.

Medina, R. and Romero, J. (1959). Estudio clinico y parasitologico de una nueva cepa de leishmania. *Archivos Venezolanos de Patologia Tropical y Parasitologia Médica*, 3, 298–326.

Medina, R., Romero, J., Goldman, C. and Espín, J. (1960). Comprobación del primer perro infectado con kala-azar en Venezuela. *Gaceta Médica de Caracas*, 69, 441–447.

Mello, G. B. (1940). Verificação da infecção natural do gato (*Felix domesticus*) por um protozoário do gênero *Leishmania*. *Brasil-Médico*, 54, 180.

Migone, L. E. (1913). Un caso de kala-azar a Assuncion (Paraguay). *Bulletin de la Société de Pathologie Exotique*, 6, 118–120.

Migone, L. E. (1935). La leishmaniosis forestal americana en el Paraguay. *Revista Argentina de Dermato-sifilogia*, 19, 46–49.

Muirhead-Thompson, R. C. (1968). "Ecology of Insect Vector Populations". Academic Press, London and New York.

Muniz, J. and Medina, H. (1948). Leishmaniose tegumentar do cobaio (*Leishmania enriettii* n. sp.). *Hospital* (*Rio de Janeiro*), 33, 7–25.

110   R. LAINSON AND J. J. SHAW

Nadim, A., Seyedi-Rashti, M. A. and Mesghali, A. (1968). Epidemiology of cutaneous leishmaniasis in Turkemen Sahar, Iran. *Journal of Tropical Medicine and Hygiene*, **71**, 238–239.

Neiva, A. and Barbará, B. (1917). Leishmaniasis tegumentaria americana. Numerosos casos autóctones en la Republica Argentina. *1° Conferencia Sud-Americana de la Sociedad de Microbiología y Patología (Buenos Aires)*, pp. 311–372.

Nicoli, R. M. (1963). Le genre *Leishmania* R. Ross, 1903. *Bulletin de la Société de Pathologie Exotique*, **56**, 408–416.

Noguchi, H., Shannon, R. C., Tilden, E. and Tyler, J. R. (1929). Etiology of Oroya fever. XIV. The insect vector of Carrion's disease. *Journal of Experimental Medicine*, **49**, 993–1008.

Nuernberger, S. P., Ramos, C. V. and Custidio, R. (1975). Visceral leishmaniasis in Honduras. Report of three proven cases and a suspected case. *American Journal of Tropical Medicine and Hygiene*, **24**, 917–920.

Nussenzweig, V., Nussenzweig, R. S. and Alencar, J. E. (1957). Leishmaniose visceral canina no arredores de Fortaleza, Estado do Ceará: inquérito sero-lógico utilizando a reação de fixação do complemento com antígeno extraído do bacilo de tuberculose. Observações sôbre o diagnóstico e epidemiologia da doença. *Hospital (Rio de Janeiro)*, **52**, 111–129.

Oliveira, A. C. (1938). Um caso de leishmaniose visceral americana. *Hospital (Rio de Janeiro)*, **13**, 465–470.

Oliveira, A. C., Batista, S. M. and Falcão, L. A. (1959). Calazar em Minas Gerais. Revisão dos dados epidemiológicos obtidos até 1958. *Hospital (Rio de Janeiro)*, **56**, 625–643.

Paraense, L. and Chagas, A. W. (1940). Transmissão experimental da leishmaniose visceral americana pelo *Phlebotomus intermedius*. Nota prévia. *Brasil-Médico*, **54**, 179–180.

Pedrosa, A. M. (1913). Leishmaniose local do cão. *Anais Paulistas de Medicina e Cirurgia*, **1**, 33–39.

Penna, H. A. (1934). Leishmaniose visceral no Brasil. *Brasil-Médico*, **48**, 949–950.

Pessôa, S. B. (1967). "Parasitologia Médica", 7th Edition. Rio de Janeiro: Guanabara and Koogan.

Pessôa, S. B. and Coutinho, J. O. (1940). Infecção natural do *Phlebotomus pessoai* por formas em leptomonas, provávelmente da *Leishmania brasiliensis*. *Revista de Biologia e Higiene (São Paulo)*, **10**, 139–142.

Pessôa, S. B. and Coutinho, J. O. (1941). Infecção natural e experimental dos flebótomus pela *Leishmania brasiliensis*, no Estado do São Paulo. *Hospital (Rio de Janeiro)*, **20**, 25–35.

Pessôa, S. B. and Pestana, B. R. (1940). Infecção natural de "*Phlebotomus migonei*" por formas em leptomonas provávelmente da "*Leishmania brasiliensis*". *Acta Medica (Rio de Janeiro)*, **5**, 106–111.

Peters, W. (1975). [Biochemical Characters of *Leishmania* of the *mexicana* complex: *in litteris*.]

Pifano, C. F. (1940a). La leishmaniasis tegumentaria en el Estado Yaracuy, Venezuela. *Revista de la Policlinica (Caracas)*, **9**, 3639–3658.

Pifano, C. F. (1940b). Sobre el desarrollo de *Leishmania tropica braziliensis* en *Phlebotomus* de Venezuela. *Gaceta Médica de Caracas*, **48**, 114–116.

Pifano, C. F. (1943). Notas sobre entomologia médica venezolana. I. Flebotomus transmisores de leishmaniasis tegumentaria en al valle del Yaracuy. *Boletín de Entomología Venezolana (Caracas)*, **2**, 99–102.

Pifano, C. F. (1949). La leishmaniasis tegumentaria en Venezuela. *Archivos Venezolanos de Patologia Tropical y Parasitologia Médica*, **1**, 170–183.

Pifano, C. F. (1956). [cited in Forattini (1959): *q.v.*]

Pifano, C. F. (1960). Algunos aspectos de la patologia comparada geografica de la leishmaniasis tegumentaria en el tropico Americano. *Gaceta Médica de Caracas*, **68**, 89–98.

Pifano, C. F. and Romero, M. J. (1964a). Investigaciones epidemiológicas sobre la leishmaniasis visceral en la Isla de Margarita, Edo Nueva Esparta, Venezuela. *Gaceta Médica de Caracas*, **72**, 425–430.

Pifano, C. F. and Romero, M. J. (1964b). Comprobación de un nuevo foco de leishmaniasis en Venezuela, Valle de Cumanacoa, Edo Sucre. *Gaceta Médica de Caracas*, **72**, 473–479.

Pifano, C. F. and Romero, M. J. (1973). Comprobación de un foco autoctóno de leishmaniasis visceral (kala-azar) en el Isla de Margarita, Edo Nueva Esparta, Venezuela. *Archivos Venezelanos de Medicina Tropical e Parasitologia Médica*, **5**, 129–144.

Pifano, C. F., Romero, M. J. and Henríquez, G. R. (1962). Comprobación de un foco de leishmaniasis visceral (kala-azar) en un sector del piedemonte andinollanero del Estado Portuguesa. *Archivos Venezelanos de Medicina Tropical e Parasitologia Médica*, **4**, 3–15.

Pifano, C. F., Kerdel-Vegas, F. and Romero, M. J. (1968). Nidos de zoonosis en la leishmaniasis tegumentaria americana. *Dermatologia Venezolana*, **11**, 520–529.

Pifano, C. F., Romero, M. J. and Alvarez, A. (1973). Comprobación de una cepa de leishmania dermotropa en *Phlebotomus flaviscutellata* Mangabeira, 1942 de La Sierra Parima, Territorio Federal Amazonas, Venezuela. *Archivos Venezolanos de Medicina Tropical y Parasitologia Médica*, **5**, 145–170.

Pine, R. H. (1973). Mammals (exclusive of bats) of Belém, Pará, Brazil. *Acta Amazônica*, **3** (2), 47–79.

Piva, N. and Barros, P. R. C. (1966). Foco autóctone de calazar em Sergipe. *Revista Brasileira de Malariologia e Doenças Tropicais*, **18**, 217–220.

Pondé, R., Mangabeira, O. and Jansen, G. (1942). Alguns dados sobre a leishmaniose visceral e doença de Chagas no Nordeste Brasileiro. (Relatório de uma excursão realizada nos Estados do Ceará, Pernambuco e Bahia). *Memórias do Instituto Oswaldo Cruz*, **17**, 333–352.

Pons, A. R. (1968). Leishmaniasis tegumentaria americana en el Asentamiento Campesino de Zipayare. Aspectos epidemiológicos clínicos e inmunológicos. Su importancia en la reforma agraria. *Kasmera*, **3**, 5–59.

Potenza, L. and Anduze, J. (1942). Kala-azar en el Estado de Bolivar, Venezuela. *Revista Policlinica (Caracas)*, **11**, 312–317.

Rassi, D. M., Oliveira, G. S. C., Auad, A. and Dias, J. B. (1972). Leishmaniose tegumentar (forma recente) na região centro oeste. *Revista da Sociedade Brasileira de Medicina Tropical*, **6**, 376–377.

Romaña, C. and Abalos, J. W. (1949). Distribucion de flebotomos y leishmaniasis en la Argentina. *Anales del Instituto de Medicina Regional (Tucumán)*, **2**, 293–302.

Romaña, C., Najera, L., Conejos, M. and Abalos, J. W. (1949). I. Leishmaniose tegumentar en perros de Tucumán. II. Foco domestico de leishmaniosis. *Anales del Instituto de Medicina Regional (Tucumán)*, **2**, 283–292.

Rutledge, L. C. and Ellenwood, D. A. (1975a). Production of phlebotomine sandflies on the open forest floor in Panama: hydrologic and physiographic relations. *Environmental Entomology*, **4**, 78–82.

Rutledge, L. C. and Ellenwood, D. A. (1975b). Production of phlebotomine sand-flies on the open forest floor in Panama: phytologic and edaphic relations. *Environmental Entomology*, **4**, 83–89.

Rutledge, L. C., Ellenwood, D. A. and Johnston, L. (1975). An analysis of sand fly light trap collections in the Panama Canal Zone (*Diptera: Psychodidae*). *Journal of Medical Entomology*, **12**, 179–183.

Rutledge, L. C., Walton, B. C., Ellenwood, D. A. and Correa, M. A. (1976). A transect study of sand fly populations in Panama (*Diptera: Psychodidae*). *Environmental Entomology*, **5**, 1149–1154.

Sabroza, P. C., Wagner, M. S. and Sobrero, N. (1975). Inquérito epidemiológico de leishmaniose tegumentar americana em Jacarepaguá, Guanabara. XI. Congresso da Sociedade Brasileira de Medicina Tropical, Rio de Janeiro.

Schneider, C. R. and Hertig, M. (1966). Immunodiffusion reactions of Panamanian *Leishmania*. *Experimental Parasitology*, **18**, 25–34.

Senekjie, C. M. (1944). American visceral leishmaniasis. The etiological agent. *Journal of Parasitology*, **30**, 303–308.

Shaw, J. J. (1964). A possible vector of *Endotrypanum schaudinni* of the sloth *Choloepus hoffmanni*, in Panama. *Nature, London*, **201**, 417–418.

Shaw, J. J. and Lainson, R. (1968). Leishmaniasis in Brazil. II. Observations on enzootic rodent leishmaniasis in the lower Amazon region—the feeding habits of the vector, *Lutzomyia flaviscutellata* in reference to man, rodents and other animals. *Transactions of the Royal Society of Tropical Medicine and Hygiene*, **62**, 396–405.

Shaw, J. J. and Lainson, R. (1972). Leishmaniasis in Brazil. VI. Observations on the seasonal variations of *Lutzomyia flaviscutellata* in different types of forest and its relationship to enzootic rodent leishmaniasis (*Leishmania mexicana amazonensis*). *Transactions of the Royal Society of Tropical Medicine and Hygiene*, **66**, 709–717.

Shaw, J. J. and Lainson, R. (1973). [cited in Lainson and Shaw (1973): *q.v.*]

Shaw, J. J. and Lainson, R. (1975). Leishmaniasis in Brazil. X. Some observations on intradermal reactions to different trypanosomatid antigens of patients suffering from cutaneous and mucocutaneous leishmaniasis. *Transactions of the Royal Society of Tropical Medicine and Hygiene*, **69**, 323–335.

Shaw, J. J. and Lainson, R. (1976). Leishmaniasis in Brazil. XI. Observations on the morphology of *Leishmania* of the *braziliensis* and *mexicana* complexes. *Journal of Tropical Medicine and Hygiene*, **79**, 9–13.

Shaw, J. J., Lainson, R. and Ward, R. D. (1972). Leishmaniasis in Brazil. VII. Further observations on the feeding habitats of *Lutzomyia flaviscutellata* (Mangabeira) with particular reference to its biting habits at different heights. *Transactions of the Royal Society of Tropical Medicine and Hygiene*, **66**, 718–723.

Sherlock, I. A. (1964). Notas sôbre a transmissão da leishmaniose visceral no Brasil. *Revista Brasileira de Malariologia e Doenças Tropicais*, **16**, 19–26.

Sherlock, I. A. and Almeida, S. P. (1970a). Observações sôbre calazar em Jacobina, Bahia. V. Resultados de medidas profilácticas. *Revista Brasileira de Malariologia e Doenças Tropicais*, **22**, 175–181.

Sherlock, I. A. and Almeida, S. P. (1970b) Notas sôbre leishmaniose canina no Estado da Bahia. *Revista Brasileira de Malariologia e Doenças Tropicais*, **22**, 231–242.

Sherlock, I. A. and Pessôa, S. B. (1966). *Leptomonas* infectando naturalmente *Phlebotomus* em Salvador (Bahia, Brasil). *Revista Latino-Americana Microbiologia e Parasitologia*, **8**, 47–50.

Sherlock, I. A. and Santos, A. C. (1964). Leishmaniose visceral na zona de Jequié, Estado da Bahia. *Revista Brasileira de Malariologia e Doenças Tropicais*, **16**, 441–448.

Sherlock, I. A. and Sherlock, V. A. (1972). Tentativa de transmissão da *Leishmania donovani* pela picada de *Lutzomyia longipalpis* entre cães. *Revista da Sociedade de Medicina Tropical*, **6**, 35–39.

Silva, J. R. (1957). "Leishmaniose visceral (calazar)". Thesis. 498 pp. Sedegra, Sociedade Editora e Gráfica Ltda., Rio de Janeiro.

Strangways-Dixon, J. and Lainson, R. (1962). Dermal leishmaniasis in British Honduras: Transmission of *L. brasiliensis* by *Phlebotomus* species. *British Medical Journal*, **1**, 297–299.

Strangways-Dixon, J. and Lainson, R. (1966). The epidemiology of dermal leishmaniasis in British Honduras. Part III. The transmission of *Leishmania mexicana* to man by *Phlebotomus pessoanus*, with observations on the development of the parasite in different species of *Phlebotomus*. *Transactions of the Royal Society of Tropical Medicine and Hygiene*, **60**, 192–207.

Strong, R. P., Tyzzer, E. E., Brues, C. T., Sellards, A. W. and Gastiaburu, J. C. (1913). Verruga Peruviana, Oroya Fever and Uta. *Journal of the American Medical Association*, **8**, 1713–1716.

Strong, R. P., Tyzzer, E. P., Brues, C. T., Sellards, A. W. and Gastiaburu, J. C. (1915). *Harvard School of Tropical Medicine. Report of the first expedition to South America*, **1913**, Cambridge, Mass., 220 pp.

Telford, S. R., Herrer, A. and Christensen, H. A. (1972). Enzootic cutaneous leishmaniasis in eastern Panama. III. Ecological factors relating to the mammalian hosts. *Annals of Tropical Medicine and Parasitology*, **66**, 173–179.

Tempelis, C. H. (1974). Host-feeding patterns of mosquitoes, with a review of advances in analysis of blood meals by serology. *Journal of Medical Entomology*, **11**, 635–653.

Tesh, R. B., Chaniotis, B. N., Aronson, M. D. and Johnson, K. M. (1971). Natural host preferences of Panamanian phlebotomine sandflies as determined by precipitin test. *American Journal of Tropical Medicine and Hygiene*, **20**, 150–156.

Tesh, R. B., Chaniotis, B. N. and Johnson, K. M. (1972). Further studies on the natural host preferences of Panamanian phlebotomine sandflies. *American Journal of Epidemiology*, **95**, 88–93.

Thatcher, V. E. (1968). Studies of phlebotomine sandflies using castor oil traps baited with Panamanian animals. *Journal of Medical Entomology*, **5**, 293–297.

Thatcher, V. E. and Hertig, M. (1966). Field studies on the feeding habits and diurnal shelters of some *Phlebotomus* sandflies (*Diptera: Psychodidae*) in Panama. *Annals of the Entomological Society of America*, **59**, 46–52.

Thatcher, V. E., Eisenmann, C. and Hertig, M. (1965). A natural infection of *Leishmania* in the kinkajou, *Potus flavus*, in Panama. *Journal of Parasitology*, **51**, 1022–1023.

Tikasingh, E. S. (1969). Leishmaniasis in Trinidad. A preliminary report. *Transactions of the Royal Society of Tropical Medicine and Hygiene*, **63**, 411.

Tikasingh, E. S. (1974). Enzootic rodent leishmaniasis in Trinidad, West Indies. *Bulletin of the Pan American Health Organization*, **8**, 232–242.

Tikasingh, E. S. (1975). Observations on *Lutzomyia flaviscutellata* (Mangabeira) (*Diptera: Psychodidae*), a vector of enzootic leishmaniasis in Trinidad, West Indies. *Journal of Medical Entomology*, **12**, 228–232.

Torrealba, J. W. (1964). Consideraciones sobre epidemiologia de la leishmaniasis visceral en Venezuela. *Gaceta Médica de Caracas*, **72**, 99–115.

Torrealba, J. W. and Torrealba, J. F. (1964). Infección experimental de *Cerdocyon thous* (zorro commún) con *Leishmania donovani*. *Gaceta Médica de Caracas*, **72**, 117–118.

Torrealba, J. W., Amaral, A. D. F., Henríquez, C. E., Kowalenko, W. and Barrios, P. A. (1961). Observaciones inciales sobre el perro (*Canis familiaris*) como reservorio de kala-azar en Venezuela. *Folia Clinica et Biologica* (*São Paulo*), **30**, 25–36.

Torrealba, J. W., Torrealba, J. F., Torrealba, R. T., Malpica, N. Z., Ramos, I. and Henríquez, C. E. (1963). Kala-azar canino, en el Estado Guarico. Resultados de una encuestra en 1,105 perros empleando la tecnica de reaccíon de fijacíon del complemento en sangre desecada, retirada con papel de filtro. Quince nuevos casos de kala-azar canino comprobados parasitologicamente. *Folio Clinica et Biologica* (*São Paulo*), **32**, 1–13.

Torrealba, J. W., Gómez-Núñez, J. C. and Ulloa, G. (1972). Isolation of *Leishmania braziliensis* by intraperitoneal inoculation of blood from a reservoir host into hamsters. *Transactions of the Royal Society of Tropical Medicine and Hygiene*, **66**, 361.

Townsend, C. H. T. (1914). The conquest of verruga. A brief statement of the results of the investigation. *Perú to-day*, **6**, 57–67.

Townsend, C. H. T. (1915). The insect vector of uta, a Peruvian disease. *Journal of Parasitology*, **2**, 67–73.

Trejos, A., Chang Peña, T. and Godoy, G. A. (1966). Vectores del kala-azar en El Salvador. *Archivos del Colegio médico de El Salvador*, **19**, 113–117.

Velez, L. R. (1913). Uta et espundia. *Bulletin de la Société de Pathologie Exotique*, **6**, 545.

Vianna, G. (1911). Sôbre uma nova especie de *Leishmania* (Nota preliminar). *Brasil-Médico*, **25**, 411.

Villalonga, J. F. (1963). Leishmaniosis tegumentaria Americana: Clinica y tratamiento. *Revista de la Facultad de Medicina de Tucumán*, **6**, 197–208.

Villaseñor, J. B., Ruiloba, J., Rojas, E., Trevião, A. and Campillo, C. (1953). Un caso de kala-azar en México. *Boletín de la Oficina Sanitaria Panamericana*, **34**, 23–30.

Walton, B. C., Person, D. A. and Bernstein, R. (1968). Leishmaniasis in the U.S. military in the Canal Zone. *American Journal of Tropical Medicine and Hygiene*, **17**, 19–24.

Walton, B. C., Chinel, L. V. and Eguia, O. E. (1973). Onset of espundia after many years of occult infection with *Leishmania braziliensis*. *American Journal of Tropical Medicine and Hygiene*, **22**, 696–698.

Walton, B. C., Shaw, J. J. and Lainson, R. (1977). Observations on the *in vitro* cultivation of *Leishmania braziliensis*. *Journal of Parasitology*, **63**, 1118–1119.

Ward, R. D. (1974). "Studies on the adult and immature stages of some phlebotomid sandflies (Diptera: Phlebotomidae) in Northern Brazil". Thesis for degree of Ph.D., pp. 327. Faculty of Science, University of London.

Ward, R. D. (1977a). New World Leishmaniasis: a review of the epidemiological changes in the last 3 decades. *Proceedings of the XVth International Congress of Entomology, Washington, D.C.*, 505–522.

Ward, R. D. (1977b). The colonization of *Lutzomyia flaviscutellata* (Diptera: Psychodidae), a vector of *Leishmania mexicana amazonensis* in Brazil. *Journal of Medical Entomology*, **14**, 469–476.

Ward, R. D. and Fraiha, H (1977). *Lutzomyia umbratilis*, a new species of sandfly from Brazil (Diptera: Psychodidae). *Journal of Medical Entomology*, **14**, 313–317.

Ward, R. D. and Ready, P. A. (1975). Chorionic sculpturing in some sandfly eggs (Diptera: Psychodidae). *Journal of Entomology, Series A*, **50**, 127–134.

Ward, R. D., Lainson, R. and Shaw, J. J. (1973a). Further evidence of the role of *Lutzomyia flaviscutellata* (Mangabeira) as the vector of *Leishmania mexicana amazonensis* in Brazil. *Transactions of the Royal Society of Tropical Medicine and Hygiene*, **67**, 608–609.

Ward, R. D., Shaw, J. J., Lainson, R. and Fraiha, H. (1973b). Leishmaniasis in Brazil. VIII. Observations on the phlebotomine fauna of an area highly endemic for cutaneous leishmaniasis, in the Serra dos Carajás, Pará State. *Transactions of the Royal Society of Tropical Medicine and Hygiene*, **67**, 174–183.

Ward, R. D., Lainson, R. and Shaw, J. J. (1977). Experimental transmission of *Leishmania mexicana amazonensis* Lainson and Shaw, between hamsters by the bite of *Lutzomyia flaviscutellata* (Mangabeira). *Transactions of the Royal Society of Tropical Medicine and Hygiene*, **71**, 265–266.

Weitz, B. (1956). Identification of bloodmeals of blood-sucking arthropods. *Bulletin of the World Health Organization*, **15**, 473–490.

Weitz, B. (1963). The feeding habits of *Glossina*. *Bulletin of the World Health Organization*, **28**, 711–729.

Wenyon, C. M. (1926). "Protozoology. A Manual for Medical Men, Veterinarians and Zoologists". Vol. I. London: Baillière, Tindall and Cox.

Wenyon, C. M. (1946). Comment in an abstract of Cunha (1942). *Tropical Diseases Bulletin*, **43**, 113–114.

Wijers, D. J. B. and Linger, R. (1966). Man-biting sandflies in Surinam (Dutch Guiana): *Phlebotomus anduzei* as a possible vector of *Leishmania braziliensis*. *Annals of Tropical Medicine and Parasitology*, **60**, 501–508.

Williams, P. (1965). Observations on the phlebotomine sandflies of British Honduras. *Annals of Tropical Medicine and Parasitology*, **60**, 393–404.

Williams, P. (1966). Experimental Transmission of *Leishmania mexicana* by *Lutzomyia cruciata*. *Annals of Tropical Medicine and Parasitology*, **60**, 365–372.

Williams, P. (1970). Phlebotomine sandflies and leishmaniasis in British Honduras (Belize). *Transactions of the Royal Society of Tropical Medicine and Hygiene*, **64**, 317–364.

Williams, P., Lewis, D. J. and Garnham, P. C. C. (1965). On dermal leishmaniasis in British Honduras. *Transactions of the Royal Society of Tropical Medicine and Hygiene*, **59**, 64–71.

Winckel, W. E. F. and Aalstein, M. (1953). Contribution to the geographical pathology of Surinam. First case of kala-azar in Surinam. *Documenta de Medicina Geographica et Tropica, Amsterdam*, **5**, 399–342.

Worth, C. B., Downs, W. G., Aitken, T. H. G. and Tikasingh, E. (1968). Arbovirus studies in Bush Bush Forest, Trinidad, W. I., September 1959–December 1964. Vertebrate populations. *American Journal of Tropical Medicine and Hygiene*, **17**, 269–275.

Zeledon, R. and Alfaro, M. (1973). Isolation of *Leishmania braziliensis* from a Costa Rican sandfly and its possible use as a human vaccine. *Transactions of the Royal Society of Tropical Medicine and Hygiene*, **67**, 416–417.

Zeledon, R., Ponce, C. and Ponce, E. (1975). The isolation of *Leishmania braziliensis* from sloths in Costa Rica. *American Journal of Tropical Medicine and Hygiene*, **24**, 706–707.

Zuckerman, A. and Lainson, R. (1977). *Leishmania. In:* "Protozoa of Veterinary and Medical Interest" (Ed. J. P. Kreier). Academic Press, New York and London.

Addendum

Since the preparation of this manuscript, we have studied the behaviour of some isolates of Peruvian *Leishmania peruviana* in laboratory-bred sandflies, *Lutzomyia longipalpis*. Development in the sandfly includes proliferation of the parasite in the hindgut, with round-oval promastigotes firmly attached to the wall of the pylorus and (to a lesser extent) the ileum. This growth is typical of leishmanias within the Section Peripylaria, as defined in this chapter, in which group *L. peruviana* clearly belongs.

Whether or not *L. peruviana* will prove to be another member of the *L. braziliensis* Complex, remains to be seen. In the meantime, however, the present observation does invalidate the theory that "uta" is merely "oriental sore", due to *L. tropica* which was imported into the Western Hemisphere in post-Columbian times, for the latter parasite shows no hindgut development in its sandfly vectors. In our opinion there is no doubt that *L. peruviana* is indigenous to the New World.

In addition, recent studies have incriminated the sandfly *Lutzomyia umbratilis* as a major vector of cutaneous leishmaniasis in the vicinity of Manaus, Amazônas State, Brazil (Arias and de Freitas, 1977). Preliminary observations suggest the causative parasite to be *L. braziliensis guyanensis*, extending the geographic range of "pian-bois" from the Guyanas, Territory of Amapá and north Pará State, Brazil, into Amazônas State and probably, therefore, the Territory of Roraima of the latter country.

Reference:

Arias, J. R. and Freitas, R. A. de (1977). On the vectors of cutaneous leishmaniasis in the Central Amazon of Brazil. I. Preliminary findings. *Acta Amazônica*, **7**, 293–294.

2

Transmission Cycles and the Heterogeneity of *Trypanosoma cruzi*

M. A. MILES

Department of Medical Protozoology,
London School of Hygiene and Tropical Medicine,
Keppel Street, London, England

I.	Introduction	118
II.	Morphological and behavioural criteria for the identification of *T. cruzi*	120
III.	Diagnosis and survey methods	121
IV.	Distribution and transmission cycles	124
	A. Distribution	124
	B. Secondary modes of transmission	125
	C. Transmission cycles	126
V.	Circumstantial evidence of the heterogeneity of *T. cruzi* . .	137
	A. Biometric comparisons	137
	B. Ultrastructure	138
	C. Virulence and histotropism	138
	D. Enteromegaly	140
	E. Drug sensitivity	141
	F. Infectivity to vectors	142
	G. Immunological differentiation	143
VI.	Biochemical characterization—enzyme electrophoresis and DNA studies	144
VII.	Prospects of Chagas' disease research	153
	A. Immune response, immunopathogenesis and vaccination .	153

B. Chemotherapy 155
C. Vector control 156

VIII. Concluding remarks 156

IX. Acknowledgements 157

X. References 157

XI. Appendix 172

Addendum 184

I. Introduction

In 1908 Carlos Chagas discovered the disease which, in recognition of his accomplishments, is called "Chagas" disease. His discovery was particularly remarkable as it was the finding of the causative organism, *Trypanosoma cruzi*, in one of the insect vectors, *Panstrongylus megistus*, which stimulated the search for the human infection.

Chagas was a prominent medical student at the Manguinhos Institute of Rio de Janeiro, which had been established by Oswaldo Cruz in 1900. He was working on the control of malaria among railway workers based at Lassance, Minas Gerais State, Brazil, when the abundance of a triatomine bug in local houses was brought to his attention. The bugs were blood-sucking and it occurred immediately to Chagas that they might transmit human disease. Dissection of the bugs revealed a flagellate infection in the hindgut. Marmosets (*Callithrix penicillata*), which were exposed to infected bugs at the Manguinhos laboratory in Rio, developed a new trypanosome in the blood, quite distinct from *T. minasense*, which Chagas had already described from marmosets. The new trypanosome was named *T. cruzi* and was infective to a variety of laboratory mammals. Chagas examined the blood of a sick child, who was living in a heavily bug-infested house. He found trypanosomes morphologically identical to *T. cruzi* and recognized the first clinical case of American trypanosomiasis. In April 1909 he gave an exhibition, at Lassance, for his colleagues, summarizing the life cycle of *T. cruzi* and describing the new human disease. Subsequently, in 1912, he reported the first reservoir host of *T. cruzi*, the armadillo—*Dasypus novemcinctus*. His work was rapidly extended by his collaborators at the Manguinhos Institute in Rio, even to the production, in 1913, of a complement fixation test for the serological diagnosis of human infection (Machado-Guerreiro test).

Chagas' discoveries were outstanding, and fundamentally correct, but not without some misconceptions. The conclusion that mammals acquired infection from the salivary glands of the vector was questioned by Brumpt, who demonstrated that transmission was by the contamination of mucous membranes or skin with infected bug faeces. Schizogony of the trypanosomes, which Chagas alleged occurred in the lungs of the infected mammal, was shown by Delanoë and Delanoë in 1912 to be due to confusion with *Pneumocystis carinii* (*vide* Hoare, 1972). Unfortunately, as well as heart defects and nervous system disorders, Chagas attributed goitre and cretinism to *T. cruzi* infection. This led to bitter criticism and ridicule, particularly by the eminent Rudolf Kraus, who failed to find Chagas' disease in bug-infested areas of Argentina. Chagas was described as "a man who searches in the forest for diseases which do not exist". Vianna (1911) had reported the intracellular reproduction of *T. cruzi* in various mammalian tissues, Brumpt (1912) had described the entire development in both mammal and vector, and the widespread distribution of *T. cruzi* in South and Central America was recognized soon after its discovery. However, criticism of Chagas was so fervent that only in the 1930's was interest revived by the work of Mazza and his collaborators in Argentina, and Dias in Brazil. The significance of Chagas' disease as a problem of public health began to be acknowledged (Romaña, 1962; Guerra, 1970; Hoare, 1972).

There are now thousands of published papers on Chagas' disease, of which a substantial proportion are listed in bibliographies (Miles and Rouse, 1970; Olivier *et al.*, 1972; Diaz Vasquez, 1971). In addition, there is a diverse literature on the triatomine vectors of *T. cruzi*, which is not readily accessible and not covered in the available bibliographies. As a result of this intensive research interest, a large volume of data has accumulated on the biology and epidemiology of American trypanosomiasis and there are several useful summaries (Cançado, 1968; Goble, 1970; Anonymous, 1972; Hoare, 1972; Brener, 1973; Anonymous, 1976). It is estimated that more than 10 million persons may be infected with *T. cruzi*, and, although clinically indeterminate infection may be more common than overt disease, there is no question that Chagas' disease is an important cause of mortality and morbidity on the South American continent (WHO, 1976). However, whilst serological diagnosis of human infection is much improved, progress with low-cost control of Chagas' disease is far from satisfactory; there is no effective vaccine or acceptable therapy, and vector control by insecticides remains problematical.

Not only is the practical control of Chagas' disease unresolved, but two pronounced enigmas have arisen from experimental research on the relationship of *T. cruzi* to its mammalian host. Firstly, it is not understood by what mechanism the organism persists, for life, in a supposedly immune animal; whether by seclusion and dormancy of the intracellular forms, mimicry of host antigens, adsorption of host antigens, or antigenic variation. Secondly, the pathogenetic mechanism of Chagas' disease is still controversial, despite the elegant work of Köberle (1968, 1974), which implies that an endotoxin released from the tissue forms of *T. cruzi* causes parasympathetic neurone destruction in the acute phase of infection; the neurone loss precipitates the mega syndromes of chronic Chagas' disease. Recent work suggests that, at least in some areas, a continuing immunopathogenesis may also be involved in chronic Chagas' disease (Teixeira, 1976).

Fundamental to an understanding, with a view to disease control, of *T. cruzi* epidemiology, and of the host–parasite relationship, is the ability to determine whether different types of *T. cruzi* exist. If such heterogeneity occurs, it is necessary to identify strains* and relate them to biological characteristics, including the form and distribution of human disease.

Evidence will be reviewed here for heterogeneity among *T. cruzi*, particularly from the recent use of isoenzyme electrophoresis to identify *T. cruzi* strains. This evidence will be presented within the broad perspective of the current status of Chagas' disease research, but without a reiteration of all published work for, within such a context, "of making many books there is no end; and much study is a weariness" (Ecclesiastes, 12:12). A synopsis of the Triatominae is included, as the vector literature is diverse, and frequently divorced from other aspects of Chagas' disease research. Emphasis is placed on the need to integrate the laboratory and field approach.

II. Morphological and behavioural criteria for the identification of T. cruzi

T. cruzi is the type species of the subgenus *Schizotrypanum*. In mammalian blood *T. cruzi* is described (Hoare, 1972) as a small, characteristically "C"-shaped, trypanosome with a large, round or oval kinetoplast (diameter about 1·2 μm) near the short pointed posterior end, a free flagellum, and an undulating membrane with 2–3 shallow convolutions. The broader "C"-shaped forms are typical, although slender, more motile forms are also seen, particularly if an early parasitaemia appears in experimental infections. The broad form has an oval nucleus, a kinetoplast which is practically terminal and a long free flagellum; whilst the slender form has an elongated nucleus, a subterminal kinetoplast and a shorter free flagellum.

Hoare (1972) summarizes available mensural data on *T. cruzi* blood forms giving the following ranges for proven *T. cruzi* from man: total length 11·7 μm–30·4 μm (means 16·3 μm and 21·8 μm); free flagellum 2·0 μm–11·2 μm; breadth 0·7 μm–5·9 μm; and nuclear index 0·9 μm–1·7 μm. Measurements of *T. cruzi*-like organisms from diverse, presump-

---

* Strain = "a set of populations originating from a group of trypanosomes of a given species or subspecies present at a given time in a given host or culture and defined by the possession of one or more designated characters". (Meeting on Characterization, Nomenclature and Maintenance of Salivarian Trypanosomes; London, 1976. See Chapter 15.)

tive reservoirs were comparable, and had the same wide range. Thus, with the exception of some bat *Schizotrypanum*, such as *T. vespertilionis*, which can possibly be distinguished from *T. cruzi* by statistical comparisons of large numbers (Hoare, 1972; Marinkelle, 1976), biometric data of blood forms does not justify division of the subgenus *Schizotrypanum* into minor taxonomic groups.

It has been assumed that, as *T. cruzi*-like organisms from (non-Chiropteran) mammals are morphologically indistinguishable from human *T. cruzi*, these mammals are reservoir hosts of the causative organism of Chagas' disease. As pointed out by Hoare (1972), it is possible that some of these organisms are not infective to man, in the same way that *T. brucei brucei* does not infect man in Africa. However, there is no evidence for this, and from a few cases of naturally acquired or experimentally induced human infection it seems that *T. cruzi*-like organisms from feral mammals can infect man (Chagas, 1936; Packchanian, 1943; Woody and Woody, 1964; Moura et al., 1969; Shaw et al., 1969).

It is obviously unacceptable to infect human volunteers, so indirect criteria have been used to identify *T. cruzi*. Barretto (1965, 1970) has used the following characters in conjunction with biometric data: growth on blood-agar media; development in triatomine bugs and production of metacyclic trypanosomes in the hindgut; and, in laboratory animals, particularly young mice and rats, infectivity, intracellular mutiplication as amastigotes, and the induction of protection against a normally lethal challenge with proven *T. cruzi*. There can be little doubt that the *T. cruzi*-like organisms from the many mammal species which Barretto has examined with these methods, are indeed *T. cruzi* and would probably infect man. The term "*T. cruzi*-like" is still used if identification is by blood form morphology alone, without the additional criteria of Barretto, or without evidence from comparison with proven *T. cruzi* by the newer biochemical methods, such as DNA analysis or enzyme electrophoresis.

III. Diagnosis and survey methods

In acute *T. cruzi* infections trypanosomes are usually common in the peripheral blood and can be detected by fresh or thick blood film examinations, or gradient and microhaematocrit centrifugation and lysis concentration methods, followed by identification in stained thin blood films (Hoff, 1974; Budzko and Kierszenbaum, 1974).

In untreated chronic infections, trypanosomes are present in peripheral blood, but are extremely rare. Xenodiagnosis, blood culture and animal inoculation are employed for the parasitological diagnosis of chronic infections and, if necessary, of acute infections with scanty blood parasitaemias. If performed correctly, xenodiagnosis is the most successful of these methods, but for optimum results an appropriate vector species and proven susceptible bug population should be used (Cerisola *et al.*, 1971b; Zeledón, 1974; Miles *et al.*, 1975; Maudlin, 1976); occasionally irritating skin reactions result in sensitized individuals. Under ideal conditions blood culture can be at least as sensitive as xenodiagnosis, but because of the need for aseptic procedure, it is impractical for routine field application (Albuquerque *et al.*, 1972; Minter-Goedbloed, 1976).

In human blood *T. cruzi* must be distinguished from the non-pathogenic *T. rangeli* (subgenus *Herpetosoma*), which may be as prevalent as *T. cruzi*, or more so, especially in areas where *Rhodnius* species are domiciliated vectors (Sousa, 1972). In other New World mammals which harbour *T. cruzi* many trypanosome species occur, for example, *T. rangeli*, *T. lewisi* (*Herpetosoma*), *T. conorhini*, *T. minasense*, *T. freitasi* and *T. legeri* (*Megatrypanum*). Mixed infections are also found. Even so, the distinction of the subgenera *Herpetosoma* and *Megatrypanum* from *Schizotrypanum* presents no problem in well-stained thin blood films (Hoare, 1972).

Identification of flagellates in naturally infected bugs or bugs used in xenodiagnosis is far more difficult than in infected blood, as morphological differences are less distinct and the intestinal contents interfere with the quality of staining. Triatomine bugs are the vectors of *T. rangeli* and *T. conorhini* and, experimentally, intestinal infections of other trypanosome species develop (e.g. *T. legeri*, Deane, 1967). Mixed infections may occur, just as in the mammal, and recognition of these species, although theoretically possible, cannot be based on the morphology of intestinal infections alone. *T. rangeli* intestinal infections usually progress to the haemolymph and salivary glands (D'Alessandro, 1976) (although apparently not in some *T. rangeli*-like trypanosomes such as *T. diasi*, or *T. saimirii*, and certainly not in all triatomine species). *T. conorhini* is usually associated with infected rats (*Rattus rattus*) and *Triatoma rubrofasciata*.

Laboratory colonies of bugs bred for xenodiagnosis must be examined periodically for the presence of *Blastocrithidia triatomae* (Cerisola *et al.*, 1971a), or other organisms, and with untrained personnel even ciliate contaminants of non-sterile diluents have led to false positive results of xenodiagnosis (Miles, unpublished observations).

Once infection is established, *T. cruzi* seems to persist for life in both man and experimental animals. After fifty years, *T. cruzi* was still detectable by xenodiagnosis of Chagas' first recorded case (Salgado *et al.*, 1962). Repeated parasitological diagnosis may be necessary to demonstrate *T. cruzi* in chronic cases, whereas serology is highly sensitive, and the best tests suffer few cross-reactions. The much-improved complement-fixation test (CFT) is still in use, but a recent comparison of methods has shown the importance of standardizing procedure (Almeida and Fife, 1976). Many new serological tests have been developed (reviewed by Voller, 1977). Of the numerous methods described, CFT, the indirect fluorescent antibody test (IFAT), indirect haemagglutination test (IHAT) (Cerisola *et al.*, 1970; Neal and Miles, 1970; Camargo and Shimizu, 1974) and enzyme-linked immunosorbent assay (ELISA) (Voller *et al.*, 1975, 1976) are reliable, if rigorous test procedures are used, and can be performed on filter paper blood samples. Even so, at least two of these methods are normally used in combination.

As IgM is only elevated in the acute phase of infection and does not traverse the placenta, IgM and IgG-specific IFAT can distinguish recent cases from chronic cases, and congenital cases from transplacental antibody transfer (but presumably with deep-frozen sera only, as IgM deteriorates rapidly on filter paper stored at 4°C) (Szarfman *et al.*, 1973; Camargo and Amato Neto, 1974).

Serology is not often used for diagnosis of *T. cruzi* in reservoir hosts. Experimentally, IFAT, IHAT, and a direct agglutination test using trypsinized epimastigotes (DAT) (Vattuone and Yanovsky, 1971; Schmunis *et al.*, 1972; Allain and Kagan, 1974) give consistent results for rodents, but for opossum (*Didelphis*) CFT, IFAT, IHAT, DAT, and skin tests, so far, have been totally unsatisfactory in experimental trials on small numbers of infected opossums and controls (Miles, Camargo, Kagan and Draper, unpublished data). This may be due to the weak immunological response of the opossum (Marx *et al.*, 1971; Major and Burrell, 1971; Prasad *et al.*, 1971; Rowlands *et al.*, 1972), or a result of a long-established equilibrium between host and parasite, as well as the inadequacy of current techniques. The ELISA test, which is extremely sensitive, may solve the problem of serological diagnosis of *T. cruzi* in marsupials, although there are many natural infections in the opossum which might give rise to serological cross-reaction (Potkay, 1970).

In human diagnosis, history of exposure to triatomine bites is usually sought but may be absent in infections acquired by blood transfusion, congenital, or oral, transmission. In the acute phase of Chagas' disease clinical features, such as unilateral conjunctivitis (Romaña's sign) or cutaneous chagoma at the portal of entry, and in the chronic phase, such as cardiomegaly, ECG changes and enteromegaly (megaoesophagus and megacolon) may substantiate serological evidence of infection, and, in some instances, are almost considered pathognomonic. However, many cases of Chagas' disease may be asymptomatic; the first recorded case showed no apparent abnormalities after fifty years of infection (Salgado *et al.*, 1962). Little is yet known of the symptomology or pathological sequels to *T. cruzi* infection in reservoir hosts, although ECG abnormalities are reported from Panamanian rats (Blandon *et al.*, 1974).

A combination of all these diagnostic methods has been used to establish our present picture of the distribution of *T. cruzi*, although, for human infection, major emphasis has been placed on serology.

IV. Distribution and transmission cycles

A. DISTRIBUTION

Apart from the *T. cruzi*-like organisms which are cosmopolitan in bats, *Schizotrypanum* is known only from the Western Hemisphere, from well over 100 species of mammals, of 8 orders. In addition there are more than 80 species of Triatominae in the Americas which may transmit *T. cruzi*.

The most important mammal hosts are among the Marsupialia (*Didelphis, Lutreolina, Marmosa*), Edentata (*Dasypus*), and Rodentia (*Coendou, Neotoma, Rattus*). The most prominent of all is the opossum of the genus *Didelphis*, which is ubiquitous within the range of *T. cruzi*, and susceptible to relatively high, persistent *T. cruzi* parasitaemias. Infections are also recorded from anthropoid primates (*Alouatta, Callithrix, Leontocebus, Saimiri*), Carnivora (*Mephitis, Nasua, Procyon, Urocyon*), Lagomorpha and Artiodactyla, as well as the Chiroptera. The significance of sylvatic Chiroptera as hosts of *T. cruzi* is unclear as characterization of the bat trypanosomes is inadequate; organisms which are morphologically indistinguishable from *T. cruzi* often do not infect experimental animals (Marinkelle, 1976). However, bats roosting in bug-infested houses are commonly infected with typical *T. cruzi*. Birds have a solid insusceptibility to *T. cruzi* (Kierszenbaum *et al.*, 1976) but some lizard species can support transient experimental infections (Ryckman, 1954).

The majority of the Triatominae, listed in the Appendix, have been found naturally infected with *T. cruzi*; others have been infected experimentally. Genetic variation in vector susceptibility may occur (Maudlin, 1976), but no insusceptible triatomine species are known.

The distribution of *T. cruzi*-like organisms in mammals and bugs (latitude 43°S to 42°N) is much wider than that in man (latitude 38°S to 25°N), despite the two human cases recorded in the USA (Hoare, 1972). For man, knowledge of distribution and prevalence is largely dependent on serology which has reached a high degree of sophistication and reliability, and can be used for detailed epidemiological studies (Mott *et al.*, 1976). For many areas, the prevalence of *T. cruzi* in man is still unclear, as it is a function of public health or research facilities. In countries where the disease is relatively well studied, prevalence estimates are 4 million (Brazil); 2·3 million (Argentina); 2 million (Colombia) and 0·56 million (Venezuela) (Hoare, 1972; Anonymous, 1972). Thus, more than 10 million cases probably exist overall and far more individuals are exposed to infection. Whilst reliable seropositivity is an index of current infection, it does not demonstrate the presence of the syndromes of the chronic disease, which are markedly discontinuous in distribution.

Several authors have reported *T. cruzi* from Asia, or from animals of reputedly Asian origin but Hoare (1972) explains all such reports as either due to *T. cruzi* transmission in captivity, which can occur experimentally by bed bugs and ticks (*Cimex lectularius, Rhipicephalus, Amblyomma*), or, in the case of the most recent report of *T. cruzi*-like simian trypanosomes from Indonesia (Weinman and Wiratmadja, 1969), as failure to recognize *T. conorhini* (but see Addendum, p. 185).

B. SECONDARY MODES OF TRANSMISSION

Several means of transmission, other than by direct contamination of mucous membranes and skin with infected faeces from a feeding vector, are known or suspected (Pipkin, 1969). These are:
1. Congenital transmission, in man, reservoir hosts and experimental animals (Miles, 1972; Bittencourt, 1976; Howard, 1976).
2. Transfusion of infected donor blood (Cerisola *et al.*, 1972a; Camargo and Leser, 1974; Becker, 1975; Rassi and Rezende, 1976).
3. Oral transmission from eating infected mammals and vectors, or accidentally ingesting fragments of them (Dias, 1940; Phillips, 1958).
4. Transmission via infected maternal milk (Miles, 1972).
5. Fly-borne contamination (Diaz-Ungria, 1968).
6. Contamination with urine or saliva from heavily infected animals (Zeledón. 1974).
7. Laboratory accident (Hanson *et al.*, 1974).

Two of these modes of transmission, congenital transmission and transmission by blood transfusion, are important in the spread of human infection, although uncommon in comparison with vectorial transmission. Transmission by blood transfusion can be prevented by serological screening of donor blood or routine storage with a 1:4000 concentration of crystal violet for 24 hours at 4°C. A more acceptable means of destroying *T. cruzi* in donor blood is urgently required, as transmission by blood transfusion is an all too frequent occurrence in South American cities, which are expanding with immigrants from rural endemic foci. It is suggested that oral transmission has resulted in two outbreaks of simultaneous acute cases in man (Shaw *et al.*, 1969; Zeledón, 1974); oral transmission is almost certainly a predominant natural infection route for other mammals, either by consumption of infected bugs, or in wild carnivores and domestic cats by feeding on infected mammal prey (Ryckman and Olsen, 1965; Yaeger, 1971; Zeledón, 1974; Miles, 1976a).

C. TRANSMISSION CYCLES

1. The significance of transmission cycle studies

The known prevalence of *T. cruzi* in sylvatic mammals depends predominantly on the examination of those caught in traps; seldom are they captured in their refuges, which are also the natural habitats and feeding sites of the triatomine vectors of *T. cruzi*. Thus, records of sylvatic reservoirs and vectors of *T. cruzi* are frequently unrelated and it is not known which bug species feed on a given mammal host. Mammal–vector associations are usually established, if at all, by indirect methods, mainly by the identification of bug blood-meals with precipitin tests. Many sylvatic bug species are known only from the intrusion of flying adults into houses or from locations uninhabited by their vertebrate hosts (see Appendix).

Even the most highly domiciliated triatomine bug species, which transmit *T. cruzi* to man and his domestic animals, have residual or widespread sylvatic ecotopes and feral hosts (see Appendix). In certain areas continuity or overlap occurs between sylvatic and domestic transmission cycles, either by dispersion, or human carriage, of a common vector species between sylvatic ecotopes and houses. Alternatively, contact between enzootic and endemic transmission may result from feral mammals entering houses in search of food or refuge sites (Barretto, 1976).

A detailed analysis of domestic *T. cruzi* transmission is of vital significance in understanding the role of vector ecology, human behaviour, and domestic animals such as dogs, cats, house mice (*Mus musculus*), guinea-pigs and chickens, and in designing a strategy for control. In addition, there are two principal reasons for determining where overlap occurs between sylvatic and domestic transmission cycles, and for encouraging what superficially might appear to be an academic interest in enzootic *T. cruzi*. Firstly, although eradication of *T. cruzi* is prohibited by the widespread sylvatic distribution, vector control in endemic regions where such transmission cycles overlap will be much more effectual if replenishment of domestic vectors from sylvatic sources is presupposed and combated. Secondly, in enzootic areas undergoing development and human settlement, knowledge of local sylvatic mammal–vector associations may allow the threat of emergent endemic foci of *T. cruzi* to be assessed. Vector species likely to adapt to houses are those with little climatic or microhabitat restrictions, a broad host specificity, a high rate of natural increase, and efficient powers of autonomous dispersion or adaptation to transport hosts.

To facilitiate epidemiological application, the *T. cruzi* zoonosis has been divided here into three main types of transmission cycle: (a) enzootic or purely sylvatic transmission cycles where there are no domiciliated triatomine bug species; (b) overlapping, or continuous sylvatic and domestic transmission cycles, in the same locality, with vector species which are common to both; and (c) non-overlapping or discontinuous sylvatic and domestic transmission cycles, in the same locality, with distinct sylvatic and domiciliated vector-species.

Examples are given of each of these three groups and methods are summarized for studying sylvatic mammal–vector associations and determining which of these types of transmission cycle occurs in a particular locality.

Unfortunately, this approach is a gross simplification of a complex epidemiological situation, which is constantly changing as a result of vector dispersion, human migration and ecological disturbance. House-adapted triatomine species are certainly transported with human belongings and, as is known for some sylvatic species, may be capable of rapid autonomous dispersion over long distances. It has been suggested that efficient domiciliated vectors, extending their range, may displace locally established vectors, or replace species weakened by insecticide control measures (Forattini, 1976).

The balance of evidence suggests that epidemiological threat from the migration of established house-adapted vector species far exceeds that from vectors newly adapting to houses.

In parallel to the approach outlined above, the Appendix summarizes the diverse and fragmentary information on the distribution, habitats and vertebrate hosts of the Triatominae. Species are divided into three groups as an indication of adaptation to human dwellings. The vast majority of species have been reported as infected with *T. cruzi*-like organisms. The excellent taxonomic reviews of Lent and his collaborators provide keys for the field identification of species (see references to the Appendix), with the exception of the largest genus, *Triatoma*, for which no up-to-date, comprehensive review is available. The taxonomy of this genus is particularly confused by the occurrence of polytypic species, or species which show hybrid development but may be morphologically or ecologically distinct, such as *T. protracta* and *T. barberi*, *T. infestans* and *T. rubrovaria* (Usinger *et al.*, 1966), and by the description of new species on single or few specimens, often with subsequent reduction to synonym status. Fortunately, a long-needed taxonomic review of the genus *Triatoma*, and a volume dealing with the taxonomy of the Triatominae as a whole, are shortly to appear (Lent and Wygodzinsky, personal communication).

2. Enzootic *T. cruzi*

(*a*) *The Amazon basin.* There is a high prevalence of *T. cruzi*-like organisms among the forest mammals and triatomine bugs of the Amazon basin. Deane (1958, 1960, 1961, 1964, 1967) and Deane and Damasceno (1961) report *T. cruzi* from *Didelphis marsupialis, Marmosa cinerea, Philander opossum, Nectomys squamipes, Dasypus novemcinctus, Tamandua tetradactyla, Saimiri sciurius* and various bat species. Many other species of trypanosome are also known in the region, including some of the subgenera *Herpetosoma* (*T. rangeli*-like) and *Megatrypanum* (*T. conorhini*) which develop in triatomine bugs.

Triatomine species reported from the Amazon basin are *Cavernicola pilosa, Eratyrus mucronatus, Microtriatoma* sp. indet,* *Panstrongylus geniculatus, P. lignarius, P. rufotuberculatus, Rhodnius amazonicus, R. brethesi, R. pictipes, R. prolixus, R. robustus, Rhodnius* sp. n., *Triatoma maculata, T. rubrofasciata* and *T. rubrovaria* (Rodrigues and Melo, 1942; Deane and Damasceno, 1949; Deane, 1961; Almeida, 1971; Almeida and Machado, 1971; Almeida *et al.*, 1973; Miles, 1976b). Adults of some of these, such as *P. geniculatus, P. lignarius* and *R. pictipes*, occasionally fly into local dwellings, but do not form colonies; the type of local housing, which is principally of wood, may be unsuitable for these vectors. No domiciliated vectors are known, at present, in the whole of the Amazon basin, with the exception of *T. rubrofasciata* which can be found throughout the tropics, especially in ports, in buildings infested by *Rattus rattus*, but rarely feeding on man or transmitting *T. cruzi*.

Surveys for *T. cruzi* infection in man and domestic animals have been negative, except for one canine infection, probably derived *per os* (Rodrigues and Melo, 1942), and the unusual discovery of four simultaneous acute cases in Belém, of unknown local origin (Shaw *et al.*, 1969).

Cavernicola pilosa and *P. geniculatus* are usually found with bats and armadillos respectively, but little is known of other natural vector-mammal associations in Amazonian forest. However, the use of a simple tracking device for tracing mammals from capture points to their refuges has recently given some preliminary results on the natural ecotopes of some of the local triatomine species (Miles, 1976b). *R. pictipes* and nymphs of an unidentified *Microtriatoma* species* were found in a nest of the opossum *D. marsupialis; P. lignarius* and a new species of *Rhodnius* were in a nest visited by both *D. marsupialis* and *Echimys chrysurus*; nymphs of an unidentified species were found in a refuge of *P. opossum*. It is likely that several more triatomine species remain to be discovered in the vast forested region of the Amazon.

The Amazon basin is being developed rapidly and migrants are arriving from endemic areas of Chagas' disease in the north east of Brazil. There is a very real threat of endemic Chagas' disease, either from adaptation of local forest vectors to houses, or by the introduction of domiciliated vectors as highways are opened. The occurrence of four acute cases in Belém, with one fatality, and the virulence of *T. cruzi*

* See Note 1, p. 195.

isolations to experimental animals (Deane, 1964) certainly suggest that *T. cruzi*, with the potential of causing disease in man, surrounds the human settlements (see Addendum, p. 186).

(b) *USA. T. cruzi*-like organisms are recorded in many feral mammals in the USA, from at least 10 states, particularly in the south-west. Principal among them are the wood rat (*Neotoma*), opossum (*Didelphis*), skunk (*Mephitis*), racoon (*Procyon*), deer mouse (*Peromyscus*), squirrel (*Ammospermophilus*), armadillo (*Dasypus*), and ring-tailed cat (*Bassariscus*) (Woody and Woody, 1964; Kagan *et al.*, 1966; Hoare, 1972).

There are numerous species and subspecies of North American triatomine bugs (see Appendix), which have been studied in depth by Usinger, Ryckman and collaborators (see references to the Appendix). *T. gerstaeckeri*, *T. lecticularius*, *T. protracta*, *T. recurva*, *T. rubida* and *T. sanguisuga* are reported from houses. In contrast to the Amazon basin, there is quite frequent contact between man and triatomine bugs, most of which carry *T. cruzi*-like organisms. Strong seasonal dispersal flights are made by species such as *T. protracta* and *T. rubida*, during which bugs commonly invade camping sites and houses in large numbers (Wood, 1950, 1975a, b; Sjogren and Ryckman, 1966). These bugs will attack man, and one species, *T. sanguisuga*, commonly forms small household colonies (Zeledón, 1974). However, none of these North American bug species can be regarded as totally domiciliated and household colonies are frequently associated with opossum or wood rat nests inside dwellings, from which bugs will attack man if the nests become uninhabited (Yaeger, 1959).

Despite the more frequent exposure of man in the USA to the bite of infected vectors, as in the Amazon basin he maintains an almost total isolation from the sylvan cycle of transmission because he rarely becomes infected with *T. cruzi*. Serological surveys have shown almost negligible antibody prevalence in areas where triatomine bugs invade houses, even among patients with heart disease.

In a survey in Texas, nine of 500 individuals had positive CF tests, the nine were said to have been bitten by *T. gerstaeckeri* but *T. cruzi* could be isolated from none. In further surveys three of 117; one of 108, including 48 allegedly bitten by bugs, and one of 1909 persons were serologically positive. In no case was *T. cruzi* isolated or clinical signs of the disease seen. In Georgia, only 2 weakly positive sera were found among 3883 examined (Woody and Woody, 1964; Kagan *et al.*, 1966; Farrar *et al.*, 1972).

T. cruzi in the USA is thus considered as purely enzootic. Excluding infections which have been acquired in the laboratory, only two clinical cases are known. Both occurred in Texas, one at Corpus Christi in 1955 in a 10-month-old child, and the second at Houston in 1955 in a 5-

month-old child, that had been hospitalized at the age of one month. The second case was unusual as the organism was isolated from the cerebro-spinal fluid during treatment of a *Salmonella* meningitis;* the child had received four blood transfusions; one of the donors, who could not be traced, may have carried *T. cruzi*.

Two principal explanations have been put forward for the low prevalence of human cases in the USA; either the local *T. cruzi*-like organisms are of low virulence to man, producing transient non-antibody-inducing infections, or the mode of feeding of the local vectors seldom cause man to be contaminated with infected faeces.

The "Houston strain" from man is reported to have a relatively low virulence to mice and dogs but the "Corpus Christi strain" was pathogenic to both. As Kagan *et al.* (1966) conclude from their experimental studies of *T. cruzi* from the USA, it is quite possible that a variety of organisms of different virulence circulate there in sylvatic cycles. However, measurement of *T. cruzi* virulence is extremely problematical; experimental infection of both animals and man has shown that material from the USA is infective, and in some cases pathogenic to a wide range of hosts (Yaeger, 1959; Kagan *et al.*, 1966). The more likely explanation of the absence of human infection is seen in the unusual feeding behaviour of the local vectors; they apparently rarely defaecate during feeding and avoid crawling on the host (Pippin, 1970; Hoare, 1972). As mentioned above (Section IV, B), sylvatic hosts such as rodents and opossum consume insects including triatomine bugs; it is possible that in the natural habitats of wood rat lodges and mammal nests, transmission is predominantly by the oral route rather than by contaminative transmission. Thus, delayed bug defaecation is unlikely to affect sylvatic *T. cruzi* transmission, while the unusual feeding behaviour and lack of total adaptation to local housing, may be the main factors preserving man in rural North America from the public health problems of endemic Chagas' disease.

3. Continuous sylvatic and domestic transmission

The highly domiciliated triatomine species, and vectors of *T. cruzi*, are listed in the Appendix (Group A). Over part of their range, some of these species are common in both sylvatic habitats and houses; examples are *T. dimidiata* in Costa Rica, *R. pallescens* in Panama, and *R. prolixus* in Venezuela. When a vector species is both sylvatic and domestic in the same region, it is often assumed that the vector migrates between sylvatic habitats and houses. In the case of *T. dimidiata* and *R. prolixus* such migration has been established from bug blood-meal identifications and bug dispersion studies.

In Costa Rica, Zeledón *et al.* (1970, 1973, 1975) report *T. dimidiata*
* See Note 2, p. 195.

within 1000 m of houses, in hollow trees inhabited by opossums (*Didelphis*). Precipitin tests revealed human blood in sylvatic bugs. Zeledón concludes that "the concurrent finding of human and/or domestic animal and opossum blood in some *T. dimidiata*, plus the natural association of the marsupial and *T. dimidiata* in Costa Rica, is strong evidence of a link between the wild and domestic cycles of *T. cruzi*". *T. dimidiata* is also a vector of *T. cruzi* in cooler, highland areas of western Panama, but *R. pallescens* is the principal domestic vector, of both *T. cruzi* and the non-pathogenic *T. rangeli* (Sousa and Johnson, 1973). *R. pallescens* has been found in opossum nests (Pipkin, 1968) and interchange between sylvatic and household bugs is implied, although this has not been demonstrated by blood-meal identification or mark-recapture of bugs. In Venezuela, *R. prolixus* is the main domestic vector but also inhabits palms with opossum and other hosts, particularly the palm *Attalea humboldtiana*, which provides roofing material for local dwellings. *R. prolixus* eggs adhere to the palm fronds, are transported to houses, and give rise to household colonies (Gamboa, 1973; Pifano, 1973). Gomez-Nunez (1969) has tagged adult *R. prolixus* with internally placed, gold-covered Co[60] wires, of about 75 microcuries, and demonstrated clearly that bugs migrate actively from palms to houses. Dispersion was thought to be motivated by starvation; movement from palm trees to houses was greater than between palms and between houses. In Colombia all three of the above vectors are found. *R. prolixus*, the most important domestic vector, also occurs in palm trees (although distinction from *R. brethesi* is not confirmed); *T. dimidiata* is found in houses and sylvatic habitats; and *R. pallescens* flys into houses (D'Alessandro *et al.*, 1971).

In Costa Rica, mammals may enhance the link between enzootic *T. cruzi* and endemic foci by entering houses, and encouraging transfer of associated vectors. *Rattus* spp. nest both inside and outside houses; *Didelphis* spp., the most notorious reservoir host of *T. cruzi*, visit and occasionally nest inside dwellings (Zeledón *et al.*, 1975; Barretto, 1976).

Although some house-adapted vectors have extended their ranges far beyond regions of their sylvatic distributions, the extent to which overlapping sylvatic and domestic transmission cycles occur is obscured by the inadequacy of investigations of enzootic *T. cruzi*. Such overlap is probably much wider than currently acknowledged, and, when sylvatic bugs re-invade houses, counteracts the efforts of vector control.

4. Discontinuous sylvatic and domestic transmission

Examples of highly domiciliated vectors of *T. cruzi*, in Brazil, which are widely distributed beyond their residual sylvatic habitats are: *P. megistus*, *T. brasiliensis* and *T. infestans*. *P. megistus* is found in opossum and rodent nests, and *T. brasiliensis* in rocky areas inhabited by rodents, but over much of their ranges they are said to occur exclusively in houses

(Leal *et al.*, 1961; Barretto *et al.*, 1964; Barretto, 1968; Silva *et al.*, 1974). In the case of *T. infestans* the sparse sylvatic ecotopes known from southern Brazil may be a secondary extension of domestic foci; it has been suggested that *T. infestans* originated from rodent-inhabited caves in Andean valleys (Barretto *et al.*, 1963; Barretto and Ferriolli, 1964; Usinger *et al.*, 1966).

The failure to find species such as *T. infestans, P. megistus* and *T. brasiliensis* outside houses in some areas might reflect the destruction of sylvatic habitats by rural agriculture and inadequate searches for cryptic sylvatic foci. However, there is good evidence that the true explanation is dispersion of these vectors, or migration with man, from transition zones of overlapping sylvatic and domestic transmission cycles. *P. megistus* appears to have migrated to the north, *T. brasiliensis* to the south-east and *T. infestans* to the north-east (Lucena, 1962; Barretto, 1963). The spread of house-adapted vectors is a continuing phenomenon. The genesis of new endemic foci of *T. cruzi* by the dissemination of domiciliated vectors beyond their natural range, will lead to independent, or discontinuous sylvatic and domestic transmission cycles in a given locality.

In North-eastern Brazil, *P. megistus* is a principal vector of Chagas' disease to man but has never been found outside houses. Conversely, south of São Paulo State, it is found in sylvatic habitats with opossum and rats but rarely invades houses, possibly due to dependence on the climatic conditions of its microhabitats (Forattini *et al.*, 1970; Rocha e Silva *et al.*, 1975; Barretto, 1976).

In *P. megistus*-infested houses at São Felipe, Bahia State, north-eastern Brazil, combined parasitological and serological diagnosis gives a *T. cruzi* prevalence of 50–60% in man, between 15 and 35% in dogs, cats, house mice (*Mus musculus*) and rats (*Rattus rattus frugivorus*). Xeno-diagnosis, with 10 fifth-instar *R. prolixus*, and experimental studies, demonstrated that up to 25% of trapped opossums (*Didelphis azarae*)[*] also carried *T. cruzi*. Apart from bats, *T. cruzi*-like organisms were not found in other sylvatic mammals examined (Miles, 1976a; Minter, 1976b; Prata, 1976).

Initially it was assumed that in São Felipe all hosts acquired *T. cruzi* infection from *P. megistus*-infested houses. Sylvatic bugs were alleged to be absent from the area, except for *Psammolestes tertius* in bird nests; *M. musculus* was only captured inside houses; infected *R. r. frugivorus* was trapped in or around houses; and it was assumed that *D. azarae* intruded into bug-infested houses for food or nesting sites. However, *D. azarae* was trapped close to bug-infested houses, but was never found nesting in them, and infected opossums were caught 1–2 km from any dwellings; on the basis of these observations a persistent search for sylvatic vectors in São Felipe was undertaken.

* See Note 3, p. 195.

It is now known that at least five sylvatic triatomine species occur in São Felipe:

(a) *Triatoma tibiamaculata* from bromeliad epiphytes (*Aechmea* sp.), associated with opossums and porcupine, and in palms inhabited by lizards.

(b) *Rhodnius domesticus*, previously unknown in Bahia State, from an opossum nest (*D. azarae*) in a bromeliad epiphyte.

(c) *Parabelminus* sp.n. from bromeliad epiphytes.

(d) An unidentified species, thought to be *Cavernicola pilosa* on the basis of first instar morphology, from a bat colony in a hollow tree.

(e) *Psammolestes tertius* from bird nests.

(Miles, 1976a; Barrett and Miles, unpublished data.)

Two of these sylvatic vector species, *T. tibiamaculata* and *R. domesticus*, were infected with a trypanosome identified as *T. cruzi* on the basis of morphology and infectivity to mice. *T. tibiamaculata* was quite common. Ten of 14 infected *D. azarae* were trapped in localities subsequently shown to support infected *T. tibiamaculata*; bromeliad epiphytes, in which this vector was typically found and excellently camouflaged, were ideal, proven, refuges for *D. azarae*. It was therefore tentatively assumed that *T. tibiamaculata* was the vector of *T. cruzi* to the opossum in São Felipe and that separate, discontinuous cycles of sylvatic and domestic transmission occurred. This was explicable, as mentioned above, if the infected domestic vector, *P. megistus* had arrived from southern Brazil. These conclusions have been amply confirmed recently by results of enzyme electrophoresis, which indicate that the *T. cruzi* circulating in the domestic cycle is enzymically quite distinct from *T. cruzi* of the sylvatic cycle (see Section VI below and Addendum, p. 188).

The observations from São Felipe emphasize the difficulty of locating residual sylvatic cycles, particularly in a cultivated rural area without a profusion of sylvatic vector habitats. A much wider distribution of sylvatic Triatominae than currently recognized is inferred, with cryptic sylvatic cycles being the main source of infection among *Didelphis* and other reservoirs, rather than their intrusion into domestic foci. *T. tibiamaculata*, which has a widespread sporadic distribution in Brazil (see Appendix) does not colonize houses and seems to be rarely light-attracted to them. This vector has been found elsewhere in opossum nests (Silveira *et al.*, 1969) and, with others such as *R. domesticus*, may be adept at survival in deforested areas, and ideally suited for maintaining residual sylvatic *T. cruzi* transmission. The occurrence of *T. tibiamaculata* in free-standing palms inhabited by lizards suggests that propagation of this species may be enhanced by efficient dispersion and the use of lizards as secondary hosts, although a proportion of the specimens from palms carried *T. cruzi*, which was presumably derived from mammals (Barrett, personal communication).

Investigations, such as those described in São Felipe, provide a basis for the development of methods to determine whether given domestic foci are replenished from residual sylvatic foci. If sylvatic and domestic cycles are discontinuous in a given locality, as in São Felipe, control of endemic Chagas' disease can proceed without the threat of immediate bug reinvasion from surrounding vegetation. In contrast, where sylvatic and domestic cycles are continuous, both cycles must be considered in control, not necessarily by wholesale ecological destruction, but possibly by the selective removal of sylvatic vector habitats, immediately adjacent to houses or around human settlements.

5. Methods of studying sylvatic Triatominae and detecting continuity between transmission cycles

As indicated above, our understanding of sylvatic *T. cruzi* transmission cycles is fragmentary (see Appendix), yet of importance in assessing their relevance to control of endemic Chagas' disease and in predicting the sylvatic vector species in rural development areas which are likely to adapt to houses. The methods in use for detecting sylvatic Triatominae and associated mammals are as follows:

(a) *Dissection of sylvatic microhabitats.* Typical microhabitats are bromeliad epiphytes, palm-trees, bird nests, rocky areas, caves, hollow and dead trees, tree bark, fence posts and burrows. In some areas certain habitats, especially palms and epiphytes, may be abundant and easily examined. However, a profusion of sylvatic vector species may be present outside the more obvious ecotopes, for example, in Amazonian forest without abundant palms or epiphytes (Miles, 1976b), or in cultivated rural areas. Microhabitat dissection can be extremely productive. In systematic studies in Venezuela, Tonn *et al.* (1976) collected 3394 bugs of nine species in 342 of 394 palms; 1240 bugs of three species in 66 of 147 bird nests; 112 bugs of 4 species in 15 of 49 groups of bromeliad epiphytes; 262 bugs of six species in 19 of 31 hollow trees; and 49 bugs of four species in 6 of 12 mammal refuges. However, inhabited mammal refuges are seldom found and, in forest, inhabited tree holes or burrows are impossible to locate without tremendous labour. Often the most easily found sylvatic Triatominae are those with easily recognizable specific ecotopes (see Appendix), for example, *Cavernicola pilosa* in bat roosts, *Psammolestes* species in *Anumbius* and *Phacellodomus* bird nests, and *Paratriatoma* spp. in wood rat lodges (*Neotoma*). Such mammal-feeding species may carry *T. cruzi*, but they are the least important epidemiologically because of their sylvan isolation.

(b) *Tracking mammals and locating sylvatic Triatominae in mammal refuges.* Triatominae feeding from sylvatic mammals are most likely to be

found in inhabited mammal refuges. Telemetry, the attachment of miniature radio transmitters to free mammals, is a routine method of locating
mammal refuges, but has not been applied to study enzootic *T.
cruzi*, probably because it is expensive, difficult to use in tree-cover, and requires close continuous tracking to find the multiple refuges of animals
such as the opossum. In Amazonian forest at Belém, Pará State, Brazil,
where microhabitat dissection and light-trapping had failed to detect
sylvatic bugs, a primitive tracking device was used to follow mammals
from points of capture to their refuges and locate associated Triatominae
(Miles, 1976b). The device contained a spindle-free spool of fine line,
carried by the released mammal, whilst the free end was fixed to vegetation, so that the line unwound under minimum tension as the mammal
proceeded; 15 of 31 mammals released within 6 to 24 hours of capture
were retrieved, after a complete night of activity, by following the line
and tracing arboreal ascents and descents with the aid of climbing irons;
23 Triatominae of three species were found with 3 of the mammals retrieved. An improved miniature tracking device based on this principle is
being developed and should allow systematic retrieval of some of the
mammalian reservoirs of *T. cruzi* during a trapping programme, the
location of sylvatic vectors, and thus the direct investigation of enzootic
transmission cycles.

(*c*) *Attraction of sylvatic Triatominae to experimental chicken houses.*
Small chicken houses constructed in sylvatic locations are a valuable
means of detecting dispersing Triatominae and also provide information
on the capacity of species to colonize these artificial ecotopes. Whilst less
informative than the direct approach of seeking vectors and mammals in
their natural habitats, the results are directly relevant to new human
settlements. So far this method has had limited application to *T. sordida*,
T. arthurneivai and *P. megistus* in Brazil, and *R. prolixus* in Venezuela
(Forrattini *et al.*, 1973, 1975; Otero *et al.*, 1976; and unpublished data of
the Wellcome London Research Group, São Felipe, Bahia, Brazil). In
each study, vector colonies were established with extraordinary rapidity
by dispersion from sylvatic ecotopes or, in the case of *P. megistus*, from
infested houses nearby. Otero *et al.* (1976) found adults, eggs and nymphs
of *R. prolixus* within 4–6 weeks of chicken house construction; adult *R.
pictipes* and *P. geniculatus* were also found but did not form colonies.

(*d*) *Attraction to light sources.* Black-light traps have been very successful
in capturing North American triatomine species such as *T. protracta* and
T. gerstaeckeri which undertake dramatic seasonal dispersion flights over
long distances (Wood, 1950; Sjogren and Ryckman, 1966; Pippin, 1970).
Elsewhere few or no specimens have been captured. In Bahia, Brazil,
small numbers of three species were caught, in Venezuela eight species,

but only 22 specimens in all, over 52 light-trap nights, and in Amazonian forest 70 trap-hours yielded none (Ventocilla and Silva, 1968; Miles, 1976b; Tonn *et al.*, 1976). Improved light-trapping may become standard future procedure for triatomine capture.

(*e*) *Trapping with resting-place traps or animal-baited traps.* Results with resting-place traps outside houses have been poor; animal-baited traps yield more bugs but are laborious for the results achieved. Tonn *et al.* (1976) captured only a single *P. rufotuberculatus* nymph after 3000 bamboo-resting-place trap-days; 46 bugs of three species were captured from 1105 rat or chicken-baited trap-days.

(*f*) *Precipitin testing of triatomine blood meal sources.* Hosts of well-fed triatomine bugs can be broadly identified by precipitin tests of the midgut contents, using antisera against local vertebrate serum components. Midgut contents can be preserved on filter paper for long periods and there is no necessity for tests to be performed at the field location (Boreham, 1975). However, sera of local vertebrates must be collected to allow preparation of the full complement of antisera, and a rigorous test procedure, with incorporation of controls, must be used. Several other methods, including haemagglutination inhibition (Tempelis and Rodrick, 1972) and haemoglobin crystallization (Washino and Else, 1972) have been applied to arthropod blood meal identification, but precipitin testing is the most practical. The same principle, using gel diffusion, can identify natural triatomine predators (Barrett, 1976). Epidemiological studies have been enhanced greatly by blood meal identification (Minter, 1976a), which should be standard procedure, together with dissection to record flagellate infections, for sylvatic Triatominae which are collected and not required alive for other purposes.

(*g*) *Detecting continuity between transmission cycles.* Continuity, between sylvatic and domestic transmission, can usually be assumed following demonstration of a vector species common to houses and sylvatic ecotopes. Confirmation can be sought, from studying bug dispersion by (i) blood meal identification; (ii) mark-recapture of bugs, to trace transfer between sylvatic habitats to houses or to artificial ecotopes; (iii) mark-recapture and telemetry of peridomestic mammals which might act as a bridge between sylvan and domestic transmission; and (iv) biochemical characterization of *T. cruzi* to establish the identity, or otherwise, of sylvan and domestic organisms.

The applicability of blood meal identification to this problem is seen, as mentioned above, in the work of Zeledón *et al.* in Costa Rica (1973) and that of Barretto (quoted in Minter, 1976a). Mark-recapture methods of vectors require further development (Rabinovich *et al.*, 1976). The variety of marking methods used includes paints, fluorescent powders, mutilation, specific agglutinins added to pre-release blood sources, or radioisotopes (Tonn *et al.*, 1976). Gomez-Nunez (1969) used radio-isotopes and Forattini *et al.* (1975) marked *T. sordida* with paint to follow dispersion from artificial ecotopes. Care is required in release of marked bugs not to prejudice local inhabitants. Mark-recapture of reservoir mammals, and telemetry, have not, as yet, been applied to establish the degree of contact between feral mammals and houses. The use of bio-chemical characterization of *T. cruzi* in this context is described in detail below (Section VI).

V. Circumstantial evidence of the heterogeneity of T. cruzi

As stated in the Introduction, if heterogeneity exists among *T. cruzi* it is important to rationalize research by identifying strain-groups and relating them to biological characters, including the pattern of human disease.

A. BIOMETRIC COMPARISONS

Although, as stated above (Section II), the range of mensural characters for blood-form *T. cruzi* is extremely wide (Barretto, 1968; Hoare, 1972), biometric comparisons have been used to infer intrinsic differences be-tween *T. cruzi* of diverse origins (Hoare, 1972; Petana, 1972). However, with the possible exception of an organism from the armadillo, which had a nuclear index of 2·7, all measurements fall within values predictable from some single *T. cruzi* populations. Furthermore, the fact that inter-mediate tissue forms may be found in the blood of experimental animals with heavy infections (Soto, 1971; Behbehani, 1972) underlines the tenu-ous nature of conclusions based on minor deviations from reported measurements.

Brener and his colleagues (Brener, 1969, 1976a; Howells and Chiari, 1975) have shown that the slender and broad blood-forms of *T. cruzi* may have distinct biological functions, slender forms rapidly penetrating tissues but broad forms passing into the blood and being more infective to the vector. Although some biochemical differences may exist between slender and broad forms, the biochemical evidence does not support a close analogy between the dimorphism of *T. cruzi* and the pleomorphism of African trypanosomes; there is no evidence of the biochemical adapta-tion of organisms preparing for uptake by vectors (Gutteridge, 1976a). It is true that patterns of dimorphism are a possible index of intrinsic differences between *T. cruzi* from diverse sources but they may simply reflect the intracellular developmental stages reaching the blood from the tissues, and thus depend on the complex overall relationship between parasite and host.

The life cycle of *T. cruzi* both in mammal and the vector is not fully understood. There may be two or more separate intracellular developmental patterns. An "orbicular cycle", in which vacuolated sphaeromastigotes unroll to form small "C"-shaped trypomastigotes, has been reported by some workers in both mammal and vector (Wood, 1951, 1953; Brack, 1968; Rodriguez and Marinkelle, 1970; Behbehani, 1972; Hoare, 1972). It is tempting to speculate that C-shaped broad bloodforms result from the unrolling process, whilst slender forms are the product of the more classical transformation by elongation and migration of the kinetoplast. However, there is no evidence to support this, and metacyclic trypanosomes in the bug rectum, which may be formed directly from sphaeromastigotes are not C-shaped but long and slender (Brack, 1968).

Dvorak (1976) in continuous *in vitro* observations of single cells has only observed the "fusiform progression" pathway. He states, "the fact that intracellular trypomastigote maturation involves the transition from a broad to a slender form of the parasite implies that the extracellular appearance of these morphologic forms may be a function of the time of escape or release of the parasites from the host cell, and not necessarily an attribute of parasite strain differences as has been previously postulated."

In conclusion, there is no unequivocal evidence from morphological comparisons that intrinsic differences exist between *T. cruzi* of diverse origins. Even so, morphological observations are usually made in parallel with other studies.

B. ULTRASTRUCTURE

Mühlpfordt (1975), in standardized electron microscope studies, observed that the kinetoplast DNA of *T. cruzi* epimastigotes had a conspicuous central band at the beginning of cell division when the basal body was duplicated, whereas this was not present in comparable forms of *T. conorhini*, *T. rangeli* and *T. lewisi*. However, *T. cruzi* from eight sources, including man and feral mammals, were indistinguishable by this character. Ultrastructural differences have been observed at the subgeneric level in the salivarian trypanosomes (Vickerman, 1974; Vickerman and Preston, 1976).

C. VIRULENCE AND HISTOTROPISM

T. cruzi of diverse histories may behave differently in experimental animals (Brener, 1973). However, virulence shows no clear correlation with the host of origin or geographical location, behaviour of the organism may change during maintenance, and there is no simple method of specifying virulence as a parameter. Vague differences in experimental virulence do suggest that distinct types of *T. cruzi* may be related to disease distribution in man, but it is impossible to exclude effects of inherent adaptability of the organism or of the complex host–parasite interaction. For intra-species comparisons of virulence, more constant, basic biological parameters are required, such as those investigated by Dvorak (1976) in his elegant *in vitro* model.

T. cruzi does not uniformly colonize all tissues of the mammal host, some tissues are more heavily invaded than others. Differences in tissue distribution ("tropism") have frequently been ascribed to *T. cruzi* of diverse origins and demonstrated in mice (Bice and Zeledón, 1970; Andrade *et al.*, 1970a). Zeledón and Ponce (1972) report that 20.9% of *T. cruzi* isolated from *Didelphis* in Costa Rica were neurotropic in mice. Such observations of histotropism, together with a general assessment of virulence, may, in the future, correlate with *in vitro* parameters. Dvorak (1976) observed that skeletal muscle was more avidly penetrated by *T. cruzi* trypomastigotes than kidney or neoplasm cells, probably due to physiological or biochemical differences in cell type, which may also operate *in vivo*. Doubling time and total number of parasites produced within a cell, are the most obvious basic *in vitro* biological parameters which might be expected to correlate with virulence *in vivo*, in a given host. Dvorak (1976) found that doubling time was dependent on a variety of factors, including source or passage history of *T. cruzi* (which emphasizes the need for a standard procedure in comparisons), but that it was independent of host cell type. The number of parasites produced within a cell was proportional to the number of parasites penetrating the cell, each producing 500 organisms or about nine generations, unless infection was excessive, when early cell death occurred with the liberation of amastigotes, transitional stages and trypomastigotes. Dvorak suggests that the number of parasites produced may be under genetic control, although generation number did vary during passage or adaptation to tissue culture.

Determination of tissue antigen distribution by immunofluorescence (Andrade and Andrade, 1969) and radioactive labelling of infective organisms (Kuhn *et al.*, 1974) are techniques which may improve upon the *in vivo* histological determination of parasite distribution by direct microscopical examination of stained preparations (Hanson and Roberson, 1974). Recently Mercado (1976) assessed the release into plasma of the distinct isoenzymes of lactate dehydrogenase, which are present in different tissues, as an indirect means of contrasting tropisms and tissue damage during acute phase infections of *T. cruzi* from Chile, Costa Rica and Nicaragua.

D. ENTEROMEGALY

The association between parasympathetic neurone destruction and mega-oesophagus and megacolon is firmly established. Köberle estimates that 90% denervation is required to produce megaoesophagus, and 55% to produce megacolon, although hyper-reactivity to cholinergic agents can be demonstrated when denervation is less (Rezende, 1976). The mechanism by which neurones are destroyed is uncertain. Köberle proposes that destruction occurs as a result of a toxin released from degenerating amastigotes at pseudocyst rupture; subsequent reduction in neurones occurs during the normal aging process, and the critical level may be reached long after the initial acute phase. The same mechanism is thought to apply to neurological lesions of the heart. However, descriptions of chronic Chagas' cardiomyopathy are not uniform. Two types are evident (Andrade, 1976): one, as described by Köberle, with little or no myocarditis, pronounced destructive lesions of the ganglion cells, thinning of the left ventricular apex with aneurysm and commonly resulting in sudden death; in the second type there is a moderate to intense chronic myocarditis with a history of progressive heart failure. It is not known if the two descriptions of cardiac pathology represent different stages in the development of the cardiomyopathy, but the absence of apical aneurysm from the second suggests two distinct pathological entities (Andrade, 1976) possibly related to heterogeneity among *T. cruzi*. Arrhythymias, megaoesophagus and megacolon are associated, as one would expect, with the cases of the first cardiac form which has pronounced ganglionic lesions. Increasing evidence suggests that autoimmune phenomena, both autoantibody and autoimmune hypersensitivity, may play a role in the pathology of Chagas' disease (see Section VII, A below). One may speculate that certain parasite types have a greater propensity to mimic host cardiac antigens, or absorb host antigens, and tend to precipitate a chronic progressive Chagas myocarditis, which, as in Venezuela, may occur without evidence of mega syndromes (Puigbo and Zisman, 1968). Other types of *T. cruzi* may be more capable of inducing neurone destruction.

Marked indirect evidence that there are, among *T. cruzi*, aetiological agents with different characters, is seen in the regional distribution of chagasic enteromegaly, recently reviewed by Rezende (1976). Mega may occur in a variety of organs, not only in the heart or digestive tract; cardiomegaly, megaoesophagus and megacolon have the greatest frequency.

In southern Brazil, mega syndromes are common; Rezende (1976) describes 1057 cases of megaoesophagus and 622 of megacolon from Goiania, Goias State; Barbosa *et al.* (1970), among 15 000 necropsies in north and central Minas Gerais, record 875 cases of cardiopathy, of which 145 had megaoesophagus, megacolon, or both. Köberle (1974) has reported large series of autopsy cases at Ribeirão Preto, São Paulo State. Mega syndromes are also well known from Chile, Peru, Uruguay and Argentina, although in Argentina they seem to be less frequent among carriers of T. cruzi than in southern Brazil (Rezende, 1976). Occasional cases are reported from Bolivia, Colombia and Paraguay.

In Venezuela and Central America mega syndromes are extremely rare or totally absent. In Venezuela, only 32 cases of megaoesophagus were noted among 85 820 clinical histories spanning 20 years. Even so, heart disease, with chronic myocardiopathy but apparently low incidence of sudden death, is a prominent feature of chronic T. cruzi infections in Venezuela (Maekelt, 1973; Moleiro et al., 1973; Rezende, 1976). In Panama mega syndromes are unknown. In Mexico, there were four cases of chronic Chagasic myocarditis among 2383 autopsies, but no cases of mega syndrome (Kagan et al., 1966). Rezende (1976) concludes his review with the hypothesis that the infecting agents in areas of mega-associated chronic Chagas' disease differ from those in regions without mega syndromes, although variable susceptibility of the human population may also be involved.

ECG abnormalities have been reported in anaesthetized Panamanian rats infected with T. cruzi (Blandon et al., 1974), but it is not known if mega syndromes occur in reservoir mammal hosts.

Mega syndromes have been observed in experimental infections of monkeys, dogs, rats and mice (Petana and Coura, 1974; Marsden et al., 1976; Rezende, 1976). There is an urgent need for the development of effective procedures of assessing the induction of ECG abnormality and mega syndromes by T. cruzi in experimental animals, preferably in mice or rats and without time-consuming ganglion counts in tissue sections.

E. DRUG SENSITIVITY

Compounds with promising in vivo activity against T. cruzi fall into eight basic chemical groups: bisquinaldines, arsenobenzenes, phenanthridines, 8-aminoquinolines, 5-nitrofurans, 5-nitroimidazoles, 5-nitrothiazoles and 2-nitroimidazoles (Gutteridge, 1976b). Most have been abandoned due to inefficacy and toxicity, but 8-aminoquinolines are still being investigated, a 2-nitroimidazole [Ro 7-1051 (Radinil)] is currently undergoing clinical trials, and a 5-nitrofuran [nifurtimox (Lampit, Bayer 2502)] is available throughout South America. Side-effects, sometimes severe, can be produced by both Lampit and Ro 7-1051 and, as nitro-compounds, they are suspected of mutagenicity and carcinogenicity (Levi et al., 1975; Schenone et al., 1975; Gutteridge, 1976b).

Lampit certainly suppresses parasitaemia and, if treatment is begun in the acute phase of infection, can effect serological reversion and persistent negativity of xenodiagnosis. However, there is extraordinary discordance among the results of published clinical trials of Lampit in chronic cases, even with closely allied schedules of administration and prolonged post-therapeutic examination of patients. In some trials success is reported as almost total, whilst in others as almost nil (Cerisola et al., 1972b; Silva et al., 1974; Cançado et al., 1975, 1976). In a recent review, Cançado et al. (1976) conclude that Lampit kills circulating T. cruzi, but not intracellular forms, and that prolonged administration may cause accumulative suppression, which very occasionally may result in total exhaustion of parasitaemias. Freeman et al. (1975) tested 78 compounds in vitro against three T. cruzi of diverse histories (Brazil, Corpus Christi, Tulahuen) and report marked differences in sensitivity of the three types of T. cruzi to 12 of the compounds tested; Brener (1976a, b) refers to similar observations. Such differences in drug sensitivity among T. cruzi may explain conflicting chemotherapeutic trials.

If, as Köberle suggests, T. cruzi-mediated neurone loss proceeds almost entirely in the acute phase of infection, the appearance of mega syndromes may be unaltered by removal of the parasite in the chronic phase. This is a daunting prospect for post-infection chemotherapy in areas with pronounced cardiac lesions, little chronic progressive myocarditis and frequent mega syndromes, as acute cases of Chagas' disease are very rarely seen. In view of this unconfirmed relation between prognosis and continued presence of the parasite in chronic T. cruzi infection, the use of the term curative in chemotherapeutic trials is optimistic and misleading.

F. INFECTIVITY TO VECTORS

It is claimed that local forms of T. cruzi are adapted to local vectors. Thus, Brazilian vectors are said to be more susceptible to infection with local T. cruzi than are R. prolixus from Venezuela. Some human infections in Costa Rica are reputedly detected only by xenodiagnosis with T. dimidiata and not by R. prolixus and T. infestans; others in Argentina only by the local T. infestans, T. pallidipennis and R. prolixus, but not by introduced colonies of T. dimidiata, P. herreri, R. pallescens and R. prolixus (Barretto, 1965; Zeledón, 1974).

Most of these observations are explicable by differences in the susceptibilities of triatomine species, or subspecific populations, to T. cruzi infection. In some cases there may be a genetic basis for such susceptibility differences (Maudlin, 1976).

Enzyme electrophoresis (see Section VI) may find application in identifying subpopulations of the triatomine vectors of T. cruzi which differ in behaviour. Attempts have been made to use electrophoresis of haemolymph in this way (Perassi, 1973), and preliminary results show promising results from enzyme electrophoresis of triatomine tissue extracts (Schofield, Kilgour and Miles, unpublished data).

Ryckman (1965) reports that, in the same species of North American triatomine, North American *T. cruzi* produced heavier infections than did South American *T. cruzi*. Such experiments are difficult to standardize; at present, intrinsic variation among *T. cruzi* of diverse histories in their capacity to infect a given vector species cannot be discounted but remains uncertain.

G. IMMUNOLOGICAL DIFFERENTIATION

Blood forms of the African trypanosome *T. brucei* vary their surface antigens during the course of infection and the molecular basis of this variation is partially understood (Bridgen *et al.*, 1976). Antigenic variants of *T. brucei* can be detected by agglutination, lysis, and neutralization in clonal, variant-specific antisera, and trypanosome stocks* can be classified by their antigenic repertoire (Gray and Luckins, 1976). Serological subdivisions correspond well with groupings from enzyme electrophoresis of lysed trypanosomes (Godfrey and Kilgour, 1976). It is not known whether blood forms of *T. cruzi* vary their surface antigens, as trypomastigotes are not readily and reproducibly agglutinated, lysed, or neutralized by immune sera, even though cultured epimastigotes are by some normal mammal sera (Goble, 1970).

Blood and culture forms of *T. cruzi* can be distinguished by agglutination with concanavalin A, lysis in immune serum or indirect fluorescence, but the basis of these differences is unclear (Alves and Colli, 1974; Kanabara *et al.*, 1974; Kloetzel *et al.*, 1975). In the same way the mechanism by which anti Y and anti Cl "strain" sera neutralize Y trypomastigotes but not Cl is not understood, although the authors conclude that "their results present for the first time a clear demonstration of antigenic differences in the bloodstream forms of two strains of *T. cruzi*" (Krettli and Brener, 1976; see also Section VII, A below). Immunoelectrophoretic analysis can differentiate between species, for example between *T. brucei*, *T. cruzi* and *L. donovani*, by the presence or absence of particular precipitin arcs, but three *T. cruzi* of different histories were indistinguishable by this method (Afchain *et al.*, 1973; Afchain, 1976).

Those subdivisions of *T. cruzi* which have emerged from agglutination

---

* Stock = "a population derived by serial passage *in vivo* or *in vitro* from a primary isolation, without any implication of homogeneity or characterization". Meeting on Characterization, Nomenclature and Maintenance of Salivarian Trypanosomes; London, 1976. See Chapter 15.)

and precipitation reactions show no correlation with geographical location or behaviour; in some cases subgroups separate material with identical combinations of isoenzyme pattern (see Section VI below) (Nussenzweig and Goble, 1966; Ketteridge, 1975a). Thus, so far immunological methods have failed as a means of intrinsic identification of *T. cruzi*.

VI. Biochemical characterization—enzyme electrophoresis and DNA studies

Newton (1976), in a recent review of the biochemical taxonomy of the Kinetoplastida, part of which is reiterated here, considers biochemical methods under two main headings: those concerned with cell phenotype, namely studies of nutrition, metabolism, cell composition, and multiple enzyme forms; and those concerned with cell genotype, that is, DNA analyses. He stresses that "ideally, organisms should be grown under 'chemostat' conditions using defined media" when they are being defined by biochemical characters. He further emphasizes the need to control developmental stages *in vitro*, and compare the same forms; different morphological types may have pronounced biochemical differences, as is certainly the case with *T. brucei*.

As far as *T. cruzi* is concerned, defined media are a recent development, not yet applied to biochemical definition of the organism (Cross *et al.*, 1975; Mundin *et al.*, 1976; Gutteridge, personal communication). Nutritional requirements are thus not established for *T. cruzi* species or subspecies definition; *Crithidia oncopelti*, which has endosymbiont-assisted biosynthesis,* is the only kinetoplastid flagellate identifiable on this basis (Newton, 1976; but see also Hutner *et al.*, this volume). Metabolic studies, of exogenous substrate utilization, end products of metabolism and oxidative pathway, have revealed differences between trypanosome species and are promising future means of species definition (Newton, 1976; see also Gutteridge and Rogerson—this volume). Goldberg *et al.* (1976) report that ^{14}C arginine and lysine uptake in *T. cruzi* of two diverse histories (Y and MR) was higher in three-day-old cultures than ten-day-old cultures, and that significant differences were also observed between the two types. Mancilla and Naquira (1964) report that the pentose-phosphate shunt was more active, and tri-carboxylic cycle less active, in culture forms of Tulahuen *T. cruzi* than the Peru *T. cruzi*. Overall analysis of cell composition is a crude means of distinction between closely related organisms, unlikely to correlate with significant biological characters, which are not readily identifiable by other means. Analysis of *T. cruzi* immuno-polysaccharides, or perhaps of lipids and sterols, may be of some use (Newton, 1976). Rigorous standardization of growth and extract preparation is required in such comparisons. There are indications of subspecies characteristics in the polysaccharide antigens of *T. cruzi*

* See Note 4, p. 195.

culture forms (Ketteridge, personal communication). Ketteridge (1975b) found differences in porphyrin residues of *T. cruzi*, grown in diphasic culture media, from man and domestic animals in São Felipe, although the organisms were believed to be derived from a single domestic cycle of transmission, and subsequently shown to have six identical electrophoretic enzyme patterns (see below). Polyacrylamide electrophoresis of polypeptides, from sodium dodecylsulphate disintegrated *T. cruzi*, suggests some variation in the constituent bands but the interpretation of results is extremely difficult (Taylor and Edwards, personal communication). Enzyme concentrations are said to be capable of distinguishing subspecies of *T. brucei* (Steiger *et al.*, 1974). A more promising aspect of the analysis of cell composition is the plausibility of biochemical definition by the presence or absence of structure or spectral properties of a single component, such as an enzyme.

In the characterization of organisms by enzyme electrophoresis, crude extracts of organisms or tissues are electrophoresed in a starch gel or other medium. The mobility of components of an enzyme can be compared, following addition of the appropriate substrate, linked to a visualization process. Since its development (Hunter and Markert, 1957), the method has had enormous application, particularly in the field of population genetics (Markert, 1975). Among the parasitic protozoa the technique has been applied to *Entamoeba*, *Plasmodium*, *Leishmania*, *Coccidia* and *Trypanosoma* (Reeves and Bischoff, 1968; Carter and McGregor, 1973; Carter and Voller, 1975; Gardener *et al.*, 1974; Kilgour *et al.*, 1974; Rollinson, 1976; Shirley, 1975; Miles *et al.*, 1977). The demonstration that the enzyme pattern correlated well with trypanosomes causing chronic, as distinct from acute, African trypanosomiasis, and with serological grouping (Godfrey and Kilgour, 1976) suggests that this is currently the most powerful, simple technique of identifying distinct strains of parasitic protozoa.

It has been demonstrated that *T. cruzi* collected from widely separated geographical areas differ in the electrophoretic patterns of aspartate aminotransferase (ASAT, E.C.2.6.1.1), alanine aminotransferase (ALAT, E.C.2.6.1.2.) and other enzymes (Toyé, 1974; Toyé, personal communication). A selection of *T. cruzi* from São Felipe, where, as described above (Section IV, C, 4), domestic and sylvatic transmission cycles were judged on general epidemiological grounds to be non-overlapping, have been examined by enzyme electrophoresis (Miles *et al.*, 1977). Eleven trypanosome stocks were from domestic acute or chronic human cases, dog, cat, house mouse, rat or guinea-pig, and six were from sylvatic opossum (*Didelphis*) or *Triatoma tibiamaculata*, the suspected vector of *T. cruzi* to the opossum (Fig. 1). The six enzymes used, in this case, were: ASAT; ALAT; glucose-6-phosphate dehydrogenase (G6PD, E.C.1.1.1.49); malate dehydrogenase (decarboxylating) (NADP+) (ME,

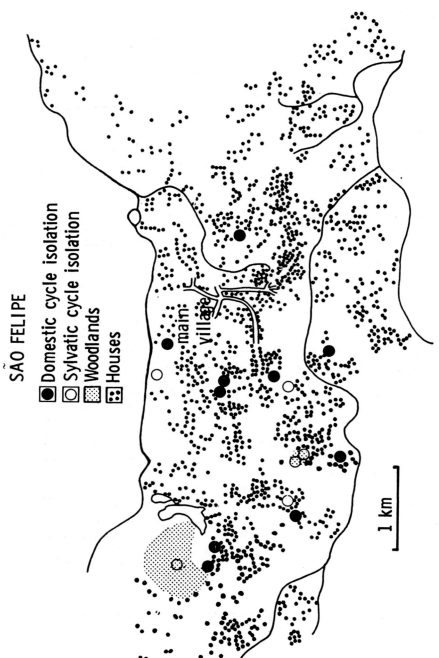

FIG. 1. The distribution of the sources of 16 out of 17 *Trypanosoma cruzi* stocks, within the district of São Felipe, which have been examined by enzyme electrophoresis. One stock is omitted as the source location is unknown. Compare with the enzyme patterns shown in Fig. 2.

SÃO FELIPE

- ● Domestic cycle isolation
- ○ Sylvatic cycle isolation
- ▨ Woodlands
- ⊞ Houses

main
village

1 km

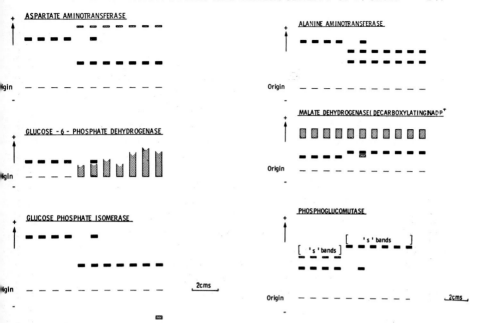

FIG. 2. Diagram summarizing electrophoretic patterns, for six enzymes, of culture forms of ten *Trypanosoma cruzi* stocks from São Felipe. The most prominent, distinct, bands are shown in black; faint or diffuse bands are stippled. "S" bands indicate the region of additional satellite bands which were too faint to be clearly resolved. All patterns were reproducible, with the exception of the G6PD patterns of sylvatic stocks which were diffuse and streaked from the origin.

Note the two distinct combinations of isoenzyme patterns, one characteristic of domestic stocks of *T. cruzi* derived from both human infections and domiciliated animals, the second characteristic of sylvatic stocks from opossums and a sylvatic triatomine species. A further seven stocks examined corresponded with this subdivision into two quite different, but enzymically homogeneous, strain-groups. Compare with Fig. 1.

The enzyme extracts are of stocks derived from the following hosts, numbered from left to right: 1. man—acute case (SF BAHIA/72/Rita/81); 2. man—chronic case (SF BAHIA/72/Phillipa/82); 3. cat (SF BAHIA/73/Cat C/36); 4. rat (SF BAHIA/72/Rat B/6); 5. sylvatic triatomine (SF BAHIA/74/*Triatoma tibiamaculata*, 3051/151); 6. extracts 4 and 5 mixed; 7. opossum (SF BAHIA/75/*Didelphis azarae*, WA301/130); 8. opossum (SF BAHIA/74/*Didelphis azarae*, WA207/191); 9. opossum (SF BAHIA/71/*Didelphis azarae*, WA6/184); 10. opossum (SF BAHIA/71/*Didelphis azarae*, WA7/183); 11. opossum (SF BAHIA/75/*Didelphis azarae*, WA250/186); (reference standard extract not shown).

"malic enzyme", E.C.1.1.1.40); glucosephosphate isomerase (GPI, E.C. 5.3.1.9); and phosphoglucomutase (PGM, E.C.2.7.5.1.)

The results of enzyme electrophoresis divided *T. cruzi* from São Felipe into two distinct strain-groups, each group enzymically homogeneous, corresponding to the eleven stocks of *T. cruzi* from the domestic cycle, and the six stocks from the sylvatic cycle (Fig. 2). The enzyme patterns were independent of the original host and the two types of culture medium used. It was concluded that the transmission cycles in São Felipe were indeed separate, and that the organisms circulating in the two cycles were quite different. Enzyme electrophoresis is thus shown to be a useful additional technique of investigating overlap of transmission cycles (Section IV, C, 5g).

We believe that the domestic form of *T. cruzi* was probably brought to São Felipe when the local domestic vector, *P. megistus*, invaded northeastern Brazil by dispersion from the south,* and that it continues to circulate independently of the possibly indigenous sylvatic form. This view was supported by the failure to find *P. megistus* in sylvatic ecotopes.

Preliminary observations suggest that the two organisms from São Felipe may behave differently in experimental mice—the sylvatic form producing less easily detectable infections in the blood than the domestic form; the full behavioural differences of the two strain-groups remain to be discovered.

It must be stressed that there is absolutely no evidence to suggest that the sylvatic organism in São Felipe is unable to infect man. On the contrary, recent examination of a few enzymes of *T. cruzi* from other, distant, localities, lead us to suppose that *T. cruzi*, like that in the sylvatic São Felipe cycle, occurs in a variety of hosts, including, and not excluding, man (Miles and Toyé, unpublished observations). Thus, for the first time, there is very sound evidence, not only that at least two enzymically distinct types of *T. cruzi* are circulating in nature, but also that they can both infect man. It is not yet known if these enzyme characters of *T. cruzi* correlate with biological behaviour, such as the pattern and distribution of human disease. However, the occurrence of distinct *T. cruzi* strain-groups infecting man is a most plausible explanation for the observed biological and clinical diversity among *T. cruzi* (Section V, A–G) (see Addendum, p. 188).

Some isoenzyme differences reflect variant genetic determinants, but, as explained below, not all genetic changes may produce new isoenzymes. If random, frequent, mutation produces new, irrelevant or physiologically-advantageous, isoenzymes, a vast array of isoenzyme combinations might be expected among *T. cruzi* in nature. However, the recurrence of indistinguishable combinations of enzyme patterns among both *T. cruzi* and *T. vespertilionis* from distant locations (Miles, unpublished data; Baker *et al.*, in preparation†), suggests that, although very few enzyme markers have been used, the number of different types of *T. cruzi* may be quite limited.

Enthusiasm for identification of *T. cruzi* strain-groups by isoenzyme electrophoresis is tempered by several provisos and pitfalls:

(a) Enzyme differences do not necessarily reflect genetic hetero-

* See Note 5, p. 195.   † See Note 6, p. 195.

geneity. Markert (1968) recognizes at least eight molecular bases for isoenzymes: once formed, enzymes may be altered by processes such as terminal amino acid deletion, polymerization, conjugation with small molecules, conformational change, and simple chemical modification such as decarboxylation or deamination of component amino acids.

(b) Chemical modification of enzymes may occur *in vitro*, during extraction, purification or exposure to mild chemical agents, giving altered mobility or multiplicity of bands; there is evidence that some simple buffer components cause such changes (Hopkinson, 1975).

(c) Enzymes are affected by storage conditions, especially temperature, causing disruption or inactivation. Optimum conditions are not the same for all enzymes.

(d) Careful development controls are required if the nature of the reactions studied are to be understood, as some enzymes have broad substrate specificities, and substrates may be unwittingly supplied with reagent contaminants.

(e) Mixed populations of organisms may give misleading multiplicity of bands unless the material used is derived from clones.

(f) Enzyme forms may vary with developmental stage of the organism, hence the need to compare identical morphological forms.

(g) It is not known to what extent interchange of *T. cruzi* enzyme repertoire may occur in nature, in response to epidemiological pressures, although in *T. vivax* Kilgour and Godfrey (1977) report stability of enzyme patterns circulating in cattle herds, after one year, and identical *T. cruzi* pattern combinations may be found in a variety of hosts and vectors (Miles, unpublished observations).

(h) Only a proportion of amino acid substitutions result in charge differences detectable by electrophoresis.

(i) Comparisons of band patterns is to some extent subjective; especially when bands corresponding in position are judged identical; enzyme concentration must be considered and reference enzyme extracts constantly used on electrophoretic plates.

Many of these objections can be overcome by control experiment and standardizing handling procedures. When bands are single, mixed populations are an unlikely complication. Even so, controlled, clonal growth of *T. cruzi* in defined media is the ideal basis for obtaining material for electrophoretic comparisons.

Subdivision of *T. cruzi* by isoenzyme combination is of little value unless related to significant biological characters. However, the presence of a large number of potential enzyme markers and the preliminary results from São Felipe promise, given reliable means of comparison in different laboratories, a meaningful classification of *T. cruzi* stocks by enzyme types. Furthermore, the technique can be used in unsophisticated laboratories. With the possible exception of slide DNA hybridization (Steinert *et al.*, 1976), the need for highly-developed laboratories is a severe limitation to other biochemical methods of characterization. Assuming that the promise of enzyme electrophoresis correlating with biological characters is fulfilled, and given adequate resources, we might, optimistically, speculate upon the following applications:

(i) the identification of *T. cruzi* strains significant to man, mapping of their enzootic and endemic distribution, and tracing of their origins;

(ii) forecasting the prognosis of particular infected individuals, or of inhabitants of a given endemic focus, based on the type of *T. cruzi* they carry;

(iii) making a more rational selection of *T. cruzi* used for chemotherapeutic or immunological comparisons;

(iv) the investigation of physiologically adaptive change in isoenzyme form during the life cycle;

(v) the initiation of genetic studies, using marker enzymes to confirm the presence or prove the absence of genetic transfer in *T. cruzi*.

Newton (1976) predicts that protozoan taxonomy, still almost entirely dependent on comparative morphology, will develop, like bacterial systematics, to use a wide range of biochemical, physiological and nutritional characters in a form of numerical taxonomy.

Ultimately, total DNA base-sequencing may be applicable to protozoal classification. Already less demanding means of crude DNA analysis are being adopted, such as: by the determination of base ratios, from either the products of DNA hydrolysis, DNA buoyant density measurement, or DNA melting temperature; and by nearest neighbour frequency analysis (Newton, 1976). In addition, DNA homologies between two organism populations can be assessed from the degree of hybridization of the two sources of heat-denatured single DNA strands, one of which is labelled with isotopes. Alternatively, labelled RNA can be synthesized on a DNA template and used to measure homologies between its template and other DNA's; this latter method is particularly promising.

Recently, of these methods, DNA analysis by cleaving doublestranded DNA with restriction endonucleases, DNA buoyant density measurements, DNA melting temperature determination, and hybridization studies, have been applied to characterization of trypanosome species. The presence of the kinetoplast provides an additional component for these investigations as kinetoplast DNA has sequence heterogeneity which can be used in comparisons. Kinetoplast DNA appears as a separate band on caesium chloride centrifugation gradients, and can be used in RNA/DNA hybridization experiments (Newton, 1976). Riou and Yot (1975) and Steinert *et al.* (1973) have used restriction endonucleases and hybridization studies to examine *T. cruzi* and indicate degrees of homology with other species. DNA buoyant density measurements in the subgenus *Trypanozoon*, although showing little variation in nuclear and kinetoplast DNA densities, do show a satellite band apparently unique to *T. brucei gambiense* (Newton, 1976). Steinert *et al.* (1976) detected considerable variation in computer analysed DNA melting profiles of kinetoplastid species, and melting profiles of *Trypanosoma mega* varied according to the history and origin of material (Steinert and Van Assel, 1974). DNA hybridization can now be performed on slides, and Steinert *et al.* (1976) distinguished subspecies of *T. brucei* by hybridization of denatured kinetoplast DNA in smears of whole organisms or lysates. However, with the exception of slide hybridization, all these techniques of DNA analysis require sophisticated laboratories and are impractical for routine use.

DNA buoyancy and restriction endonuclease analysis have been applied to subspecies characterization of *T. cruzi*. Six of the domestic trypanosome stocks from São Felipe, which had the same combination of enzyme patterns (Fig. 2), were indistinguishable by nuclear and kinetoplast DNA buoyant densities (Newton, 1976). The sylvatic trypanosome stocks from São Felipe have not yet been examined by DNA buoyancy but *T. cruzi* from elsewhere, with similar enzyme patterns, did not give significant differences in buoyant density measurements (Newton and Ketteridge, personal communication). Enzyme electrophoresis is thus perhaps a more sensitive means of strain distinction, but without the advantage of direct DNA analysis. Gradient centrifugation in caesium chloride can only detect density differences of about 0·001 gm/ml, or 1 %, in overall guanine and cytosine composition, and gives no information on base sequences (Newton, 1976). The gross nature of distinctions by DNA buoyance is emphasized by recurrence of the same density readings in nuclear and kinetoplast DNA of flagellates thought to be distant relatives and placed in separate genera (Newton, 1976). Using restriction endonuclease analysis of kinetoplast DNA Brack *et al.* (1976) and Riou (1976) were able to show subspecies differences among *T. cruzi*; in Riou's case these were found to be associated with drug resistance. With the same technique, Mattei *et al.* (1977) found pronounced differences between four *T. cruzi* of different histories.

In combination, DNA buoyant density and enzyme electrophoresis have transformed taxonomic studies of the genus *Leishmania* and slide hybridization studies have begun (Chance *et al.*, 1974; Gardener *et al.*, 1974; Chance, 1976); correspondence with biological and epidemiological observations of *Leishmania*, implicit to the value of such methods, has been good (Lainson and Shaw, this volume). We have recently been able to compare DNA buoyancy with enzyme electrophoresis for selected representatives of the genus *Schizotrypanum* from bats in Europe and South America (Baker *et al.*, in preparation). DNA buoyant density separated *T. dionisii* from *T. vespertilionis* of Europe and *T.*

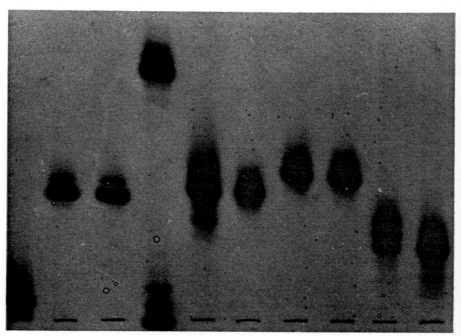

FIG. 3. An example of a zymogram of *Schizotrypanum* stocks from European and South American bats. The enzyme is glucose phosphate isomerase. From left to right enzyme extracts are derived from 1: *T, dionisii*—Europe; 2 and 3: *T. vespertilionis*—Europe; 4 to 10: *T. vespertilionis*—South America. DNA buoyancy separates *T. dionisii* from European *T. vespertilionis* and South American *T. vespertilionis*. Enzyme electrophoresis has so far confirmed these three DNA buoyancy groups but given many additional enzyme subdivisions within South American *T. vespertilionis*. Investigations are too incomplete to allow comparisons between South American *T. vespertilionsis* and *T. cruzi* (from Baker *et al.*, in preparation).

vespertilionis of South America. Results of enzyme electrophoresis corresponded with the 3 groups but with subdivisions within each (Fig. 3). *T. cruzi* was closely similar but separable from South American *T. vespertilionis* by buoyant densities. Enzyme comparisons of *T. cruzi* and *T. vespertilionis* are too incomplete to allow relationships to be assessed.

The degree of discordancy in observed and experimental Chagas' disease seems to be at least partially due to the heterogeneity of *T. cruzi*, now clearly demonstrated by enzyme electrophoresis. Biochemical methods of intrinsic taxonomy are in their infancy as applied to the parasitic protozoa. However, it is abundantly clear that enzyme electrophoresis and improved means of DNA analysis will revolutionize classical systematics, rationalize experimental subspecies comparisons, and counteract confusion, which in the past has occurred even at species level (Deane and Kloetzel, 1974). Some of these methods, such as enzyme electrophoresis, slide hybridization, and possibly restriction endonuclease analysis, should find routine epidemiological applications.

VII. Prospects of Chagas' disease research

A. IMMUNE RESPONSE, IMMUNOPATHOGENESIS AND VACCINATION

Despite the recent explosion of interest in *T. cruzi*, understanding of the organism and the relationship to its vertebrate host remains diffuse; control of Chagas' disease, whether by vaccination, therapy or suppression of vectors, is a distant objective.

The mechanism whereby the vertebrate immune response modulates infections of the salivarian trypanosome *T. brucei* is well known. Successive surface antigenic variants produce peaks of parasitaemia which are principally destroyed by variant-specific antibodies. *In vitro* these antibodies agglutinate, lyse and neutralize trypanosomes of the appropriate variant; *in vivo* persistently elevated IgM and IgG levels occur (Bridgen *et al.*, 1976; Gray and Luckins, 1976; and others).

In *T. cruzi* infection antibody is consistently present, as shown by serological testing of patients and most experimental hosts (see III above), but serum IgM is apparently only elevated in the initial phase of infection (Camargo and Amato Neto, 1974; Hanson *et al.*, 1974). Attempts to demonstrate *in vitro* effects of immune sera against *T. cruzi* have been conflicting (WHO, 1974). Complement-mediated lysis of cultured epimastigotes of *T. cruzi* occurs *in vitro* in some normal mammalian sera (Goble, 1970), and of haematozoic trypomastigotes *in vitro* and *in vivo* in normal chicken serum (Kierszenbaum *et al.*, 1976). Agglutination of enzyme-treated epimastigotes by immune sera has been used as a diagnostic test (Vattuone and Yanovsky, 1971; and others). Budzko *et al.* (1975) report that complement depletion *in vivo* by cobra venom factor exacerbates *T. cruzi* infection; *in vitro* trypomastigotes were lysed by immune human or mouse sera in the presence of active complement. Kierszenbaum and Howard (1976) correlated antibody-forming capacity in low-responding Ab/L and high-responding AbH mice with their susceptibility to infection with both Y and Tulahuén *T. cruzi*; Ab/L mice could be effectively protected by passive transfer of immune plasma. Krettli and Brener (1976) report that Y trypomastigotes were agglutinated, and their infectivity was decreased, by anti-Y or anti-Cl immune mouse sera, and by sera from chronic cases of Chagas' disease, whereas Cl trypomastigotes were totally unaffected by the same treatment (see Section V, G). In contrast, Kierszenbaum (1976) demonstrated, *in vitro*, lytic cross-reactivity of antibodies against Y and Tulahuén *T. cruzi* trypomastigotes. Finally, Teixeira (1976), using *Ernestina* trypomastigotes *in vitro*, found that "humoral antibodies have no demonstrable effect on trypomastigotes of *T. cruzi* in the presence or absence of serum complement factors."

The conflicting data summarized above, is reconcilable if, as several authors suggest, intrinsically different types of *T. cruzi* have been used in these investigations, or if antigenic variation, as yet unproven in *T. cruzi*, is complicating the interpretation of the experiments.

Cell mediated immunity in *T. cruzi* infection, reviewed recently by Hoff (1976), has been demonstrated *in vitro* by lymphoblast transformation, peripheral leucocyte migration inhibition, inhibition of peritoneal exudate cell migration, and macrophage spreading inhibition. *In vivo* the infiltration of lesions of Chagas' disease with lymphocytes and macrophages is characteristic of cell mediated immunity, but there are conflicting reports of skin test reactivity, possibly due to the different patterns of Chagas' disease or because standardized antigen preparations have not been used. While still not conclusively demonstrated, the balance of the evidence from thymectomy, adoptive transfer and cross-immunity experiments strongly suggests that cell mediated immunity plays a role in protective immunity.

Immunocytotoxic assays have recently been used to demonstrate complement-dependent lysis of *T. cruzi* in immune sera (Kühn and Vaughn, 1976). A similar method has shown the interaction of humoral and cell mediated immunity in the complement-independent lysis of *T. (Schizotrypanum) dionisii* by normal lymphocytes plus antiserum (Mkwananzi *et al.*, 1976).

Because of the difficulties, outlined above, in studying the *in vitro* effects of antibody against *T. cruzi* trypomastigotes only a single author (Dzbenski, 1974) presents, equivocal evidence that any antigenic variation occurs in the course of *T. cruzi* parasitaemia; other workers suggest, on the basis of indirect evidence, that it does not (Gonzalez-Cappa, 1976). If antigenic variation does not occur in *T. cruzi*, there are several other mechanisms which may explain the persistence of the *T. cruzi* in an apparently immune host:

(a) Intracellular forms may be protected from the immune response, and some trypomastigotes emerging from pseudocysts may rapidly penetrate nearby cells, without leaving the tissue.

(b) Circulating trypomastigotes may mimic host antigens by adsorption of serum proteins.

(c) Some trypomastigotes may possess or derive antigens which are common to, or indistinguishable from, host tissue components and therefore be unrecognizable by the immune response.

A series of recent publications implicates the second and third of these factors in the persistence of *T. cruzi* in its host irrespective of the occurrence of trypomastigote antigenic variation. With at least some of the heterogeneous *T. cruzi* infecting man, these same factors may generate an immuno-pathogenesis, either in addition to, or involved in, the neurone destruction which precipitates mega syndromes. Anti-nuclear, anti-neuronal, anti-skeletal muscle, anti-endocardial and anti-endothelial antibodies have been demonstrated in *T. cruzi* infections (Szarfman *et al.*, 1975; Laguens *et al.*, 1975; Hubsch *et al.*, 1976; Santos and Oliveira, 1976; and others). Furthermore, an autoimmune-type delayed hypersensitivity can be produced *in vivo* by administration of certain *T. cruzi* antigens, and *T. cruzi*-sensitized rabbit lymphocytes will destroy allogeneic heart cells *in vitro* (reviewed by Teixeira, 1976). The cross-reaction of heart antigens and *T. cruzi* antigens *in vitro* has also been reported in leucocyte migration inhibition tests (Vega *et al.*, 1976).

Animals which have suffered a mild *T. cruzi* infection can be superinfected with excessive challenge of highly virulent *T. cruzi* from a different source (Andrade *et al.*, 1970b). Even so, using unnatural challenge routes, and principally haematozoic trypomastigotes, cross-protection against normally lethal challenge is a consistent feature of experimental comparisons between *T. cruzi* of diverse origins. This gives rise to considerable optimism over vaccination prospects. In view of the versatile behaviour of *T. cruzi* during maintenance, it is unlikely that the attenuated live vaccines, recorded in the literature (Menezes, 1971) even of well-characterized organisms, will readily become acceptable. However, irradiated vaccines and various antigen preparations show a promising degree of protection (Hanson *et al.*, 1976; Gonzalez-Cappa, 1976; Gonzalez-Cappa *et al.*, 1976; Segura *et al.*, 1976; and others). The absence of induced immuno-pathogenesis will be an essential criterion for any prospective vaccine.

Evidence of sensitization to triatomine bites, which prevents successful subsequent feeding, presents a novel research avenue for vaccination using vector antigens (Gardiner and Maddrell, 1972).

B. CHEMOTHERAPY

Rapid progress in comprehension of *T. cruzi* metabolism, and perhaps a rational biochemical approach to chemotherapy, should result from the recent development of defined culture media for *T. cruzi* (Cross *et al.*,

1975; Scott and Krassner, 1975; Mundin *et al.*, 1976; Gutteridge, personal communication). The drug available at present, Lampit, is certainly of use in treating acute Chagas' disease, but there is an urgent need for a safe, non-toxic agent of indisputable efficacy in eradicating the organism from chronic cases, and for an improved additive to transfusion blood. Acute cases of Chagas' disease are extremely rarely seen, and, at least in *T cruzi* infections which induce mega syndromes, a pathogenic role, beyond the acute phase, for the persistent low-grade parasitaemia has been questioned. Thus, a new chemotherapeutic agent may not be a "cure-all" for the Chagas' disease problem, although, if routinely distributed, it may eradicate the human source of infection to the vector.

C. VECTOR CONTROL

Suppression of triatomine infestation by insecticides is the mainstay of Chagas' disease control; in the absence of "miracle" low-cost measures, such as vaccines, or elevation of socio-economic conditions for the rural population of South America, this is likely to remain the case. Penetration of insecticide sprays into deeply creviced walls, residual effect on a variety of surfaces, ovicidal properties, and avoidance of insecticide resistance, are desirable attributes, which, in ideal combination, have not yet been found among the variety of compounds tested (Fomm and Gandini, 1971; Gonzalez *et al.*, 1971; Schenone *et al.*,1972, Cockburn, personal communication). There is evidence that, unless frequently applied, insecticides often do not eradicate household bugs, and it has been suggested that rapid recrudescence of infestation may occur due to destruction of natural predators (Berti and Gonzalez, 1969; Forattini *et al.*, 1969; Barrett, 1976; Barrett and Miles, unpublished observations). Biological control by juvenile hormones, microhymenopteran or other vector parasites are possible future adjuncts to insecticides (Barrett, 1976; Gilbert, 1976). However, the main prospects for improvement in vector control seem to lie in a systematic re-examination of the performance of the compounds currently in use and the selection of their desirable properties. Dias and Garcia (1976) have shown that, given careful use, insecticides combined with surveillance and self-reliant control measures can successfully, and continuously, suppress household triatomine infestation.

VIII. Concluding remarks

In a simplification of the complex *T. cruzi* zoonosis, I have classed localities as enzootic or, alternatively, as having continuous or discontinuous sylvatic and domestic transmission cycles. Rural development areas are threatened by sylvatic Triatominae, and by the spread of discontinuous transmission as house-adapted vectors extend their range. Isoenzyme electrophoresis provides a method of assessing where cycle continuity occurs and if the same *T. cruzi* strain-group is both sylvatic and domestic. The identification of at least two enzymically distinct *T. cruzi* strain-groups, both of which may infect a variety of hosts, including man, confirms the manifold, circumstantial evidence of the heterogeneity of *T. cruzi*. The biochemical identification of trypanosomes should give a rational basis for subspecies comparisons and be a considerable impetus to research. However, there is an essential need to relate such novel development to the epidemiology and aetiology of the human disease.

IX. Acknowledgements

I am grateful to all collaborators and friends, who have contributed, directly or indirectly, to some of the research included here. In particular, I thank: in Brazil; Professor A. Prata and his colleagues (now at Brazilia University) for the invitation to participate in his project at São Felipe, Bahia; Dr. P. D. Marsden for an introduction to Chagas' disease beyond the laboratory bench; members of the Wellcome, London research group in Salvador, Bahia; Dr. R. Lainson and colleagues of the Wellcome Parasitology group at the Instituto Evandro Chagas, Belém, Pará; and, in London, staff of the Department of Medical Protozoology at the School of Hygiene and Tropical Medicine, especially Dr. D. G. Godfrey's Trypanosomiasis Research Group. I thank the editors of the Pan American Health Organization research publications, the Transactions of the Royal Society of Tropical Medicine and Hygiene and the American Journal of Tropical Medicine and Hygiene for permission to reproduce published material. I am indebted to the Wellcome Trust for financial support.

X. References

Afchain, D. (1976). Le caractère antigénique des *Trypanosomatidae* heteroxenes parasites de l'homme: *Trypanosoma (S.) cruzi, Trypanosoma (T.) b. gambiense* et *Leishmania donovani*. Thesis, Lille.

Afchain, D., Le Ray, D., Capron, A. and Jadin, J. (1973). Analyse antigenique comparée, par immunoelectrophorèse, des formes de culture de *Trypanosoma (Schizotrypanum) cruzi, Trypanosoma (Trypanozoon) brucei* et *Leishmania donovani*. Conséquences taxomomiques et diagnostiques. *Protistologica*, **9**, 213–220.

Albuquerque, R. D. R., Fernandes, L. A. R., Funayama, G. K., Ferriolli, F. F. and Siqueira, A. F. (1972). Hemoculturas seriadas com o meio de Warren em pacientes com reação de Guerreiro Machado positiva. *Revista do Instituto de Medicina Tropical de São Paulo*, **14**, 1–5.

Allain, D. S. and Kagan, I. G. (1974). An evaluation of the direct agglutination test for Chagas' disease. *Journal of Parasitology*, **60**, 179–184.

Almeida, F. B. (1971). Triatomineos da Amazonia. Encontro de tres especies naturalmente infectadas por *Trypanosoma* semelhante ao *cruzi*, no estado do Amazonas (Hemiptera, Reduviidae). *Acta Amazonica*, 1, 89–93.

Almeida, F. B. and Machado, P. A. (1971). Sôbre a infecção do *Panstrongylus geniculatus* pelo *Trypanosoma cruzi* em Manaus, Amazonas, Brasil. *Acta Amazonica*, 1, 71–75.

Almeida, F. B. de, Santos, E. I. and Sposina, G. (1973). Triatomineos da Amazonia. III. *Acta Amazonica*, 3, 43–46.

Almeida, J. O. and Fife, E. H. Jr. (1976). Quantitatively standardized complement-fixation methods for critical evaluation of antigens prepared from *Trypanosoma cruzi*. *Pan American Health Organization, Scientific Publication* 319.

Alves, M. J. M. and Colli, W. (1974). Agglutination of *Trypanosoma cruzi* by concanavalin A. *Journal of Protozoology*, 21, 575–578.

Andrade, S. G., Carvalho, M. L. and Figueira, R. M. (1970a). Caracterização morfo-biológica e histopatológica de diferentes cêpas do *Trypanosoma cruzi*. *Gazeta Medica da Bahia*, 70, 32–42.

Andrade, S. G., Carvalho, M. L., Figueira, R. M. and Andrade, Z. A. (1970b). Recuperação e caracterização de tripanosomas inoculados em animais imunes. (Reinoculação com diferentes cêpas do *T. cruzi*). *Revista do Instituto de Medicina Tropical de São Paulo*, 12, 395–402.

Andrade, Z. A. (1976). Chagas' disease: Pathology of the cardiac lesions. *In:* "New Approaches in American Trypanosomiasis Research". Proceedings of an International Symposium, Belo Horizonte, Minas Gerais, Brazil, 18–21 March 1975. Pan American Health Organization, Washington. Scientific Publication No. 318, 146–151.

Andrade, Z. A. and Andrade, S. G. (1969). Estudo imunocitoquimico da doença de Chagas experimental. *Revista do Instituto de Medicina Tropical de São Paulo*, 11, 44–47.

Anonymous (1972). Proceedings: Simposio internacional sobre enfermedad de Chagas. Buenos Aires, December 1972. Secretaria de Estado de Salud Publica, Buenos Aires, Argentina.

Anonymous (1976). *In:* "New approaches in American Trypanosomiasis Research". Proceedings of an International Symposium, Belo Horizonte, Minas Gerais, Brazil, 18–21 March 1975. Pan American Health Organization, Washington. Scientific Publication No. 318, 410 pp.

Barbosa, A. J. A., Pittella, J. E. H. and Tafuri, W. L. (1970). Incidência da cardiopatia chagasica em 15,000 necropsias consecutivas e sua associação com os "megas". *Revista da Sociedade Brasileira de Medicina Tropical*, 4, 219–223.

Barrett, T. V. (1976). Parasites and predators of Triatominae. *In:* "New Approaches in American Trypanosomiasis Research". Proceedings of an International Symposium, Belo Horizonte, Minas Gerais, Brazil, 18–21 March 1975. Pan American Health Organization, Washington. Pan Scientific Publication No. 318, 24–32.

Barretto, M. P. (1963). Reservatórios e vectores do *Trypanosoma cruzi* no Brasil. *Arquivos de Higiene e Saúde Pública*, 28, 43–66.

Barretto, M. P. (1965). Tripanossomos semelhantes ao *Trypanosoma cruzi* em animais silvestres e sua identificação com o agente etiologico da doença de Chagas. *Revista do Instituto de Medicina Tropical de São Paulo*, 7, 305–315.

Barretto, M. P. (1968). Transmissores do *Trypanosoma cruzi*: os triatomineos. *In:* "Doença de Chagas" (Ed. J. R. Cancado), pp. 189–224. Belo Horizonte, 1968.

Barretto, M. P. (1970). Estudos sôbre reservatórios e vectores silvestres do *Trypanosoma cruzi*. XLIII. Sôbre a validade das especies americanas de flagelados incluidos no subgenero *Schizotrypanum* Chagas 1909 do genero *Trypanosoma* Gruby 1843. *Revista do Instituto de Medicina Tropical de São Paulo*, 12, 272–278.

Barretto, M. P. (1976). Possible role of wild mammals and triatomines in the transmission of *Trypanosoma cruzi* to man. *In:* "New Approaches in American Trypanosomiasis Research". Proceedings of an International Symposium, Belo Horizonte, Minas Gerais, Brazil, 18–21 March 1975. Pan American Health Organization, Washington. Scientific Publication No. 318, 307–318.

Barretto, M. P. and Ferriolli, F. Filho (1964). Estudos sôbre reservatórios e vectores silvestres do *Trypanosoma cruzi*. IV. Infecção natural do *Triatoma infestans*, encontrado em ecótopos silvestres, por tripanossomo semelhante ao *T. cruzi*. *Revista do Instituto de Medicina Tropical de São Paulo*, **6**, 219–224.

Barretto, M. P., Siqueira, A. F. and Correa, F. M. A. (1963). Estudos sôbre reservatórios e vectores silvestres do *Trypanosoma cruzi*. I. Encontro do *Triatoma infestans* (Hemiptera, Reduviidae) em ecótopos silvestres. *Revista do Instituto de Medicina Tropical de São Paulo*, **5**, 289–293.

Barretto, M. P., Siqueira, A. F. and Freitas, J. L. P. (1964). Estudos sôbre reservatórios e vectores silvestres do *Trypanosoma cruzi*. II. Encontro do *Panstrongylus megistus* em ecótopos silvestres no Estado de São Paulo (Hemiptera, Reduviidae). *Revista do Instituto de Medicina Tropical de São Paulo*, **6**, 56–63.

Becker, P. F. L. (1975). Moléstia de Chagas aguda acidental. (Por transfusão de sangue de doador chagasico). *Revista do Instituto de Medicina Tropical de São Paulo*, **17**, 187–198.

Behbehani, M. K. (1972). Interactions between *Trypanosoma* (*Schizotrypanum*) *cruzi* and cells of vertebrate hosts *in vitro* and *in vivo*. Ph.D. Thesis, London, April 1972.

Berti, A. L. and Gonzalez Valdivieso, F. (1969). Control de triatomineos en Venezuela. *Boletin Informativo de la Direccion de Marariologia y Saneamiento Ambiental*, **9**, 3–14.

Bice, D. E. and Zeledón, R. (1970). Comparison of infectivity of strains of *Trypanosoma cruzi* (Chagas 1909). *Journal of Parasitology*, **56**, 663–670.

Bittencourt, A. L. (1976). Pathologic aspects of congenital transmission of *T. cruzi*. *In:* "New Approaches in American Trypanosomiasis Research". Proceedings of an International Symposium, Belo Horizonte, Minas Gerais, Brazil, 18–21 March 1975. Pan American Health Organization, Washington. Scientific Publication No. 318, 216–222.

Blandon, R., Edgecomb, J. H., Guevara, J. F. and Johnson, C. M. (1974). Electrocardiographic changes in Panamanian *Rattus rattus* naturally infected by *Trypanosoma cruzi*. *American Heart Journal*, **88**, 758–764.

Boreham, P. F. L. (1975). Some applications of bloodmeal identifications in relation to the epidemiology of vector-borne tropical diseases. *The Journal of Tropical Medicine and Hygiene*, **78**, 83–91.

Brack, C. (1968). Elektronenmikroskopische untersuchungen zum leben szyklus von *Trypanosoma cruzi*. Unter besonderer Berücksichtigung der entwicklungsformen im uebertrãger *Rhodnius prolixus*. *Acta Tropica*, **25**, 289–356.

Brack, C. L., Bickle, T. A., Yuan, R., Barker, D. C., Foulkes, M., Newton, B. A. and Jenni, L. (1976). The use of restriction endonucleases for the investigation of kinetoplast DNA. *In:* "Biochemistry of Parasites and Host–Parasite Relationships" (Ed. H. Van den Bossche), pp. 211–218. Janssen Research Foundation. Elsevier/North Holland Biomedical Press, Amsterdam.

Brener, Z. (1969). The behaviour of slender and stout forms of *Trypanosoma cruzi* in the blood-stream of normal and immune mice. *Annals of Tropical Medicine and Parasitology*, **63**, 215–220.

Brener, Z. (1973). Biology of *Trypanosoma cruzi*. *Annual Review of Microbiology*, **27**, 347–382.

160   M. A. MILES

Brener, Z. (1976a). Significance of morphologic variation of bloodstream forms. *In:* "New Approaches in American Trypanosomiasis Research". Proceedings of an International Symposium, Belo Horizonte, Minas Gerais, Brazil, 18–21 March 1975. Pan American Health Organization, Washington. Scientific Publication No. 318, 127–131.

Brener, Z. (1976b). Summarization. *In:* "New Approaches in American Trypanosomiasis Research". Proceedings of an International Symposium, Belo Horizonte, Minas Gerais, Brazil, 18–21 March 1975. Pan American Health Organization, Washington. Scientific Publication No. 318, 403–410.

Bridgen, P. J., Cross, G. A. M. and Bridgen, J. (1976). N-terminal amino acid sequences of variant-specific surface antigens from *Trypanosoma brucei*. *Nature, London*, **263**, 613–614.

Brumpt, E. (1912). Le *Trypanosoma cruzi* évolue chez *Conorhinus megistus, Cimex lectularius, Cimex boueti* and *Ornithodorus moubata*. Cycle évolutif de ce parasite. *Bulletin de la Société de Pathologie Exotique*, **5**, 360–367.

Budzko, D. B. and Kierszenbaum, F. (1974). Isolation of *Trypanosoma cruzi* from blood. *Journal of Parasitology*, **60**, 1037–1038.

Budzko, D. B., Pizzimenti, M. C. and Kierszenbaum, F. (1975). Effects of complement depletion in experimental Chagas' disease: immune lysis of virulent blood forms of *Trypanosoma cruzi*. *Infection and Immunity*, **11**, 86–91.

Camargo, M. E. and Amato Neto, V. (1974). Anti-*Trypanosoma cruzi* IgM antibodies as serological evidence of recent infection. *Revista do Instituto de Medicina Tropical de São Paulo*, **16**, 200–202.

Camargo, M. E. and Lesser, P. G. (1974). Diagnostico acidental de laboratorio de infecções chagasicas agudas pós-transfusionais não suspeitadas. *Revista da Associação Medica do Brasil*, **20**, 335–336.

Camargo, M. E. and Shimizu, S. H. (1974). Metodologia sorológica na infecção pelo *Trypanosoma cruzi*. *Revista Goiana de Medicina*, **20**, 47–65.

Cançado, J. R. (Ed.) (1968). Doença de Chagas. Belo Horizonte, Minas Gerais, Brazil.

Cançado, J. R., Salgado, A. de A., Marra, U. D., Alvares, J. M. and Machado, J. R. (1975). Ensaio terapêutico clinico na doença de Chagas crônica com o nifurtimox em três esquemas de duração prolongada. *Revista do Instituto de Medicina Tropical de São Paulo*, **17**, 111–125.

Cançado, J. R., Salgado, A. A., Cardoso dos Santos, J. F., Batista, S. M. and Chiari, Clea (1976). Clinical trails in Chagas' disease. *In:* "New Approaches in American Trypanosomiasis Research". Proceedings of an International Symposium, Belo Horizonte, Minas Gerais, Brazil, 18–21 March 1975. Pan American Health Organization, Scientific Publication No. 318, 266–272.

Carter, R. and McGregor, I. A. (1973). Enzyme variation in *Plasmodium falciparum* in the Gambia. *Transactions of the Royal Society of Tropical Medicine and Hygiene*, **67**, 830–837.

Carter, R. and Voller, A. (1975). The distribution of enzyme variation in populations of *Plasmodium falciparum* in Africa. *Transactions of the Royal Society of Tropical Medicine and Hygiene*, **69**, 371–376.

Cerisola, J. A., Alvarez, M. and Rissio, A. M. (1970). Imunodiagnóstico da doença de Chagas. Evolução sorológica de pacientes com doença de Chagas. *Revista do Instituto de Medicina Tropical de São Paulo*, **12**, 403–411.

Cerisola, J. A., Del Prado, C. E., Rohwedder, R. and Bozzini, J. P. (1971a). *Blastocrithidia triatomae* n. sp. found in *Triatoma infestans* from Argentina. *Journal of Protozoology*, **18**, 503–506.

Cerisola, J. A., Rohwedder, R. W. and Del Prado, C. E. (1971b). Rendimiento del xenodiagnóstico en la infección chagásica crónica humana utilizanto ninfas de diferentes especies de triatominos. *Boletin Chileno de Parasitologia*, **26**, 57–58.

Cerisola, J. A., Rabinovich, A., Alvarez, M., Di Corleto, C. A. and Pruneda, J. (1972a). Enfermedad de Chagas y la transfusion de sangre. *Boletin de la Oficina Sanitaria Panamericana*, Washington, **73**, 203–221.

Cerisola, J. A., Lugones, H. and Rabinovich, L. B. (1972b). Tratamiento de la enfermedad de Chagas. Asociacion de Caballeros Argentinos de la Soberana Orden Militar de Malta, Avenida de Mayo 633, Buenos Aires. 75 pp.

Chagas, E. (1936). Infecção experimental do homen pelo *Schizotrypanum cruzi*. 9. Reunion de la Sociedad Argentina de Patologia Regional (Mendoza), **1**, 136–159.

Chance, M. L. (1976). DNA relationships in the genus *Leishmania*. In: "Biochemistry of Parasites and Host-Parasite Relationships" (Ed. H. Van den Bossche), pp. 229–235. Janssen Research Foundation, Elsevier/North Holland Biomedical Press, Amsterdam.

Chance, M. L., Peters, W. and Shchory, L. (1974). Biochemical taxonomy of *Leishmania*. I. Observations on DNA. *Annals of Tropical Medicine and Parasitology*, **68**, 307–316.

Cross, G. A. M., Klein, R. A. and Baker, J. R. (1975). *Trypanosoma cruzi*: growth, amino acid utilization and drug action in a defined medium. *Annals of Tropical Medicine and Parasitology*, **69**, 513–514.

D'Alessandro, A. (1976). Biology of *Trypanosoma* (*Herpetosoma*) *rangeli* Tejera 1920. In: "Biology of the Kinetoplastida" (Eds W. H. R. Lumsden and D. A. Evans), Vol. 1, pp. 327–434. Academic Press, London, New York, San Francisco.

D'Alessandro, A., Barretto, P. and Duarte, C. A. (1971). Distribution of triatomine-transmitted trypanosomiasis in Colombia and new records of the bugs and infections. *Journal of Medical Entomology*, **8**, 159–172.

Deane, L. M. (1958). Novo hospedeiro de tripanossomos dos tipos *cruzi* e *rangeli* encontrado no Estado do Pará: o marsupial *Metachirops opossum opossum*. *Revista Brasileira de Malariologia e Doenças Tropicais*, **10**, 531–542.

Deane, L. M. (1960). Sôbre um tripanossomo do tipo *cruzi* encontrado num rato silvestre, no Estado do Pará. *Revista Brasileira de Malariologia e Doenças Tropicais*, **12**, 87–102.

Deane, L. M. (1961). Tripanosomideos de mamiferos da Região Amazonica. I. Alguns flagelados encontrados no sangue de mamiferos silvestres do Estado do Pará. *Revista do Instituto de Medicina Tropical de São Paulo*, **3**, 15–28.

Deane, L. M. (1964). Tripanosomideos de mamiferos da Região Amazonica. III. Hemoscopia e xenodiagnostico de animais silvestres dos arredores de Belém, Pará. *Revista do Instituto de Medicina Tropical de São Paulo*, **6**, 225–232.

Deane, L. M. (1967). Tripanosomideos de mamiferos da Região Amazonica. IV. Hemoscopia e xenodiagnostico de animais silvestres da Estrada Belém-Brasilia. *Revista do Instituto de Medicina Tropical de São Paulo*, **9**, 143–148.

Deane, L. M. and Damasceno, R. G. (1961). Tripanosomideos de mamiferos da Região Amazonica. II. Tripanosomas de macacos da Zona do Salgado, Estado do Pará. *Revista do Instituto de Medicina Tropical de São Paulo*, **3**, 61–70.

Deane, M. P. and Damasceno, R. M. G. (1949). Encontro de *Panstrongylus lignarius* naturalmente infectado por tripanosoma do tipo *cruzi* e algumas notas sôbre a biologia. *Revista do Serviço Especial de Saúde Pública*, **2**, 809–814.

Deane, M. P. and Kloetzel, J. (1974). Lack of protection against *Trypanosoma cruzi* by multiple doses of *T. lewisi* culture forms. A discussion on some strains of "lewisi". *Experimental Parasitology*, **35**, 406–410.

Dias, E. (1940). Transmissão do *Schizotrypanum cruzi* entre vertebrados, por via digestiva. *Brasil-Medico*, **54**, 775.

Dias, J. C. P. and Garcia, A. L. R. (1976). Vigilancia epidemiologica con participacion comunitaria: un programa de enfermedad de Chagas. *International Journal of Health Education*, **19**, 29–44.

Diaz-Ungria, C. (1968). Estudio experimental del *Trypanosoma cruzi* en el perro y outros vertebrados. El problema de la transmision. *Kasmera*, **3**, 73–88.

Diaz Vazquez, A. (1971). Enfermedad de Chagas: bibliografía Venezolana. Dirreccíon de Malariología y Saneamiento Ambiental, Ministerio de Sauidad y Asistencia Social, Caracas, Venezuela. 100 pp.

Dvorak, J. A. (1976). New *in vitro* approach to quantitation of *Trypanosoma cruzi*–vertebrate cell interactions. *In:* "New Approaches in American Trypanosomiasis Research". Proceedings of an International Symposium, Belo Horizonte, Minas Gerais, Brazil, 18–21 March 1975. Pan American Health Organization, Washington. Scientific Publication No. 318, 109–120.

Dzbenski, T. H. (1974). Exoantigens of *Trypanosoma cruzi in vivo*. *Tropenmedizin und Parasitologie*, **25**, 485–491.

Farrar, W. E. Jr., Gibbins, S. D. and Whitfield, S. T. (1972). Low prevalence of antibody to *Trypanosoma cruzi* in Georgia. *American Journal of Tropical Medicine and Hygiene*, **21**, 404–406.

Fomm, A. S. and Gandini, P. (1971). Adsorção do isomero gama do BHC por diferentes tipos de barro. Avaliação biologica com *T. infestans*. *Revista Brasileira de Malariologia e Doenças Tropicais*, **23**, 111–123.

Forattini, O. P. (1976). Effects of control measures on vector population dynamics. *In:* "New Approaches in American Trypanosomiasis Research". Proceedings of an International Symposium, Belo Horizonte, Minas Gerais, Brazil, 18–21 March 1975. Pan American Health Organization, Washington. Scientific Publication No. 318, 21–23.

Forattini, O. P., Juarez, E., Rabello, E. X., Pattoli, D. and Correa, R. R. (1969). Infestação domiciliar por *Triatoma infestans* e alguns aspectos epidemiologicos da tripanossomose americana em area do Estado de São Paulo, Brasil. *Revista de Saúde Pública*, **3**, 159–172.

Forattini, O. P., Rabello, E. X., Castanho, M. L. S. and Pattoli, D. G. B. (1970). Aspectos ecologicos da tripanossomose americana. I. Observações sôbre *Panstrongylus megistus* e suas relações com focos naturais da infecção, em area urbana da cidade de São Paulo, Brasil. *Revista de Saude Publica*, **4**, 19–30.

Forattini, O. P., Ferreira, O. A., Rocha e Silva, E. O. da, and Rabello, E. X. (1973). Aspectos ecologicos da tripanossomose americana. V. Observações sôbre colonização espontânea de triatomineos silvestres em ecótopos artificiais, com especial referencia ao *Triatoma sordida*. *Revista de Saúde Pública*, **7**, 219–239.

Forattini, O. P., Ferreira, O. A., Rocha e Silva, E. O. da, and Rabello, E. X. (1975). Aspectos ecologicos da tripanossomose americana. VII. Permanencia e mobilidade do *Triatoma sordida* em relação aos ecótopos artificiais. *Revista de Saude Publica*, **9**, 467–476.

Freeman, F., Wilson, Peggy L. and Kazan, Betty H. (1975). *Trypanosoma cruzi*: Antimicrobial activity and strain differentiating properties of some five- and six-membered heterocyclic compounds on trypomastigotes. *Experimental Parasitology*, **38**, 181–190.

Gamboa, C. J. (1973). La poblacion silvestre de *Rhodnius prolixus* en Venezuela. *Archivos Venezolanos de Medicina Tropical y Parasitologia Medica*, **5**, 321–352.

Gardener, P. J., Chance, M. L. and Peters, W. (1974). Biochemical taxonomy of *Leishmania*. II. Electrophoretic variations of malate dehydrogenase. *Annals of Tropical Medicine and Parasitology*, **68**, 317–325.

Gardiner, B. O. C. and Maddrell, S. H. P. (1972). Techniques for routine and large-scale rearing of *Rhodnius prolixus* Stal (Hemiptera, Reduviidae). *Bulletin of Entomoligical Research*, **61**, 505–515.

Gilbert, B. (1976). Possible use of juvenile hormone mimics in vector control. *In:* "New Approaches in American Trypanosomiasis Research". Proceedings of an International Symposium, Belo Horizonte, Minas Gerais, Brazil, 18–21 March 1975. Pan American Health Organization, Washington. Scientific Publication No. 318, 282–288.

Goble, F. C. (1970). South American trypanosomes. *In:* "Immunity to Parasitic Animals" (Eds G. J. Jackson, R. Herman and I. Singer), Vol. 2, pp. 579–689. Appleton, New York.

Godfrey, D. G. and Kilgour, V. (1976). Enzyme electrophoresis in characterizing the causative organism of Gambian trypanosomiasis. *Transactions of the Royal Society of Tropical Medicine and Hygiene*, **70**, 219–224.

Goldberg, S. S., Silva Pereira, A. A., Chiari, E., Mares-Guia, M. and Gazzinelli, G. (1976). Comparative kinetics of arginine and lysine transport by epimastigotes and trypomastigotes from two strains of *Trypanosoma cruzi*. *Journal of Protozoology*, **23**, 179–186.

Gomez-Nunez, J. C. (1969). Resting places, dispersal and survival of Co_{60}-tagged *Rhodnius prolixus*. *Journal of Medical Entomology*, **6**, 83–86.

Gonzalez-Cappa, S. M. (1976). Antigenic variation, antigenic typing, exoantigens, and prospects for vaccines. *In:* "New Approaches in American Trypanosomiasis Research". Proceedings of an International Symposium, Belo Horizonte, Minas Gerais, Brazil, 18–21 March 1975. Pan American Health Organization, Washington. Scientific Publication No. 318, 170–173.

Gonzalez-Cappa, S. M., Cantarella, A. I., Lajmanovich, S. and Segura, E. S. (1976). Experimental Chagas' disease: Studies on the stability of a protective antigen. *Journal of Parasitology*, **62**, 130–131.

Gonzalez Valdivieso, F., Sanchez Diaz, B. and Nocerino, F. (1971). Susceptibilidad de *R. prolixus* a los insecticidas clorados en Venezuela. *Boletin Informativo de la Direccion de Malariologia y Saneamiento Ambiental*, **11**, 47–52.

Gray, A. R. and Luckins, A. G. (1976). Antigenic variation in Salivarian trypanosomes. *In:* "Biology of the Kinetoplastida" (Eds W. H. R. Lumsden and D. A. Evans), Vol. 1, 493–542. Academic Press, London and New York.

Guerra, F. (1970). American Trypanosomiasis. An historical and a human lesson. *Journal of Tropical Medicine and Hygiene*, **73**, 83–118.

Gutteridge, W. E. (1976a). Biochemistry of *Trypanosoma cruzi*. *In:* "New Approaches in American Trypanosomiasis Research". Proceedings of an International Symposium, Belo Horizonte, Minas Gerais, Brazil, 18–21 March 1975. Pan American Health Organization, Washington. Scientific Publication No. 318, 135–143.

Gutteridge, W. E. (1976b). Chemotherapy of Chagas' disease: The present situation. *Tropical Diseases Bulletin*, **73**, 699–705.

Hanson, W. L. and Roberson, E. L. (1974). Density of parasites in various organs and the relation to numbers of trypomastigotes in the blood during acute infections of *Trypanosoma cruzi* in mice. *Journal of Protozoology*, **21**, 512–517.

Hanson, W. L., Devlin, R. F. and Roberson, E. L. (1974). Immunoglobulin levels in a laboratory-acquired case of human Chagas' disease. *Journal of Parasitology*, **60**, 532–533.

Hanson, W. L., Chapman, W. L. Jr., and Waits, V. B. (1976). Immunization of mice with irradiated *Trypanosoma cruzi* grown in cell culture: relation of numbers of parasites, immunizing injections and route of immunization to resistance. *International Journal for Parasitology*, **6**, 341–347.

Hoare, C. A. (1972). "The Trypanosomes of Mammals". Blackwell, Oxford.

Hoff, R. (1974). A method for counting and concentrating living *Trypanosoma cruzi* in blood lysed with ammonium chloride. *Journal of Parasitology*, **60**, 527–528.

Hoff, R. (1976). Recent advances in cell-mediated immunity to *Trypanosoma cruzi*. *In:* "New Approaches in American Trypanosomiasis Research". Proceedings of an International Symposium, Belo Horizonte, Minas Gerais, Brazil, 18–21 March 1975. Pan American Health Organization, Washington. Scientific Publication No. 318, 162–169.

Hopkinson, D. A. (1975). The use of thiol reagents in the analysis of isoenzyme patterns. *In:* "Isoenzymes" (Ed. C. L. Markert), Vol. 1, pp. 489–508. Academic Press, New York and London.

Howard, J. E. (1976). Clinical aspects of congenital Chagas' disease. *In:* "New Approaches in American Trypanosomiasis Research". Proceedings of an International Symposium, Belo Horizonte, Minas Gerais, Brazil, 18–21 March 1975. Pan American Health Organization, Washington. Scientific Publication No. 318, 212–215.

Howells, R. E. and Chiari, C. A. (1975). Observations on two strains of *Trypanosoma cruzi* in laboratory mice. *Annals of Tropical Medicine and Parasitology*, **69**, 435–448.

Hubsch, R. M., Sulzer, A. J. and Kagan, I. G. (1976). Evaluation of an autoimmune type antibody in the sera of patients with Chagas' disease. *Journal of Parasitology*, **62**, 523–527.

Hunter, R. L. and Markert, C. L. (1957). Histochemical demonstration of enzymes separated by zone electrophoresis in starch gels. *Science*, **125**, 1294–1295.

Kagan, I. G., Norman, L. and Allain, D. (1966). Studies on *Trypanosoma cruzi* isolated in the United States: A Review. *Revista de Biologia Tropical*, **14**, 55–73.

Kanabara, H., Enriquez, G. and Inoki, S. (1974). The membrane characters of different forms of *Trypanosoma cruzi*. *Japanese Journal of Parasitology*, **23**, 268–274.

Ketteridge, D. (1975a). Differentiation of newly isolated strains of *Trypanosoma (Schizotrypanum) cruzi* by agglutination and precipitation reactions. *Acta Tropica*, **32**, 173–189.

Ketteridge, D. (1975b). A fluorescent character distinguishing strains of *Trypanosoma (Schizotrypanum) cruzi* isolated from animals. *Transactions of the Royal Society of Tropical Medicine and Hygiene*, **69**, 486–487.

Kierszenbaum, F. (1976). Cross-reactivity of lytic antibody against blood forms of *Trypanosoma cruzi*. *Journal of Parasitology*, **62**, 134–135.

Kierszenbaum, F. and Howard, J. G. (1976). Mechanisms of resistance against experimental *Trypanosoma cruzi* infection: the importance of antibodies and antibody-forming capacity in the Biozii high and low responder mice. *Journal of Immunology*, **116**, 1208–1211.

Kierszenbaum, F., Ivanyi, J. and Budzko, Delia B. (1976). Mechanisms of natural resistance to trypanosomal infection: Role of complement in avian resistance to *Trypanosoma cruzi* infection. *Immunology*, **30**, 1–6.

Kilgour, V. and Godfrey, D. G. (1977). The persistence in the field of two characteristic isoenzyme patterns in Nigerian *Trypanosoma vivax*. *Annals of Tropical Medicine and Parasitology*, **71**, 387–389.

Kilgour, V., Gardener, P. J., Godfrey, D. G. and Peters, W. (1974). Demonstration of electrophoretic variation of two aminotransferases in *Leishmania*. *Annals of Tropical Medicine and Parasitology*, **68**, 245–246.

Kloetzel, J., Camargo, M. E. and Giovannini, V. L. (1975). Antigenic differences between epimastigotes, amastigotes and trypomastigotes of *Trypanosoma cruzi*. *Journal of Protozoology*, **22**, 259–261.

Köberle, F. (1968). Chagas' disease and Chagas' syndromes: the pathology of American trypanosomiasis. *Advances in Parasitology*, **6**, 63–110.

Köberle, F. (1974). Pathogenesis of Chagas' disease. *In:* "Trypanosomiasis and Leishmaniasis with Special Reference to Chagas' disease". *Ciba Symposium*, **20**, 137–158.

Krettli, A. U. and Brener, Z. (1976). Protective effects of specific antibodies in *Trypanosoma cruzi* infections. *Journal of Immunology*, **116**, 755–760.

Kühn, R. E. and Vaughn, R. T. (1976). An immunocytotoxic assay for *Trypanosoma cruzi*. *International Journal for Parasitology*, **6**, 129–134.

Kühn, R. E., Vaughn, R. T. and Iannuzzi, N. P. (1974). The *in vivo* distribution of ^{51}Cr-labelled *Trypanosoma cruzi* in mice. *International Journal for Parasitology*, **4**, 585–588.

Laguens, R. P., Cossio, P. M., Diez, C., Segal, A., Vasquez, C., Kreutzer, E., Khoury, E. and Arana, R. M. (1975). Immunopathologic and morphologic studies of skeletal muscle in Chagas' disease. *American Journal of Pathology*, **80**, 153–159.

Leal, H., Ferreira Neto, J. A. and Martins, C. M. (1961). Dados ecológicos sôbre os triatomíneos silvestres na ilha de Santa Catarina (Brasil). *Revista do Instituto de Medicina Tropical de São Paulo*, **3**, 213–220.

Levi, G. C., Amato Neto, V. and Sant'anna, I. F. de A. B. (1975). Análise de manifestações colaterais devidas ao uso do medicamento Ro 7–1051, nitroimidazólico preconizado para tentativas de tratamento específico da doença de Chagas. *Revista do Instituto de Medicina Tropical de São Paulo*, **17**, 49–54.

Lucena, D. D. de (1962). Ecologia dos triatomineios do Brasil. *Anais do Congresso Internacional sôbre a doença de Chagas, Rio de Janeiro*, **3**, 771–851.

Maekelt, G. A. (1973). Evaluacion estadistica de los resultados de encuestas epidemiologicas realizadas en Venezuela respecto a la etiologia chagasica de las miocardiopatias cronicas rurales. *Archivos Venezolanos de Medicina Tropical y Parasitologia Medica*, **5**, 107–115.

Major, P. C. and Burrell, R. (1971). Induction of acquired tolerance in neonatal opossums. *The Journal of Immunology*, **106**, 1690–1691.

Mancilla, R. and Naquira, C. (1964). Comparative metabolism of ^{14}C-glucose in two strains of *Trypanosoma cruzi*. *Journal of Protozoology*, **11**, 509–513.

Marinkelle, C. J. (1976). Biology of the trypanosomes of bats. *In:* "Biology of the Kinetoplastida" (Eds W. H. R. Lumsden and D. A. Evans), Vol. 1, pp. 175–216. Academic Press, London, New York, San Francisco.

Markert, C. L. (1968). The molecular basis for isozymes. *Annals of the New York Academy of Science*, **151**, 14–40.

Markert, C. L. (Ed.) (1975). "Isozymes". I. Molecular Structure. Academic Press, New York, San Francisco, London. 856 pp.

Marsden, P. D., Seah, S. K. K., Draper, C. C., Pettitt, L. E., Miles, M. A. and Voller, A. (1976). Experimental *Trypanosoma cruzi* infections in rhesus monkeys. II. The early chronic phase. *Transactions of the Royal Society of Tropical Medicine and Hygiene*, **70**, 247–251.

Marx, J. J. Jr., Burrell, R. and Fisher, S. Q. (1971). A study of the afferent and efferent limbs of the immune response in opossums. *The Journal of Immunology*, **106**, 1043–1049.

Mattei, Denise M., Goldenberg, S., Morel, C., Azevedo, H. P. and Roitman, I. (1977). Biochemical strain characterization of *Trypanosoma cruzi* by restriction endonuclease cleavage of kinetoplast DNA. *FEBS Letters*, **74**, 264–268.

166   M. A. MILES

Maudlin, I. (1976). Inheritance of susceptibility of *Trypanosoma cruzi* infection in *Rhodnius prolixus*. *Nature*, **262**, 214–215.

Menezes, H. (1971). Aplicação de vacina viva avirulenta de *Trypanosoma cruzi* em seres humanos. (Nota previa). *Revista do Instituto de Medicina Tropical de São Paulo*, **13**, 144–154.

Mercado, T. I. (1976). *Trypanosoma cruzi*: lactate dehydrogenase isoenzymes and infections in mice. *Experimental Parasitology*, **40**, 411–420.

Miles, M. A. (1972). *Trypanosoma cruzi*—milk transmission of infection and immunity from mother to young. *Parasitology*, **65**, 1–9.

Miles, M. A. (1976a). Distribution and importance of Triatominae as vectors of *T. cruzi*. In: "New Approaches in American Trypanosomiasis Research". Proceedings of an International Symposium, Belo Horizonte, Minas Gerais, Brazil, 18–21 March 1975. Pan American Health Organization, Washington. Scientific Publication No. 318, 24–32.

Miles, M. A. (1976b). A simple method of tracking mammals and locating triatomine vectors of *Trypanosoma cruzi* in Amazonian forest. *American Journal of Tropical Medicine and Hygiene*, **25**, 671–674.

Miles, M. A. and Rouse, Jean E. (1970). Chagas' Disease (South American Trypanosomiasis); A Bibliography. Supplement to *Tropical Diseases Bulletin*, **67**, 209.

Miles, M. A., Patterson, J. W., Marsden, P. D. and Minter, D. M. (1975). A comparison of *Rhodnius prolixus*, *Triatoma infestans* and *Panstrongylus megistus* in the xenodiagnosis of a chronic *Trypanosoma* (*Schizotrypanum*) *cruzi* infection in a rhesus monkey (*Macaca mullatta*). *Transactions of the Royal Society of Tropical Medicine and Hygiene*, **69**, 377–382.

Miles, M. A., Toyé, P. J., Oswald, Sarah C. and Godfrey, D. G. (1977). The identification by isoenzyme patterns of two distinct strain-groups of *Trypanosoma cruzi* circulating independently in a rural area of Brazil. *Transactions of the Royal Society of Tropical Medicine and Hygiene*, **71**, 217–225.

Minter, D. M. (1976). Feeding patterns of some triatomine vector species. In "New Approaches in American Trypanosomiasis Research". Proceedings of an International Symposium, Belo Horizonte, Minas Gerais, Brazil, 18–21 March 1975. Pan American Health Organization, Washington. Scientific Publication No. 318, 33–47.

Minter, D. M. (1976). Epidemiology of Chagas' disease. *Transactions of the Royal Society of Tropical Medicine and Hygiene*, **70**, 124.

Minter-Goedbloed, E. (1976). Hemoculture compared with xenodiagnosis for the detection of *T. cruzi* infection in man and in animals. In: "New Approaches in American Trypanosomiasis Research". Proceedings of an International Symposium, Belo Horizonte, Minas Gerais, Brazil, 18–21 March 1975. Pan American Health Organization, Washington. Scientific Publication No. 318, 245–252.

Mkwananzi, J. B., Franks, D. and Baker, J. R. (1976). Cytotoxicity of antibody-coated trypanosomes by normal human lymphoid cells. *Nature*, London, **259**, 403–404.

Moleiro, F., Pifano, C. F., Anselmi, A. and Ruestra, V. (1973). La dinamica epidemiologica de la enfermedad de Chagas en el Valle de los Naranjos, Estado Carabobo, Venezuela. III. Evaluacion longitudinal del dano miocardico en casos de enfermedad de Chagas en fase cronica del Valle de los Naranjos, Estado Carabobo, Venezuela. *Archivos Venezolanos de Medicina Tropical y Parasitologia Medica*, **5**, 47–83.

Mott, K. E., Lehman, J. S. Jr., Hoff, R., Morrow, R. H., Muniz, T. M., Sherlock, I., Draper, C. C., Pugliese, C. and Guimaraes, A. C. (1976). The epidemiology and household distribution of seroreactivity to *Trypanosoma cruzi* in a rural community in the north east Brazil. *American Journal of Tropical Medicine and Hygiene*, **25**, 552–562.

Moura, A., Luz, E., Cotrrea Lima, E., Borba, A. M., De Christan, A. and Veiga, A. A. (1969). Cardiopatia chagásica de origem silvestre no litoral paranaense. Estudo epidemiológico da área. *Revista do Instituto de Medicina Tropical de São Paulo*, **11**, 408–424.

Mühlpfordt, H. (1975). Vergleichende kinetoplastmorphologie verschiedener Trypanosomenarten unter besonderer Berücksichtigung von *Trypanosoma cruzi*. *Tropenmedizin und Parasitologie*, **26**, 239–246.

Mundin, M. H., Azevedo, H. P., Roitman, C., Gama, M. I. C., Manaia, A. C., Previato, J. O. and Roitman, I. (1976). Cultivation of *Trypanosoma cruzi* in defined medium. *Revista do Instituto de Medicina Tropical de São Paulo*, **18**, 143.

Neal, R. A. and Miles, R. A. (1970). Indirect haemagglutination test for Chagas' disease, with a simple method for survey work. *Revista do Instituto de Medicina Tropical de São Paulo*, **12**, 325–332.

Newton, B. A. (1976). Biochemical Approaches to the Taxonomy of Kinetoplastid Flagellates. *In:* "Biology of the Kinetoplastida" (Eds W. H. R. Lumsden and D. A. Evans), Vol. 1, pp. 405–434. Academic Press, London, New York, San Francisco.

Nussenzweig, V. and Goble, F. C. (1966). Further studies on the antigenic constitution of strains of *Trypanosoma* (*Schizotrypanum*) *cruzi*. *Experimental Parasitology*, **18**, 224–230.

Olivier, Margaret, C., Olivier, L. J. and Segal, D. B. (1972). A bibliography on Chagas' Disease (1909–1969). U.S. Government Printing Office, Washington, D.C. 20402.

Otero, M. A., Tonn, R. J., Jimenez, J. and Rosales, M. (1976). El uso de pequenos gallineros como método de estudio de triatominos selvaticos. *Boletin de la Direccion de Malariologia y Saneamiento Ambiental*, *XVI*, 46–49.

Packchanian, A. (1943). Infectivity of the Texas strain of *Trypanosoma cruzi* to man. *American Journal of Tropical Medicine*, **23**, 309–314.

Perassi, Ruth (1973). Female specific proteins in *Triatoma infestans* haemolymph. *Journal of Insect Physiology*, **19**, 663–671.

Petana, W. B. (1972). A revision of *Trypanosoma* (*Schizotrypanum*) *cruzi* strains from British Honduras, and the importance of strain characteristics in experimental chemotherapy of Chagas' disease. *Transactions of the Royal Society of Tropical Medicine and Hygiene*, **66**, 463–470.

Petana, W. B. and Coura, J. R. (1974). Experimental studies on *Trypanosoma* (*Schizotrypanum*) *cruzi* isolated from man, from animals and from triatomine bugs in Brazil. *Revista da Sociedade Brasileira de Medicina Tropical*, **8**, 315–323.

Phillips, N. R. (1958). Experimental studies on epidemiological factors in the transmission of American human trypanosomiasis. Thesis, University of London.

Pifano, C. F. (1973). La epidemiologia de la enfermedad de Chagas en Venezuela. *Archivos Venezolanos de Medicina Tropical y Parasitologia Medica*, **5**, 171–184.

Pipkin, A. C. Sr. (1968). Domiciliary reduviid bugs and the epidemiology of Chagas' disease in Panama. (Hemiptera, Reduviidae, Triatominae). *Journal of Medical Entomology*, **5**, 107–124.

Pipkin, A. C. (1969). Transmission of *Trypanosoma cruzi* by arthropod vectors: anterior versus posterior route infection. *International Revue of Tropical Medicine*, **3**, 1–47.

Pippin, W. F. (1970). The biology of vector capability of *Triatoma sanguisuga texana* Usinger and *Triatoma gerstaeckeri* (Stål) compared with *Rhodnius prolixus* (Stål) (Hemiptera, Triatominae.) *Journal of Medical Entomology*, **7**, 30–45.

Potkay, S. (1970). Diseases of the opossum (*Didelphis marsupialis*): A Review. *Laboratory Animal Care*, **20**, 502–511.

Prasad, N., Bushong, S. C. and Barton, H. L. (1971). Opossum lymphocytes in short-term culture with phytohemagglutinin. *Experimental Cell Research*, **69**, 425–429.

Prata, A. R. (1976). Natural history of chagasic cardiomyopathy. *In:* "New Approaches in American Trypanosomiasis Research". Proceedings of an International Symposium, Belo Horizonte, Minas Gerais, Brazil, 18–21 March 1975. Pan American Health Organization, Washington. Scientific Publication No. 318, 191–193.

Puigbo, J. J. and Zisman, E. (1968). Descripcion y evaluacion critica de la patogenia de las lesiones cardiacas en la enfermedad de Chagas. *Acta Medica da Venezuela*, **15**, 310–319.

Rabinovich, J. E., Carcavallo, R. U. and Barretto, M. P. (1976). Ecologic methods: marking, trapping and sampling for vector studies in the field. *In:* "New Approaches in American Trypanosomiasis Research". Proceedings of an International Symposium, Belo Horizonte, Minas Gerais, Brazil, 18–21 March 1975. Pan American Health Organization, Washington. Scientific Publication No. 318, 16–20.

Rassi, A. and Rezende, J. M. de (1976). Prevention of transmission of *T. cruzi* by blood transfusion. *In:* "New Approaches in American Trypanosomiasis Research". Proceedings of an International Symposium, Belo Horizonte, Minas Gerais, Brazil, 18–21 March 1975. Pan American Health Organization, Washington. Scientific Publication No. 318, 273–278.

Reeves, R. E. and Bischoff, J. M. (1968). Classification of *Entamoeba* species by means of electrophoretic properties of amoebal enzymes. *Journal of Parasitology*, **54**, 594–600.

Rezende, J. F. M. de (1976). Chagasic mega syndromes and regional differences. *In:* "New Approaches in American Trypanosomiasis Research". Proceedings of an International Symposium, Belo Horizonte, Minas Gerais, Brazil, 18–21 March 1975. Pan American Health Organization, Washington. Scientific Publication No. 318, 195–205.

Riou, G. (1976). Establishment and characterization of *Trypanosoma cruzi* strains resistant to ethidium bromide. *In:* "Biochemistry of Parasites and Host–Parasite Relationships" (Ed. H. Van den Bossche), pp. 237–244. Janssen Research Foundation. Elsevier/North Holland Biomedical Press—Amsterdam.

Riou, G. and Yot, P. (1975). Etude de l'ADN kinetoplastique de *Trypanosoma cruzi* a l'aide d'endonucleases de restriction. *Comptes rendus, Academie des Sciences, Paris*, **280**, Serie D, 2701–2704.

Rocha e Silva, E. O., Andrade, J. C. R. and Lima, A. R. (1975). Importância dos animais sinantrópicos no controle da endemia chagásica. *Revista de Saúde Pública*, **9**, 371–381.

Rodrigues, B. A. and Melo, G. B. (1942). Contribução ao estudo da tripanosomiase americana. *Memorias do Instituto Oswaldo Cruz*, **37**, 77–90.

Rodriguez, E. and Marinkelle, C. J. (1970). *Trypanosoma cruzi* development in tissue culture. *Experimental Parasitology*, **27**, 78–87.

Rollinson, D. (1976). Electrophoretic variation of enzymes in mammalian coccidia. *Transactions of the Royal Society of Tropical Medicine and Hygiene*, **70**, 21–22.

Romana, C. (1962). Epidemiologia e distribuição geográfica da doença de Chagas. *Revista Brasileira de Malariologia e Doenças Tropicais*, **14**, 549–563.

Rowlands, D. T. Jr., Blakeslee, D. and Lin, H. H. (1972). The early immune response and immunoglobulins of opossum embryos. *Journal of Immunology*, **108**, 941–946.

Ryckman, R. E. (1954). Lizards: a laboratory host for Triatominae and *Trypanosoma cruzi* Chagas (Hemiptera, Reduviidae) (Protomonadida, Trypanosomidae). *Transactions of the American Microscopical Society, LXXIII*, 215–218.

Ryckman, R. E. (1965). Epizootiology of *Trypanosoma cruzi* in south-western North America. B. Host parasite specificity between *Trypanosoma cruzi* and Triatominae (Kinetoplastida, Trypanosomatidae) (Hemiptera, Triatominae). *Journal of Medical Entomology*, **2**, 96–99.

Ryckman, R. E. and Olsen, L. E. (1965). Epizootiology of *Trypanosoma cruzi* in south-western North America. VI. Insectivorous hosts of Triatominae—the epizootiological relationship to *Trypanosoma cruzi*. *Journal of Medical Entomology*, **2**, 99–104.

Salgado, J. A., Garez, P. N., Oliveira, C. A. de and Galizzi, J. (1962). Revisão clinica atuel do primeiro caso humano descrito da doença de Chagas. *Revista do Instituto de Medicina Tropical de São Paulo*, **4**, 330–337.

Santos, R. B. dos and Oliveira, J. C. de (1976). Antibodies to neurons in chronic Chagas' disease. *Transactions of the Royal Society of Tropical Medicine and Hygiene*, **70**, 167.

Schenone, H., Zomosa, E., Villarroel, F., Rojas, A., Alfaro, E. and Quiroz, M. (1972). Inaction of 7 insecticide preparations on laboratory-raised *Triatoma infestans*. *Boletin Chileno de Parasitologia*, **27**, 14–22.

Schenone, H., Concha, L., Aranda, R., Rojas, A., Alfaro, E. and Knierim, F. (1975). Actividad quimioterapica de un derivado de la nitroimidazolacetamida en la infeccion chagasica cronica. *Boletin Chileno de Parasitologia*, **30**, 91–93.

Schmunis, G. A., Szarfman, A. and Vattuone, N. (1972). Direct agglutination test in the detection of anti-*Trypanosoma cruzi* antibodies in mice. *Journal of Parasitology*, **58**, 1006–1007.

Scott, J. A. and Krassner, S. M. (1975). Axenic culture of *Trypanosoma cruzi* in a chemically defined medium. *Journal of Parasitology*, **6**, 144–145.

Segura, E. L., Paulone, I., Cerisola, J. and Gonzalez-Cappa, S. M. (1976). Experimental Chagas' disease: Protective activity in relation with subcellular fractions of the parasite. *Journal of Parasitology*, **62**, 131–133.

Shaw, J. J., Lainson, R. and Fraiha, H. (1969). Considerações sôbre a epidemiologia dos primeiros casos autoctones de doença de Chagas registrados em Belém, Pará, Brasil. *Revista de Saude Publica, São Paulo*, **3**, 153–157.

Shirley, M. W. (1975). Isoenzymes in the coccidia. 28th Annual Meeting of the Society of Protozoologists. Abstract 162, pp. 55A. *Journal of Protozoology*, **22**.

Silva, N. N., Kuhn, G., Santos, J. F. C., Von Eye, G. and Chaher, J. A. B. (1974). Eficácia e tolerânciá do nitrofurfurilidena na fase cronica do moléstia de Chagas. *Revista da Sociedade Brasileira de Medicina Tropical*, **8**, 325–334.

Silveira, C. da, Luz, E., Borva, A. M. and Costa, Maria R. T. da (1969). Sôbre o diagnostico especifico de sangue encontrado em triatomineos capturados em ninho de gamba. *Anais da Faculdade de Medicine da Universidade Federal do Parana*, **12**, 173–177.

Sjogren, R. D. and Ryckman, R. E. (1966). Epizootiology of *Trypanosoma cruzi* in south-western North America. VIII. Nocturnal flights of *Triatoma protracta* (Uhler) as indicated by collections at black light traps (Hemiptera, Reduviidae, Triatominae). *Journal of Medical Entomology*, **3**, 81–92.

Soto, S. T. (1971). Hallazgo de formas evolutivas intermedias de *Trypanosoma cruzi* Chagas 1909, em la sangre periferica de ratones blancos (*Mus musculus*). *Revista da Faculdade de Medicina de Maracaibo*, **4**, 138–146.

Sousa, O. E. (1972). Anotaciones sôbre la enfermedad de Chagas en Panama. Frecuencia y distribucion de *Trypanosoma cruzi* y *Trypanosoma rangeli*. *Revista de Biologia Tropical*, **20**, 167–179.

Sousa, O. E. and Johnson, C. M. (1973). Prevalence of *Trypanosoma cruzi* and *Trypanosoma rangeli* in triatomines (Hemiptera, Reduviidae) collected in the Republic of Panama. *American Journal of Tropical Medicine and Hygiene*, **22**, 18–23.

Steiger, R., Krassner, S. M. and Jenni, L. (1974). Comparison of specific and relative alanine and aspartate aminotransferases of *Trypanosoma brucei* subgroup trypanosomes. *Acta Tropica*, **31**, 202–218.

Steinert, M. and Van Assel, S. (1974). Base composition heterogeneity in kinetoplast DNA from four species of hemoflagellates. *Biochemical and Biophysical Research Communications*, **61**, 1249–1255.

Steinert, M., Van Assel, S., Borst, P., Mol, M. N. M., Kleisen, C. M. and Newton, B. A. (1973). Specific detection of kinetoplast DNA in cytological preparations of trypanosomes by hybridization with complementary RNA. *Experimental Cell Research*, **76**, 175–185.

Steinert, M., Van Assel, S., Borst, P. and Newton, B. A. (1976). The genetic function of mitochondrial DNA. *In:* Proceedings of the 10th International Bari Conference on Genetic Function of DNA, Riva dei Tessali, Italy, 25–29 May 1976 (Eds C. Saccone and A. M. Kroon). Amsterdam, North Holland.

Szarfman, A., Otatti, L., Schmunis, G. A. and Vilches, A. M. (1973). A simple method for the detection of human congenital Chagas' disease. *Journal of Parasitology*, **59**, 723.

Szarfman, A., Cossio, P. M., Laguens, R. P., Segal, A., de la Vega, M. T., Arana, R. M. and Schmunis, G. A. (1975). Immunological studies in Rockland mice infected with *T. cruzi*. Development of antinuclear antibodies. *Biomedicine*, **22**, 489–495.

Teixeira, A. R. L. (1976). Autoimmune mechanisms in Chagas' disease. *In:* "New Approaches in American Trypanosomiasis Research". Proceedings of an International Symposium, Belo Horizonte, Minas Gerais, Brazil, 18–21 March 1975. Pan American Health Organization, Washington. Scientific Publication No. 318, 98–108.

Tempelis, C. H. and Rodrick, Mary L. (1972). Passive hemagglutination inhibition technique for the identification of arthropod blood meals. *American Journal of Tropical Medicine and Hygiene*, **21**, 238–245.

Tonn, R. J., Carcavallo, R. U., Ortega, R. and Carrasquero, B. (1976). Metodos de estudio de triatominos en el medio silvestre. *Boletin de la Direccion de Malariologia y Saneamiento Ambiental*, **XVI**, 146–152.

Toyé, P. J. (1974). Isoenzyme variation in isolates of *Trypanosoma cruzi*. *Transactions of the Royal Society of Tropical Medicine and Hygiene*, **68**, 147.

Usinger, R. L., Wygodzinsky, P. and Ryckman, R. E. (1966). The biosystematics of Triatominae. *Annual Review of Entomology*, **11**, 309–331.

Vattuone, N. H. and Yanovsky, J. F. (1971). *Trypanosoma cruzi*: agglutination activity of enzyme-treated epimastigotes. *Experimental Parasitology*, **30**, 349–355.

Vega, M. T. de la, Damilano, G. and Diez, C. (1976). Leucocyte migration inhibition test with heart antigens in American Trypanosomiasis. *Journal of Parasitology*, **62**, 129–130.

Ventocilla, J. A. and Silva, P. (1968). Triatomineos capturados em armadilha luminosa na área cacaueira da Bahia. *Revista Brasileira de Malariologia e Doenças Tropicais*, **20**, 161–169.

Vianna, G. (1911). Beitrag zum Studium der pathologischen Anatomie der krankheit von Carlos Chagas. *Memorias do Instituto Oswaldo Cruz*, **3**, 276–279.

Vickerman, K. (1974). The ultrastructure of pathogenic flagellates. *In:* "Trypanosomiasis and Leishmaniasis", pp. 171–190. Ciba Foundation Symposium 20 (New Series), Elsevier, Amsterdam.

Vickerman, K. and Preston, T. M. (1976). Comparative cell biology of the Kinetoplastid flagellates. *In:* "Biology of the Kinetoplastida" (Eds W. H. R. Lumsden and D. A. Evans), Vol. 1, pp. 35–113. Academic Press, London and New York.

Voller, A. (1977). Serological methods in the diagnosis of Chagas' disease. *Transactions of the Royal Society of Tropical Medicine and Hygiene*, **71**, 10–11.

Voller, A., Draper, C., Bidwell, D. E. and Bartlett, Ann (1975). Microplate enzyme-linked immunosorbent assay for Chagas' disease. *The Lancet*, 22 February 1975, pp. 426–428.

Voller, A., Bartlett, Ann and Bidwell, D. E. (1976). Enzyme immunoassays for parasitic diseases. *Transactions of the Royal Society of Tropical Medicine and Hygiene*, **70**, 98–106.

Washino, R. K. and Else, J. G. (1972). Identification of blood meals of hematophagous arthropods by the hemoglobin crystallization method. *American Journal of Tropical Medicine and Hygiene*, **21**, 120–122.

Weinman, D. and Wiratmadja, N. S. (1969). The first isolates of trypanosomes in Indonesia and in history from primates other than man. *Transactions of the Royal Society of Tropical Medicine and Hygiene*, **63**, 497–506.

Wood, S. F. (1950). Dispersal flight of *Triatoma* in southern Arizona. *Journal of Parasitology*, **36**, 498–499.

Wood, S. F. (1951). Development of Arizona *Trypanosoma cruzi* in mouse muscle. *American Journal of Tropical Medicine*, **31**, 1–11.

Wood, S. F. (1953). Hematologic differentiation of the intra-muscular development forms of *Trypanosoma cruzi* Chagas. *American Journal of Tropical Medicine and Hygiene*, **2**, 1015–1033.

Wood, S. F. (1975a). *Trypanosoma cruzi*: New foci of enzootic Chagas' disease in California. *Experimental Parasitology*, **38**, 153–160.

Wood, S. F. (1975b). Home invasions of conenose bugs (Hemiptera, Reduviidae) and their control. *National Pest Control Operator News, March*, 16–18.

Woody, N. C. and Woody, H. B. (1964). Chagas' Disease in the United States of North America. *Anais do Congresso Internacional sobre a Doença de Chagas*, **V**, 1699–1724.

World Health Organization (1974). Immunology of Chagas' disease. *Bulletin of the World Health Organization*, **50**, 459–472.

World Health Organization (1976). Trypanosomiasis. I. African Trypanosomiasis. II. Chagas' disease. Special Programme for Research and Training in Tropical Diseases. TDR/WP/76.12.

Yaeger, R. G. (1959). Chagas' disease in the United States. *Revista Goiana de Medicina*, **5**, 461–470.

Yaeger, R. G. (1971). Transmission of *Trypanosoma cruzi* infection to opossums via the oral route. *Journal of Parasitology*, **57**, 1375–1376.

Zeledón, R. (1972). Los vectores de la enfermedad de Chagas en America. Simposio internacional sôbre enfermedad de Chagas, Buenos Aires, December 1975, pp. 327–345. Secretaria de Estado de Salud Publica, Buenos Aires, Argentina.

Zeledón, R. (1974). Epidemiology, modes of transmission and reservoir hosts of

Chagas' disease. *In:* "Trypanosomiasis and Leishmaniasis with special reference to Chagas' disease". Ciba Foundation Symposium 20 (New Series), pp. 51–85.

Zeledón, R. and Ponce, C. (1972). Neurotropism in Costa Rican strains of *Trypanosoma cruzi. Journal of Parasitology*, **58**, 180–181.

Zeledón, R., Soegano, Georgina, Saem, G. S. and Swartzwelder, J. C. (1970). Wild reservoirs of *Trypanosoma cruzi* with special mention of the opossum, *Didelphis marsupialis*, and its role in the epidemiology of Chagas' disease in an endemic area of Costa Rica. *Journal of Parasitology*, **56**, 38.

Zeledón, R., Solgano, G., Zuniga, A. and Swartzwelder, J. C. (1973). Biology and ethology of *Triatoma dimidiata* (Latreille 1811). III. Habitat and blood sources. *Journal of Medical Entomology*, **10**, 363–370.

Zeledón, R., Solgano, G., Burstin, L. and Swartzwelder, J. C. (1975). Epidemiological pattern of Chagas' disease in an endemic area of Costa Rica. *American Journal of Tropical Medicine and Hygiene*, **24**, 214–225.

XI. Appendix

Distribution and Habitats of the Triatominae (Western Hemisphere)
Explanation

This Appendix attempts to summarize what is known of the distribution and principal habitats of Triatomine species. Information is based on the selected sources given in the references to this Appendix.

The Appendix deals only with Triatominae of the Western Hemisphere and therefore excludes the following species: *Linshocosteus carnifex* Distant, 1904, *Triatoma africana* Neiva, 1911, *Triatoma amicitiae* Lent, 1951, *Triatoma bouvieri* Larrousse, 1924, *Triatoma howardi* Neiva, 1911, *Triatoma leopoldi* (Schouteden, 1933), *Triatoma migrans* (Breddin, 1903) and *Triatoma pugasi* Lent, 1953 (see Addendum, p. 185).

Classification is based on: Lent and Jurberg (1969b, 1975) for *Rhodnius* and *Panstrongylus*; Usinger *et al.* (1966) for North American species; and otherwise upon Lent (1962), with the addition of more recently described species, and 2 species not yet described (*Rhodnius* species and *Parabelminus* species; Sherlock *et al.* in press, Lent *et al.* in preparation). Subspecies, which may differ in degree of domiciliation, are not given, nor are species synonyms, some of which are still used by various authors (see Addendum, p. 186).

Groupings of species into sections A, B, and C gives a broad indication of domiciliation and adaptation to man and domestic animals. However, the divisions are somewhat artificial; as indicated some species may colonize houses but probably feed predominantly on reptilian or avian hosts (e.g. *Belminus peruvianus*, *Triatoma arthurneivai* and *Triatoma platensis*). The distinction between bugs forming small household colonies and bugs attracted by light into houses is sometimes unclear. The paper of Zeledón (1972) should be consulted for further information on household records of species in groups A and B.

Key to Distribution
1 Argentina, 2 Belize, 3 Bolivia, 4 Brazil (a, Acre; b, Alagoas; c, Amazonas; d, Bahia; e, Ceará; f, Espirito Santo; g, Goiás; h, Guanabara; i, Maranhão; j, Mato Grosso; k, Minas Gerais; l, Pará; m, Paraíba; n, Paraná; o, Pernambuco; p, Piauí; q, Rio de Janeiro; r, Rio Grande do Norte; s, Rio Grande do Sul; t, Santa Catarina; u, São Paulo; v, Sergipe) 5 Chile, 6 Colombia, 7 Costa Rica, 8 Cuba, 9 Ecuador, 10 El Salvador, 11 French Guiana, 12 Guatemala, 13 Guyana, 14 Honduras, 15 Mexico, 16 Nicaragua, 17 Panama, 18 Paraguay, 19 Peru, 20 Surinam, 21 Trinidad, 22 USA, 23 Uruguay, 24 Venezuela.

A. *Domestic and Sylvatic species*

Panstrongylus herreri Wygodzinsky, 1948
   19: man and domestic animals. Some authors do not distinguish this species from *Panstrongylus lignarius* (Walker 1873); but see Lent and Jurberg (1975) for comparative descriptions.
Panstrongylus megistus (Burmeister, 1835)
   1, 3, 4 (b, d, e-v), 13, 18, 23: man, chicken, dog, cat and rodents; also Bromeliaceae, trees (*Cryptomeria japonica*), rocks and palms (*Orbignya martiana, Acrocomia macrocarpa, Mauritia vinifera, Scheelea phalerata, Arecastrum, Syagrus*) with opossum (*Didelphis, Marmosa*) rodents, armadillo, birds and bats.
Rhodnius ecuadoriensis Lent and León 1958
   9, 19: man and chicken.
Rhodnius nasutus Stal 1859
   4 (e, p, r): man and domestic animals.
Rhodnius pallescens Barber 1932
   6, 17 (19?): man, chicken, dog, cat and pig; also burrows and trees with armadillo, sloth and opossum.
Rhodnius prolixus Stål 1859
   3, 4 (c, k, l), 6, 7, 9, 10, 11, 12, 13, 14, 15, 16, 17, 20, 24: man and domestic animals; also palms (*Attalea humboldtiana, Acrocomia sclerocarpa, Copernicia tectorum, Leopoldinia piassaba, Sabal, Scheelea*) trees and burrows with paca, armadillo, porcupine and birds (*Jabiru mycteria, Mycteria americana*).
Triatoma brasiliensis Neiva, 1911 (3 subspecies)
   4 (b, d, e, k, m, o, p, r): man and domestic animals; also rocks with rodents (mocó = *Kerodon rupestris*).
Triatoma carrioni Larrousse 1926
   9, 19: man and horse.
Triatoma dimidiata (Latreille, 1811) (3 subspecies)
   2, 6, 7, 9, 10, 12, 14, 15, 16, 17, 19, 24: man, dog, cat, chicken, rodents;

also trees with opossum and rodents.

Triatoma eratyrusiforme   Del Ponte, 1929

1:    man and domestic animals; also trees and rocks near rodent and edentate burrows.

Triatoma guasayana   Wygodzinsky and Abalos, 1949

1, 3, 18: man and domestic animals; also goat enclosures, trees, fallen trees and rocks (with lizards, toads and birds).

Triatoma infestans   (Klug, 1834)

1, 3, 4 (d, g, j, k, n, o, q, s, t, u), 5, 18, 19, 23: man, cat, chicken and rodents; also palms (*Acrocomia macrocarpa*) (and possibly caves) with birds, opossum and rodents.

Triatoma maculata   (Erichson, 1848)

and *Triatoma pseudomaculata*   Correia and Espinola, 1964

4 (b, d, e, g, k, m, o, p, r, Roraima), 6, 13, 20, 24: man and domestic animals; also rocks with rodents (mocó = *Kerodon rupestris*) (*Triatoma maculata*), and rocks and hollow trees with opossum and rodents (*Triatoma pseudomaculata*). Galvão (1973) discusses the separation of these two, similar, species and their comparative distributions.

Triatoma patagonica   Del Ponte, 1929

1: man and domestic animals, also rocks and burrows with rodents (*Microcavia; Graomys*).

Triatoma phyllosoma   (Burmeister, 1835) (6 subspecies)

15, 22: man and domestic animals.

Triatoma rubrofasciata   (De Geer, 1773)

Ports in the tropics, associated with *Rattus* spp. and rarely attacking man.

Triatoma sordida   (Stål, 1859)

1 3, 4 (d, e, g, j, k, n, o, p, s, t, u), 5, 18, 23: man and domestic animals; also palms (*Orbignya martiana*, *Acrocomia sclerocarpa*, *Mauritia vinifera*, *Scheelea phalerata*, *Arecastrum*, *Syagrus*, *Copernicia*), trees, Bromeliaceae and fences with birds (*Phacellodomus*, *Anumbius*), opossum, rodents and bats.

Triatoma spinolai   Porter, 1933

5: man and domestic animals; also sylvatic with rodents and canids.

B. *Sylvatic species, small colonies occasionally reported in houses*

Belminus peruvianus   Herrer, Lent and Wygodzinsky, 1954

19: although reported from houses this species probably feeds on lizard or birds, not man.

Eratyrus cuspidatus   Stål, 1859

6, 9, 12, 17, 24: forest, goat enclosures and bat roosting sites.

Eratyrus mucronatus   Stål, 1859

3, 4 (c, l), 6 (9?), 11, 13 (17?), 19, 24: houses in Venezuela; also forest and palms.

Panstrongylus chinai   (Del Ponte, 1929)
    9, 19: houses in Ecuador; also forest.
Panstrongylus geniculatus   (Latreille, 1811)
    1, 3, 4 (a, c, d, e, f, g, h, i, j, k, l, n, q, u, Amapa Rondonia), 6, 7, 9,
11, 13, 17, 18, 19, 21, 23, 24: only a single colony reported from houses
(Rodrigues and Melo, 1942); also burrows, rocks, palms and Bromeli-
aceae with armadillo, opossum, rodents, paca and bats.
Panstrongylus rufotuberculatus   (Champion, 1898)
    3, 4 (c, l), 6, 7, 9, 17, 19, 24: houses in Ecuador; also forest, burrows
and hollow trees (with *Potos flavus* in 4 (l)).
Rhodnius brethesi   Matta, 1919
    4 (c, l), 6, 24: palms (*Leopoldinia piassaba*).
Rhodnius neglectus   Lent, 1954
    4 (d, g, k, u), 24: palms (*Orbignya martiana, Acrocomia macrocarpa,
Mauritia vinifera, Scheelea phalerata, Arecastrum, Syagrus*), trees and
hollow trees with birds (*Anumbius, Phacellodomus*) opossum, rodents
and bats.
Rhodnius neivai   Lent, 1953
    24: palms (*Copernicia tectorum*) and hollow trees.
Rhodnius pictipes   Stål, 1872
    3, 4 (c, g, j, l), 6, 9, 11, 13, 19, 20, 21, 24: palms (*Attalea, Scheelea,
Copernicia*) and Bromeliaceae (*Aechmea*) with birds, bats and opossum
(*Didelphis marsupialis*, in 4 (l)).
Rhodnius robustus   Larrousse, 1927
    3, 4 (c, l), 6, 9, 11, 19, 24: palms (*Attalea, Scheelea*) and Bromeliaceae
(*Aechmea*).
Triatoma arthurneivai   Lent and Martins, 1940
    4 (k, p): rocks with lizards (*Tropidurus torquatus*).
Triatoma gerstaeckeri   (Stål, 1859)
    15, 22: in rodent lodges (*Neotoma, Ammospermophilus*).
Triatoma lecticularius   (Stål, 1859) (3 subspecies)
    15, 22: in rodent lodges (*Neotoma, Ammospermophilus*).
Triatoma lenti   Sherlock and Serafim, 1967
    4 (d): rocks.
Triatoma nigromaculata   (Stål, 1872)
    24: trees with birds and opossum.
Triatoma nitida   Usinger, 1939
    12, 14
Triatoma pessoai   Sherlock and Serafim, 1967
    4 (d): rocks.
Triatoma platensis   Neiva, 1913
    1: colonizes chicken houses, also sylvatic with birds.
Triatoma protracta complex   (Uhler, 1894)
    5 subspecies of *Triatoma protracta* and *Triatoma barberi* Usinger, 1939,

Triatoma incrassata Usinger, 1939, *Triatoma peninsularis* (Usinger, 1940), *Triatoma sinaloensis* Ryckman, 1962.

15, 22: the complex is typically sylvatic in rodent lodges (*Neotoma, Peromyscus*), and is also associated with racoons, but *Triatoma barberi* is found in houses in Mexico.

Triatoma recurva (Stal, 1868)
15, 22: in rodent lodges (*Neotoma, Peromyscus, Citellus*).

Triatoma rubida (Uhler, 1894) (3 subspecies)
15, 22: typically sylvatic in rodent lodges (*Neotoma, Peromyscus*) but *Triatoma rubida uhleri* Neiva, 1911 and *Triatoma rubida sonoriana* Del Ponte, 1930 are reported from houses.

Triatoma rubrovaria (Blanchard, 1843)
1, 4 ((c?), d, s), 5, 18, 23: only stone houses in Uruguay; also rocks and hollow trees with rodents (*Cavia*) and lizards (*Tupinambis*).

Triatoma sanguisuga (Leconte, 1855) (5 subspecies)
15, 22: hollow and dead trees with rodents, opossum, racoon and skunk.

Triatoma venosa (Stål, 1872)
3, 6, 7, 9.

Triatoma vitticeps (Stål, 1859)
4 (f, h, k, q, s).

Triatoma williami Galvao, Honorato and Lima, 1965
4 (g).

C. *Sylvatic species or rare species presumed to be light attracted into houses*

Belminus costaricensis Herrer, Lent and Wygodzinsky, 1954
7: Bromeliaceae (with sloths?).

Belminus rugulosus Stål, 1859
6, 24.

Bolbodera scabrosa Valdés, 1910
8.

Cavernicola pilosa Barber, 1937
4 (f, j, l) 6, 17, 24: hollow trees and caves with bats.

Dipetalogaster maximus (Uhler, 1894)
15: rocks, with lizards and mammals.

Microtriatoma mansosotoi Prosen and Martinez, 1952
3, 6: trees.

Microtriatoma trinidadensis (Lent, 1951)
19, 21, 4 (l): nest of opossum (*Oidelphis* marsupialis).

Neotriatoma—See *Triatoma circummaculata*.

Nesotriatoma flavida (Neiva, 1911)
8.

Panstrongylus diasi Pinto and Lent, 1946
3, 4 (d, g, k, u).

Panstrongylus guentheri   Berg, 1879
  1, 3, 18: burrows with rodents.
Panstrongylus howardi   (Neiva, 1911)
  9.
Panstrongylus humeralis   (Usinger, 1939)
  17: forest.
Panstrongylus lenti   Galvao and Palma, 1968
  4 (g?).
Panstrongylus lignarius   (Walker, 1873)
  4 (c, l), 13, 20, 24: forest, with opossum or rodents (*Didelphis marsu-pialis* or *Echimys chrysurus*, 4 (1)).
Panstrongylus lutzi   (Neiva and Pinto, 1923)
  4 (d, e, m, o, r).
Panstrongylus tupinambai   Lent, 1942
  4 (s), 23.
Parabelminus carioca   Lent, 1943
  4 (q, t): palms (*Attalea indaya*) with opossum (*Didelphis aurita*).
Parabelminus species
  4 (d): Bromeliaceae (*Aechmea*).
Paratriatoma hirsuta   Barber, 1938 (5 subspecies)
  15, 22: rodent lodges (*Neotoma*).
Psammolestes arthuri   (Pinto, 1926)
  24: birds nests (*Phacellodomus*).
Psammolestes coreodes   Bergroth, 1911
  1, 3, 4 (d, e, g, j, k, o), 7, 18: birds nests (*Anumbius, Phacellodomus, Myopsitta*).
Psammolestes tertius   Lent and Jurberg, 1965
  4 (d, k): palms (*Mauritia vinefera*) and birds nests (*Anumbius, Phacello-domus*), and with rodents and opossum.
Rhodnius amazonicus   Almeida, Santos and Sposina, 1973
  4 (c).
Rhodnius dalessandroi   Carcavallo and Barretto, 1976
  6.
Rhodnius domesticus   Neiva and Pinto, 1923
  4 (d, f, n, q, t, u): Bromeliaceae (*Aechmea*) and hollow trees with rodents (*Phyllomys dasylhrix*) and opossum (*Didelphis azarae*).
Rhodnius species (not *Rhodnius domesticus*, as stated by Miles (1976))*
  4 (l): hollow tree with opossum or rodents (*Didelphis marsupialis* or *Echimys chrysurus*).
Triatoma breyeri   Del Ponte, 1929
  1: wooden enclosures with rodents.
Triatoma circummaculata   (Stål, 1859) (2 subspecies)

---

* See Note 7, p. 195.

(= *Neotriatoma circummaculata/limai*)
1, 4 (s), 23: rocks and hollow trees with rodents.
Triatoma costalimai   Verano and Galvao, 1958
4 (d, g): rocks with rodents (mocó = *Kerodon rupestris*).
Triatoma deanei   Galvao, Honorato and Lima, 1967
4 (g).
Triatoma delpontei   Romana and Abalos, 1947
1: birds nests (*Myopsitta monacha cotorra*).
Triatoma dispar   Lent, 1950
7, 9, 17: in trees (with sloths).
Triatoma garciabesi   Carcavallo, Martinez, Prosen and Cichero, 1964
1: with rodents (*Microcavia; Graomys*) and birds (*Myopsitta*).
Triatoma hegneri   Mazotti, 1940
15.
Triatoma mattogrossensis   Leite and Barbosa, 1953.
4 (j).
Triatoma melanocephala   Neiva and Pinto, 1923
4 (d, o).
Triatoma mexicana   (Herrich and Schaeffer, 1848)
15.
Triatoma neotomae   Neiva, 1911
15, 22: in rodent lodges (*Neotoma*).
Triatoma ninioi   Carcavallo, Martinez, Prosen and Cichero, 1964
1: burrows with rodents (*Microcavia*).
Triatoma oliveirai   Neiva, Pinto and Lent, 1939
4 (s).
Triatoma petrochii   Pinto and Barretto, 1925
4 (d, o, r): rocks with rodents (mocó = *Kerodon rupestris*).
Triatoma ryckmani   Zeledón and Ponce, 1972
14.
Triatoma tibiamaculata   (Pinto, 1926)
4 (d, f, h, k, n, q, r, t, u, v): Bromeliaceae (*Aechmea*) with opossum
(*Didelphis azarae*) rodents and porcupine (and lizards?).
Triatoma wygodzinskyi   Lent, 1951
4 (k).

Sources and Selected Bibliography of the Triatominae

Abalos, J. W. (1972). Distribucion de vectores en la Argentina. Symposio internacional sôbre enfermedad de Chagas. Buenos Aires, December 1972. Secretaria de Estado de Salud Publica; Buenos Aires, Argentina.
Abalos, J. W. and Wygodzinsky, P. (1951). Las Triatominae argentineas (Reduviidae, Hemiptera). Tucuman: Universidad Nacional de Tucuman. Instituto de Medicina Regional. Publication No. 601, 178 pp.

Almeida, F. B. de (1971). Triatomineos da Amazonia. Encontro de tres especies naturalmente infectadas por trypanosoma semelhante ao *cruzi*, no Estado do Amazonas (Hemiptera, Reduviidae). *Acta Amazonica*, **1**, 84–93.

Almeida Rodrigues, B. de and Brito Melo, G. de (1942). Contribuição ao estudo da tripanosomiase americana. *Memorias do Instituto Oswaldo Cruz*, **37**, 77–90.

Almeida, F. B. de and Almeida Machado, P. de (1971). Sôbre a infecção do *Panstrongylus geniculatus* pelo *Trypanosoma cruzi* em Manaus, Amazonas, Brasil. *Acta Amazonica*, **1**, 71–75.

Almeida, F. B. de, Santos, E. I. and Sposina, G. (1973). Triatomineos da Amazonia III. *Acta Amazonica*, **3**, 43–46.

Barretto, M. P. (1963). Reservatórios e vectores do *Trypanosoma cruzi* no Brasil. *Arquivos de Higiene e Saúde Pública*, **28**, 43–66.

Barretto, M. P. (1968). Reservatórios de *Trypanosoma cruzi*. *In:* "Doença de Chagas" (Ed. J. R. Cançado), pp. 163–188. Belo Horizonte.

Barretto, M. P. (1968). Transmissores do *Trypanosoma cruzi*: os triatomineos. *In:* "Doença de Chagas" (Ed. J. R. Cançado), pp. 189–224. Belo Horizonte, 1968.

Barretto, M. P. (1968). Estudos sôbre reservatórios e vectores silvestres do *Trypanosoma cruzi*. XXXI. Observações sôbre a associação entre reservatórios e vectores com especial referencia a região nordeste do estado de São Paulo. *Revista Brasileira de Biologia*, **28**, 481–494.

Barretto, M. P. (1971). Estudos sobre reservatórios e vectores silvestres do *Trypanosoma cruzi*. XLV. Inquerito preliminar sobre triatomineos silvestres no sul do Estado de Mato Grosso, Brasil (Hemiptera, Reduviidae). *Revista Brasileira de Biologia*, **31**, 225–233.

Barretto, M. P. (1976). Possible role of wild mammals and triatomines in the transmission of *Trypanosoma cruzi* to man. *In:* "New Approaches in American Trypanosomiasis Research". Proceedings of an International Symposium, Belo Horizonte, Minas Gerais, Brazil, 18–21 March 1975. Pan American Health Organization, Washington. Scientific Publication No. 318, pp. 307–318.

Barretto, M. P. and Siqueira, A. F. (1963). Estudos sôbre reservatórios e vectores silvestres do *Trypanosoma cruzi*. I. Encontro do *Triatoma infestans* (Hemiptera, Reduviidae) em ecótopos silvestres. *Revista do Instituto de Medicina Tropical de São Paulo*. **5**, 289–293.

Barretto, M. P., Siqueira, A. F. and Freitas, J. L. P. (1964). Estudos sôbre reservatórios e vectores silvestres do *Trypanosoma cruzi*. II. Encontro do *Panstrongylus megistus* em ecótopos silvestres no Estado de São Paulo (Hemiptera, Reduviidae). *Revista do Instituto de Medicina Tropical de São Paulo*, **6**, 56–63.

Barretto, M. P. and Ferriolli, F. Filho (1964). Estudos sôbre reservatórios e vectores silvestres do *Trypanosoma cruzi*. IV. Infecção natural do *Triatoma infestans*, encontrado em ecótopos silvestres, por tripanossomo semelhante ao *T. cruzi*. *Revista do Instituto de Medicina Tropical de São Paulo*, **6**, 219–224.

Barretto, M. P. and Carvalheiro, J. da Rocha (1968). Estudos sôbre reservatórios e vectores silvestres do *Trypanosoma cruzi*. XXVIII. Sôbre o encontro de *Triatoma sordida* Stål, 1859 e de *Rhodnius neglectus* Lent, 1954 em ninhos de passaros da familia Furnariidae (Hemiptera Reduviidae). *Revista Brasileira de Biologia*, **28**, 289–293.

Barretto, M. P., Albuquerque, Rosa, D. R. and Funayama, G. K. (1969). Estudos sôbre reservatórios e vectores silvestres do *Trypanosoma cruzi*. XXXVI. Investigações sôbre triatomineos de palmeiras no municipio de Uberaba, Minas Gerais, Brasil. *Revista Brasileira de Biologia*, **29**, 577–588.

Carcavallo, R. U., personal communication.

Carcavallo, R. U. (1976). Aspects of the epidemiology of Chagas' disease in

Venezuela and Argentina. *In:* "New Approaches in American Trypanosomiasis Research". Proceedings of an International Symposium, Belo Horizonte, Minas Gerais, Brazil, 18–21 March 1975. Pan American Health Organization, Washington. Scientific Publication No. 318, 347–358.

Carcavallo, R. U., Martinez, A., Prosen, A. F. and Cichero, J. A. (1964). Una nueva especie de *Triatominae* de la Republica Argentina. *Anales del Instituto de Medicina Regional* (Suplemento), **6**, 151–157.

Carcavallo, R. U. and Martinez, A. (1968). Comunicaciones cientificas entomoepidemiologia de la Republica Argentina. *Junta del Investigaciones Cientificas de las Fuerzas Armadas Argentinas*, **13**, 1–144.

Carcavallo, R. U. and Celis, M. R. de (1972). La enfermedad de Chagas en la provincia de Buenos Aires. Bases para el diagnostico epidemiologico y formulacion del programa de control. Provincia de Buenos Aires, Ministero de Bienestar Social, Argentina.

Carcavallo, R. U., Otero, M. A., Tonn, R. J. and Ortega, R. (1975). Notas sobre la biologia, ecologia y distribucion geografica de *Psammolestes arthuri* (Pinto) 1926 (Hemiptera, Reduviidae). Descripcion de los estadios preimagales. *Boletin de la Direccion de Malariologia y Saneamiento Ambiental, XV*, 231–239.

Carcavallo, R. U., Tonn, R. J. and Jimenez, J. C. (1976). Notas sôbre la biologia, ecologia y distribucion geografica de *Rhodnius neivai* Lent, 1953 (Hemiptera, Reduviidae). *Boletin de la Direccion de Malariologia y Saneamiento Ambiental, XVI*, 169–171.

Carcavallo, R. U., Tonn, R. J., Gonzalez, J. and Otero, M. A. (1976). Notas sôbre la biologia, ecologia y distribucion geografica de *Cavernicola pilosa* Barber, 1937 (Hemiptera, Reduviidae). *Boletin de la Direccion de Malariologia y Saneamiento Ambiental, XVI*, 172–175.

Carcavallo, R. U. and Barreto, P. (1976). Una nueva especie de *Rhodnius* Stål (Hemiptera, Reduviidae, Triatominae) de Colombia. *Boletin de la Direccion de Malariologia y Saneamiento Ambiental, XVI*, 176–183.

Cichero, J. A. and Carcavallo, R. U. (1967). Notas sôbre bioecologia del *Triatoma breyeri* Del Ponte, 1929. *Neotropica*, **13**, 52–53.

Correa, R. R., Rochae Silva, E. O. and Schiavi, A. (1963). Observações sôbre o *Panstrongylus megistus*, transmissor da molestia de Chagas (Hemiptera, Reduviidae). *Arquivos de Higiene e Saúde Pública*, **28**, 165–174.

D'Alessandro, A. (1972). Epidemiologia de la enfermedad de Chagas en Colombia. Simposio internacional sôbre enfermedad de Chagas, Buenos Aires, December 1972. Secretaria de Estado de Salud Publica, Buenos Aires, Argentina.

D'Alessandro, A., Barreto, P. and Duarte, R. (1971). Distribution of triatomine-transmitted trypanosomiasis in Colombia and new records of the bugs and infections. *Journal of Medical Entomology*, **8**, 159–172.

Del Ponte, E. (1961). Importancia sanitaria de la biologia de los triatomineos argentinos en la enfermedad de Chagas. *Anais do Congresso Internacional sobre a doença de Chagas, II*, 459–477.

Dias, E. (1951). Doença de Chagas nos Americas. II. Mexico. *Revista Brasileira de Malariologia e Doenças Tropicais*, **3**, 555–570.

Forattini, O. P., Rabello, E. X., Castanho, M. L. S. and Pattoli, D. G. B. (1970). Aspectos ecologicos da tripanossomose americana. I. Observações sôbre *Panstrongylus megistus* e suas relações com focos naturais da infecção, em area urbana da cidade de São Paulo, Brasil. *Revista da Saúde Pública*, **4**, 19–30.

Forattini, O. P., Rabello, E. X. and Pattoli, D. B. G. (1972). Aspectos ecologicos da tripanossomose Americana. IV. Mobilidade de *Triatoma arthurneivai* em seus ecótopos naturais. *Revista de Saúde Pública*, **6**, 183–187.

Freitas, J. L. P. de, Siqueira, A. F. and Ferreira, O. A. (1961). Investigações epidemiologicas sôbre triatomineos de habitos domesticos e silvestres com auxilio da reação de precipitina. *Anais do Congresso Internacional sôbre a doença de Chagas, II,* 525–556.

Galvao, A. B. (1973). Contribução ao conhecimento do *Triatoma maculata* (Erichson, 1848) e do *Triatoma pseudomaculata* Correia e Espinola, 1964 (Hemiptera, Reduviidae). *Revista da Sociedade Brasileira de Medicina Tropical,* 7, 367–380.

Galvao, A. B. and Fuentes, F. B. (1971). Descrição das ninfas de *Triatoma williami* (B. Galvao e col., 1965) e *T. deanei* (B. Galvao e col., 1967). *Revista Goiana de Medicina,* 17, 141–145.

Gomez-Nunez, J. C. (1969). Resting places, dispersal and survival of CO^{60}-tagged adult *Rhodnius prolixus. Journal of Medical Entomology,* 6, 83–86.

Herrer, A. (1959). La enfermedad de Chagas en el Peru. *Revista Goiana de Medicina,* 5, 389–409.

Herrer, A., Lent, H. and Wygodzinsky, P. (1954). Contribucion al conocimiento del genero *Belminus* Stål, 1859 (Triatominae, Reduviidae, Hemiptera). *Anales del Instituto de Medicina Regional de la Universidade Nacional de Tucuman,* 4, 85–106.

Jauregui, L. R. and Valdivia, C. J. B. (1972). Epidemiologia de la enfermedad de Chagas en Bolivia. Simposio internacional sôbre enfermedad de Chagas, Buenos Aires, December 1972. Secretaria de Estado de Salud Publica, Buenos Aires, Argentina.

Leal, H., Ferreira Neto, J. A. and Martins, C. M. (1961). Dados ecologicos sôbre os triatomineos silvestres na ilha de Santa Catarina (Brasil). *Revista do Instituto de Medicina Tropical de São Paulo,* 3, 213–220.

Lent, H. (1943). Novo transmissor da doença de Chagas na cidade do Rio de Janeiro, D. F. Estudo dos generos *Belminus* Stål, 1859, *Bolbodera* Valdes, 1910 e descrição de *Parabelminus carioca* n.g., n sp. (Hemiptera, Triatomidae). *Memorias do Instituto Oswaldo Cruz,* 38, 497–516.

Lent, H. (1950). Nova especie de *Triatoma* Laporte, 1833 (Hemiptera, Reduviidae). *Revista Brasileira de Biologia,* 10, 437–440.

Lent, H. (1953). Nova especie de *Triatoma* da região oriental (Hemiptera, Reduviidae). *Revista Brasileira de Biologia,* 13, 315–319.

Lent, H. (1962). Estado atual dos estudos sôbre os transmissores da doença de Chagas (Relatorio). *Anais do Congresso Internacional sôbre doença de Chagas, III,* 739–760.

Lent, H. and Jurberg, J. (1967). Algumas informações sôbre *Triatoma spinolai* Porter, 1934, com um estudo sôbre as genitalias externas (Hemiptera, Reduviidae). *Revista Brasileira de Biologia,* 27, 273–288.

Lent, H. and Jurberg, J. (1968). Estudo morphologico comparativo de *Panstrongylus geniculatus* (Latreille, 1811) e *Panstrongylus megistus* (Burmeister, 1835) e suas genitalias externas (Hemiptera, Reduviidae, Triatominae). *Revista Brasileira de Biologia,* 28, 499–520.

Lent, H. and Jurberg, J. (1969a). O genero "*Cavernicola*" Barber, 1937, com um estudo sôbre a genitalia externa (Hemiptera, Reduviidae, Triatominae). *Revista Brasileira de Biologia,* 29, 317–327.

Lent, H. and Jurberg, J. (1969b). O genero "*Rhodnius*" Stål, 1859, com um estudo sôbre a genitalia das especies (Hemiptera, Reduviidae, Triatominae). *Revista Brasileira de Biologia,* 29, 487–560.

Lent, H. and Jurberg, J. (1970). O genero "*Eratyrus*" Stål, 1859, com um estudo sôbre a genitalia externa (Hemiptera, Reduviidae, Triatominae). *Revista Brasileira de Biologia,* 30, 297–312.

Lent, H. and Jurberg, J. (1971). O genero *"Paratriatoma"* Barber, 1938, com um estudo sôbre a genitalia externa (Hemiptera, Reduviidae, Triatominae). *Revista Brasileira de Biologia*, **31**, 39–48.

Lent, H. and Jurberg, J. (1972). O genero *"Dipetalogaster"* Usinger, 1939, com um estudo sôbre a genitalia externa (Hemiptera, Reduviidae, Triatominae). *Studia Entomologica*, **15**, 465–484.

Lent, H. and Jurberg, J. (1975). O genero *"Panstrongylus"* Berg, 1879, com um estudo sôbre a genitalia externa das especies (Hemiptera, Reduviidae, Triatominae). *Revista Brasileira de Biologia*, **35**, 379–438.

Lent, H. and Valderrama, A. (1973). Hallazgo en Venezuela del Triatomino *Rhodnius robustus* Larrousse, 1927, en la palma *Attalea maracaibensis* Martins (Hemiptera, Reduviidae). *Boletin Informativo Direccion de Malariologia y Saneamiento Ambiental, XIII*, 175–179.

Lucena, D. T. de (1962). Ecologia dos triatomineos do Brasil. *Anais do Congresso Internacional sôbre a doença de Chagas, Rio de Janeiro*, **3**, 771–851.

Lucena, D. T. de and Marques, R. J. (1955). Subsidios para o estudo ecologico do *Triatoma rubrofasciata* no Brasil. *Anais da Faculdade de Medicina da Universidade do Recife*, **15**, 19–31.

Marinkelle, C. J. (1976). Epidemiology of Chagas' disease in Colombia. *In:* "New Approaches in American Trypanosomiasis Research". Proceedings of an International Symposium, Belo Horizonte, Minas Gerais, Brazil, 18–21 March 1975. Pan American Health Organization, Washington. Scientific Publication No. 318, 340–346.

Miles, M. A. (1976). A simple method of tracking mammals and locating triatomine vectors of *Trypanosoma cruzi* in Amazonian forest. *American Journal of Tropical Medicine and Hygiene*, **25**, 671–674.

Miles, M. A. (1976). Distribution and importance of Triatominae as vectors of *T. cruzi*. *In:* "New Approaches in American Trypanosomiasis Research". Proceedings of an International Symposium, Belo Horizonte, Minas Gerais, Brazil, 18–21 March 1975. Pan American Health Organization, Washington. Scientific Publication No. 318, 48–56.

Minter, D. M. (1976). Feeding patterns of some triatomine vector species. *In:* "New Approaches in American Trypanosomiasis Research". Proceedings of an International Symposium, Belo Horizonte, Minas Gerais, Brazil, 18–21 March 1975. Pan American Health Organization, Washington. Scientific Publication No. 318, pp. 33–47.

Monteith, G. B. (1974). Confirmation of the presence of Triatominae (Hemiptera, Reduviidae) in Australia, with notes on Indo-Pacific species. *Journal of the Australian Entomological Society*, **13**, 89–94.

Naquira, F., Cordova, E., Neira, M. and Valdivia, L. (1972). Epidemiologia de la enfermedad de Chagas en el Peru. Simposio internacional sôbre enfermedad de Chagas, Buenos Aires, December 1972. Secretaria de Estado de Salud Publica, Buenos Aires, Argentina.

Neiva, A. and Lent, H. (1936). Notas e commentarios sôbre triatomideos. Lista de especies e sua distribuição geographica. *Revista de Entomologia*, **6**, 153–190.

Neiva, A. and Lent, H. (1941). Sinopse dos Triatomideos. *Revista de Entomologia*, **12**, 61–92.

Olsen, P. F. (1966). Epizoology of Chagas' disease in the southeastern United States. *Wildlife Disease*, **47**, 1–108. (Supplement).

Ortiz, I. (1971). Sôbre algunos arreglos taxonomicos en el orden de los Hemiptera (insecta) com referencia especial a la identificacion de la Familia Triatomidae Pinto, 1931, revision del genero *Panstrongylus* Berg, 1875 y descripcion de una nueva especie. *Revista del Instituto Nacional de Higiene*, **4**, 49–90.

Osimani, J. J. (1942). *Haemogregarina triatomae* n. sp. from a South American lizard *Tupinambis teguixin* transmitted by the reduviid *Triatoma rubrovaria*. *Journal of Parasitology*, **28**, 147–154.

Osimani, J. J. (1959). Enfermedad de Chagas: Importante flagelo de las zonas rurales del Uruguay. *Revista Goiana de Medicina*, **5**, 339–356.

Osimani, J. J. (1972). Epidemiologia de la enfermedad de Chagas en Uruguay. Simposio Internacional sôbre enfermedad de Chagas, Buenos Aires, December 1972. Secretaria de Estado de Salud Publica, Buenos Aires, Argentina.

Otero, M. A., Jimenez, J. C., Carcavallo, R. U., Ortega, R. and Tonn, R. J. (1975). Actualizacion de la distribucion geografica de *Triatominae* (Hemiptera, Reduviidae) en Venezuela. *Boletin de la Direccion de Malariologia y Saneamiento Ambiental*, *XV*, 217–230.

Otero, M. A. A., Carcavallo, R. U. and Tonn, R. J. (1976). Notas sôbre la biologia, ecologia y distribucion geografica de *Rhodnius pictipes* Stål, 1872 (Hemiptera, Reduviidae). *Boletin de la Direccion de Malariologia y Saneamiento Ambiental*, *XVI*, 163–168.

Pifano, F. C. (1972). La epidemiologia de la enfermedad de Chagas en Venezuela. Simposio Internacional sôbre enfermedad de Chagas. Buenos Aires, December 1972. Secretaria de Estado de Salud Publica, Buenos Aires, Argentina.

Pinto, C. (1931). Valor do rostro e antenas na caracterização dos generos de Triatomideos, Hemiptera, Reduvidioidea. *Boletim Biologico*, **19**, 45–136.

Rodrigues, B. A. and Melo, G. B. (1942). Contribução ao estudo da tripano-somiase americana. *Memorias do Instituto Oswaldo Cruz*, **37**, 77–90.

Rodriguez, J. D. M. (1959). Epidemiologia de la enfermedad de Chagas en la republica del Ecuador. *Revista Goiana de Medicina*, **5**, 411–438.

Ryckman, R. E. (1971). The genus *Paratriatoma* in Western North America (Hemiptera, Reduviidae). *Journal of Medical Entomology*, **8**, 87–97.

Ryckman, R. E., personal communication.

Schenone, H., Rojas, A., Villarroel, F. and Knierim, F. (1972). Epidemiologia de la enfermedad de Chagas en Chile. Simposio Internacional sôbre enfermedad de Chagas, Buenos Aires, December 1972. Secretaria de Estado de Salud Publica; Buenos Aires, Argentina.

Sherlock, I. A. and Guitton, N. (1967). Sôbre o *Triatoma petrochii* Pinto e Barretto, 1925 (Hemiptera, Reduviidae). *Revista Brasileira de Malariologia e Doenças Tropicais*, *XIX*, 625–632.

Sherlock, I. A. and Serafim, E. M. (1967). *Triatoma lenti* sp. n. *Triatoma pessoai* sp. n. e *Triatoma bahiensis* sp. n. do estado da Bahia, Brasil (Hemiptera, Reduviidae). *Gazeta Medica da Bahia*, **67**, 75–92.

Sherlock, I. A. and Serafim, E. M. (1972). Fauna triatominae do estado da Bahia, Brasil. I. As especies e distribução geografica. *Revista da Sociedade Brasileira de Medicina Tropical*, **6**, 265–297.

Sherlock, I. A. and Guitton, N. (1974). Fauna triatominae do estado da Bahia, Brasil. III. Notas sôbre ecótopos silvestres e o genero *Psammolestes*. *Memorias do Instituto Oswaldo Cruz*, **72**, 91–101.

Sousa, O. E. (1972). Anotaciones sobre la enfermedad de Chagas en Panama. Frecuencia y distribucion de *Trypanosoma cruzi* y *Trypanosoma rangeli*. *Revista de Biologia Tropical*, **20**, 167–179.

Sousa, O. E. and Galindo, P. (1972). Natural infections of *Triatoma dispar* Lent, 1950, with *Trypanosoma cruzi* in Panama. *American Journal of Tropical Medicine and Hygiene*, **21**, 293–295.

Tonn, R. J., Carcavallo, R. U. and Ortega, R. (1976). Notas sôbre la biologia, ecologia y distribucion geografica de *Rhodnius robustus* Larrousse, 1927

184   M. A. MILES

(Hemiptera, Reduviidae). *Boletin de la Direccion de Malariologia y Saneamiento Ambiental, XVI*, 158–162.

Torrealba, J. F. (1964). Apuntes para la geografia de la enfermedad de Chagas en Venezuela. *Anais do Congresso Internacional sôbre a doença de Chagas, V*, 1599–1611, Rio de Janeiro.

Torrico, R. A. M. (1959). Enfermedad de Chagas en Bolivia. *Revista Goiana de Medicina*, **5**, 375–387.

Usinger, R. L. (1944). The triatominae of North and Central America and the West Indies and their public health significance. *Public Health Bulletin No.* **288**.

Usinger, R. L., Wygodzinsky, P. and Ryckman, R. E. (1966). The biosystematics of Triatominae. *Annual Review of Entomology*, **11**, 309–331.

Vargas, V. M. and Montero-Gei, F. (1971). *Triatoma dispar* Lent, 1950, in Costa Rica (Hemiptera, Reduviidae). *Journal of Medical Entomology*, **8**, 454–455.

Velazquez, C. J. and Gonzalez, G. (1964). Estado actual de la enfermedad de Chagas en el Paraguay. *Anais do Congresso Internacional sôbre a doença de Chagas, V*, 1671–1692.

Woody, N. C. and Woody, H. B. (1964). Chagas' disease in the United States of North America. *Anais do Congresso Internacional sôbre a doença de Chagas, V*, 1699–1724.

Wygodzinsky, P. (1949). Elenco sistematico de los reduviiformes Americanos. Tucuman: Universidad Nacional de Tucuman. Instituto de Medicina Regional. Publication No. 473.

Yaeger, R. G. (1959). Chagas' disease in the United States. *Revista Goiana de Medicina*, **5**, 461–470.

Zeledón, R. (1972). Los vectores de la enfermedad de Chagas en America. Simposio internacional sôbre enfermedad de Chagas, Buenos Aires, December 1972, pp. 327–345. Secretaria de Estado de Salud Publica, Buenos Aires, Argentina.

Zeledón, R. (1976). Effects of triatomine behaviour on trypanosome transmission. *In:* "New approaches in American Trypanosomiasis Research". Proceedings of an International Symposium, Belo Horizonte, Minas Gerais, Brazil, 18–21 March 1975. Pan American Health Organization, Washington. Scientific Publication No. 318, 326–329.

Zeledón, R. and Ponce, C. (1972). Descripcion de una nueva especie de *Triatoma* de Honduras, America Central (Hemiptera, Reduviidae). *Revista de Biologia Tropical*, **20**, 275–279.

Zeledón, R., Solano, G., Zúniga, A. and Swartzwelder, J. C. (1973). Biology and ethology of *Triatoma dimidiata* (Latreille, 1811). III. Habitat and blood sources. *Journal of Medical Entomology*, **10**, 363–370.

Addendum

The chapter above was written in January-February 1977. Since then many additional, relevant publications have appeared. Furthermore, we have been able to apply isoenzyme characterization of *Trypanosoma cruzi* widely in Brazil, in localities with enzootic, continuous or discontinuous transmission cycles. The addendum which follows briefly updates the text, as far as early 1978, and also refers to work in press on the epidemiological significance of *T. cruzi* strain-groups, as identified by isoenzyme electrophoresis. The subdivisions of the text are followed and principal references are given.

I. Kean (1977) has produced a lucid account of Carlos Chagas' discoveries.

II. The sensitivity of blood culture is reported to compare favourably with that of xenodiagnosis (Neal and Miles, 1977; Minter-Goedbloed, 1978; Minter-Goedbloed *et al.*, 1978); in first instar triatomine bugs, fed experimentally on a *T. cruzi*-infected rhesus monkey, a relationship between estimated size of blood-meal and the subsequent development of *T. cruzi* infection is described (Minter *et al.*, 1977). Molyneux (1977) succinctly reviews the pathogenic relationship between *T. rangeli* and its principal vector *Rhodnius prolixus*; *Blastocrithidia* infections are reported from both *Panstrongylus megistus* and *Triatoma sordida* collected in São Paulo State, Brazil (Rocha e Silva *et al.*, 1977).

Lopes *et al.* (1978) have successfully diagnosed *T. cruzi* infection at human post-mortem by applying IFAT, CFT and IHAT serological tests to pericardial fluid; Guimaraes *et al.* (1978) find that, by storing at −20°C, both IgG and IgM are preserved in serum or filter paper eluates, at essentially equivalent levels, for at least 10 weeks after collection of blood samples.

In a detailed description of the clinical features of Chagas' disease, not referred to previously, Marsden (1971) draws attention to the experimental observation of Lumbreras *et al.* (1959) that Romaña's sign may be induced, in sensitive individuals, by the bite of uninfected triatomine bugs. Hoff *et al.* (1978b) demonstrate, by culture, that *T. cruzi* is frequently present in human cerebrospinal fluid (CSF) during acute infections, and is associated with other CSF abnormalities.

IV A. Further to the possible occurrence of *T. cruzi* in Asia, Arambulo and Cabrera (1977) found no trypanosomes in 200 adult Philippine monkeys (*Macaca philippensis*) examined by blood smears and blood cultures. However, Weinman *et al.* (1978) show, without question, that trypanosomiasis is enzootic in the simians of the Asian mainland and Indonesia, but that the trypanosomes involved are previously undescribed organisms and are quite distinct from *T. cruzi*; the organisms will multiply in *Rhodnius prolixus* and *Triatoma rubrofasciata*, producing infective forms in the faeces, but the natural mode of transmission is unknown.

IV B. Hoff *et al.* (1978c) describe congenital *T. cruzi* infection in premature dizygotic twins, detected during an investigation of the congenital transmission of Chagas' disease in an urban population of Salvador, Bahia, Brazil.

IV C.

1 and Appendix—A checklist and bibliography of the *Triatominae* of Western North America is given by Ryckman and Casidin (1976); Ghauri (1976) revises the genus *Linshcosteus* and describes two new

species—*L. confumus* and *L. costalis*—from rocky localities in Bangalore, India; a new species of cave-dwelling triatomine—*Triatoma cavernicola*— is described from Perlis, northern Malaysia by Else *et al.* (1977). The comprehensive taxonomic treatise of Lent and Wygodzinsky, revising the genus *Triatoma*, and giving descriptions of several new triatomine species not included in the Appendix, is to appear shortly (Lent, personal communication).

2a—In Amazonian Brazil, the isoenzyme characters of *T. cruzi* responsible for the first autochthonous cases of Chagas' disease have confirmed the sylvatic origin of the organisms responsible; the arrival of domiciliated triatomine bug species from other regions is seen as the main threat of introducing endemic Chagas' disease to the Amazon basin (Miles *et al.*, 1978b). Lainson *et al.* (1979) review the current status of the *T. cruzi* zoonosis in the Amazon basin with much new information in the reservoir hosts, sylvatic triatomine species, and clinical cases of Chagas' disease, and with records of sylvatic bugs invading houses in Pará State, Brazil. The new species of *Rhodnius* associated with *Didelphis marsupialis* and *Echimys chrysurus*, on the outskirts of the city of Belém, has been described as *Rhodnius paraensis* (Sherlock *et al.*, 1977).

2b—In Texas, new emphasis has been placed on the local occurrence of enzootic *T. cruzi* by the reports of nine fatal cases of *T. cruzi* infection in domestic dogs and the endemic infection of a primate research colony (*Macaca mulatta*) (Williams *et al.*, 1977; Kasa *et al.*, 1977).

4—The sylvatic ecotopes and potential of *P. megistus* to invade dwellings in São Paulo State, Brazil have been discussed at length by Forattini *et al.* (1977a, b); experimental chicken houses were readily colonized (1977c).

5b—A much improved version of the spool-and-line mammal tracking device, using precision-wound thread, is currently under trial at Belém, Brazil; the device has given 50–60% retrieval of mammals released and proved fundamental to the identification of the sylvatic ecotopes of local triatomine species (Miles, Souza and Povoa, unpublished work).

V D—Among many recent publications on the pathology of Chagas' disease, an elegant histopathological study of 25 human cases of chagasic myocarditis has appeared, which employed complete serial sections mounted on continuous transparent plastic tape (Andrade *et al.*, 1978). A clear correlation was demonstrated between clinical electrocardiographic abnormalities and the extensive and variable histopathological changes in the cardiac conducting tissue found after death. Puigbo *et al.* (1977) give a detailed account of the clinical and pathological manifestations of chagasic heart disease, classified according to acute, latent and chronic phases (3). Hernandez-Pieretti (1977) reports that echocardiographic changes in chronic chagasic patients are non-specific and similar to those occurring in non-specific congestive cardiomyopathy; in a single clinical case, an expatriate Swede infected in Colombia, pyrophosphate scinti-graphy revealed extensive cardiac fibrosis (Lessem and Persson, 1977). Machado *et al.* (1978) found cardiac norepinephrine depletion, by fluorometric assay, in acute experimental infections in rats, with partial recovery in the chronic phase, and suggest that this is associated with destruction and regeneration of sympathetic neurones. Padovan *et al.* (1977) find a disturbance of acid and pepsin production in chagasic patients, which is believed to be due to degeneration of intramural para-sympathetic ganglia in the stomach; Almeida *et al.* (1977) describe a dramatic reduction in the total number of dense vesicles in the Auer-bach's plexus of acutely infected mouse colon, which is concomitant with a significant reduction in substance P activity. Burnstock (1977) suggests that disturbance of a recently discovered third component of the autonomic nervous system—the purinergic nerves—may play a role in the pathogenesis of Chagas' disease. Carvalhal (1977) reviews the history of studies of the pathogenesis of chronic Chagas' disease.

An autoantibody reacting with the plasma membrane of striated muscle fibres and endothelial cells (EVI antibody) is shown to commonly occur in, but not to be pathognomonic for, *T. cruzi* infection in Argentina (Cossio *et al.*, 1977; Szarfman *et al.*, 1977a; Khoury *et al.*, 1978). The evidence for such autoimmune involvement in the pathogenesis of Chagas' disease has been reviewed recently (Anon, 1977).

V E—Brener *et al.* (1976) find different *in vivo* sensitivities to 3 chemo-therapeutic agents among 3 *T. cruzi* stocks of diverse origins. Andrade and Figueira (1977) report different *in vivo* sensitivities of "Peru strain" and "Colombian strain" *T. cruzi* to the drug Ro 7-1051. Dvorak and Howe (1976) demonstrate the remarkable ease with which a Lampit resistant strain of *T. cruzi* can be produced *in vitro*. Continuous perfusion of *T. cruzi*–vertebrate cell culture, with low concentrations of Lampit, rapidly produced a stable strain resistant *in vitro* to 100-fold greater concentrations of the drug than the parent strain.

V F—Experimental work of Urdaneta-Morales and Rueda (1977) sug-gests that a Venezuelan *T. cruzi* ("EP strain") is better adapted to de-velop in the local vector *Rhodnius prolixus* than Brazilian *T. cruzi* ("Y strain").

V G—Milder *et al.* (1977) find that the capacity of *T. cruzi* "Y strain" bloodstream forms to survive, differentiate and multiply *in vitro* in ham-ster peritoneal macrophages is much greater than that of *T. cruzi* "F strain". Kloetzel and Deane (1977) further report "immunological differences between bloodstream trypomastigotes of the F and Y strains"; attached IgG and IgM host mouse immunoglobulins were not demonstrated in the "Y strain", by direct immunofluorescence, but were demonstrated in the "F strain". (However, there seems to be no evidence that these differences are not due simply to the harvesting of the

"Y strain" on day 7 and the "F strain" on days 30–40.) Reis *et al.* (1976) report greater leucocyte migration inhibition in mice inoculated with predominantly stout trypomastigotes ("CL strain" and "PNM strain") than in mice inoculated with predominantly slender trypomastigotes ("Y strain"). Gonzales-Cappa *et al.* (1977) found that the action of rabbit immune sera on epimastigote cultures was "strain-independent".

VI—A multiple biochemical approach has become appropriate to the intrinsic characterization of parasitic protozoa, using a selection of the available techniques of restriction endonuclease analysis, DNA buoyant density measurement, DNA melting curve analysis, DNA hybridization, SDS polyacrylamide electrophoresis, amino acid analysis, protein and isoenzyme electrofocussing and starch or polyacrylamide gel enzyme electrophoresis (Riou and Yot, 1977; Frank-Kamenetskii and Vologodskii, 1977; Gibson *et al.*, 1978; Ebert *et al.*, 1978). The impact of isoenzyme electrophoresis continues to be most pronounced (Godfrey, 1978) for example, for the identification of *Leishmania* (Al-Taqi and Evans, 1978), *Coccidia* (Long *et al.*, 1977; Shirley and Lee, 1977) and rodent *Plasmodia* in Africa (Carter and Walliker, 1977; Carter, 1978).

We have continued our collaborative studies of *Trypanosoma cruzi* strain-groups in Brazil, which henceforth, when identified on the basis of isoenzyme patterns, we have elected to call "zymodemes" (Barrett *et al.*, 1979b, in press; Lumsden and Ketteridge—this volume). Zymodeme corresponds with "strain-group" and "type" of Miles *et al.* (1978b). Three *T. cruzi* zymodemes, 1, 2 and 3 are widely distributed in a variety of mammals and vectors in northeastern and northern Brazil. An epidemiological correlation between the distribution of the 3 zymodemes and patterns of local transmission has become apparent. Thus:

(a) the separation of zymodeme 1 (sylvatic) and zymodeme 2 (domestic), as described in São Felipe—which has predominantly discontinuous sylvatic and domestic transmission cycles—has been confirmed in other, similar, localities (Barrett *et al.*, 1979b; Miles *et al.*, unpublished data).

(b) Following the recent incursion of enzootic *T. cruzi* into an established domestic cycle of transmission, causing an outbreak of acute Chagas' disease, both zymodemes 1 and 2 were identified in man and his domestic animals. Thus, as predictable, continuous sylvatic and domestic transmission in a locality was confirmed by the zymodeme distribution (Hoff *et al.*, 1978a; Barrett *et al.*, 1979a, b).

(c) In the Amazon basin, characterization of *T. cruzi* from sylvatic mammals and vectors and the first autochthonous cases of Chagas' disease, confirm the capacity of the local zymodemes 1 and 3 to produce acute infection in man (Miles *et al.*, 1978a, b).

It is known that at least these 3 *T. cruzi* zymodemes can infect man in

Brazil and are responsible for acute disease; zymodeme 2 certainly causes cardiomyopathy and mega syndromes in Bahia State. A relationship between infecting zymodemes and the form and severity of human disease has yet to be demonstrated. 10 and 7 of 18 enzymic characters have separated sample Brazilian *T. cruzi* stocks of zymodemes 1 and 2 and 1 and 3, respectively; so far no genetic interaction has been observed when mixtures of zymodemes 1 and 2 are cyclically transmitted (Miles, Souza and Povoa, unpublished work). Nevertheless, during prolonged maintenance, Y "strain" (uncloned) can exhibit variable enzymic patterns (Neal and Miles, unpublished work; Romanha, personal communication); it is conceivable that some clonal enzymic characters of *T. cruzi* may yet prove unstable or subject, experimentally and in nature, to genetic induction or repression; minor banding differences are best interpreted initially with caution.

VII, A—Investigations, *in vitro* and *in vivo*, of the immune response to *T. cruzi* infection is the most prolific area of current research. Kress *et al.* (1977) confirm the enhanced destruction of *T. Cruzi* in BCG-activated macrophages. Nogueira and Cohn (1977) review the uptake and intracellular fate of *T. cruzi* in normal and activated cells. Significant trypomastigote destruction was found only in macrophages activated by secondary challenge with specific antigen. Kuhn and Murnane (1977) demonstrate that spleen cells from infected, but not immunized, mouse donors "effect significant cytolysis of parasitized syngeneic fibroblasts"; however, in parallel with the work of Teixeira, previously referred to, they did not find autoimmune destruction of normal fibroblasts. Sanderson (1977) using a ^{3}H-uridine, RNA labelled, cytotoxicity test demonstrates that eosinophils destroy *T. cruzi* epimastigotes *in vitro*.

Partial protection, in the form of surviving virulent challenge, has been confirmed, in mice, using live epimastigotes (Szarfman *et al.*, 1977b), killed epimastigotes or trypomastigotes with saponin as adjuvant (Neal and Johnson, 1977), or flagellar antigens (Pereira *et al.*, 1977; Segura *et al.*, 1977). McHardy (1977) finds passive protection against death in mice treated with convalescent serum. The immunosuppressive effect of acute *T. cruzi* infection has been demonstrated (Reed *et al.*, 1977; Schmunis *et al.*, 1977, Szarfman *et al.*, 1977b) and strain dependent recrudescence of *T. cruzi* infection was induced by challenge with *Plasmodium berghei* (Krettli, 1977). A lipoprotein *T. cruzi* antigen has been implicated as having special immunogenic and pathogenic properties (Ketteridge, 1978; Lederkremer *et al.*, 1977). Teixeira (1977a, b) reviews the immune and autoimmune response to *T. cruzi* and the prospects for immunoprophylaxis.

VII B. Gaborak *et al.* (1977) find *in vitro* drug sensitivities of *T. cruzi* and *T. dionisii* to be similar. Morrow *et al.* (1977) suggest that prolonged treatment with Lampit eradicated *T. cruzi* infection from mice (but this was assessed only by the relatively insensitive methods of X-irradiation and animal inoculation). Kinnamon *et al.* (1977) and Neville and Verge (1977) describe drugs with *T. cruzi* suppressive activities, detected during drug screening programmes.

VIII C. Maudlin (1976) describes the inheritance of radiation-induced sterility in *Rhodnius prolixus*.

In addition to the above, the growth and isolation of the life cycle stages of *T. cruzi* has progressed further: Gutteridge *et al.* (1978) describe the efficient separation of intracellular forms of *T. cruzi* from infected rodents; Kanbara *et al.* (1977) confirm that cultured epimastigotes and trypomastigotes can be separated on anion exchangers. Pudney and Lanar (1977) have established a cell line from *Triatoma infestans* which may provide an alternative avenue for mass production of metacyclic trypomastigotes. Enders *et al.* (1977) review the growth requirements of *T. cruzi* and its mass production for immunogenic and biochemical investigations.

A series of fundamental biochemical papers on *T. cruzi* have also recently appeared (see Boveris and Stoppani, 1977; Flombaum *et al.*, 1977; Funayama *et al.*, 1977; Juan and Cazzulo, 1977 and Gutteridge and Rogerson—this volume).

References

Almeida, H. O., Tafuri, W. L., Cunha-Melo, J. R., Freire-Maia, L., Raso, P. and Brener, Z. (1977). Studies on the vesicular component of the Auerbach's plexus and the substance P content of the mouse colon in the acute phase of the experimental *Trypanosoma cruzi* infection. *Virchows Archiv-Abteilung A: Pathology, Anatomy and Histology*, **376**, 353–360.

Al-Taqi, Muna and Evans, D. A. (1978). Characterization of *Leishmania* spp. from Kuwait by isoenzyme electrophoresis. *Transactions of the Royal Society of Tropical Medicine and Hygiene*, **72**, 56–65.

Andrade, Sonia G. and Figueira Rozalia M. (1977). Estudo experimental sobre a ação terapêutica da droga Ro 7–1051 na infecção por diferentes cepas do *Trypanosoma cruzi*. *Revista do Instituto de Medicina Tropical de São Paulo*, **19**, 335–341.

Andrade, Z. A., Andrade, Sonia, G., Oliveira, G. B., Alonso, D. R. (1978). Histopathology of the conducting tissue of the heart in Chagas' myocarditis. *American Heart Journal*, **95**, 316–324.

Anonymous (1977). Autoimmunity in Chagas' disease. *British Medical Journal*, **2**, 1243–1244.

Arambulo, P. V. III and Cabrera, B. D. (1977). On the examination of Philippine monkeys for trypanosomes. *South East Asian Journal of Tropical Medicine and Public Health*, **8**, 277.

Barrett, T. V., Hoff, R., Mott, K. E., Guedes, F. and Sherlock, I. A. (1979a). An outbreak of acute Chagas' disease in the São Francisco valley region of Bahia, Brazil. I. Triatomine vectors and animal reservoirs of *Trypanosoma cruzi. Transactions of the Royal Society of Tropical Medicine and Hygiene.* In press.

Barrett, T. V., Hoff, R. H., Mott, K. E., Miles, M. A., Godfrey, D. G., Teixeira, R., Almeida de Souza, J. A. and Sherlock I. A. (1979b). Epidemiological aspects of three *Trypanosoma cruzi* zymodemes in Bahia state, Brazil. *Transactions of the Royal Society of Tropical Medicine and Hygiene.* In press.

Boveris, A. and Stoppani, A. O. M. (1977). Hydrogen peroxide generation in *Trypanosoma cruzi. Experientia,* 33, 1306–1308.

Brener, Z., Costa, C. A. G. and Chiari, C. (1976). Differences in the susceptibility of *Trypanosoma cruzi* strains to active chemotherapeutic agents. *Revista do Instituto de Medicina Tropical de São Paulo,* 18, 450–455.

Burnstock, G. (1977). The purinergic nerve hypothesis. *In:* "Purine and Pyrimidine Metabolism". Ciba Foundation Symposium 48 (new series), Elsevier. Excerpta Medica. North-Holland. Amsterdam, Oxford, New York, pp. 295–314.

Carter, R. (1978). Studies on enzyme variation in the murine malaria parasites *Plasmodium berghei, P. yoelii, P. vinckei* and *P. chabaudi* by starch gel electrophoresis. *Parasitology,* 76, 241–267.

Carter, R. and Walliker, D. (1977). Biochemical markers for strain differentiation in malarial parasites. *Bulletin of the World Health Organization,* 55, 339–345.

Carvalhal, S. (1977). Considerações em torno da patogênese da moléstia de Chagas. Especial ênfase em relação à fase crônica. *Revista da Associação Medica do Brasil,* 23, 139–142.

Cossio, P. M., Laguens, R. P., Kreutzer, E., Diez, C., Segal, A. and Arana, R. M. (1977). Chagasic Cardiopathy. Immunopathologic and morphologic studies in myocardial biopsies. *American Journal of Pathology,* 86, 533–544.

Dvorak, J. A. and Christine L. Howe. (1977). The effects of Lampit (Bayer 2502) on the interaction of *Trypanosoma cruzi* with vertebrate cells *in vitro. The American Journal of Tropical Medicine and Hygiene,* 26, 58–63.

Ebert, F., Schudnagis, R. and Muhlpfordt, H. (1978). Protein typing by disc electrophoresis of some species of trypanosomes with special emphasis to *Trypanosoma cruzi. Tropenmedizin und Parasitologie,* 29, 115–118.

Else, J. G., Cheong, W. H., Mahadevan, S. and Zarate, L. G. (1977). A new species of cave-inhabiting *Triatoma* (Hemiptera: Reduviidae) from Malaysia. *Journal of Medical Entomology,* 14, 367–369.

Enders, B., Brauns, F. and Zwisler, O. (1977). Biochemical and technical considerations regarding the mass production of certain parasitic protozoa. *Bulletin of the World Health Organization,* 55, 393–402.

Flombaum, Maria A. Cataldi de, Cannata, J. J. B., Cazzulo, J. J. and Segura, E. L. (1977). CO_2-fixing enzymes in *Trypanosoma cruzi. Comparative Biochemistry and Physiology,* 58B, 67–69.

Forattini, O. P., Ferreira, O. A., Rocha e Silva, E. O. da and Rabello, E. X. (1977a). Aspectos ecológicos da tripanossomíase americana. VIII. Domiciliação de *Panstrongylus megistus* e sua presença extradomiciliar. *Revista de Saúde Pública,* 11, 73–86.

Forattini, O. P., Rocha e Silva, E. O. da, Ferreira, O. A., Rabello, E. X., Santos, J. L. Ferreira and Lima, A. Ribeiro de (1977b). Aspectos ecológicos da tripanossomíase americana. XI. Domiciliação de *Panstrongylus megistus* e potencial enzoótico. *Revista de Saúde Pública,* 11, 527–550.

Forattini, O. P., Santos, J. L. F., Ferreira, O. A., Rocha e Silva, E. O. da and Rabello, E. X. (1977c). Aspectos ecológicos da tripanossomíase americana. X. Dados populacionais das colônias de *Panstrongylus megistus* e de *Triatoma sordida* espontaneamente desenvolvidas em ecótopos artificiais. *Revista de Saúde Pública*, **11**, 362–374.

Frank-Kamenetskii, N. D. and Vologodskii, A. V. (1977). The nature of the fine structure of DNA melting curves. *Nature*, London, **269**, 729.

Funayama, S., Funayama, S., Ito, Isabel Y. and Veiga, L. A. (1977). *Trypanosoma cruzi*: Kinetic properties of glucose-6-phosphate dehydrogenase. *Experimental Parasitology*, **43**, 376–381.

Gaborak, M., Darling, J. L. and Gutteridge, W. E. (1977). Comparative drug sensitivities of culture forms of *Trypanosoma cruzi* and *Trypanosoma dionisii*. *Nature*, London, **268**, 339–340.

Ghauri, M. S. K. (1976). The Indian triatomine genus *Linshcosteus* (Reduviidae). *Systematic Entomology*, **1**, 183–187.

Gibson, Wendy C., Parr, C. W., Swindlehurst, Christine A. and Welch, S. G. (1978). A comparison of the isoenzymes, soluble proteins, polypeptides and free amino acids from ten isolates of *Trypanosoma evansi*. *Comparative Biochemistry and Physiology*, **60B**, 137–142.

Godfrey, D. G. (1978). Identification of economically important parasites. *Nature*, London, **273**, 600–604.

Gonzalez-Cappa, S. M., Pesce, U. J., Cantarella, A. I. and Schmunis, G. A. (1977). *Trypanosoma cruzi*: Acción de inmunosueros de conejo sobre el cultivo de epimastigotes en medios bifásicos. *Revista do Instituto de Medicina Tropical de São Paulo*, **19**, 221–231.

Guimarães, Maria C. S., Camargo, M. E., Ferreira, A. W., Castilho, E. A. de and Nakahara, O. S. (1978). Comparison of IgG and IgM contents in serum and filter paper blood eluates. *The American Journal of Tropical Medicine and Hygiene*, **27**, 350–353.

Gutteridge, W. E., Cover, B. and Gaborak, Maria (1978). Isolation of blood and intracellular forms of *Trypanosoma cruzi* from rats and other rodents and preliminary studies of their metabolism. *Parasitology*, **76**, 159–176.

Hernandez-Pieretti, O. (1977). Echocardiographic diagnosis and evaluation of cardiomyopathies: idiopathic hypertrophic subaortic stenosis, Chagas' heart disease and endomyocardial fibrosis. *Postgraduate Medical Journal*, **53**, 533–536.

Hoff, R., Barrett, T., Miles, M., Godfrey, D., Sherlock, I., Teixeira, R. and Mott, K. (1978a). Tipos de isoenzimas de *T. cruzi* isolado do homem em duas regiões do Estado da Bahia. *XIV Congresso da Sociedade Brasileira de Medicina Tropical*, João Pessoa, 19–23 February.

Hoff, R., Teixeira, R. S., Carvalho, J. S. and Mott, K. E. (1978b). *Trypanosoma cruzi* in the cerebrospinal fluid during the acute stage of Chagas' disease. *The New England Journal of Medicine*, **298**, 604–606.

Hoff, R., Mott, K. E., Milanesi, Maria L., Bittencourt, Achilea L. and Barbosa, Helenemarie S. (1978c). Congenital Chagas's disease in an urban population: investigation of infected twins. *Transactions of the Royal Society of Tropical Medicine and Hygiene*, **72**, 247–250.

Juan, S. M., Cazzulo, J. J. and Segura, E. L. (1977). The citrate synthase from *Trypanosoma cruzi*. *The Journal of Parasitology*, **63**, 921–922.

Kanbara, H., Fukuma, T. and Nakabayashi, T. (1977). Separation with CM-cellulose of the trypomastigote form of *Trypanosoma cruzi* from the forms grown in fibroblast cell cultures. *Biken Journal*, **20**, 147–149.

Kasa, T. J., Lathrop, G. D., Dupuy, H. J., Bonney, C. H. and Toft, J. D. (1977). An endemic focus of *Trypanosoma cruzi* infection in a subhuman primate research colony. *Journal of the American Veterinary Medical Association*, **171**, 850–854.

Kean, B. H. (1977). Carlos Chagas and Chagas' disease. *The American Journal of Tropical Medicine and Hygiene*, **26**, 1084–1087.

Ketteridge, D. S. (1978). Lipopolysaccharide from *Trypanosoma cruzi*. *Transactions of the Royal Society of Tropical Medicine and Hygiene*, **72**, 101–102.

Khoury, E. L., Cossio, P. M., Szarfman, Ana, Marcos, J. C., Morteo, O. G. and Arana, R. M. (1978). Immunofluorescent vascular pattern due to EVI antibody of Chagas' disease. *American Journal of Clinical Pathology*, **69**, 62–65.

Kinnamon, K. E., Steck, E. A., Hanson, W. L. and Chapman, W. L. Jr. (1977). In search of anti-*Trypanosoma cruzi* drugs: New leads from a mouse model. *Journal of Medicinal Chemistry*, **20**, 741–744.

Kloetzel, Judith and Deane, Maria P. (1977). Presence of immunoglobulins on the surface of bloodstream *Trypanosoma cruzi*. Capping during differentiation in culture. *Revista do Instituto de Medicina Tropical de São Paulo*, **19**, 397–402.

Kress, Yvonne, Tanowitz, H., Bloom B. and Wittner, M. (1977). *Trypanosoma cruzi*: Infection of normal and activated mouse macrophages. *Experimental Parasitology*, **41**, 385–396.

Krettli, Antoniana U. (1977). Exacerbation of experimental *Trypanosoma cruzi* infection in mice by concomitant malaria. *Journal of Protozoology*, **24**, 514–518.

Kuhn, R. E. and Murnane, J. E. (1977). *Trypanosoma cruzi*: Immune destruction of parasitized mouse fibroblasts *in vitro*. *Experimental Parasitology*, **41**, 66–73.

Lainson, R., Shaw, J. J., Fraiha, H., Miles, M. A. and Draper, C. C. Chagas' disease in the Amazon basin. I. *Trypanosoma cruzi* infections in silvatic mammals, triatomine bugs and man, in the State of Pará, north Brazil. *Transactions of the Royal Society of Tropical Medicine and Hygiene*, 1979. In press.

Lederkremer, Rosa M. de, Tanaka, Cecelia T., Alves, Maria J. M. and Colli, W. (1977). Lipopeptidophosphoglycan from *Trypanosoma cruzi*. *European Journal of Biochemistry*, **74**, 263–267.

Lessem, J. and Persson, B. (1977). Myocardial scintigraphy in Chagas' disease. *The Lancet*, 6 August, p. 310.

Long, P. L., Millard, B. J. and Shirley, M. W. (1977). Strain variation within *Eimeria meleagrimitis* from the turkey. *Parasitology*, **75**, 177–182.

Lopes, E. R., Chapadeiro, E., Batista, S. M., Cunha, J. G., Rocha, A., Miziara, L., Ribeiro, J. U. and Patto, R. J. (1978). Post-mortem diagnosis of chronic Chagas's disease: comparative evaluation of three serological tests on pericardial fluid. *Transaction of the Royal Society of Tropical Medicine and Hygiene*, **72**, 244–246.

Lumbreras, H., Flores, W. and Escallón, A. (1959). Allergische reaktionen auf stiche von reduviiden und ihre bedeutung bei der Chagaskrankheit. *Tropenmedizin und Parasitologie*, **10**, 6–19.

Machado, Conceição R. S., Machado, A. B. M. and Chiari, Cléa A. (1978). Recovery from heart norepinephrine depletion in experimental Chagas' disease. *The American Journal of Tropical Medicine and Hygiene*, **27**, 20–24.

Marsden, P. D. (1971). South American Trypanosomiasis (Chagas' disease). *International Review of Tropical Medicine*, **4**, 97–121.

Maudlin, I. (1976). The inheritance of radiation induced semi-sterility in *Rhodnius prolixus*. *Chromasoma (Berl)*, **58**, 285–306.

McHardy, N. (1977). Passive immunization of mice against *Trypanosoma cruzi* using convalescent mouse serum. *Tropenmedizin und Parasitologie*, **28**, 195–201.

Milder, Regina, Kloetzel, Judith and Deane, Maria P. (1977). Observation on the interaction of peritoneal macrophages with *Trypanosoma cruzi*. II. Intracellular fate of bloodstream forms. *Revista do Instituto de Medicina Tropical de São Paulo*, **19**, 313–322.

Miles, M. A., Souza, A., Povoa, M., Shaw, J. J., Lainson, R. and Fraiha, H. (1978a). Três tipos distintos de *Trypanosoma cruzi*, identificados por electroforese de enzímas, infetam o homen no Brasil. *XIV Congresso da Sociedade Brasileira de Medicina Tropical*, João Pessoa, 19–23 February.

Miles, M. A., Souza, A., Povoa, M., Shaw, J. J., Lainson, R. and Toyé, P. J. (1978b). Isozymic heterogeneity of *Trypanosoma cruzi* in the first autochthonous patients with Chagas' disease in Amazonian Brazil, *Nature*, London, **272**, 819–821.

Minter, D. M., Minter-Goedbloed, E. and Ferro Vela, C. (1977). Quantitative studies with first-instar triatomines in the xenodiagnosis of *Trypanosoma (Schizotrypanum) cruzi* in experimentally and naturally infected hosts. *Transactions of the Royal Society of Tropical Medicine and Hygiene*, **71**, 530–541.

Minter-Goedbloed, E. (1978). The primary isolation by haemoculture of *Trypansoma (Schizotrypanum) cruzi* from animals and from man. *Transactions of the Royal Society of Tropical Medicine and Hygiene*, **72**, 22–30.

Minter-Goedbloed, E., Minter, D. M. and Marshall, T. F. de C. (1978). Quantitative comparison between xenodiagnosis and haemoculture in the detection of *Trypanosoma (Schizotrypanum) cruzi* in experimental and natural chronic infections. *Transactions of the Royal Society of Tropical Medicine and Hygiene*, **72**, 217–225.

Molyneux, D. H. (1977). Vector relationships in the Trypanosomatidae. *Advances in Parasitology*, **15**, 1–82.

Morrow, D. T., Wescott, R. B. and Davis, W. C. (1977). Effect of length of treatment with Bayer 2502 on isolation of *Trypanosoma cruzi* and resistance to challenge in the mouse. *The American Journal of Tropical Medicine and Hygiene*, **26**, 382–386.

Neal, R. A. and Johnson, Pauline (1977). Immunization against *Trypanosoma cruzi* using killed antigens and with saponin as adjuvant. *Acta Tropica*, **34**, 87–96.

Neal, R. A. and Miles, R. A. (1977). The sensitivity of culture methods to detect experimental infections of *Trypanosoma cruzi* and comparison with xenodiagnosis. *Revista do Instituto de Medicina Tropical de São Paulo*, **19**, 170–176.

Neville, M. C. and Verge, J. P. (1977). Antiprotozoal thiazoles. 2. 2-(5-Nitro-2-furyl-, thiazolyl-, and 1-methylimidazolyl-) thiazoles. *Journal of Medicinal Chemistry*, **20**, 946–949.

Nogueira, N. and Cohn, Z. (1977). *Trypanosoma cruzi*: uptake and intracellular fate in normal and activated cells. *The American Journal of Tropical Medicine and Hygiene*, **26**, 194–203.

Padovan, W., Meneghelli, U. G. and Godoy, R. A. de (1977). Gastric secretory and motility studies in chronic chagasic patients. *American Journal of Digestive Diseases*, **22**, 618–622.

Pereira, N. M., Souza, W. de, Machado, R. D. and Castro, F. T. de (1977). Isolation and properties of flagella of Trypanosomatids. *Journal of Protozoology*, **24**, 511–514.

Pudney, Mary and Lanar, D. (1977). Establishment and characterization of a cell line (BTC-32) from the triatomine bug, *Triatoma infestans* (Klug) (Hemiptera: Reduviidae). *Annals of Tropical Medicine and Parasitology*, **71**, 109–118.

Puigbó, J. J., Valecillos, R., Hirschhaut, E., Giordano, H. M., Boccalandro, I., Suárez, Claudia and Aparicio, J. M. (1977). Diagnosis of Chagas' cardiomyopathy. Non-invasive techniques. *Postgraduate Medical Journal*, **53**, 527–532.

Reed, S. G., Larson, C. L. and Speer, C. A. (1977). Suppression of cell-mediated immunity in experimental Chagas' disease. *Zeitschrift fur Parasitenkunde*, **52**, 11–17.

Reis, A. P., Chiari, C. A., Tanus, R. and Andrade, I. M. (1976). Cellular immunity to *Trypanosoma cruzi* infection in mice. *Revista do Instituto de Medicina Tropical de São Paulo*, **18**, 422–426.

Riou, G. F. and Yot, P. (1977). Heterogeneity of the kinetoplast DNA molecules of *Trypanosoma cruzi*. *Biochemistry*, **16**, 2390–2396.

Rocha e Silva, E. O. da, Pattoli, D. B. G., Corrêa, R. R. and Andrade, J. C. R. de (1977). Observações sobre o encontro de tripanossomatídeos do género *Blastocrithidia*. Infectando naturalmente triatomíneos em insetário e no campo. *Revista de Saúde Pública*, **11**, 87–96.

Ryckman, R. E. and Casdin, Margaret A. (1976). The Triatominae of western north America, a checklist and bibliography. *California Vector Views*, **23**, 35–52.

Sanderson, C. J., Lopez, A. F. and Bunn Moreno, Marlene M. (1977). Eosinophils and not lymphoid K cells kill *Trypanosoma cruzi* epimastigotes. *Nature, London*, **268**, 340–341.

Schmunis, G. A., Szarfman, A., Pesce, U. J. and Gonzales-Cappa, S. M. (1977). The effect of acute infection by *Trypanosoma cruzi* upon the response of mice to sheep erythrocytes. *Revista do Instituto de Medicina Tropical de São Paulo*, **19**, 323–331.

Segura, E. L., Vazquez, C., Bronzina, A., Campos, J. M., Cerisola, J. A. and Gonzales-Cappa, S. M. (1977). Antigens of the subcellular fractions of *Trypanosoma cruzi*. II. Flagellar and membrane fraction. *Journal of Protozoology*, **24**, 540–543.

Sherlock, I. A., Guitton, N. and Miles, M. A. (1977). *Rhodnius paraensis*, especie nova do Estado do Pará, Brasil (Hemiptera, Reduviidae, Triatominae). *Acta Amazonica*, **7**, 71–74.

Shirley, M. W. and Lee, D. L. (1977). Isoelectric focusing of Coccidial enzymes. *The Journal of Parasitology*, **63**, 390–392.

Szarfman, Ana, Cossio, P. M., Schmunis, G. A. and Arana, R. M. (1977a). The EVI antibody in acute Chagas' disease. *Journal of Parasitology*, **63**, 149.

Szarfman, A., Schmunis, G. A., Vattuone, N. H., Yanovsky, J. F., Cossio, P. M. and Arana, R. M. (1977b). Protection against challenge of mice experimentally infected with *Trypanosoma cruzi*. *Tropenmedizin und Parasitologie*, **28**, 333–341.

Teixeira, A. R. L. (1977a). Immunoprophylaxis in Chagas' disease. *Advances in Experimental Medicine and Biology*, **93**, 243–280.

Teixeira, A. R. L. (1977b). Evidência de imunidade na doença de Chagas. O papel da imunidade celular. *Revista Goiana de Medicina*, **23**, 15–22.

Urdaneta-Morales, S. and Rueda, Irma G. (1977). A comparative study of the behaviour of Venezuelan and Brazilian strains of *Trypanosoma* (*Schizotrypanum*) *cruzi* in the Venezuelan invertebrate host (*Rhodnius prolixus*). *Revista do Instituto de Medicine Tropical de São Paulo*, **19**, 241–250.

Weinman, D., Wallis, R. C., Cheong, W. H. and Mahadevan, S. (1978). Triatomines as experimental vectors of trypanosomes of Asian monkeys. *The American Journal of Tropical Medicine and Hygiene*, **27**, 232–237.

Williams, Gail D., Adams, L. G., Yaeger, R. G., McGrath, R. K., Read, W. K. and Bilderback, W. R. (1977). Naturally occurring trypanosomiasis (Chagas' disease) in dogs. *Journal of the American Veterinary Medical Association*, **171**, 171–177.

Notes

1. Now identified as *M. trinidadensis* (Lent, 1951).
2. See Hoff *et al.* (1978b) referred to in the Addendum, p. 185.

3. Now renamed *Didelphis albiventris*.
4. See Carmargo, E. P. and Freymuller, E. (1977). *Nature, Lond.*, **270**, 52–53.
5. This hypothesis has not been confirmed by our recent results.
6. Now published—Baker, J. R., Miles, M. A., Godfrey, D. G. and Barrett, T. V. (1978). *American Journal of Tropical Medicine and Hygiene*, **27**, 483–491.
7. = *R. paraensis* Sherlock, Guillon and Miles, 1977. See Addendum, p. 186.

3

Epidemiology of Leishmaniasis in the USSR

V. P. SERGIEV

Department of Epidemiology,
Main Board of Sanitation and Epidemiology,
Ministry of Health of the USSR,
Moscow, USSR

I.	Zoonotic cutaneous leishmaniases	198
II.	Anthroponotic cutaneous leishmaniasis	206
III.	Visceral leishmaniasis	208
IV.	Conclusion	209
V.	References	209

All three of the kinds of Old World leishmaniasis—zoonotic cutaneous, anthroponotic cutaneous and visceral—have been observed in the southern regions of the Soviet Union. The northern borderline of these infections is determined by the distribution of the vectors (42–46° North latitude). Within the endemic area, foci of different kinds of leishmaniasis often overlapped. For example, both anthroponotic and zoonotic cutaneous leishmaniases occurred in the suburbs of Ashkhabad. Anthroponotic cutaneous and visceral leishmaniases occurred simultaneously in Samarkand, Tashkent and Kirovabad. At the same time, the ecology and epidemiology of each kind of leishmaniasis was specific.

Nowadays, after control campaigns have been carried out, only zoonotic cutaneous leishmaniasis has retained epidemiological significance.

I. Zoonotic cutaneous leishmaniases

The Soviet investigator Latyshev was the first to discover the natural focality of cutaneous leishmaniasis. He found great gerbils—*Rhombomys opimus*—infected with *Leishmania* in 1937 in southern Turkmenia (Latyshev and Krjukova, 1941). Later, Kojevnikov *et al.* (1947), on the basis of a profound investigation, predicted that cutaneous leishmaniasis should have natural reservoirs not only in rural areas of the south of the USSR, but also in some other countries, including Israel and Tunisia. The correctness of this prediction was proved by the detection of leishmanial infection in *R. opimus* in Afghanistan (Eliseev and Kellina, 1963), in *R. opimus, Meriones libycus, M. persicus* in Iran (Ansari and Faghih, 1953; Neronov and Farang-Azad, 1973), in *Psammomys obesus* in Israel (Gunders *et al.*, 1968) and in Africa (Bray, 1972).

In the USSR leishmanial infection was detected in nine species of mammals—*R. opimus, M. libycus, M. meridianus, Spermophilopsis leptodactilus, Mus musculus, Allactaga severtzovi, Mustela nivalis, Vormela peregusna, Hemiechinus auritus*—by microscopic investigation. Five other species of mammals—*Allactaga elater, Dipus sagitta, M. tamariscinus, Nesokia indica, Hystryx leucura*—are also suspected to be involved in the epizootiology of cutaneous leishmaniasis in the USSR (Kojevnikov *et al.*, 1947; Petrishcheva and Safyanova, 1969; Dubrovsky, 1974). These 14 species of mammals are not equally important as reservoirs of *Leishmania tropica major*. Conditions most favourable for the parasite exist in the skin of the ears of great gerbils. On average, a lesion (as a rule, a non-ulcerated infiltration) persists for 11 months after inoculation in spring by sandflies of the first generation, and 23 months after the inoculation, in July-August, by sandflies of the second generation (Shishlyaeva-Matova, 1966). Thus, leishmanias survive in great gerbils during an interepizootic (winter) season, and sometimes even during two such seasons. Other hosts are less suitable for *Leishmania tropica major*; in their lesions parasites are extremely scanty.

It is of interest to note that, after an artificial inoculation into the skin of the back or the base of the tail of *R. opimus* or *M. libycus*, the appearance of the lesions developed was unusual. The lesions resembled human cutaneous leishmaniasis with rapid ulceration. After 17 to 98 days a scar appeared. The same picture was observed in gerbils that had spontaneous lesions in the ears (Krjukova, 1941). The difference in pathogenesis probably depends on the difference between the skin temperature of the ears and the temperature of the hairy parts of the body. The skin temperature of the ears of *R. opimus* is 6–8°C lower than the skin temperature of the back, and 5–6°C lower than the skin temperature of the head, with the air temperature 20–30°C. The differences for *M. libycus* are 8–9°C and

6–8°C, respectively (in the same conditions) (Eliseev and Strelkova, 1966).

Sandflies are closely linked with gerbils' burrows. There they find all the necessary conditions for life and breeding (Vlassov, 1941). As a rule, other desert animals are much less numerous than great gerbils and fail to create conditions suitable for sandflies. Besides *R. opimus*, only *M. libycus* produces numerous holes, thus giving rise to significant numbers of sandflies in some areas (Artemiev *et al.*, 1972). At present it is recognized that the following four species of the genus *Phlebotomus*—*P. papatasi*, *P. caucasicus*, *P. andrejevi*, *P. mongolensis*—play a major part in the dissemination of *Leishmania tropica major* in the USSR. Each of these species is the principal vector in the different parts of the enzootic area (Safyanova, 1967, 1974). *R. opimus* is the preferred host for bloodsucking by the genus *Phlebotomus*. Other leishmania hosts (except *H. auritus*) are rarely bitten by sandflies (Strelkova and Djabarov, 1971).

Thus, the difference in effectiveness of various animals as reservoirs of *Leishmania tropica major* is a result of different adaptation to them of both the parasite and the vectors.

The natural foci of cutaneous leishmaniasis in the USSR are widespread in the deserts of Turkmenia, Uzbekistan, southern Kazakhstan and southern Tadjikistan. The northern boundary of the zoonotic cutaneous leishmaniasis area coincides with the northern boundary of the distribution of great gerbils—the main reservoir of this infection in the USSR (Dubrovsky, 1973a, b). In the eastern part of the Surkhan Darya geographical district, the main reservoir is *M. libycus* (Latyshev *et al.*, 1971). The same rodent served as the reservoir of cutaneous leishmaniasis in the now eliminated foci in the south of Tadjikistan (Latyshev *et al.*, 1951; Gozodova *et al.*, 1967) and around the town of Nurek (Tadjikistan), where cases are occasionally observed.

The spatial structure of the zoonotic cutaneous leishmaniasis distribution area in the USSR was investigated by Dubrovsky (1973a, 1976). He recognized 12 regions and 35 separate groups of natural foci in the desert zone of the USSR (Fig. 1). Depending on the main animal reservoir concerned, the natural foci fall into two groups—the eastern part of the Surkhan Darya geographical district (the main reservoir is *M. libycus*) and all the others (the main host is *R. opimus*). The latter are of two kinds, depending on the presence of additional hosts: monohostal simple foci (no additional host is known) are foci of the northern deserts from 42–43° to 47–48° North latitude (Fig. 1: 1–7, 10.1, 10.2); monohostal complex foci (additional hosts are present) are foci of the southern deserts (all other groups of foci). Several complex foci have some polyhostal features. Thus, *Leishmania tropica major* persists in populations of *M. libycus* in Tedzhen Valley, where the density of *R. opimus* is low (Artemiev *et al.*, 1972). In the western part of the Kara Kum desert, *M.*

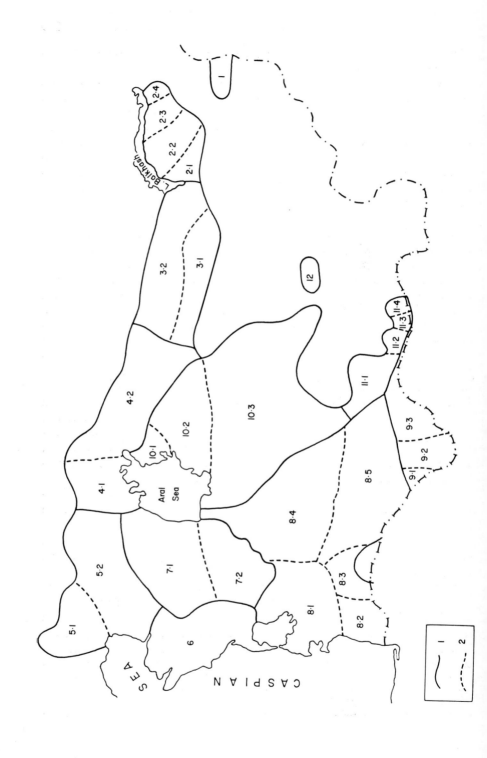

libycus are often involved in epizootiology as well as *R. opimus* and increase dissemination of *Leishmania* (Remyannikova, 1968).

According to the number of the species of sandflies present and according to the most widespread species, natural foci fall into three groups: monovectoral—one species present, *P. mongolensis* (Fig. 1: 5.1, 5.2, probably 4.1); oligovectoral—5–6 species present, the most widespread being *P. mongolensis* (Fig. 1: 2.3, 4.2, probably 6, 7.1, 7.2, 10.1, 10.2); and polyvectoral (all other foci)—10–12 species with 3–4 most widespread, changing with the type of the soil. *P. andrejevi* predominates in sand soil, *P. causasicus* in the loess soil of elevation and *P. papatasi* in humid soil of valleys and oases (Dergacheva and Zherikhina, 1974; Remyannikova, 1970).

The survival of *Leishmania tropica major* in monovectoral monohostal natural foci testifies to the stability of the parasite system of the infection even in the simplest variant with one reservoir and one vector.

The abundance of sandflies in great gerbils' burrows does not differ appreciably between the northern and southern groups of natural foci. The intensity of epizootiology does not differ from one group of natural foci to another, either. Both in the north and the south of the epizootic area, a severe epizootiology can be detected with more than 50% of gerbils infected.

In the deserts and semideserts of Central Asia human cases of zoonotic cutaneous leishmaniasis are extremely rare in spite of the widespread intensive epizootiology in gerbils. Most human cases are due to the infection in oases located in the river valleys and foothill plains of southern Turkmenia and Uzbekistan, where sufficient numbers of *P. papatasi* (the species responsible for the transmission of *Leishmania tropica major* to man) are present. However, the epidemiological activity of natural foci depends not only on the density of *P. papatasi* but also on the number of biotic and abiotic factors influencing the level of transmission. Therefore, it is impossible to detect the endemicity level on the basis of

FIG. 1. Epizootiological structure of the zoonotic cutaneous leishmaniasis area of the USSR (after Dubrovsky, 1973a, 1976). I: Boundaries of regions; II: Boundaries of groups of natural foci.

Regions and Groups of Natural Foci: 1. Ily (5 groups of foci); 2. Near Lake Balkhash; 2.1. Taukum; 2.2. Saryishikotrau; 2.3. Lukkum; 2.4. Aralkum; 3. Chu; 3.1. Mujnkum; 3.2. Betpakdala; 4. Near Aral Sea; 4.1. Northern Aral; 4.2. Kara Kum—Transaral; 5. Near Caspian Sea; 5.1. Ural-Amba; 5.2. Preusturt; 6. Mangyslak; 7. Usturt; 7.1. Northern Usturt; 7.2. Southern Usturt; 8. Turkmenian; 8.1. Krasnovodsk; 8.2. Atrek; 8.3. Western Kopetdag; 8.4. Sarykamysh-Zaungyth; 8.5. Kara-Kum; 9. South-eastern Kara-Kum; 9.1. Serakhs; 9.2. Tedzhen-Murgab; 9.3. Murgab-Amu Darya; 10. Kzyl-Kum; 10.1. Bozkol; 10.2. Northern Kzyl-Kum; 10.3. Central Kzyl-Kum; 10.4. Golodnaya Steppe; 11. Karshi; 11.1. Karshi (Kashka darya); 11.2. Sharabaddarya; 11.3. Termez; 11.4. Southern Tadjikistan; 12. Fergana.

epizootiological data alone. This should be done only after calculating the epidemiological parameters. The proper choice of criteria is very important.

The morbidity from zoonotic cutaneous leishmaniasis cannot serve as an indicator of the endemicity level. The disease produces stable resistance to a secondary (repeat) infection. Therefore, the morbidity among the population in the foci is limited by the level of collective (herd) immunity and does not reflect the intensity of transmission (here and later only the foci with negligible migrations of the inhabitants are taken into account). Zoonotic cutaneous leishmaniasis is a children's disease in foci with a high level of transmission because of the immunity developed by older people. The morbidity in such foci depends on the birth rate.

The pervasiveness (the proportion of persons with a cutaneous leishmaniasis history in the population) cannot be considered to be a reliable criterion of the endemic level either. This criterion can be as great in foci with a low level of transmission and a low birth rate as in foci with a high level of transmission but a high birth rate.

Belyaev (1973) proposed a method for quantitative determination of the degree of endemicity. The method is based on the model of malaria transmission by Moshkovski (1950) plus an additional demographic parameter. According to the model the age-specific distribution of persons who have not suffered from zoonotic cutaneous leishmaniasis among the inhabitants of a focus is described by the function:

$$f(x) = e^{-(n + p)x}$$

where n = natality; p = loimopotential (number of acts of transmission per head per unit of time = force of infection; after Muench, 1959) and x = age in years. The model is close to reality in the following conditions: the population is characterized by a high or moderate coefficient of natural growth; the intensity of migration is negligible; the risk of infection of non-immunes does not depend on the age; the loimopotential is more or less constant.

Using the model, the mean loimopotential for x years can be calculated. The value of the loimopotential for any specific (a particular) year is calculated from the proportion of zoonotic cutaneous leishmaniasis cases among the non-immunes who have spent the whole season of transmission at risk of infection. An analysis of the model shows the "critical" value of the loimopotential when endemicity changes qualitatively. Accordingly, three degrees of endemicity of zoonotic cutaneous leishmaniasis can be distinguished: hyper-endemicity (loimopotential is more than 0·25 per annum), meso-endemicity (loimopotential fluctuates between 0·05 and 0·25), and hypo-endemicity (loimopotential is less than 0·05).

Other epidemiological parameters depend on the value of the loimo-potential. Thus, foci with different degrees of endemicity have certain peculiarities. According to the model and investigations of the foci, all persons who have never been affected by zoonotic cutaneous leishmani-asis or persons in the acute stage of the disease are children in an *hyper-endemic focus*. Among the persons with acute leishmaniasis at least 25% are children under one year old and at least 85% are pre-school children (from 0 to 6 years old). In ordinary years the number of cases is close to the number of newborn infants, and the morbidity approximately equals the natality. The level of transmission is high every year. However, in occasional years, with extremely unusual weather, a noticeable decrease of the level of transmission can take place. Such a picture was observed in 1969 in Turkmenia after an exceptionally cold winter and a rainy spring (Belyaev, 1973). In an *hypo-endemic focus*, among the persons who have never been affected by the disease or were in the acute stage of zoonotic cutaneous leishmaniasis there are not a few adults (at least 20% of acute cases are older than 15 years). The morbidity is noticeably lower than the birth rate. The level of transmission fluctuates. *Meso-endemic foci* are located between hyper- and hypo-endemic ones.

Using Belyaev's method, we divided the zoonotic cutaneous leish-maniasis area in the USSR according to the main epidemiological parameter—the level of transmission (Fig. 2). The degree of endemicity was determined for irrigated regions—the most epidemiologically danger-ous territories. As our analysis has shown, the most epidemiologically active territories are situated in the Turkmen SSR. Hyper-endemic regions were found in Turkmenia alone, in the river-valleys of the Tedzhen and the Murgab. The further from the hyper-endemic Ted-zhen, Serakhs and Takhta-Bazar oases, the lower is the endemicity. In the Murgab and Ateck oases, the nearest to this "epicentre of endemicity" of zoonotic cutaneous leishmaniasis in the USSR, meso-endemicity is observed. Hypo-endemicity was found in more remote oases in the Amu-Darya Valley and at the foothills of Kopetdag between the cities of Kzil-Arvat and Ashkhabad (Akhal-Tekin oasis). In Uzbekistan, meso-endemicity of zoonotic cutaneous leishmaniasis was observed only in the irrigated region of the Kashka Darya Valley. In the rest of the territory of the Republic, only hypo-endemic regions were found. No reliable local human cases of zoonotic cutaneous leishmaniasis were reported in areas north of the border-line of the *P. papatasi* distribution (Fig. 2).

Inside oases the intensity of transmission is not equal from settlement to settlement, its level depending on the size of the village, its age and how far it is situated from gerbils' burrows. In the hyper-endemic Tedzhen oasis which is the most active in Turkmenia, the loimopotential fluctuates between 0·30 and 1·00 in different villages. In Kashka Darya

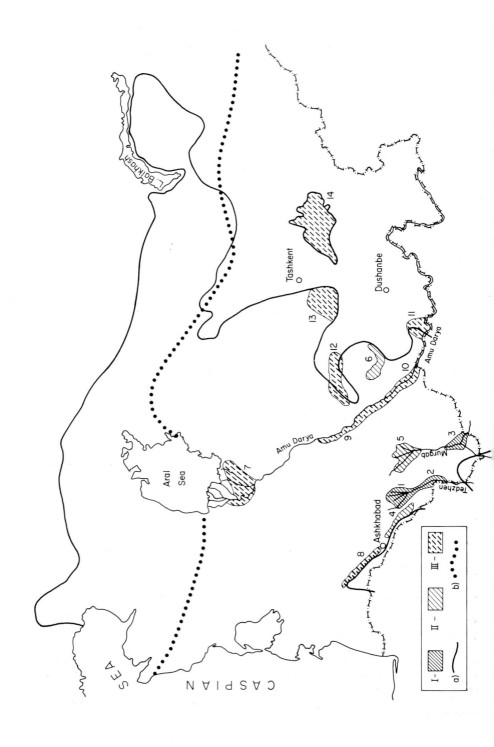

CASPIAN SEA

Aral Sea

L. Balkhash

Tashkent ○

Dushanbe ○

Amu Darya

Amu Darya

Murgab

Tedzhen

Ashkhabad ○

1
2
3
4
5
6
7
8
9
10
11
12
13
14

I -
II -
III -
a)
b)

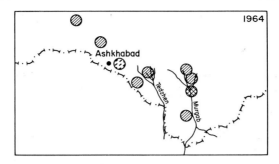

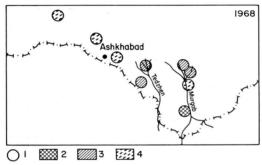

○ 1   ▦ 2   ▨ 3   ▦ 4

FIG. 3. Level of zoonotic cutaneous leishmaniasis transmission to man in Southern Turkmenia in 1964 and 1968. 1. Level of transmission in a single settlement. 2. Loimopotential is more than 0·25 per annum. 3. Loimopotential fluctuates between 0·05 and 0·25 per annum. 4. Loimopotential is less than 0·05 per annum.

oasis which is the most active in Uzbekistan the differences are wider—from 0·005 up to 0·4 per annum.

At the same time the level of transmission of zoonotic cutaneous leishmaniasis in a settlement is not constant, but fluctuates from year to year (Sergiev et al., 1974). These changes in the level of transmission are not

FIG. 2. Epidemiological structure of the zoonotic cutaneous leishmaniasis area of the USSR. 1: Hyper-endemicity (loimopotential is more than 0·25 per annum); II: Meso-endemicity (loimopotential fluctuates between 0·05 and 0·25 per annum); III: Hypo-endemicity (loimopotential is less than 0·05 per annum).

Irrigated regions (oases): 1. Tedzhen; 2. Serakhs; 3. Takhta-Bazar; 4. Ateck; 5. Murgab; 6. Kashka Darya; 7. Southern Sea of Aral zone; 8. Akhal-Tekin; 9. Chardzou; 10. Kerki; 11. Surkhan Sharabad Darya; 12. Bukhara; 13. Goldnaja Steppe; 14. Ferghana.

[a] Northern limit of distribution of *Rhombomys opimus*; [b] Northern limit of distribution of *Phlebotomus papatasi*.

synchronous in different parts of the endemic area (Fig. 3). The epidemiological situation in a village may change noticeably after agricultural development of the surrounding area (Neronov and Gunin, 1971; Sergiev *et al.*, 1973) or as a result of preventive measures. It was shown that rodent control within a limited area with a high possibility of inward movement of rodents from untreated territory is epidemiologically ineffective. At the same time control of gerbils within the natural boundaries of individual populations is an effective method of protection of local inhabitants from zoonotic cutaneous leishmaniasis (Sergiev, 1974). Artificial immunization can be used as a preventive measure to protect small groups of newcomers, seasonal workers, and so on (P. G. Sergiev *et al.*, 1974).

The choice of proper preventive measures is invariably a subject for a special investigation. Only on the basis of information about the natural foci, the level of transmission of the infection, the immunological structure of the population and the time of exposure to the risk of infection can an epidemiologically effective and inexpensive (in the given conditions) system of zoonotic cutaneous leishmaniasis control be evolved.

II. Anthroponotic cutaneous leishmaniasis

This type of cutaneous leishmaniasis was widespread in cities and towns of Central Asia and Transcaucasia in the USSR. Ashkhabad, Tashkent, Kokand (Central Asia) Barda, Kirovabad (Azerbaijan) were the notorious foci of urban cutaneous leishmaniasis, although cases of the disease were registered in a number of other towns. According to Kojevnikov *et al.* (1947), Rodiakin (1957) and other Soviet scientists, the differences between anthroponotic and zoonotic types of cutaneous leishmaniasis are represented in Table 1.

As a rule, anthroponotic cutaneous leishmaniasis lasts approximately one year. But in some cases there appears leishmaniasis recidiva on the edge of the scar and the process becomes chronic. A patient in the acute stage of anthroponotic cutaneous leishmaniasis or with leishmaniasis recidiva is the sole source of infection in the USSR. The main vector is *P. sergenti*, an additional one in some foci being *P. papatasi*.

The cases were distributed unevenly throughout a city or town. Surveys showed that the source of infection lay either in the same courtyard or in a neighbouring one. The microfocal distribution of new cases not far from the patient depended on the short radius of migration of sandflies within the city or town (Moshkovski and Nosina, 1933).

The control measures against anthroponotic cutaneous leishmaniasis carried out in the foci were as follows: case finding and effective treatment of the source of infection; elimination of vectors in the microfoci by the use of insecticides (Nadjafov, 1966).

In all the cities and towns—the foci of the infection in the USSR—

Table 1. Differences between the anthroponotic and zoonotic types of cutaneous leishmaniasis or oriental sore [According to Kojevnikov *et al.* (1947), Rodiakin (1957) and others]

	Anthroponotic type	Zoonotic type
Synonyms	Leishmaniasis cutanea tarde exulcerans. Dry type, Urban type	Leishmaniasis cutanea cito necrotisans, moist type, Rural type
ECOLOGY		
Agent	*Leishmania tropica minor*	*Leishmania tropica major*
Virulence for white mice	Low	High
Reservoir (Host)	Man	Wild mammals (mainly rodents)
Main vector	*Phlebotomus sergenti*	*Phlebotomus papatasi*
Distribution	Mainly in towns	Mainly in villages in open country (desert, semi-desert), occasionally in city and town suburbs
Seasonal occurrence	Perennial	Aestivo-autumnal
Epidemic outbreaks	Rare	Common
Immunity	One attack protects against homologous infection but not completely against heterologous infection	One attack or artificial inoculation protects against both types of infection
CLINICAL PICTURE		
Incubation period	Long (2–6 months)	Short (1–3 weeks)
Course of disease	Chronic; unbroken "dry" papules persisting several months; ulceration retarded. Duration up to 12 months or longer	Acute; "moist" lesions ulcerating rapidly (after 5–10 days). Duration 3–5 months
Lymphangitis	Rare	Common
Parasites in lesions	Numerous	Scanty

transmission has been controlled as a result of using the complex of measures (Petrishcheva and Safyanova, 1969). The government-sponsored malaria eradication programme has also played an important part in the elimination of anthroponotic cutaneous leishmaniasis. At present only sporadic cases of leishmaniasis recidiva can be found in the former foci of anthroponotic cutaneous leishmaniasis. This is due to the fact that such cases are extremely hard to cure.

III. Visceral leishmaniasis

In the USSR, visceral leishmaniasis occurred in the Central Asian Republics (Turkmenia, Uzbekistan, Tadjikistan and Kirgizia), in the south of Kazakhstan and in the Transcaucasian Republics (Azerbaidjan, Georgia and Armenia). The disease affected mainly children, but not infrequently cases of visceral leishmaniasis were also reported among adults (Khodukin et al., 1932; Maruashvili, 1968; Mirzojan, 1957). *P. kandelaki* and *P. chinensis* in Transcaucasia and *P. caucasicus, P. chinensis* and *P. mongolensis* in Central Asia and Kazakhstan were considered to be the main vectors of the causal agent of the disease (Lisova and Vavilova, 1955; Chun-Sun, 1962; Saladze, 1963; Dursunova et al., 1965; Nadjafov, 1968). Dogs were the primary source of infection in the cities and towns (Khodukin, 1959). Jackals (*Canis aureus*) and foxes (*Vulpes vulpes* and *Vulpes corsak*) are the natural carriers of visceral leishmaniasis in rural foci, in addition to dogs if any (Latyshev et al., 1951; Maruashvili and Bardzadze, 1966; Lysenko and Lubova, 1974).

At present human cases have become sporadic everywhere within the former endemic area of the USSR except the Kzyl-Orda oblast (province) of the Kazakh SSR (Lysenko and Lubova, 1974). The control measures against visceral leishmaniasis consisted of detection and destruction of all infected dogs, effective treatment of human cases and residual insecticide spraying (Nadjafov, 1966). Visceral leishmaniasis control was facilitated since it coincided with a campaign for destroying homeless dogs under the government-sponsored rabies control plan (Petrishcheva and Safyanova, 1969).

Sporadic cases of visceral leishmaniasis have recently been detected in rural areas. As a rule, they have contracted the infection either from a natural reservoir or from dogs which themselves got the infection from natural reservoirs. In Central Asia, watering-places in deserts are dangerous in this respect. In such places the density of sandflies is a little higher than in deserts. Wild reservoirs of visceral leishmaniasis (mainly *Canidae*) often visit watering-places. The *Phlebotomus* that have fed on their blood, can if *Leishmania* is present in them, serve as a source of infection for sheep-dogs, which, in their turn, may pass the infection to people. In some foci, jackals and foxes pay visits to villages at night in search of food. Sandflies can acquire *Leishmania* from them and then transmit the infection to dogs and people. Thus the ecological chain of a rural focus of visceral leishmaniasis is more complicated than an urban one and can be represented as follows:

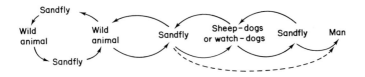

IV. Conclusion

Planned leishmaniasis control has led to remarkable changes in the epidemiological situation in the USSR. Since the successful carrying out of the control measures in the cities and towns human cases of leishmaniasis are restricted exclusively to contacts with natural foci. When man intrudes on such an area, where both the reservoir and the vector thrive, and where the vector will take human as well as animal blood, transmission to man can and generally does occur. Natural foci of cutaneous leishmaniasis are widely distributed in Central Asia. Therefore the problem of zoonotic cutaneous leishmaniasis is more important for Soviet regional public health authorities than that of visceral leishmaniasis. The study of the epidemiology of zoonotic cutaneous leishmaniasis was intensified in connection with the cultivation of deserts, the irrigation of vast land tracts and the creation of new rural communities in the south of the USSR. Large numbers of people have begun to arrive in a number of rural communities or even in previously unsettled areas of Central Asia, where natural cutaneous leishmaniasis foci exist; the need has arisen to work out complex leishmaniasis control measures to eliminate natural foci within the area being developed. The control of gerbils—the natural reservoir of the disease—was regularly carried out in Golodnaja and Karshi Steppes and the Surhan Sherabad Daryas zone—the reclamation areas of Uzbekistan. This method has sharply decreased the risk of being infected with zoonotic cutaneous leishmaniasis in all these regions.

V. References

Ansari, N. and Faghih, M. (1953). Cutaneous leishmaniasis from *L. tropica* in *Rhombomys opimus*. *Annales de Parasitologie Humaine et Comparée, France* **28**, 241–246.

Artemiev, M. M., Flerova, O. A. and Belyaev, A. E. (1972). Quantitative evaluation of productivity of breeding places of sandflies in nature and villages. *Meditsinskaya Parazitologiya i Parazitarnie Bolezni, USSR*, **41**, 31–35.

Belyaev, A. E. (1973). System of epidemetric magnitudes for investigation of geography of zoonotic cutaneous leishmaniasis. *In:* "Research in Medical Geography". Moscow Branch of the Geographical Society of the USSR, Moscow, 7–9 (In Russian).

Bray, R. S. (1972). Leishmaniasis in the Old World. *British Medical Bulletin*, **28**, 39–43.

Chun-Sun, F. (1962). Study on visceral leishmaniasis in Kzyl-Orda oblast of the

Kazakh SSR. Conference on Leishmaniases and Sandfly Fever. Abstracts, Moscow, 65–68 (In Russian).

Dergacheva, T. I. and Zherikhina, I. I. (1974). Regularities of distribution of sandflies of the Genus *Phlebotomus* in colonies of great gerbils in Karshinskaya Steppe. *Meditsinskaya Parazitologia i Parazitarnie Bolezni, USSR,* **43,** 423–428.

Djabarov, L. N. (1969). Prevalence of cutaneous leishmaniasis in *Mus musculus* in Termez. Proceedings of the 3rd Conference on Leishmaniasis and other Human Vector-borne Tropical Diseases with Natural Focality in Central Asia and Kazakhstan, Moscow, 71–72 (In Russian).

Dubrovsky, Y. A. (1973a). Some data on the spatial structure of area of natural nidality of cutaneous leishmaniasis. "Research in Medical Geography". Moscow Branch of the Geographical Society of the USSR, Moscow, 35–37 (In Russian).

Dubrovsky, Y. A. (1973b). Materials on natural focality of cutaneous leishmaniasis in the subzone of northern deserts of the USSR. *Meditsinskaya Parazitologia i Parazitarnie Bolezni, USSR,* **42,** 646–655.

Dubrovsky, Y. A. (1974). Mammals as reservoirs in natural nidi of cutaneous leishmaniasis with special references to great gerbils. "Terriology", *Science,* Novosibirsk, part 2, 202–217.

Dubrovsky, Y. A. (1976). Materials on the spatial structure of zoonotic cutaneous leishmaniasis distribution area. *Meditsinskaya Parazitologia i Parazitarnie Bolezni, USSR,* **45,** 274–284.

Dubrovsky, Y. A., Neronov, V. M., Belova, E. M. and Komarova, L. V. (1968). On the role of different species of mammals in natural foci of cutaneous leishmaniasis in the Murgab Valley and adjoining areas. *Meditsinskaya Parazitologia i Parazitarnie Bolezni, USSR,* **37,** 60–65.

Dursunova, S. M., Karapetyan, A. B. and Ponirovsky, E. N. (1965). Some data of investigation of visceral leishmaniasis in the Turkmen SSR. *Meditsinskaya Parazitologia i Parazitarnie Bolezni, USSR,* **34,** 303–309.

Eliseev, L. N. and Kellina, O. I. (1963). Cutaneous leishmaniasis in Afghanistan. *Meditsinskaya Parazitologia i Parazitarnie Bolezni, USSR,* **32,** 728–735.

Eliseev, L. N. and Strelkova, M. V. (1966). The effect of environmental temperature upon the temperature of the skin and the course of cutaneous leishmaniasis in *Rhombomys opimus* Licht. and *Meriones libicus* Licht. *Meditsinskaya Parazitologia i Parazitarnie Bolezni, USSR,* **35,** 696–705.

Gozodova, G. E., Martynova, Z. I., Kondrashin, A. V. and Barkov, V. N. (1967). The spatial structure of the cutaneous leishmaniasis distribution area in the Western Pamirs. Proceedings of the 1st Inter-republic Scientific Conference of the Central Asian Republics and the Kazakh SSR on the problem "The main parasitic diseases, their prevention and treatment", *Medicine,* Tashkent, 20–22 (In Russian).

Gunders, A. E., Foner, A. and Motilio, B. (1968). Identification of *Leishmania* species isolated from rodents in Israel. *Nature,* London, **219,** 85.

Khodukin, N. I. (1959). The basic problems of leishmaniasis in the USSR. "Khodukin's selected papers", Academy of Science of the Uzbek SSR, Tashkent, 180–188 (In Russian).

Khodukin, N. I., Petrov, V. P. and Kevorkov, N. P. (1932). Epidemiology of Kala-azar in Tashkent. Transactions of the Institute of Epidemiology and Micro-Biology, Tashkent, **1,** 74–145 (In Russian).

Kojevnikov, P. V., Dobrotvorskaya, N. V. and Latyshev, N. I. (1947). Studies on cutaneous leishmaniasis, "Medgyz", Moscow. (In Russian).

Krjukova, A. P. (1941). Le leishmaniose cutanée expérimentale des rongeurs sauvages de la Turkmenie. Conference Interrepublicaine sur la Leishmaniose Cutanée at le Problème des Phlebotomes. Ashkhabad, 241–248.

Latyshev, N. I. and Krjukova, A. P. (1941). L'epidémiologie de la leishmaniose cutanée dans les conditions du desert sablonneux. Conference Interrepublicaine sur la Leishmaniose Cutanée et le Problème des Phlebotomes. Ashkhabad, 55–73.

Latyshev, N. I., Krjukova, A. P. and Povalishina, T. P. (1951). Essays on the regional parasitology of Middle Asia. 1. Leishmaniases in Tadjikistan. Materials for the medical geography of Tadjik SSR (Results of expeditions in 1945–47). Problems of Regional, General and Experimental Parasitology and Medical Zoology. Transactions of Gamaleya Institute, Moscow, 7, 35–62 (In Russian).

Latyshev, N. I., Krjukova, A. P., Povalishina, T. P. and Ivashkina, K. A. (1971). Cutaneous leishmaniasis in Termez. Conference on Medical Parasitology. Samarkand. Abstracts, 178–183 (In Russian).

Lisova, A. U. and Vavilova, M. P. (1955). The infection incidence of *Phlebotomus papatasi* and *Phlebotomus caucasicus* with a form of *Leishmania infantum* and *Leishmania canis*. Problems of Regional Pathology. Academy of Science of the Uzbek SSR, Tashkent, 215–220 (In Russian).

Lysenko, A. Y. and Lubova, V. V. (1974). Epidemiology and geography of the visceral leishmaniasis in the USSR. International Symposium on Leishmaniasis Ecology, Montpellier, France.

Maruashvili, G. M. (1968). Visceral leishmaniasis, "Sabchota Sakartvelo", Tbilisi (In Russian).

Maruashvili, G. M. and Bardzhadze, B. G. (1966). Natural focality of visceral leishmaniasis in Georgia. *Meditsinskaya Parazitologia i Parazitarnie Bolezni, USSR,* 35, 462–463.

Mirzojan, N. A. (1957). Some data of distribution of visceral leishmaniasis in the USSR (abstract). *Meditsinskaya Parazitologia i Parazitarnie Bolezni, USSR,* 26, suppl., 47.

Moshkovski, Sh. D. (1950). The Main Natural Laws of Malaria Epidemiology, "Academy of Medical Science" of the USSR, Moscow (In Russian).

Moshkovski, Sh. D. and Nosina, V. D. (1933). The staining of sandflies as a method of studying certain features of their biology and ecology. *Meditsinskaya Parazitologia i Parazitarnie Bolezni, USSR,* 2, 407–409.

Muench, H. (1959). Catalytic models in epidemiology. Cambridge.

Nadjafov, A. Y. (1966). The status of leishmaniasis incidence and their control in Azerbaijan SSR. *Meditsinskaya Parazitologia i Parazitarnie Bolezni, USSR,* 35, 463–470.

Nadjafov, A. Y. (1968). Leishmaniasis, its vectors and appropriate control measures applied in Azerbaidjan SSR. 8th International Congresses on Tropical Medicine and Malaria. Teheran, Iran. *Abstracts and Reviews,* 296–297.

Neronov, V. M. and Farang-Azad, A. (1973). Cutaneous leishmaniasis in Iran, its reservoirs and vectors (Literature Survey). *Meditsinskaya Parazitologia i Parazitarnie Bolezni, USSR,* 42, 666–674.

Neronov, V. M. and Gunin, P. D. (1971). The structure of natural foci of zoonotic cutaneous leishmaniasis and its dependence on landscape morphology. *Bulletin of the World Health Organization,* 44, 575–581.

Petrishcheva, P. A. and Safyanova, V. M. (1969). Leishmaniases. *In:* "Geography of Diseases with Natural Focality in connection with their Prevention", *Medicine,* Moscow (In Russian)

Remyannikova, T. P. (1968). The dissemination of *Leishmania tropica major* in the Kara-Kum desert. "Parasites of Animals and Plants in Turkmenia", Ashkhabad, 32–39 (In Russian).

Remyannikova, T. P. (1970). Distribution of sandflies in natural foci of cutaneous leishmaniasis in different landscape of Turkmenia, *Parazitologia, USSR*, **4**, 418–422.

Rodiakin, N. F. (1951). Problems of Immunity and Specific Prophylaxis in Borowsky's Disease (cutaneous leishmaniasis). Ministry of Health of the Turkmen SSR, Ashkhabad (In Russian).

Safyanova, V. M. (1967). *Phlebotominae* and *Leishmania. In:* "Biological Relationships between Blood-Sucking Insects and Pathogens of Human Diseases". *Medicine*, Moscow, 246–285 (In Russian).

Safyanova, V. M. (1974). Typification of leishmaniases nidi on the basis of transmissible factor. *Parazitologia, USSR*, **8**, 336–347.

Saladize, I. D. (1963). Sandfly species in Eastern Georgia and some features of the biology of *P. chinensis* and *P. kandelaki*. Transactions of Virsaladze Institute of Medical Parasitology and Tropical Medicine, Tbilisi, **4**, 155–163.

Sergiev, V. P. (1974). The efficiency of different control measures against cutaneous leishmaniasis. International Symposium on Leishmaniasis Ecology, Montpellier, France.

Sergiev, P. G., Beislekhem, R. I., Moshkovsky, Sh. D., Demina N. A., Kellina, O. I., Shuikina, E. E., Sergiev, V. P., Dukhanina, N. N., Triers, I. I., Scherbakov, V. A., Yarmukhamedov, M. A., Uskov, N. E., Losikov, I. N. and Nedospelova, E. I. (1970). Results of mass vaccination against zoonotic cutaneous leishmaniasis. *Meditsinskaya Parazitologia i Parazitarnie Bolezni, USSR*, **39**, 541–551.

Sergiev, V. P., Shuikina, E. E. and Uzbekov, M. K. (1973). Features of the study of epidemiology of cutaneous leishmaniasis in newly developing territories. *Meditsinskaya Parazitologia i Parazitarnie Bolezni, USSR*, **42**, 273–279.

Sergiev, V. P., Vdovin, D. G., Scherbakov, V. A. and Yarmukhamedov, M. A. (1974). Dynamics of the epidemic activity of zoonotic cutaneous leishmaniasis nidi and variations in the population morbidity. *Meditsinskaya Parazitologia i Parazitarnie Bolezni, USSR*, **42**, 663–666.

Shishlyaeva-Matova, Z. S. (1966). Duration of cutaneous leishmaniasis in *Rhombomys opimus* Licht. and its dependence upon the season in which the animals acquire the infection. *Meditsinskaya Parazitologia i Parazitarnie Bolezni, USSR*, **35**, 85–91.

Strelkova, M. V. and Djabarov, L. N. (1971). Unequal role of different mammals as a host for bloodsucking by sandflies. Conference on Medical Parasitology, Samarkand. Abstracts, 226–228 (In Russian).

Vlassov, J. P. (1941). Le terrier du spermophil (*Spermophilopsis leptodactylus* Licht.) et de la grosse gerbille (*Rhombomys opimus* Licht.) comme biotope original dans les environs de le ville d'Ashkhabad. Conference Interrepublicaine sur la Leishmaniose Cutanée et le Problème des Phlébotomes, Ashkhabad, 74–89.

4

Biology of the Kinetoplastida
of Arthropods

F. G. WALLACE

Department of Zoology,
University of Minnesota,
Minneapolis, Minnesota, USA

I.	Introduction	213
II.	Morphology	215
III.	Life cycles	216
IV.	Transmission	218
V.	Site in host and pathogenicity	219
VI.	Endosymbionts	219
VII.	Methods of study	221
VIII.	Systematics	224
	A. Genus *Leptomonas* Kent, 1880	225
	B. Genus *Herpetomonas* Kent, 1880	226
	C. Genus *Crithidia* Léger, 1902	230
	D. Genus *Blastocrithidia* Laird, 1959	233
	E. Genus *Rhynchoidomonas* Patton, 1910	235
IX.	References	235

I. Introduction

The kinetoplastid parasites of arthropods are mainly in the family *Try-panosomatidae* though there are a few records of *Bodo* and *Karotomorpha* which will not be considered here. The *Trypanosoma* and *Leishmania* of vertebrates, which have stages in arthropods, are considered elsewhere in these volumes. Thus this chapter is devoted to the genera *Leptomonas*, *Crithidia*, *Herpetomonas*, *Blastocrithidia*, and *Rhynchoidomonas*. They are parasites of invertebrates exclusively and the vast majority are parasites of insects, along with a few in arachnids. But there are also records from nematodes (Goodey and Triffitt, 1927; Bovien, 1937), molluscs (Porter, 1914; Mello, 1921), rotifers (Chatton, 1938) and protozoa (Gillies and Hanson, 1963). There is no taxon that includes only the five genera concerned so they can be referred to only by the circumlocution that forms the title of this chapter or, as do many of my colleagues, as the "lower trypanosomatids". More precisely they might be called "trypanosomatids of lower hosts" though if one accepts Szidat's law, which states that in any parasitic group the more primitive parasites are found in the more primitive hosts, the two terms would coincide.

Throughout its history the study of the lower trypanosomatids has been pervaded by the realization of the similarity of these organisms to the trypanosomes and the leishmanias. Though the earliest discoverers of insect flagellates (Burnett, 1851 and Leidy, 1856) did not mention a possible relationship to parasites of vertebrates, Kent (1880) placed the housefly parasite in the same genus (*Herpetomonas*) as the rat trypanosome. Most of the studies of the early twentieth century on taxonomy and life histories were undertaken because the insect flagellates were thought to be stages of trypanosomes or because they might provide models that would clarify the succession of stages in the heteroxenous members of the family.

The solution of some intricate problems in the differentiation of lower trypanosomatids from parasites of plants or of higher animals has come only recently. The stage by stage comparison of *Leptomonas oncopelti* and *Phytomonas elmassiani* in the insect, *Oncopeltus fasciatus*, by McGhee and Hanson (1964) was a major milestone in this field. The recognition of *Blastocrithidia triatomae* by Cerisola *et al.* (1971) in the insect host of *T. cruzi* was a recent taxonomic achievement of great practical significance.

Other reasons for the study of lower trypanosomatids are found in their possible immunological applications, their possible use as control agents against vectors or pathogens and in their use as models in the study of nutrition, chemotherapy and symbiosis.

The close relationship between insect trypanosomatids and *Trypanosoma* and *Leishmania* suggests that there may be an immunological relationship and this has been put to use in a few instances. Zeledon *et al.* (1961) used *Crithidia oncopelti* as an antigen for the diagnosis of cutaneous leishmaniasis. The advantage of a non-pathogen in the preparation of a live antigen for skin testing is obvious. Johnson *et al.* (1963) found that *Crithidia fasciculata* and *Leptomonas collosoma* with saponin adjuvant gave some protection to experimental animals against *Trypanosoma cruzi*. Souza *et al.* (1974) found that *Leptomonas pessoai* (probably the strain now identified as *Herpetomonas samuelpessoai*) conferred protection against *T. cruzi* injected into mice.

Any parasite of an insect comes into consideration as a possible agent for biological control but trypanosomatids offer scant encouragement for this as they are usually non-pathogenic. *Herpetomonas* in flies is pathogenic under certain circumstances (Kramer, 1961; Bailey and Brooks, 1972).

There has been no inquiry at all into the possible effects of lower trypanosomatids on other protozoa, bacteria or viruses in insects although I have found two references to the effect of other pathogens on trypanosomatids. Smirnoff and Lipa (1970) found that *Herpetomonas swainei* had no effect on the development of *Borrelinavirus swainei* in the same insect host though the flagellates died when the polyhedral virus filled the host nuclei. Lushbaugh *et al.* (1976) redescribed a yeastlike fungus, *Coccidiascus legeri* Chatton, 1913 in *Drosophila melanogaster*. *Herpetomonas* sp. in the same flies was normally in the intestinal lumen but in the presence of the fungus it penetrated the cells of the intestinal wall.

As trypanosomatids are easily cultivated axenically and easily established experimentally in insects their effect on concomitant infections with other organisms should be investigated.

II. Morphology

The morphology of the *Kinetoplastida* is covered very thoroughly in Chapters 1 and 2 of Volume I of this book. Only a few points peculiar to the lower trypanosomatids need be mentioned here.

Longitudinal superficial lines (myonemes, costae, striae) are seen in some trypanosomes, particularly some of the species of the subgenus *Megatrypanum* and many of the larger forms from fish, amphibia, reptiles and birds. Baker (1976) said that electron microscopy reveals no fibrillar structures that could be called myonemes and suggested that the visible lines may be surface foldings of the pellicle. These myonemes or striae have been described in only one insect flagellate—*Leptomonas jaculum* by Porter (1910).

Lwoff and Lwoff (1931) described what is probably another type of "striae" in *Crithidia fasciculata* and *C. oncopelti*. These longitudinal helical lines stained with aniline fuchsin and were twelve in number. No one since has used the same technique or has described the same structures. Electron micrographs of transverse sections and the reconstructions of the unitary mitochondrion of certain other trypanosomatids (Paulin, 1975) suggest strongly that the Lwoffs' striae in *Crithidia* spp. are arms of the mitochondrion.

Chatton (1913) noted that several species of *Leptomonas*, particularly those of fleas, attached themselves to the host tissues or to the slide by the flagellar end and that the flagellum became short, broad and brush-like, the "mèche muqueuse". This adaptation has been noted in a number of species, for example *L. arctocorixae*, *L. ctenocephali* var. *chattoni*, *L. drosophilae*, *L. craggi*, *L. roubaudi*, *L. legerorum* and *L. pattoni*. Lwoff and Lwoff (1931) took this as characteristic of the genus *Leptomonas sensu stricto* while their subgenus *Strigomonas*, now considered to be *Crithidia*, attached itself by the end of the flagellum without its transformation into the "mèche muqueuse". Electron microscopy shows that in both genera the broadened tip of the flagellum attaches to the host or other substrates by desmosomes (see Vickerman and Preston, 1976). Brooker (1971) made thin sections of *C. fasciculata* attached to the rectal wall of *Anopheles gambiae* and studied them with the electron microscope. He said that the flagellum varied in length, sometimes hardly extending beyond the opening of the flagellar pocket. But in all cases the tip was wider than the more proximal part and the axoneme was present, reaching to 170 nm from the end. Brun (1974) presented electron micrographs of *L. mirabilis* attached to the wall of the posterior midgut of the fly host. The entire flagellum was broadened and the axoneme and intraflagellar structure were lacking. These differences may explain the difference noted by the Lwoffs with the light microscope. They suggest that the flagellum of *Leptomonas* is more highly modified for attachment than that of *Crithidia* which are usually attached to the hindgut cuticle while *Leptomonas* are usually attached to the midgut lining.

III. Life cycles

The cell cycle of the individual trypanosomatid is very simple. Denied the attribute of sex it has only to divide, though with small variations impressed on this elementary process. In a few instances (*L. mirabilis*, see Wallace and Todd, 1964, and *Phytomonas elmassiani*, see McGhee and Hanson, 1964) cytokinesis is unequal and one daughter cell is several times larger than the other. Unequal cytokinesis with the daughter cells attached to the same flagellum has been thought to be the first step in the formation of flagellar cysts. Division of the kinetoplast and formation of a new flagellum generally precede nuclear division. In some species of *Herpetomonas* replication of the mastigont appears to follow immediately after cell division so that cells with two flagella are the rule. The remarkable *Leptomonas oestrorum* of oestrid flies, described by Rodhain and Bequaert (1916), repeat this process and normally boast four flagella each, with eight in dividing individuals.

Population cycles in trypanosomatids, with differentiation of various stages, become complex in the heteroxenous forms. In the monoxenous lower trypanosomatids true cyclic development with different stages is much less marked and is often non-existent. A major and recurring problem has been that of distinguishing between stage differences that are due to an obligate cycle and differences in form or behaviour that are impressed on the organism by external factors.

Ross (1906) made the very important observation that the *Crithidia* of mosquitoes were short, stubby and motionless while they were attached to the wall of the relatively undisturbed host intestine but promptly became elongate, free and active when the gut was teased apart in water. French authors applied the words grégarinien and monadien to the attached and swimming forms respectively while haptomonad (Minchin and Thompson, 1915) and nectomonad (Woodcock, 1914) have been used similarly.

Many of the presumed cycles that have been described for lower trypanosomatids have been based on such environmentally caused transformations or to mixed infections. But in the genus *Herpetomonas* the promastigote–opisthomastigote transformation appears to be a natural part of the life cycle. While a predictable occurrence of these two stages in different parts of the cycle in the host or in culture has not yet been shown it appears that opisthomastigotes become more numerous with the end of rapid reproduction (Cosgrove, 1971; Janovy *et al.*, 1974).

The cysts of lower trypanosomatids require much more investigation. In fact there are no studies that correlate drying experiments or other demonstrations of resistance to environmental conditions beyond the resistance that is characteristic of the active stages with morphological cysts. Amastigotes or haptomonads of *Crithidia* have often been called cysts with no evidence that they were surrounded by any kind of protective cyst wall.

Three kinds of cysts have been described. Flagellar cysts, the "straphangers" of McGhee and Hanson (1962), are thought to originate from an unequal division of a flagellate. The smaller daughter cell remains attached to the flagellum of the larger and then moves distally along the flagellum, becoming more rounded and compact as it does so. *Blastocrithidia triatomae* has flagellar cysts more frequently and in greater numbers per flagellate than any other trypanosomatid. They become compact bacillus-like cysts about 2 μm in length. The smaller more compact cysts are proximal on the flagellum to the longer pointed cells so the process of formation can hardly be explained by the unequal division hypothesis.

Flagellar cysts are reported (see Wallace, 1966) in *Leptomonas lygaei*, *L. oncopelti*, *Blastocrithidia euschisti*, *B. familiaris*, *B. leptocoridis*, *B. ortheae*, *B. sandoni* and *B. triatomae*. They have not been reported from other genera.

Internal buds, which may form cysts, were described by McCulloch

(1917) in *B. euryophthalmi*. They looked like amastigotes with the nucleus and kinetoplast present but with no evidence of a cyst wall. From one to 13 of these "buds" were found embedded in the cytoplasm. McCullough saw many smaller, more compact "spores", exhibiting nucleus and kinetoplast, among the flagellates and she suggested that they might be enclosed in a protective coat because they were slower to destain than the "buds". Studies on their development and possible relation to the flagellar cysts are in progress.

Gibbs (1951) graphically described the formation of cysts in *L. capsularis* by a process that we may call enclosure. An elongate promastigote bends double and a jelly-like substance appears between the two arms of the bend, holds the organism in the doubled position as it increases in quantity and finally encloses the organism completely. When such cysts are fully formed the organisms can be seen bending and turning inside.

Accompanying many species of *Leptomonas* and *Blastocrithidia* there have been found small rounded forms either attached to the wall of the hindgut or free. While many authors have called them cysts there is no evidence either that they belong to the species being described or that they possess cyst walls. Among those for which such "cysts" have been described are various species of *Leptomonas* from fleas, *L. legerorum*, *L. lygaei*, *L. mirperi*, *L. tortum*, *B. euryophthalmi*, *B. pulicis*, *B. raabei* and *B. vagoi*. The identity of these "cysts" can be determined only from observation of experimental infections of parasite-free, laboratory reared insect hosts with clone cultures.

IV. Transmission

There is ample evidence that intestinal flagellates of arthropods are transmitted from host to host contaminatively by ingestion of faecal material from infected hosts. While it has sometimes been assumed that this manner of transmission requires cysts it is clear that species for which cysts are unknown (*Herpetomonas muscarum*, *Blastocrithidia culicis*, *Crithidia fasciculata*) may be transmitted by contamination. All records of experimental transmission were tabulated by Wallace (1966). Since that time further experiments on transmission of *H. muscarum* have been conducted by Bailey and Brooks (1971), Rogers and Wallace (1971), Carvalho and Deane (1974) and Brun (1974). Daggett *et al.* (1972) reported experimental infections with *H. megaseliae*. Bailey and Brooks (1971) showed that *H. muscarum* passed from larva to larva and from adult to adult in the insect host *Hippelates pusio*. They also found that insects infected in the larval stage retained the infection through the pupal stage to the adult. Insectivorous insects may become infected from their prey. Carvalho and Deane (1974) pointed out that *C. luciliae* and *H. muscarum* found in the reduviid bug, *Zelus leucogrammus*, were probably parasites of the flies on which the *Zelus* fed.

V. Site in host and pathogenicity

Most of the lower trypanosomatids occur in the intestine of the host. There is a distinct tendency for *Crithidia* to live in the hindgut or rectum where haptomonads attach to the wall. *L. mirabilis* is usually attached to the wall of the midgut just anterior to the openings of the Malpighian tubules. Most species of *Leptomonas, Herpetomonas* and *Blastocrithidia* are free and active in the lumen. Whether or not they are within (endotrophic) or outside (peritrophic) the peritrophic membrane has been a subject of some concern, particularly to Chatton (see Wenyon, 1926 for a summary of Chatton's numerous papers on the parasites of *Drosophila*). Chatton found that *L. drosophilae* Chatton and Alilaire 1908 were endotrophic in the larva and peritrophic in the adult. An unnamed *Herpetomonas* was endotrophic in the adult. Lushbaugh *et al.* (1976) found an unidentified *Herpetomonas* in *Drosophila melanogaster*; it was both endotrophic and peritrophic.

In many insects the peritrophic membrane is secreted by the entire inner wall of the midgut (Richards and Richards, 1977). Among the blood sucking Nematocera the peritrophic membrane of the adult appears after a blood meal (or after an experimental enema that distends the gut). In mosquitoes flagellates are found in unfed insects where no peritrophic membrane exists or outside the membrane after a blood meal. In many higher Diptera, including *Drosophila* and *Glossina*, the peritrophic membrane is secreted by a ring of cells at the anterior end of the midgut so it is a cylinder attached anteriorly around its circumference but ending freely in the posterior end of the midgut. In these flies some parasites (*Herpetomonas*) are endotrophic for the most part, a few individuals occurring in the peritrophic space. Those flagellates that attach to the intestinal wall are, of course, peritrophic. Certain flagellates, particularly *Rhynchoidomonas*, are usually in the Malpighian tubules. Two species of *Blastocrithidia* in ticks and four species of *Leptomonas* in insects occur in the haemocoel. Three species of *Leptomonas* and one species of *Blastocrithidia* have been found in the salivary glands, all in Hemiptera.

The only known cases of pathogenicity were mentioned in the Introduction.

VI. Endosymbionts

Bacteria-like endosymbionts are found in a few trypanosomatids and, as the host organisms can be cultivated in defined media and can be cured of the symbionts, these systems are very valuable for analytical studies on symbiosis.

In their description of *Blastocrithidia culicis* from mosquitoes, Novy *et al.* (1907) described the diplosome, an elongate bacillus-like body 1 to 2 μm in length with a constriction in the middle, located either anterior or posterior to the nucleus and dividing just before division of the host cell. Subsequent studies by Indurkar (1965), Brueske (1967) and Chang (1974) show that its ultrastructure is that of a typical bacterium. Newton and Horne (1957) using electron microscopy found bacteria-like bodies in *Crithidia oncopelti*. This flagellate, described by Noguchi and Tilden (1926), was said to come from the milkweed bug, *Oncopeltus fasciatus*, but the source of the extant culture is unknown (see Wallace 1966). As seen with the light microscope the stained symbionts were darker at the ends than in the middle and were called bipolar bodies. Mundim *et al.* (1974) found similar bodies in *C. deanei*, a recently described parasite of flies (see below). These three forms occur in 100% of their host protozoa and thus fulfil one of the criteria of a true mutual (Brooks, 1975).

Wenyon (1913) described bacillus-like inclusions in *H. muscarum* from Bagdad. Brun (1974) confirmed their occurrence in the same protozoon from East African flies and made electron micrographs that support the hypothesis that they are bacteria. In this case about 40% of the host cells carry the inclusions in infected populations and the same species of flagellate is often found with no inclusions at all. Weinman and Cheong (1978) found bacterium-like inclusions in an unnamed *Herpetomonas* from *Aedes aegypti* and *A. albopictus* from Malaysia. The symbionts were found in 35 to 46% of the flagellates.

Analysis of the function of endosymbionts of trypanosomatids began with Lwoff (1940) and Newton (1956) who found that *Crithidia oncopelti* did not require haematin and that its biosynthetic capabilities surpass those of all other trypanosomatids that have been studied. Mundim *et al.* (1974) found that *C. deanei* also had simple requirements, needing only two amino acids, methionine and tyrosine, and no purine source or haemin. These observations, comparing species with symbionts to other species without symbionts, are highly suggestive but firm evidence that a symbiont contributes to the nutrition of the host must come from a comparison of symbiont-containing and symbiont-free (aposymbiotic) cultures of the same species. Early studies of presumed "cured" *Crithidia oncopelti* are of doubtful validity. The reader is referred to Newton (1968) for a critical review.

Brueske (1967) cured *Blastocrithidia culicis* of its symbiont by adding chloramphenicol to the culture medium. He found that while normal *B. culicis* grew on a synthetic medium the aposymbiotic strain did not.

Chang and Trager (1974) repeated Brueske's cure of *B. culicis* and also obtained an aposymbiotic culture of *C. oncopelti* by using similar methods.

Both the normal and aposymbiotic strains of the two species grew in Trager's defined medium, which contains haemin, when liver fraction was added. If haemin was left out the cured strains did not grow while the normal strains did. Chang *et al.* (1975) found that aposymbiotic flagellates require at least 0·1 μg/ml of haemin. Protoporphyrin IX and iron can be substituted for haemin, indicating that symbionts are not necessary for the last step in haemin synthesis, i.e. the addition of iron to protoporphyrin. They presented evidence that the symbionts supply uroporphyrinogen I synthetase, an enzyme used in an earlier step in the biosynthetic chain. Thus the host cell and the symbiont share a single sequence of enzymatic reactions, each providing different steps, and a most intimate inter-dependence and control is demonstrated.

Trypanosomatids cannot synthesize haemin as can most other organisms, with the exception of rickettsiae, a few bacteria, a fungus and certain hematophagous insects. Chang *et al.* (1975) stated that the only trypanosomatids that are capable of synthesizing haemin are those that contain symbionts. An exception to this is *Crithidia fasciculata* var. *culicis*, which was isolated from *Culex* larvae by Noguchi and Tilden (1926) and was found by Lwoff (1935) not to require haemin.

Mundim and Roitman (1977) compared aposymbiotic and normal *Crithidia deanei* and found that the former required a purine, haemin, ten amino acids and seven vitamins in addition to the nutrients required by the latter.

Camargo and Freymuller (1977) presented histochemical as well as biochemical evidence of the presence of an essential enzyme in the endosymbiont of *C. deanei*. All species of *Crithidia* tested, except for those that contain endosymbionts, require either arginine or citrulline. Normal symbiont-containing *C. deanei* and *C. oncopelti* require neither of these amino acids. The enzyme, ornithinecarbamoyl transferase (OCT), which catalyses the synthesis of citrulline from ornithine, was found in symbiont-containing *Crithidia* by biochemical analysis and was found localized in the endosymbiont when an electron microscopic histochemical test for OCT was applied.

VII. Methods of study

While trypanosomatids are usually sought when dissecting the insect hosts, they may be found in the faeces from the living insect. *Triatoma* often expel liquid faeces a few minutes after a blood meal. McGhee and Hanson (1962) imprisoned *Oncopeltus* in chambers made of glass slides so that faecal droplets could be stained and examined directly.

For the dissection of insects one should use fine watchmakers' forceps, iridectomy scissors, and fine needles or number 11 (straight pointed) disposable scalpel blades. Legs and wings should be removed first. In the case of small insects, particularly mosquitoes, the entire alimentary tract can be drawn out through the posterior end after the head is removed. The entire dorsum should be removed from larger insects. The intestine should be placed in a drop of 0·5 % saline, and should be straightened out and freed from other tissues. It can then be examined intact after it is covered with a cover slip, and later compressed or uncovered and teased apart for further examination. Haemolymph, salivary glands, and Malpighian tubules should also be examined.

Dried smears may be stained with Giemsa's stain diluted in water buffered to pH 7·0. A minute drop of mammalian blood mixed with the insect material, or dried on the slide before the smear is prepared, often improves the quality of the staining. A procedure that gives good results in our laboratory in staining cultured haemoflagellates is the following.

1. Fix 5 minutes in Ponselle's fixative (tincture of iodine 1 part, methyl alcohol 5 parts).
2. Rinse with methyl alcohol.
3. Hydrolyse or wash either in
    (a) 1 N HCl at 60°C for 5 minutes or
    (b) $M/15$ KH$_2$PO$_4$ at room temperature for 5 minutes.
4. Rinse in buffered water (pH 7)
5. Dry
6. Stain for 20 minutes in Giemsa's stain diluted 1 to 20 in buffered water, pH 7 ($M/15$ Na$_2$HPO$_4$ 61·1 ml; $M/15$ KH$_2$PO$_4$ 38·9 ml; distilled water 900 ml).

The flagellum stains better after Ponselle's fixation than after methyl alcohol fixation. Step 3 washes out most cytoplasmic granules, leaving the nucleus, kinetoplast, flagellum, and endosymbionts. It may be omitted.

Isolation of trypanosomatids from insects in culture requires an aseptic technique. Antibiotics are usually added to the culture medium but many were isolated and cultured before the advent of antibiotics. Slides, cover slips, petri dishes, filter paper circles, 0·5 % saline, and cotton-plugged Pasteur pipettes are all sterilized beforehand. Dissecting instruments may be sterilized repeatedly as one works by immersion in 70 % alcohol, dipping in sterile water and drying on sterile filter paper. Ordinary forceps, used to handle insects, slides, and cover slips may be sterilized in 95 % alcohol, which is burned off. The instruments are passed through the flame only to ignite the alcohol but not long enough to heat the metal. Fine instruments should not be flamed at all.

The insect is killed with ether or CO$_2$ and then immersed in zephiran chloride for ten minutes or more, washed in sterile water, and laid on sterile filter paper, or a slide, for dissection. The intestine or other internal organ is covered with a sterile cover slip and examined. If flagellates are found the material is transferred to a culture tube to which penicillin (1000 to 2000 units per ml) and streptomycin (1000 to 2000 micrograms per ml) are added.

The original culture medium for lower trypanosomatids was NNN. Numerous modifications have been developed and each laboratory has its favourite. Usually diphasic media, i.e. a blood agar slant to which a liquid component is added, are better for isolation than all liquid, monophasic, media. For isolation, media with 20 to 30% blood in the solid phase are advisable but established cultures may be maintained with 10% blood.

Three diphasic media that can be recommended follow:

(A). NNN medium.

Agar	24 g
NaCl	6 g
Distilled water	900 ml

Dissolve the agar and salt in the water by boiling, put about 3 ml in each culture tube and autoclave the tubes. Cool the agar to 48°C in a water bath and add 1 ml of fresh defibrinated rabbit blood. Chill the tubes in cracked ice. The few drops of condensate at the bottom of each tube provide the liquid phase. Screw cap tubes should be used.

(B). SNB9 medium (Diamond and Herman, 1954)

Neopeptone (Difco)	9 g
NaCl	2·5 g
Agar	9 g
Distilled water	450 ml

Dissolve the solid ingredients in the water with heat, put 5 ml in each tube and autoclave. Cool the tubes to 48°C and add 1 ml fresh defibrinated rabbit blood per tube for isolation or 0·5 ml blood per tube for maintenance. A broth of the same composition as the medium above but without the agar is prepared, autoclaved, and added to the slanted agar tubes, 0·5 ml per tube.

(C). McConnell's medium (McConnell, 1963)

| Bacto beef (Difco) | 2·5 g |
| Distilled water | 100 ml |

Boil together and filter through filter paper. Then add and dissolve

Neopeptone (Difco)	2 g
NaCl	0·5 g
Agar	2·0 g

Adjust the pH to 7·2 to 7·4 and then autoclave. To the melted tubes, cooled to 48°C, add 15% defibrinated rabbit blood and cool the tubes in a slanted position. A broth of the same composition as the medium but without the agar is added, 0·5 ml per tube.

(D). Ho Mem medium (Berens et al., 1976)

This is a monophasic medium made from commercially available ingredients. It has been tested for a number of lower trypanosomatids and will probably be very useful for mass production. The following formula is modified slightly, according to a letter from Dr. Brun, from the published formula.

For 1 L water

SMEM Minimum Essential Medium (Eagle) for suspension culture with Spinner's salts (Gibco)	10·6 g
MEM Amino acids 50x (Gibco)	10·0 ml
MEM Non-essential Amino acids 100x (Gibco)	10·0 ml
Na pyruvate 100x (Gibco)	11·0 ml
Na bicarbonate	2·2 g
Glucose	3 g
Biotin	0·1 mg
Para amino benzoic acid	1·0 g
Haemin solution (2 mg/ml in NaOH)	3·0 ml
Hepes buffer (pH 7·2 to 7·4)	·060 M

Sterilize by filtration. Add 5 to 10% foetal calf serum. Gibco = Grand Island Biologicals Company.

A number of lower trypanosomatids have been found to grow well in culture only at low pH, 5 to 5·5 (see Section VIII, Systematics). With very few exceptions the lower trypanosomatids grow in culture at room temperature (20°C to 26°C) and a common difficulty, at least in North American laboratories, is that of losing cultures in overheated rooms. Temperature control is essential for continued and consistent work.

Definitive studies of life cycles require clone cultures. McGhee et al (1969), Rogers and Wallace (1971), Weinman (1972) and Podkulski et al. (1974) present techniques for cloning trypanosomatid cultures. The clone cultures then may be used to infect insect hosts under controlled conditions. The many techniques that have been developed for rearing and feeding insects in the laboratory cannot be reviewed here but it is essential that laboratory-reared, flagellate-free insects be used.

VIII. Systematics

Wallace (1966) listed and characterized nearly all of the species of trypanosomatids in arthropods then in the literature. The reader is referred to that review for host lists, species not mentioned here and author citations which are not included here. In this chapter only certain selected species are discussed plus subsequently described species, and a few that were inadvertently omitted before. Vickerman (1976) gives generic diagnoses so they will not be repeated though additional remarks for some of the genera will be made.

A. GENUS *LEPTOMONAS* KENT, 1880

The type species, *L. bütschlii*, was found in a marine nematode, *Tobrilus gracilis*. This has nearly always been cited as *Trilobus* but Nicoli *et al.* (1971) noted that the name had been changed in 1959 as *Trilobus* was already in use.

They said that the genus *Leptomonas* should be suppressed because the type species was a euglenoid, not a Trypanosomatid, and named the new genus *Nematodomonas* for other flagellates from nematodes. They proposed no other name for the promastigote parasites of arthropods. As the type species of *Leptomonas* has not been restudied and as host alone is a tenuous ground for defining a genus of parasitic protozoa the author prefers to retain the name *Leptomonas* for all promastigote parasites of invertebrates.

L. jaculum (Léger, 1902b) Woodcock, 1914
   Synonym: *Herpetomonas jaculum* Léger, 1902
   Hosts: *Nepa cinerea, Ranatra linearis* (Hemiptera: Nepidae)
   Location: Intestine
   Locality: France, England
   Remarks: This parasite of water scorpions was the first representative of the genus *Leptomonas* to be described from an insect host. Porter (1910) described the life history and mentioned the presence of "myonemes" which, though common in many trypanosomes, are otherwise unknown in the lower trypanosomatids. Length 13 μm to 33 μm, free flagellum about the same length. Relatively broad and blunt.

L. ctenocephali (Fantham, 1912) Wenyon, 1926
   Synonyms: *H. ctenocephali* Fantham, 1912
            H. pseudoleishmania Brumpt, 1913
   Host: *Ctenocephalides canis* (Siphonaptera)
   Location: Intestine
   Locality: Europe, USA, India, New Zealand
   Remarks: Length 6 μm to 17 μm; flagellum up to 16 μm. In the attached forms the flagellum is transformed into a brush-like structure. *L. ctenocephali* var. *chattoni* Laveran and Franchini 1920 from Tunis was studied by Chatton (1913) and was the subject of a classic morphological study by Lwoff and Lwoff (1931).

L. oxyuri Nöller, 1931
   Host: *Ceratophyllus gallinae* (Siphonaptera)
   Location: Intestine
   Locality: Germany

Remarks: This species was omitted from Wallace (1966) and is there-fore included in this paper. It differs from other flagellates of fleas in having a long pointed posterior end resembling the next species.

L. mirabilis Roubaud, 1908
Synonyms: *Cercoplasma mirabilis* Roubaud, 1911
　　　　　 Herpetomonas graphomyiae Franchini, 1922
Hosts: Many species of *Calliphoridae* and other muscoid flies
Locality: Congo, India, Italy, Guatemala, Tanzania
Remarks: The anterior end is rounded and the posterior end drawn out into a slender "tail". Length up to 198 μm. Body twisted into a very regular helix with as many as 24 gyres. Roubaud (1911) and Brun (1974) believed that opisthomastigotes found in the same flies were conspecific with *L. mirabilis*. Roubaud (1911) named a new genus, *Cercoplasma*, for these giant leptomonas and the opisthomastigotes which were said to be the characteristic stages for the genus. There is further discussion below under *H. muscarum*.

L. pessoai Galvão et al., 1970
See *H. samuelpessoai*

L. samueli Carvalho, 1973
Host: *Zelus leucogrammus* (Hemiptera: Reduviidae)
Location: Intestine
Locality: Belo Horizonte, Brazil
Remarks: Length 7·8 μm to 20 μm (average 7·4 μm); width 0·8 μm to 2·5 mμ (average 1·4 μm). Posterior end pointed, body twisted. The host is insectivorous and some other flagellates found in it have been identified as being parasites of the flies on which the *Zelus* feeds.

B. GENUS *HERPETOMONAS* KENT, 1880

The rather involved history of this genus, which is characterized by the presence of opisthomastigotes, is discussed by Wallace (1966). It has been the subject of a number of important recent studies. With both promastigote and opisthomastigote stages this genus offers the best example of morphological transformation among the lower trypano-somatids. And the frequent occurrence of biflagellate promastigotes re-sulting from precocious replication of the flagellum adds a third morphological type. We do not yet have precise information on the conditions, extrinsic or intrinsic, which govern the appearance of these three forms but it appears that opisthomastigotes and paramastigotes (those with the kinetoplast beside the nucleus) increase in cultures as the rate of multiplication decreases (Cosgrove, 1971; Janovy et al., 1974).

Cultivation at 37°C (Roitman *et al.*, 1976), addition of 2-Deoxy-D-glucose to the medium (Angluster *et al.*, 1977) and increased osmolarity (DeAlmeida and De Souza, 1978) raised the proportion of paramastigotes and opisthomastigotes. However, in these studies the relative numbers of the different stages were not related to total population curves. Studies of differentiation in *Herpetomonas* should include the population dynamics of the culture.

Rogers and Wallace (1971) cloned two strains, named as subspecies of *H. muscarum*, and found that in the two subspecies the pro- and opistho-mastigote stages occurred in different proportions under the same conditions. *H. muscarum ingenoplastis* occurs almost exclusively as long biflagellate promastigotes and opisthomastigotes are almost never found in culture, though they constitute a substantial percentage of the parasites found in laboratory-reared flies infected from clone cultures. *H. muscarum muscarum* has very few biflagellate promastigotes, either in the host or in culture, and exhibits up to 39 per cent opisthomastigotes in older cultures.

Brun (1974) studied the flagellate parasites of the fly *Chrysomyia chloropyga* in East Africa. His excellent electron micrographs show the two types of kinetoplast (types A and B of Vickerman and Preston, 1976) that are characteristic of the two subspecies of *H. muscarum*. His photomicrographs and drawings show forms typical of *Crithidia luciliae* and *Leptomonas mirabilis* and the manner of attachment of their haptomonads. On the basis of cultures and experimental infections he concluded that *C. luciliae* is different from the others but that the two types of *H. muscarum* free in the midgut and *L. mirabilis* attached in the pyloric region belong to one species.

Brun assumed that the *H. muscarum* with the two types of kinetoplast were the same. Type B kinetoplast was characteristic of the midgut forms and Type A of culture forms. He demonstrated oral transmission of *H. muscarum* and *C. luciliae* to clean flies with faeces of infected flies placed on fresh meat. *L. mirabilis*, however, did not produce infections in this manner. *H. muscarum* was isolated in culture from flies in which only endotrophic *H. muscarum* was seen. *L. mirabilis* attached to the midgut appeared in one to two days in flies fed these cultures. After three to six days there were in addition free opisthomastigotes. Midgut opistho-mastigotes were found in 90·8% of flies from one locality and attached pyloric promastigotes (*L. mirabilis*) were in 20%. There were double infections in 17%. Thus the two types of infection did not occur together more often than would be expected from chance and there was no evidence that one was derived from the other in the same fly. Brun proposed a hypothesis that midgut forms in order to transform into the attached pyloric forms that we call *L. mirabilis* require a stimulus. This stimulus is provided outside the fly, either in culture or on meat. When stimulated flagellates from one fly are ingested by another they are capable of transforming into the pyloric forms, which develop only when they are in contact with the pyloric epithelium. The attached pyloric forms are not infectious and are apparently a blind alley in development.

These results differ from those of Rogers and Wallace (1971) and Wallace and Todd (1964). Rogers cloned strains of *H. muscarum* (now designated as subspecies) with type A and type B kinetoplasts. These strains retained their individual characteristics in culture and in laboratory-reared experimentally infected flies. When the two clones were mixed the one with type B kinetoplast predominated in the fly midgut while the one with type A kinetoplast predominated in culture. These results suggest an alternative explanation for the kinetoplast transformation that Brun postulated.

Wallace and Todd (1964) cultured *L. mirabilis* and found that the species retained its characteristic morphology in culture. However, we did not attempt to infect flies with the culture. On the other hand Rogers and Wallace (1971) fed flies on various strains of *H. muscarum* and never recovered *L. mirabilis* in the experimental flies. Brun transferred infections of *C. luciliae* and *H. muscarum* from fly to fly by feeding them faeces or intestinal contents. When he fed flies on a culture of *H. muscarum* the recipients in 12% of the cases had *L. mirabilis* but none had *H. muscarum*. There is no explanation for this discrepancy.

H. muscarum muscarum Rogers and Wallace, 1971
    Host: *Musca domestica*
    Location: Endotrophic in midgut
    Locality: Minnesota, USA
    Remarks: Body length 10 μm to 25 μm (average 19·7 μm), free flagellum twice the body length. The type A kinetoplast is unremarkable, the nucleoid being a disc 150 to 200 nm in thickness. A few biflagellates are seen among the more numerous monoflagellate promastigotes. The number of opisthomastigotes in culture varies widely but may reach 15% in old cultures.

H. muscarum ingenoplastis Rogers and Wallace, 1971
    Host: *Phormia regina* (Diptera: Calliphoridae)
    Location: Midgut
    Locality: Minnesota, USA
    Remarks: Length of biflagellate promastigotes 20 μm to 30 μm (average 27·9 μm). Opisthomastigotes, which are 9 μm to 11 μm long, appear in infected flies, constituting up to 39% of the population in old infections, but are very rare (less than 1%) in cultures. The kinetoplast is type B, pyriform or tear-drop shaped and up to 2·5 μm in length.

H. megaseliae Daggett, Dollahon and Janovy, 1972
    Host: *Megaselia scalaris* (Diptera: Phoridae)
    Location: Intestine
    Locality: Nebraska, USA
    Remarks: Relatively wide and truncate. Small type A kinetoplast.
Length 8 μm to 22 μm (average 13 μm), width up to 5 μm. Flagellum
8 μm to 30 μm (average 14 μm). Opisthomastigotes made up 22% in a
seven day culture. Biflagellate forms uncommon. No opisthomastigotes
in experimentally infected flies. This *Herpetomonas* produced apparently
transitory infections in lizards in the laboratory where they fed on
naturally infected flies.

H. samuelpessoai Roitman, Brener and Roitman, 1976
    Synonyms: *L. pessoai* Galvão *et al.*, 1970 in part
              H. muscarum Carvalho 1973
    Host: *Zelus leucogrammus* (Hemiptera: Reduviidae) but it may be
        normally parasitic in flies which the *Zelus* eat
    Location: Intestine
    Locality: Goiania, Brazil
    Remarks: Promastigotes 5·7 μm to 15·2 μm long (average 10·7 μm).
Average length of flagellum 10·4 μm. Opisthomastigotes 5·4 μm to
10·2 μm long (average 7·8 μm), free flagellum 1·1 μm to 4·5 μm (average
3 μm). These measurements are from Carvalho's (1973) description of
the culture that was isolated by Galvão *et al.* (1970). Galvão *et al.*
described a new flagellate, *Leptomonas pessoai*, from the insectivorous
bug, *Zelus leucogrammus*. They found epimastigotes (see *Blastocrithidia
triatomae galvoi* below), promastigotes and amastigotes. Only promastigotes were seen in culture and the new species was based upon them.
Carvalho, one of the coauthors of the original description, reported
further studies in 1973. She found opisthomastigotes in the original culture and concluded that the organism was *H. muscarum* which was
parasitic in the flies on which the *Zelus* fed. She concluded that the name
L. pessoai was invalid. Roitman *et al.* (1976) studied the same culture and
found that it could grow indefinitely at 37°C and on this basis named it
as a new species different from *H. muscarum*.

H. swainei Smirnoff and Lipa, 1970
    Host: *Neodiprion swainei* (Hymenoptera: Tenthridinidae)
    Location: Intestine, Malpighian tubules, haemocoel
    Locality: Quebec, Canada.
    Remarks: Opisthomastigotes 7·5 μm to 13 μm in length (average
9·05 μm) and 3 μm to 4 μm in width. Flagellum 0·5 μm to 10 μm in
length (average 5·6 μm). Promastigotes 11 μm to 19 μm (average 13·8 μm)

in length by 1·5 μm to 3 μm (average 2·2 μm) in width. Flagellum 6 μm to 14 μm (average 9·5 μm). Often attached to gut wall by flagellar end. In the haemolymph 38 % were opisthomastigotes. There was no evidence of disease in naturally infected insects but when larvae were infected experimentally in the first or second instars they showed 20 % mortality on reaching the fourth and fifth instars. Infections acquired in larval stages persisted into the adult stage.

C. GENUS *CRITHIDIA* LÉGER, 1902

Features characteristic of this genus in addition to those given by Vickerman (1976) are the 12 striae and the presence of a free flagellum rather than a brush or "mèche muqueuse" on attached forms (see Section II, Morphology). As Lwoff and Lwoff (1931) pointed out, most members of the genus have greater synthetic ability and grow more readily in culture than other trypanosomatids.

Morphological differences between the various species of *Crithidia* are slight and it is often impossible to describe species so that they can be distinguished from other species when they are encountered again. Still, most species have been described on the basis of morphology, especially measurements, and the identity of the host. Even Noguchi (1926), who first used serological tests and the utilization of carbohydrates to characterize trypanosomatids, described his species (Noguchi and Tilden, 1926) on morphological grounds.

The only attempts to use biological characters along with morphology in describing new species were those of Langridge and McGhee (1967) and McGhee *et al.* (1969). They compared growth rates in a modified Cowperthwaite's medium and a diphasic medium. They also found that certain species had particular pH requirements in Cowperthwaite's medium. McGhee *et al.* (1969) also characterized species by their growth rates in the chorioallantoic cavity of the chick embryo, the haemocoel of *Drosophila virilis* and *Acheta domesticus*, and the intestine of *Oncopeltus fasciatus*.

There have been a number of comparative studies on nutritional differences, DNA characterization and other biochemical criteria for differentiating previously described *Crithidia* species as well as other lower trypanosomatids. These have been summarized by Newton (1976). Clearly, biochemical criteria are of little use in systematics if each investigator uses different criteria.

C. fasciculata Léger, 1902

Remarks: Synonyms, hosts, localities and the characteristics of four subspecies for this cosmopolitan parasite of mosquitoes are given by Wallace (1966). This species utilizes lactose but not sorbitose and some of the subspecies differ in their utilization of ribose and xylose (Newton, 1976). *C. fasciculata culicis* was found by Lwoff (1935) to be able to synthesize haemin, a unique ability for a haemoflagellate without a symbiont.

C. oncopelti (Noguchi and Tilden, 1926) Wallace, 1966.
   Remarks: The history of this confused species is given in Wallace (1966). Reasons are there given for the author's belief that Noguchi's strain number 4, which was preserved in culture and has been the subject of all subsequent research on the species, did not come from the milkweed as claimed and is of unknown origin. The species is of particular interest because of its symbiont.

C. lucilia (Strickland, 1911) Wallace and Clark, 1959
   Synonyms: *H. luciliae* Strickland (in part)
                      L. luciliae Wenyon, 1926
   Hosts: *Lucilia* spp., *Phaenicia sericata* (Calliphoridae), *Musca domestica* (experimental), *Zelus leucogrammus*
   Location: Hindgut, rectum, occasionally other parts of the alimentary tract.
   Locality: England, United States, Brazil
   Remarks: Length 8·5 μm to 13·6 μm; flagellum 10 μm to 14 μm.
This typical *Crithidia* was once thought to include opisthomastigotes, which probably belonged to *Herpetomonas* sp. from the same hosts.

C. deanei Carvalho, 1973
   Host: *Zelus leucogrammus* (Hemiptera: Reduviidae)
   Location: Intestine
   Locality: Belo Horizonte, Brazil
   Remarks: Length 3·7 μm to 6·4 μm (average 4·7 μm). Flagellum 0·1 μm to 7·4 μm (average 3·6 μm). Nuclear index 0·1 to 0·5 (average 0·2). This is distinguished from *C. luciliae* by its smaller size. Mundim and Roitman (1974) found bacterial endosymbionts in this species.

C. arili McGhee, Hanson and Schmittner, 1969
   Host: *Arilus cristatus* (Hemiptera: Reduviidae)
   Location: Intestine
   Locality: Georgia, USA
   Remarks: Length 6·1 μm and width 2·4 μm. This species grows slowly in Cowperthwaite's medium but very vigorously in the chick embryo, in *Drosophila* and in *Oncopeltus*.

C. harmosa McGhee, Hanson and Schmittner, 1969
   Host: *Euryophthalmus davisi*
   Location: Intestine

Locality: Georgia, USA

Remarks: Length 6·8 μm and width 2·4 μm. The posterior tip is pointed. Growth in Cowperthwaite's medium is best at pH 5. In the chick embryo growth is minimal. It is pathogenic in *Drosophila virilis* when injected into the haemocoel.

C. acidophili McGhee, Hanson and Schmittner, 1969

Host: *Oncopeltus fasciatus* (Hemiptera: Lygaeidae)
Location: Intestine
Locality: Virginia, USA
Remarks: Length 5·8 μm and width 2·2 μm. This is a fastidious organism that grew on diphasic medium but on Cowperthwaite's medium only at pH 5.

C. epedana McGhee, Hanson and Schmittner, 1969

Host: *Euschistus servus* (Hemiptera: Pentatomidae)
Location: Intestine
Locality: Georgia, USA
Remarks: Length 6·22 μm and width 1·8 μm. This species grew very feebly in all media tried.

C. cimbexi Lipa and Smirnoff, 1971

Host: *Cimbex americana* (Hymenoptera, Tenthredinidae)
Location: not given
Locality: St. Honoré, Quebec, Canada
Remarks: Length 11 μm to 17 μm (average 14·5 μm). Width 6 μm to 8 μm (average 7 μm). Length of flagellum 4 μm to 19 μm (average 13μ5 μm). Kinetoplast 2 μm to 3 μm from anterior end. This is unusually large for a *Crithidia*. In the description the meaning of the word epimastigote is apparently misapplied but it is clear that this description applies to choanomastigotes and refers to *Crithidia* in the modern sense.

C. mellificae Langridge and McGhee, 1967

Synonym: *Leptomonas apis* Lotmar, 1946
Host: *Apis mellifera* (Hemiptera: Apidae)
Location: Rectum, ileum in heavy infections
Locality: New South Wales and Victoria, Australia; Europe.
Remarks: Length 3·4 μm to 10·8 μm (average 7·04 μm) and width 2·87 μm to 9 μm (average 5·48 μm). In culture the measurements were 4·5 μm to 9·6 μm (average 6·5 μm) by 1·6 μm to 4·2 μm (average 3·2 μm). This is a fastidious organism that was cultivated only with difficulty. The addition of sugars and honey to the culture medium did not improve growth but a culture was established in Cowperthwaite's medium at pH 5·2. Bees were infected experimentally and the organism was transmitted among bees housed together. There was no evidence of pathogenicity.

D. GENUS *BLASTOCRITHIDIA* LAIRD, 1959

Blastocrithidia, the epimastigote parasites of arthropods, must be distinguished on the one hand from *Herpetomonas*, whose opisthomastigotes resemble it in the position of the kinetoplast on the longitudinal axis, but differ in the course of the flagellum and in the absence of the undulating membrane. On the other hand *Blastocrithidia* must be distinguished from epimastigotes of trypanosomes, which occur in haematophagous arthropod hosts and establish themselves in appropriate vertebrate hosts under the proper experimental conditions. Some *Blastocrithidia* are fastidious and can be isolated in culture only with difficulty.

B. gerridis (Patton, 1908) Laird, 1959. Type species
    Synonym: *C. gerridis* Patton, 1908
    Hosts: Water striders of the hemipteran family *Gerridae*
    Location: Intestine
    Locality: World wide
    Remarks: Length 17·5 μm to 70 μm (average 48·6 μm) and width 1·25 μm to 2·75 μm. Flagellum 1·75 μm to 15 μm (average 7·8 μm). This elongate flagellate does not grow on media that support most other lower trypanosomatids. No cysts or stages other than the epimastigotes have been attributed to this species with certainty.

B. culicis (Novy, MacNeal and Torrey) Wallace and Johnson, 1961
    Synonyms: *Trypanosoma (Herpetomonas) culicis* Novy, MacNeal and
            Torrey, 1907
            T. culici Mezincescu, 1908
            C. culicis Woodcock, 1914
    Hosts: Mosquitoes of many species
    Location: Midgut
    Locality: USA, Europe
    Remarks: Length 12 μm to 35 μm. Free flagellum 5 μm to 10 μm. No cysts. A bacillus-like endosymbiont, which is usually transversely constricted and thus looks like a double body, is always present (except in "cured" strains). See the discussion of endosymbionts in Section VI above.

B. raabei Lipa, 1966
    Host: *Mesocerus marginatus* (Hemiptera: Coreidae)
    Location: Intestine and haemocoel
    Locality: Poland
    Remarks: Length including the flagellum 21·3 μm to 31·7 μm (average 26·5 μm) and width 3 μm to 4·1 μm (average 3·4 μm). Free flagellum 4 μm to 13 μm (average 7·8 μm). Amastigotes, cysts and promastigotes

were described by Lipa but may well belong to other species found in the same hosts.

B. vagoi Tuzet and Laporte, 1965
Host: *Eurydema ventralis* (Hemiptera: Pentatomidae)
Location: Midgut
Locality: Southern France
Remarks: Length up to 24 μm and width 1·5 μm to 2 μm. Free flagellum up to 28 μm. Promastigotes and cysts that were described as stages of this species are possibly other species of trypanosomatids.

B. triatomae Cerisola *et al.*, 1971
Host: *Triatoma infestans* (Hemiptera: Reduviidae)
Location: Midgut and hindgut
Locality: Argentina
Remarks: Length 14·8 μm to 32 μm (average 25 μm). Width 2·2 μm to 2·9 μm (average 2·6 μm). Free flagellum 19·5 μm to 28·5 μm (average 22·5 μm). The flagellar cysts are 2·8 μm by 0·9 μm.

This species was found in a colony of *Triatoma infestans* that was used for xenodiagnosis of *Trypanosoma cruzi* infections. Its presence could obviously be a source of error in xenodiagnosis. The flagellar cysts exceed in frequency and in number per parent organism those of any other trypanosomatid. The cysts apparently begin as elongate amastigotes 3·4 μm or more in length in which the nucleus and kinetoplast can be distinguished. They then become "condensed" cysts, 2·8 μm or less in length, constricted in the middle and showing no detail in stained preparations. It is probable that this organism was the subject of observations on what were thought to be cysts of *T. cruzi* (Silva, 1958). This organism is very difficult to cultivate but after many attempts a few cultures have been established in this laboratory in media at pH 5·5 to 6·5.

B. triatomae galvaoi Carvalho, 1973
Host: *Zelus leucogrammus* (Hemiptera: Reduviidae)
Location: Intestine; female reproductive tract
Locality: Brazil
Remarks: Length 9.1 μm to 22·8 μm (average 15·6 μm); width 1·1 μm to 3·7 μm (average 2·1 μm). Flagellum 1·4 μm to 22·8 μm (average 3·3 μm). This is smaller than *B. triatomae*. It was found in 100% of the hosts, which also harboured, though less frequently, *C. luciliae*, *C. deanei*, *H. samuelpessoai* and *L. samueli*. These last four species were thought to be parasites of the flies which serve as prey for the *Zelus*. After many attempts Carvalho succeeded in cultivating this organism from the host ovaries in McConnell's medium.

B. apiomerusi Floch and Abonnenc, 1941
Host: *Apiomerus* sp. (Hemiptera: Reduviidae)
Location: Intestine
Locality: French Guiana
Remarks: Measurements of a typical epimastigote were length 34 μm, width 5 μm and free flagellum 20 μm. Amastigotes 6 μm to 7 μm by 4 μm to 5 μm were often in fan-shaped groups. No flagellar cysts were described.

E. GENUS *RHYNCHOIDOMONAS* PATTON, 1910

These are trypomastigotes with the flagellum closely adherent to the body surface so there is no undulating membrane. They are usually in the Malpighian tubules and always in Diptera. Wenyon (1926) regarded them as stages of *Herpetomonas muscarum*. This author prefers to accept *Rhynchoidomonas* as a separate genus for the following reasons: (1) these characteristic forms have been described separately by a number of investigators in different countries; and (2) many investigators, including the author, have studied, isolated, and infected hosts with *H. muscarum* without encountering *Rhynchoidomonas*. Nothing new on this genus has been published since 1966.

IX. References

Angluster, J. M., Bunn, M. and De Souza, W. (1977). Effect of 2-Deoxy-D-glucose on differentiation of *Herpetomonas samuelpessoai*. *Journal of Parasitology*, **63**, 922–924.
Bailey, C. H. and Brooks, W. M. (1971). Transmission of the flagellate, *Herpetomonas muscarum*, in laboratory cultures of the eye gnat, *Hippelates pusio* (Diptera: Chloropidae). *Proceedings of the Fourth International Colloquium on Insect Pathology and the Society of Invertebrate Pathology*. College Park Md., pp. 60–65.
Bailey, C. H. and Brooks, W. M. (1972). Effects of *Herpetomonas muscarum* on development and longevity of the eye gnat, *Hippelates pusio* (Diptera: Chloropidae). *Journal of Invertebrate Pathology*, **20**, 31–36.
Baker, J. R. (1976). *In:* "Biology of the Kinetoplastida" (W. H. R. Lumsden and D. A. Evans, eds), Vol. I, pp. 131–174.
Berens, R., Brun, R. and Krassner, S. M. (1976). A simple monophasic medium for axenic culture of hemoflagellates. *Journal of Parasitology*, **62**, 360–365.
Bovien, P. (1937). Some types of association between nematodes and insects. *Videnskabelige Meddelelser fra Dansk Naturhistorisk Forening*, **101**, 1–144.
Brooker, B. E. (1971). Flagellar attachment and detachment of *Crithidia fasciculata* to the gut wall of *Anopheles gambiae Protoplasma*, **73**, 191–202.
Brooks, M. A. (1975). *In:* "Pathobiology of Invertebrate Vectors of Disease" (L. A. Bulla and T. C. Cheng, eds), pp. 166–172. *Annals of the New York Academy of Science*, Vol. 266.

Brueske, W. A. (1967). The diplosome of *Blastocrithidia culicis* (Novy MacNeal and Torrey, 1907). *Ph.D. Thesis, University of Minnesota*, iv + 73 pp.

Brumpt, E. (1913). Evolution de *Trypanosoma lewisi, duttoni nabiasi, blanchardi* chez les puces et les punaises. Transmission par les déjections. Comparison avec *T. cruzi. Bulletin de la Société de Pathologie Exotique*, **6**, 167–171.

Brun, R. (1974). Ultrastruktur und Zyklus von *Herpetomonas muscarum, Herpetomonas mirabilis* und *Crithidia luciliae* in *Chrysomyia chloropyga. Acta Tropica,* **31**, 219–290.

Burnett, W. J. (1851). The organic relations of some of the infusoria, including investigations concerning the structure of the genus *Bodo* (Ehr.). *Proceedings of the Boston Society of Natural History*, **4**, 124–125.

Camargo, E. P. and Freymuller, E. (1977). Endosymbiont as supplier of ornithine carbamoyl transferase in a trypanosomatid. *Nature, London*, **270**, 52–53.

Carvalho, A. L. de M. (1973). Estudos sobre a posição sistemática a biologia e a transmissão de tripanosomatideos encontrados em *Zelus leucogrammus* (Perty, 1834) (Hemptera: Reduviidae). *Revista de Patologia Tropica*, **2**, 223–274.

Carvalho, A. L. de M. and Deane, M. P. (1974). Trypanosomatidae isolated from *Zelus leucogrammus* (Perty, 1834) (Hemiptera: Reduviidae) with a discussion of flagellates of insectivorous bugs. *Journal of Protozoology*, **21**, 5–8.

Cerisola, J. A., Del Prado, C. E., Rohwedder, R. and Bozzini, J. P. (1971). *Blastocrithidia triatomae* n. sp. found in *Triatoma infestans* from Argentina. *Journal of Protozoology*, **18**, 503–506.

Chang, K. P. (1974). Ultrastructure of symbiotic bacteria in normal and antibiotic-treated *Blastocrithidia culicis* and *Crithidia oncopelti. Journal of Protozoology*, **21**, 699–707.

Chang, K. P. and Trager, W. (1974). Nutritional significance of symbiotic bacteria in two species of hemoflagellates. *Science*, **183**, 531–532.

Chang, K. P., Chang, C. S. and Sassa, S. (1975). Heme biosynthesis in bacterium-protozoon symbioses. Enzymic defects in host hemoflagellates and complemental role of their intracellular symbiotes. *Proceedings of the National Academy of Science*, **72**, 2979–2983.

Chatton, E. (1913). L'ordre, la succession et l'importance relative des stades dans l'evolution des trypanosomides chez les insects. *Comptes Rendus des Séances de la Société de Biologie et des ses Filiales*, **74**, 1145–1147.

Chatton, E. (1938). Titres et travaux scientifiques (1906–1937). Imprimerie Sottano, Sète.

Chatton, E. and Alilaire, E. (1908). Coexistence d'un *Leptomonas (Herpetomonas)* et d'un *Trypanosoma* chez un muscide non vulnérant, *Drosophila confusa* Staeger. *Comptes Rendus des Séances de la Société de Biologie et des ses Filiales*, **64**, 1004–1006.

Cosgrove, W. B. (1971). *In:* "Developmental aspects of the Cell Cycle" (E. L. Cameron, G. M. Padilla and A. M. Zimmerman, eds), pp. 1–21. Academic Press, New York and London.

Daggett, P. M., Dollahon, N. and Janovy, J. (1972). *Herpetomonas megaseliae* sp. n. (Protozoa: Trypanosomatidae) from *Megaselia scalaris* (Loew, 1866) Schmitz, 1929 (Diptera: Phoridae). *Journal of Parasitology*, **58**, 946–949.

De Almeida, D. F. and De Souza, W. (1978). Morphological changes of *Herpetomonas samuelpessoai. Journal of Parasitology*, **64**, 17–22.

Diamond, L. S. and Herman, C. M. (1954). Incidence of trypanosomes in the Canada goose as revealed by bone marrow culture. *Journal of Parasitology*, **40**, 195–202.

Fantham, H. B. (1912). Some insect flagellates and the problem of the transmission of *Leishmania. British Medical Journal*, (2705), **2**, 1196–1197.

Floch, H. and Abonnenc, E. (1941). Flagellé parasite du tube digestif de reduvidé du genre *Apiomerus*. *Institut Pasteur de la Guyane et du Territoire de l'Inini.* Publication 24, pp. 1–5.

Franchini, G. (1922). Protozoaires de muscides divers capturés sur des euphorbes. *Bulletin de la Société de Pathologie Exotique*, **15**, 970–978.

Galvão, A. B., Oliveira, R. L., Carvalho, A. and Veiga, G. P. (1970). *Leptomonas pessoai* sp. n. (Trypanosomatidae, Kinetoplastida, Protozoa). *Revista Goiana de Medicina*, **16**, 229–236.

Gibbs, A. J. (1951). *Leptomonas capsularis* n. sp. and other flagellates parasitic in *Cletus ochraceus* (Hemiptera). *Parasitology*, **41**, 128–133.

Gillies, C. and Hanson, E. (1963). A new species parasitizing the macronucleus of *Paramecium trichius*. *Journal of Protozoology*, **10**, 467–473.

Goodey, T. and Triffitt, M. J. (1927). On the presence of flagellates in the intestine of the nematode *Diplogaster longicauda Protozoology, A supplement to the Journal of Helminthology*, No. 3, pp. 47–58.

Indurkar, A. K. (1965). Studies on the kinetoplast of three species of flagellates (*Trypanosoma lewisi*, *Blastocrithidia culicis* and *Bodo saltans*]. Ph.D. Thesis, University of Wisconsin, 148 pp.

Janovy, J., Lee, K. W. and Brumbaugh, J. A. (1974). The differentiation of *Herpetomonas megaseliae*: ultrastructural observations. *Journal of Protozoology*, **21**, 53–59.

Johnson, P., Neal, R. A. and Gall, D. (1963). Protective effect of killed trypanosome vaccines with incorporated adjuvants. *Nature, London*, **200**, 83.

Kent, W. S. (1880). "A Manual of the Infusoria". Bogue, London.

Kramer, J. P. (1961). *Herpetomonas muscarum* (Leidy) in the haemocoel of larval *Musca domestica* L. *Entomological News*, **72**, 165–166.

Laird, M. (1959). *Blastocrithidia* n.g. (Mastigophora; Protomonadina) for *Crithidia* (in part) with a subarctic record for *B. gerridis* (Patton). *Canadian Journal of Zoology*, **37**, 749–752.

Langridge, D. F. and McGhee, R. B. (1967). *Crithidia mellificae* n. sp., an acidophilic trypanosomatid of the honey bee, *Apis mellifera*. *Journal of Protozoology*, **14**, 485–487.

Léger, L. (1902a). Sur un flagellé parasite de l'*Anopheles maculipennis*. *Comptes Rendus des Séances de la Société de Biologie et des ses Filiales*, **54**, 354–356.

Léger, L. (1902b). Sur la structure et le mode de multiplication des flagellés du genre *Herpetomonas* Kent. *Comptes Rendus des Séances de la Société de Biologie et des ses Filiales*, **54**, 398–400.

Leidy, J. (1856). A synopsis of Entozoa and some of their ectocongeners observed by the author. *Proceedings of the Academy of Natural Sciences, Philadelphia*, **8**, 42–58.

Lipa, J. J. (1966). *Blastocrithidia raabei* sp. n., a flagellate parasite of *Mesocerus marginatus* L. (Hemiptera: Coreidae). *Acta Protozoologica*, **4**, 19–23.

Lipa, J. J. and Smirnoff, W. A. (1971). *Crithidia cimbexi* sp. n., a new Flagellate Parasite of *Cimbex americana* Leach (*Hymenoptera, Tenthredinidae*). *Bulletin de l'Academie Polonaise des Sciences. Serie des Sciences biologiques* Cl. 2, **19**, 269–274.

Lushbaugh, W. B., Rowton, E. D. and McGhee, R. B. (1976). Redescription of *Coccidiascus legeri* Chatton, 1913 (Nematosporacea: Hemiascomycetidae), an intracellular parasitic yeast-like fungus from the intestinal epithelium of *Drosophila melanogaster*. *Journal of Invertebrate Pathology*, **28**, 93–107.

Lwoff, M. (1935). Le pouvoir de synthèse des trypanosomides des culicides. *Comptes Rendus des Séances de la Société de Biologie et des ses Filiales*, **119**, 969–971.

Lwoff, M. (1940). Recherches sur le pouvoir de synthèse des flagellés trypano-somides. *Monographie de l'Institut Pasteur*, Masson, Paris.

Lwoff, M. and Lwoff, A. (1931). Recherches sur la morphologie de *Leptomonas oncopelti* Noguchi et Tilden et *Leptomonas fasciculata* Novy McNeal et Torrey. *Archives de Zoologie Expérimentale et Générale*, **71**, Notes et Revue No. 1, pp. 21–37.

McConnell, E. (1963). Leptomonads of wildcaught Panamanian *Phlebotomus*: culture and animal inoculation. *Experimental Parasitology*, **14**, 123–128.

McCulloch, I. (1917). *Crithidia euryophthalmi* sp. nov. from the hemipteran bug, *Euryophthalmus convivus* Stal. *University of California Publications in Zoology*, **18**, 75–88.

McGhee, R. B. and Hanson, W. L. (1962). Growth and reproduction of *Leptomonas oncopelti* in the milkweed bug, *Oncopeltus fasciatus*. *Journal of Protozoology*, **9**, 488–493.

McGhee, R. B. and Hanson, W. L. (1964). Comparison of the Life cycle of *Leptomonas oncopelti* and *Phytomonas elmassiani*. *Journal of Protozoology*, **11**, 555–562.

McGhee, R. B., Hanson, W. L. and Schmittner, S. M. (1969). Isolation, cloning and determination of biologic characteristics of five new species of *Crithidia*. *Journal of Protozoology*, **16**, 514–520.

Mello, I. F. (1921). Protozoaires parasites du *Pachylabra moesta* Reeve. *Comptes Rendus des Séances de la Société de Biologie et des ses Filiales*, **84**, 341–342.

Mezincescu, D. (1908). Les trypanosomes des moustiques et leurs relations avec les *Haemoproteus* des oiseaux. *Comptes Rendus des Séances de la Société de Biologie et des ses Filiales*, **64**, 975–976.

Minchin, E. A. and Thomson, J. D. (1915). The rat trypanosome *Trypanosoma lewisi* in its relation to the rat flea, *Ceratophyllus fasciatus*. *Quarterly Journal of Microscopical Science*, **60**, 463–692.

Mundim, M. H. and Roitman, I. (1977). Extra nutritional requirements of arti-ficially aposymbiotic *Crithidia deanei*. *Journal of Protozoology*, **24**, 329–331.

Mundim, M. H., Roitman, I., Hermans, M. A. and Kitajima, E. W. (1974). Simple nutrition of *Crithidia deanei*, a reduviid trypanosomatid with an endosym-biont. *Journal of Protozoology*, **21**, 518–521.

Newton, B. A. (1956). A synthetic growth medium for the trypanosomatid flagel-late *Strigomonas* (*Herpetomonas*) *oncopelti*. *Nature, London*, **177**, 279–280.

Newton, B. A. (1968). Biochemical peculiarities of trypanosomatid flagellates. *Annual of Review of Microbiology*, **22**, 109–130.

Newton, B. A. (1976). *In:* "Biology of the Kinetoplastida" W. H. R. Lumsden and D. A. Evans, eds), Vol. I, pp. 405–434.

Newton, F. A. and Horne, R. W. (1957). Intracellular structures in *Strigomonas oncopelti*. I. Cytoplasmic structures containing ribonucleoprotein. *Experimental Cell Research*, **13**, 563–574.

Nicoli, R. M., Penaud, A. and Timon-David, P. (1971). Recherches systématiques sur les trypanosomides 1. Le genre *Nematodomonas* N. gen. *Bulletin de la Société Zoologique de France*, **96**, 405–415.

Noguchi, H. (1926). Comparative studies of herpetomonads and leishmanias. II. Differentiation of the organisms by serological reactions and fermentation tests. *Journal of Experimental Medicine*, **44**, 327–337.

Noguchi, H. and Tilden, E. B. (1926). Comparative studies of herpetomonads and leishmanias. I. Cultivation of herpetomonads from insects and plants. *Journal of Experimental Medicine*, **44**, 307–325.

Nöller, W. (1925). Die nächsten Verwandten des Blutflagellaten und ihre Bezie-hungen zu den blutbewohnenden Formen. *In:* "Handbuch der Pathogenen Protozoen" (S. von Prowazek and W. Nöller, eds), Vol. 3, 1969. Leipzig.

Novy, F. G., MacNeal, W. J. and Torrey, H. N. (1907). The trypanosomes of mosquitoes and other insects. *Journal of Infectious Diseases*, **4**, 223–276.

Patton, W. S. (1908). The life cycle of a species of *Crithidia* parasitic in the intestinal tract of *Gerris fossarum* Fabr. *Archiv für Protistenkunde*, **12**, 131–146.

Patton, W. S. (1910). *Rhynchomonas luciliae*, nov. gen., nov. sp. A new flagellate parasitic in the Malpighian tubes of *Lucilia serenissima* Walk. *Bulletin de la Société de Pathologie exotique*, **3**, 300–303 and note of correction 433.

Paulin, J. (1975). The chondriome of selected trypanosomatids. *Journal of Cell Biology*, **66**, 404–413.

Podkulski, K., Sullivan, W., Bacchi, C. J. and Hutner, S. H. (1974). Cloning drug resistant populations of a *Leptomonas*. *Journal of Protozoology*, **21**, (3) Abstract 63.

Porter, A. (1910). The life-cycle of *Herpetomonas jaculum* (Léger), parasitic in the alimentary tract of *Nepa cinerea*. *Parasitology*, **2**, 367–391.

Porter, A. (1914). The morphology and biology of *Herpetomonas patellae* n. sp. parasitic in the limpet, *Patella vulgata*, together with remarks on the pathogenic significance of certain flagellates found in invertebrates. *Parasitology*, **7**, 322–329.

Richards, A. G. and Richards, P. A. (1977). The peritrophic membranes of insects. *Annual Review of Entomology*, **22**, 219–240.

Rodhain, J. and Bequaert, J. (1916). Materiaux pour une étude monographique des diptères parasites de l'Afrique. Revision des Oestrinae. *Bulletin biologique de la France et de la Belgique*, **50**, 53–165.

Rogers, W. E. and Wallace, F. G. (1971). Two new subspecies of *Herpetomonas muscarum* (Leidy, 1856) Kent, 1880. *Journal of Protozoology*, **18**, 645–649.

Roitman, I., Brener, Z., Roitman, C. and Kitajima, E. W. (1976). Demonstration that *Leptomonas pessoai* Galvão, Oliveira, Carvalho, and Veiga, 1970 is a *Herpetomonas*. *Journal of Protozoology*, **23**, 291–292.

Ross, R. (1906). Notes on the parasites of mosquitoes found in India between 1895 and 1899. *Journal of Hygiene*, **6**, 101–109.

Roubaud, E. (1908). Sur un nouveau flagellé, parasite de l'intestin des muscides au Congo français. *Comptes Rendus des Séances de la Société de Biologie et des ses Filiales*, **64**, 1106–1108.

Roubaud, E. (1911). *Cercoplasma* (n. gen.) *caulleryi* (n. sp.): nouveau flagellé à formes trypanosomiennes de l'intestin d'*Auchmeromyia luteola* Fabr. (Muscidae). *Comptes Rendus des Séances de la Société de Biologie et des ses Filiales*, **71**, 570–573.

Silva, I. I. (1958). Forma quistica del *Trypanosoma* (*Schizotrypanum*) *cruzi*. *Revista de la Faculdad de Medicina de Tucuman* (*Argentina*), **1**, 39–66.

Smirnoff, W. A. and Lipa, J. J. (1970). *Herpetomonas swainei* sp. n., a new flagellate parasite of *Neodiprion swainei* (Hymenoptera: Tenthredinidae). *Journal of Invertebrate Pathology*, **16**, 187–195.

Souza, M. C., Reis, A. P., da Silva, W. D. and Brener, Z. (1974). Mechanism of acquired immunity induced by *Leptomonas pessoai* against *Trypanosoma cruzi*. *Journal of Protozoology*, **21**, 579–584.

Strickland, C. (1911). Description of a *Herpetomonas* parasitic in the alimentary tract of the common green bottle fly, *Lucilia* sp. *Parasitology*, **4**, 222–236.

Tuzet, O. and Laporte, M. (1965). *Blastocrithidia vagoi* n. sp. parasite de l'Hemiptère Hétéroptère *Eurydema ventralis* Kol. *Archives de Zoologie Expérimentale et Générale*, **105**, 77–81.

Vickerman, K. (1976). *In:* "Biology of the Kinetoplastida" (W. H. R. Lumsden and D. A. Evans, eds), Vol. I, pp. 1–34. Academic Press, New York and London.

Vickerman, K. and Preston, T. M. (1976). *In:* "Biology of the Kinetoplastida"

(W. H. R. Lumsden and D. A. Evans, eds), Vol. I, pp. 35–130. Academic Press, New York and London.

Wallace, F. G. (1966). The trypanosomatid parasites of insects and arachnids. *Experimental Parasitology*, **18**, 124–193.

Wallace, F. G. and Clark, T. B. (1959). Flagellate parasites of the fly, *Phaenicia sericata* (Meigen). *Journal of Protozoology*, **6**, 58–61.

Wallace, F. G. and Johnson, A. (1961). The infectivity of old cultured strains of mosquito flagellates. *Journal of Insect Pathology*, **3**, 75–80.

Wallace, F. G. and Todd, S. R. (1964). *Leptomonas mirabilis* Roubaud 1908 in a Central American blowfly. *Journal of Protozoology*, **11**, 502–505.

Weinman, D. (1972). *Trypanosoma cyclops* n. sp.: a pigmented trypanosome from the Malayan primates *Macaca nemestrina* and *M. ira*. *Transactions of the Royal Society of Tropical Medicine and Hygiene*, **66**, 628–636.

Weinman, D. and Cheong, W. H. (1978). *Herpetomonas* with bacterium-like inclusions, in Malaysian *Aedes aegypti* and *Aedes albopictus*. *Journal of Protozoology*, **25**, 167–169.

Wenyon, C. M. (1913). Observations on *Herpetomonas muscae domesticae* and some allied flagellates. *Archiv für Protistenkunde*, **31**, 1–36.

Wenyon, C. M. (1926). "Protozoology: A Manual for Medical Men, Veterinarians and Zoologists", Vols I and II. Ballière, Tindall and Cox, London.

Woodcock, H. M. (1914). Further remarks on the flagellate parasites of *Culex*. Is there a generic type, *Crithidia*? *Zoologischer Anzeiger*, **44**, 26–33.

Zeledon, R., Hidalgo, W. and Hidalgo, H. (1961). Consideraciones cuantitativas sobre la intradermo-reaccion de Montenegro con antigeno homologo (leishmanina) y antigeno de *Strigomonas oncopelti*. *Programa y Resumen de Trabajos del segundo Congreso Latinoamericano* (Ciudad Universitaria, Costa Rica).

5

Lizard *Leishmania*

VANESSA C. L. C. WILSON*
and B. A. SOUTHGATE
London School of Hygiene and Tropical Medicine,
London, England

I. Historical aspects and evolutionary trends   242

II. Species   243
   A. Lizard parasites   243
   B. Reptilian hosts   243

III. Morphology and life cycle   245
   A. Lizard parasite   245
   B. Transmission and vector   247

IV. Relationship of lizard and mammalian leishmanias   .   .   .   248
   A. Susceptibility of lizards to promastigotes of *Leishmania* species   248
   B. Susceptibility of mammals to lizard leishmanias   .   .   250

V. Leishmanias of lizards and human leishmaniasis   .   .   .   253
   A. Serology   253
   B. Cross immunity between leishmanias of lizards and man   .   256
   C. Lizard *Leishmania* and human epidemiology   .   .   .   260

VI. Physiology and biochemistry   261

VII. References   263

* Former lecturer in Medical Protozoology.

I. Historical aspects and evolutionary trends

It seems probable that the family Trypanosomatidae, to which the genus *Leishmania* belongs, arose from the arthropod flagellates: the ancestral form was *Leptomonas*, Kent 1880, a monoxenous parasite which inhabited the lumen of the gut and was transmitted from one arthropod host to another by the ingestion of encysted amastigote-like forms passed with the faeces.

The majority of the Trypanosomatidae still continue to produce their infective stages in the posterior station of an invertebrate host; however, the genera *Phytomonas* (in which the infective stage is passed to a plant host as a result of an insect bite, and is subsequently ingested by the insect host) and *Leishmania* can complete their development in the foregut or anterior station of the invertebrate host.

Hoare (1948) postulated that the lizard leishmaniae provide convincing evidence of a transitory stage of evolution in which an invertebrate parasite has become adapted to life in a vertebrate host. Both he and Baker (1965) felt it reasonable to assume that, although promastigote forms have been reported from the intestine of reptilian vertebrates (Bayon, 1915; Léger, 1918; Wenyon, 1921; Franchini, 1921) they do occur more rarely in vertebrate than in invertebrate hosts and that if they are genuine intestinal promastigotes they have been acquired secondarily —first, for example, via the ingestion of infected arthropods by ancestral saurians and subsequently by their adaptation to the intestinal environment within the vertebrate host. It seems reasonable to suppose that subsequent invasion of the blood and other tissues took place; and in most modern *Leishmania* species of lizards the parasite has become restricted to the blood and viscera.

Léger (1918) described the promastigote form of a parasite which he found in both the blood and intestine of the lizard genus *Anolis*; this finding supported the suggestion of a possible evolutionary route towards the development of mammalian leishmaniae, a view held in the early part of this century by Minchin (1908) initially [who later, (1912, 1914) changed his mind], Mesnil (1918) and later by Lavier (1943), Hoare (1948) and Cameron (1956). This view was rejected by the majority of protozoologists who believed that the haemoflagellates arose from intestinal flagellates of invertebrates, without an intervening phase in the gut of a vertebrate. Hoare (1948) advanced a working hypothesis by which evolutionary events, based on the known life-cycles of various lizard species, could be traced: *Leishmania chamaeleonis*, the most primitive of the lizard leishmanias, is restricted to the intestine and cloaca of chameleons in the promastigote form. The subsequent stage is represented by *L. henrici* of iguanas in which promastigotes are found in the cloaca but have also invaded the blood in small numbers whereas *L. hemidactyli* promastigotes appear to inhabit the blood in large numbers thus providing a route by which cyclical development in a phlebotomine can occur if it bites an infected lizard. Additional evidence to support this hypothesis has been shown (see pp. 250–1) by the ability of promastigotes of *L. adleri*, *L. gymnodactyli* and *L. tarentolae* to form amastigotes when inoculated into warm-blooded hosts. Presumably, a similar event took place in nature and the mammalian genus *Leishmania* arose, i.e. the parasites became phagocytosed by the vertebrate mononuclear phagocyte and intracellular multiplication occurred; a phlebotomid vector ingested these forms from the mammalian skin, transformation to the promastigote stage took place in the insect gut and cyclical development was completed by their anterior migration to the mouth parts of the vector. *L. adleri* also provides an example of a saurian leishmania which has undergone this latter evolutionary step in the vector *Sergentomyia clydei* (Heisch, 1958).

II. Species

A. LIZARD PARASITES

Saurian species of *Leishmania*, with the exception of *L. henrici*, are entirely confined to the Old World; cultures of blood taken from lizards in North and Central America, Venezuela and Brazil have consistently proved negative for promastigotes (Dollahon and Janovy, 1974).

One of the first reports of reptilian promastigotes was that of Sergent *et al.* (1914), who obtained cultures of typical *Leishmania* promastigotes from 16% of NNN media inoculated with either blood or organs of the gecko, *Tarentola mauritanica* in Algeria. They assumed that they had discovered an important natural reservoir of cutaneous leishmaniasis. Since then the natural occurrence of ten species of lizard *Leishmania* has been described from different parts of the world, in five families (Agamidae, Gekkonidae, Scinciidae, Lacertidae and Iguanidae) and located at different sites within the body of the vertebrate host (Table 1).

B. REPTILIAN HOSTS

Belova (1971), in an excellent review, has listed the reptilian species from different parts of the Turkmenian SSR which were found to be infected with promastigotes of reptilian *Leishmania* (Table 2). She cites the first report of a natural infection of *Leishmania* promastigotes in geckoes in the USSR by Sahsuvarli (1934), and also cites subsequent studies of natural infections by the Russian workers, Zmeyev (1936), Khodukin and Sofiev (1940), Latysev and Pozyvaj (1937), Latysev (1949), Popov (1941), Andrusko and Markov (1955) and herself.

Table 1. *Leishmania* species in lizards (Adapted from Garnham, 1971).

Species	Vertebrate host	Site in vertebrate host	Suspected phlebotomine host	Region	Author
L. henrici	Anolis sp.	Blood, cloaca	Unknown	Martinique	Léger, 1918
L. tarentolae	Tarentola mauritanica	Blood, spleen	Sergentomyia minuta, S. minuta minuta	Malta, S. France, North Africa	Wenyon, 1921
L. chamaeleonis	Chamaeleon pumilus	Cloaca, intestine	Unknown	Egypt, Israel, Uganda and Madagascar	Wenyon, 1921
L. hemidactyli	Hemidactylus brooki	Blood	Unknown	India	Mackie et al., 1923
L. agamae	Agama stellio, A. sanguinolenta	Blood	Phlebotomus papatasi, P. caucasicus S. sintoni	Eastern Mediterranean, Turkmenian SSR	David, 1929
L. ceramodactyli	Ceramodactylus doriae	Blood	P. papatasi, P. caucasicus S. sintoni	Eastern Mediterranean, Turkmenian SSR	Adler and Theodor, 1929
L. gymnodactyli	Gymnodactylus caspius	Blood	P. papatasi, P. caucasicus S. sintoni	Turkmenian SSR	Khodukin and Sofiev, 1940
L. zmeevi	Eremias intermedia grammica	Blood	P. papatasi, S. sintoni	Turkmenian SSR	Andrusko and Markov, 1955
L. adleri	Latastia longicaudata	Blood, skin	S. clydei	Kenya	Heisch, 1958
L. hoogstraali	Hemidactylus turcicus	Blood	? S. clydei	S. Sudan	McMillan, 1965
Unnamed	Alsophylax pipiens	Blood, liver	Sergentomyia sp.	Mainland China	

Table 2. Species of lizards examined for promastigote infection in the Turkmenian SSR.

Family	Species	No. of specimens examined	No. of specimens with promastigotes
Agamidae	*Phrynocephalus interscapularis*	926	17
	Agama sanguinolenta	683	41
	Phrynocephalus mystaceus	99	1
	Agama caucasica	39	0
	Phrynocephalus raddei raddei	20	2[a]
	Phrynocephalus helioscopus	4	0
Lacertidae	*Eremias velox*	354	11[a]
	E. intermedia	277	3
	E. guttulata guttulata	169	3
	E. lineolata	113	5[a]
	E. grammica	88	2
	E. scripta scripta	4	0
Gekkonidae	*Gymnodactylus caspius*	907	139
	Teratascincus scincus	101	1[a]
	Gymnodactylus russowi	3	0
	Crossobamon eversamani	4	0
Anguidae	*Opisaurus apodus*	13	0
	Mabuya aurata	7	0
Varanidae	*Varanus griseus*	4	0
Scinciidae	*Eumeces taeniolatus*	1	0
	E. schneideri princeps	2	0

[a] New World record as a promastigote carrier. (Adapted from Belova, 1971)

III. Morphology and life cycle

A. LIZARD PARASITE

Lizard leishmanias have been the subject of very few morphological studies, either within the vector or the vertebrate host. They live predominantly as promastigotes, which are similar morphologically to those of the mammalian species, within the cloaca, intestine or blood of the vertebrate host; in most species the parasite is found exclusively in the blood where it may also assume an amastigote form. Garnham (1971) cites the observations of Avakyan (at the Gameleja Institute for Epidemiology and Microbiology, Moscow) in which he noted a striking ultrastructural difference between promastigotes of the reptilian and mammalian species. In the former, the subpellicular tubules lie 58–67 nm apart whereas in the latter they are only 35–42 nm apart. The difference in the spacing of these organelles, between reptilian and mammalian species, has been confirmed by Lewis (1975); he used promastigotes of *L. agamae*, *L. hoogstraali*, *L. adleri* and *L. mexicana mexicana* and found a mean separation of 45·6 nm and 26·5 nm respectively.

The amastigote form has never been described in detail and has been seen only on rare occasions in reptiles. Shortt and Swaminath (1928) described the presence of amastigote forms in saurian species of *Leishmania* for the first time. Six amastigotes, measuring 2·5 μm in diameter, were found within a peripheral blood leucocyte and others were extracellular in the blood. Previously, the parasite had been demonstrated in the promastigote form only by Mackie *et al.* (1923) and named *Herpetomonas hemidactyli*. These typical leishmania-like amastigotes provided the necessary evidence for placing the gecko parasite in the genus *Leishmania*, a taxonomic position into which it had already been placed by Wenyon (1926) on the grounds that it underwent part of its life-cycle in a vertebrate host.

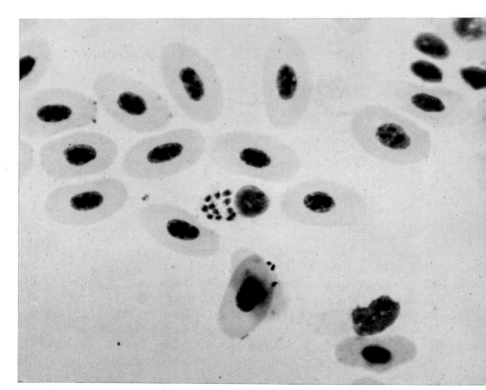

FIG. 1.   Amastigotes of *Leishmania* in a monocyte in peripheral blood of *Agama stellio* from Lebanon. (Specimen photographed by courtesy of Dr J. F. B. Edeson and Professor P. C. C. Garnham.)

In 1929 David isolated *L. agamae* from cultures of the cardiac blood of *Agama stellio* in Palestine; on examination of stained blood films she eventually discovered a single amastigote within a monocyte. This finding was confirmed almost fifty years later by Edeson and Himo (1973) who examined Giemsa-stained blood films from *A. stellio*, caught in the Bekaa and Roumieh districts of Lebanon, and demonstrated the presence of amastigotes (Fig. 1) in 8% (16/200) of the lizards.

The fourth and only other occasion to our knowledge that amastigote forms of *Leishmania* have been demonstrated in the blood of a naturally infected lizard was during an epidemiological study by Rioux *et al.* (1969). They found amastigote forms of *L. tarentolae* in the peripheral blood of geckoes caught in the district of Banyuls-sur-mer (P-O), Southern France; from 3 to 10 parasites were seen within individual monocytes and others were extracellular.

B. TRANSMISSION AND VECTOR

The problem of transmission has been reviewed by Adler and Theodor (1957). The possibility of transovarial transmission was excluded by Belova (1971) as the result of an experiment in which leishmanial infection could not be detected in young *Gymnodactylus caspius* bred from the eggs of females known to be naturally infected with promastigotes. It is now generally accepted that infection of the phlebotomine host follows the ingestion of a blood meal, that multiplication of lizard *Leishmania* occurs within this host and that the promastigotes develop typically (Hertig *et al.*, 1969), but not always (Adler, 1964), at the posterior station in the hindgut of the sandfly. Furthermore, such posterior development suggests that transmission to the saurian host is by ingestion of an infected sandfly.

The behaviour of lizard *Leishmania* within the sandfly and the ability of the latter to feed on saurian hosts are of major relevance to the problem of transmission, which has been poorly studied. Lainson *et al.* (1977) were unable to establish *L. hoogstraali* (isolated in 1965 and maintained in blood agar medium) in *Lutzomyia longipalpis*; they suggested that either the parasites had lost their infectivity to the phlebotomine host or that the sandfly environment was unfavourable. David (1929) and Adler and Theodor (1929) found, respectively, that *L. agamae* and *L. ceramodactyli* adopted a posterior position in the sandfly *Phlebotomus papatasi*. In 1935 conflicting evidence was provided by Adler who recorded the development of an experimental infection of *L. tarentolae* at the anterior station in *S. minuta*, whereas Parrot (1935) recorded the development of the same parasite at the posterior station of *S. minuta minuta*. However, Heisch (1958) described a new parasite, *L. adleri*, from the blood of *Latastia longicaudata* from Kenya and presented evidence that the natural vector of this parasite was *S. clydei* in which the promastigotes developed at the anterior station. It thus became clear that the position of the promastigotes in the invertebrate host does not provide a certain clue as to the vertebrate host. On the other hand, evidence of the anterior development of a saurian *Leishmania* does indicate the possibility of transmission to the lizard by the bite of an infected fly.

The first report of the ability of sandflies to feed on reptiles was that of Simic (1930) in Yugoslavia. Petrisceva (1949), as cited by Belova (1971), observed female *P. papatasi* and sandflies of the genus *Sergentomyia* sucking blood from geckoes. Minter and Wijers (1963) stated that both *S. clydei* and *S. schwetzi* fed mainly on the blood of reptiles and the former observation was confirmed by Dr. B. McMillan during studies in the Malakal area of the Sudan (Hoogstraal and Heyneman, 1969). Nadim *et al.* (1968) and Seyedi-Rashti *et al.* (1971) have presented evidence to show that *S. sintoni* is probably the vector of a lizard parasite in the Iranian Turkmen Sahara. In France, Reynal (1954) found that *S. minuta* was feeding only on snakes and lizards (cf. Rioux *et al.*, 1969). Belova (1971) provided experimental evidence to show that three species of sandfly *P. papatasi*, *P. caucasicus* and *S. sintoni* (formerly *S. arpaklensis*) were all able to feed on the lizards *Agama sanguinolenta* and *Gymnodactylus caspius*.

IV. Relationship of lizard and mammalian leishmanias

A. SUSCEPTIBILITY OF LIZARDS TO PROMASTIGOTES OF *LEISHMANIA* SPECIES

It has been shown that under natural conditions *Leishmania*-infected lizards do live in close association with sandflies and rodents and that certain sandfly species are both saurian and mammalian (including man) biters. However, in order to determine the epidemiological importance of reptilian promastigotes and their possible relationship to the leishmaniae of man, it is necessary to investigate the susceptibility of lizards to promastigotes of different origin and, conversely that of mammalian hosts to lizard leishmanias.

Kandelaki (1939) reported successful infection of seven *Agama caucasica* in Georgian SSR with strains isolated from cases of visceral leishmaniasis. Khodukin and Sofiev (1940) obtained negative results in *Gymnodactylus caspius* inoculated with strains of *Leishmania* isolated from lizards and a dog.

During the period 1963–1966, Belova (1971) sought to clarify the relationship of reptilian *Leishmania* species to those of man by investigating the susceptibility of lizards to promastigote cultures of different origin. She carried out inoculation experiments with fourteen species of lizard;

cultures of the causative agent of zoonotic cutaneous leishmaniasis isolated from humans and gerbils, of human and canine visceral leishmaniasis and promastigotes of sandfly (*P. caucasicus*) and reptilian (*A. sanguinolenta, G. caspius, Phyrynocephalis interscapularis, Eremias intermedia* and *E. velox*) origin were used. Positive results were obtained from inoculation with the reptilian strains in only five of the lizard hosts, with visceral strains in four genera of lizards and with sandfly strains in only *G. caspius* (Table 3). These experimental infections of lizards by *Leishmania* species from warm-blooded animals were considered proof of a genetic affinity between reptilian and mammalian species of *Leishmania*.

Table 3. The susceptibility of 14 lizard species to promastigote cultures of different origin.[a]

Species of lizard	Isolated positive infections with promastigote cultures		
	Reptilian strains	Visceral leishmaniasis strains	Sandfly strains
Agama sanguinolenta	+	+	—
Gymnodactylus caspius	+	+	+
Phrynocephalus interscapularis	—	+	—
Eremias intermedia	+	+	—
E. velox	+	—	N.T.
E. lineolata	+	—	—
P. mystaceus	—	—	—
A. caucasica	—	—	N.T.
Tetrascincus scincus	—	—	N.T.
E. guttulata	N.T.	N.T.	—
E. grammica	—	N.T.	N.T.
Mabuya aurata	N.T.	—	N.T.
Eumeces schneideri	N.T.	N.T.	—
Varanus griseus	N.T.	N.T.	N.T.

[a] Adapted from Belova (1971). N.T. = not tested.

Mohiuddin (1959) studied the behaviour of 9-day cultures of *L. adleri* in four species of lizards (*Mabuya striata,** A. mutabilis, Lacerta viridis* and *Acanthodactylus boskianus asper*) some of which came from a different geographic region to that of the parasite's East African host. He showed that the first three species could be infected only by intracardiac inoculation; the infections were occult and could be demonstrated only by the culture of heart blood from the lizard for up to two months post-inoculation. Cultures of recently isolated mammalian strains of *L. donovani* and *L. tropica* failed to infect these lizards; the latter observation

* It is of interest to note that McMillan (1965) did not recover a single strain of *Leishmania* from the culture of cardiac blood from 350 specimens of the skink, *M. striata* in the Upper Nile province of the Sudan.

is of some significance when related to the suggestion of earlier workers (Laveran, 1915) that the gecko, *Tarentola mauritanica*, was a host of *L. tropica* in North Africa.

The work of Medina (1966, 1968) in Venezuela supported the findings and conclusions of Belova (1971); he was able to infect seven species of saurians with each of the four species of mammalian leishmania: *L. braziliensis braziliensis*, *L. m. pifanoi*, *L. m. mexicana* and *L. tropica*. The lizards were inoculated intraperitoneally and became infected from 4–63 days post-inoculation, in the following order of decreasing susceptibility: *Cnemidophorus lemniscatus*, *Thecadactylus rapicauda*, *Ameiva ameiva*, *Polychrus marmoratus*, *Tupinambis nigropinctatus*, *Iguana iguana*, *Tropidoactylus onca*. In some hosts there was a high percentage of hepato-splenic involvement and occasionally myocardial invasion was detected; the majority of lizards developed visceral amastigote infections and the subsequent intraperitoneal inoculation of this material into hamsters produced an almost 100% infection of the viscera from 10–39 days post-inoculation. However, in those lizards in which amastigote infection of the liver could not be demonstrated microscopically, the inoculation of the saurian liver tissues into hamsters produced positive visceral infections in 65% of the animals and demonstrated the presence of cryptic infections in the reptilian hosts. *Hemidactylus* sp. could not be infected with any of the mammalian species of *Leishmania*, and in *Gonatodes vittatus* and *Mabuya mabouya* hepato-splenic infections could be obtained only with *L. m. pifanoi* and *L. m. mexicana*.

Dollahon and Janovy (1973) described the *in vitro* phagocytosis of *L. adleri* promastigotes by iguanid lizard (*Dipsosaurus dorsalis*) leucocytes and peritoneal exudate cells. This interaction was observed using wet mount preparations, and found to be remarkably similar to that of mammalian leishmanias with mammalian macrophage cultures (Miller and Twohy, 1967; Akiyama and Haight, 1971) under similar *in vitro* conditions. Similar cell cultures prepared from *Basilicus vittatus* were also inoculated with *L. adleri* promastigotes; intracellular amastigotes were observed for up to 36 h at 25° and 35°C.

B. SUSCEPTIBILITY OF MAMMALS TO LIZARD LEISHMANIAE

Young and Hertig (1927) produced visceral, followed by cutaneous, lesions in the chinese hamster (*Cricetus griseus*) as a result of inoculating, intraperitoneally, promastigotes of the gecko parasite, *L. tarentolae*. In recent years, Manson-Bahr and Heisch (1961) obtained transient infections in man by inoculating five-day promastigote cultures of *L. adleri* (grown on NNN) into four volunteers. Three of the volunteers developed small skin nodules at the site of infection and amastigotes were demonstrated in smears made from them for up to five days after inoculation. A positive culture of *L. adleri* was obtained from one nodule after seven days; subsequently the nodule faded rapidly and had disappeared after one month.

During the period 1963–1966, Belova (1971) carried out experiments to determine whether a variety of mammals (white mice, golden hamsters and red-tailed gerbils) were susceptible to seven promastigote reptilian strains isolated from *G. caspius*, *Agama sanguinolenta*, *Phrynocephalus interscapularis*, *E. intermedia*, *E. velox* and *E. guttulata guttulata* in the Turkmenian SSR. Subcutaneous and intraperitoneal inoculations were made and the experimental animals were observed for from two to three and a half months. The results were negative in all cases, but supported the work of the previous Russian workers Khodukin and Sofiev (1940), who obtained negative results following the inoculation of promastigote cultures from three central Asian species of lizard into human volunteers, monkeys, hamsters and white mice; and also that of Krjukova (1941), as cited by Belova (1971), who studied the pathogenicity of a strain from *G. caspius* in gerbils, mice and human volunteers.

However, Adler (1962a) using a culture of *L. adleri* shortly after isolation, inoculated adult and baby hamsters and baby mice and obtained transient infections; in hamsters the infection was always cryptic and splenic infections, lasting up to five weeks, were detected only on culture whereas in mice inoculated during their suckling period, amastigotes could be detected in stained smears for a period of ten days after which the infection became cryptic and was demonstrated, in cultures of dermis only, for up to five weeks after inoculation.

Confirmation of the transformation of lizard promastigotes to amastigotes in the skin of mammals, other than humans, has been histologically demonstrated by Gleyberman (Belova, 1971). Intradermal inoculation of *Leishmania* promastigotes from *G. caspius* produced similar results in both gerbils and white mice; the experimental gerbils were killed at 2–4 h, 24–27 h, 2–4 days and 5–7 days post-inoculation and portions of skin processed for the examination of histological changes. Promastigotes became intracellular amastigotes at 2–4 h post-inoculation; this was accompanied by moderate infiltration, oedema and loosening of the dermis. Within 24 h both typical amastigotes and degenerating parasite forms showing pycnotic nuclei were present. The parasites did not survive for more than 4 days, when only chromatic granules from disintegrating parasites were observed. The inflammatory reaction gradually disappeared. These interesting results of both Adler (1962a) and the Russian workers (Belova, 1971) provide further evidence of a certain affinity between reptilian promastigotes and mammalian leishmaniae.

Scheiber (1972) examined the *in vitro* interaction of hamster peri-

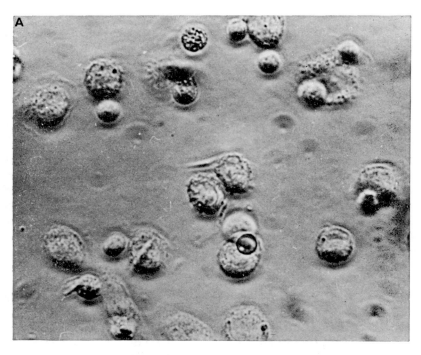

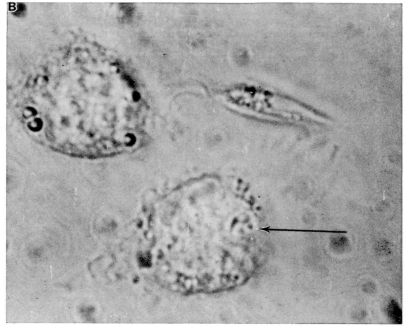

toneal macrophages (maintained at 28° and 37°C) and promastigotes of *L. adleri* by phase contrast microscopy and Giemsa-stained monolayer preparations; he showed that the parasites were readily engulfed by the mammalian macrophages. The infected macrophage monolayer was observed at 15, 30, 60, 120 min and at 14, 24, 48, 60 and 72 h. Approximately 46% of the promastigotes were attached to cells, by either the flagellum or the body, within 15 min of the initial inoculation; at 30 min a few intracellular amastigote forms were seen and 50% of the cells contained engulfed parasites whilst the remaining promastigotes were "rounding off" (Figs 2 and 3). At 14–48 h, although 65% of the macrophages were parasitized, it appeared that at least 50% of these were degenerating. This was the first time that the *in vitro* intracellular transformation of lizard *Leishmania* promastigotes had been demonstrated in mammalian cells and is in agreement with the *in vivo* observations of Gleyberman (Belova, 1971) and Manson-Bahr and Heisch (1961).

V. Leishmanias of lizards and human leishmaniasis

The identification of *Leishmania* species, particularly those which originate from areas where two or more species are present, has until recently been difficult. In the past, a number of biological methods have been used: morphology, cultural characteristics, response of the vertebrate host to natural or experimental infections, the behaviour of the parasite in natural or experimental invertebrate infections, drug sensitivity and serological reactions. These characteristics were combined to form a useful and comprehensive trinomial classification of *Leishmania* species (Lainson and Shaw, 1972). The most important of these methods are serology, vertebrate host response and, with the recent establishment of closed laboratory colonies of *Lu. longipalpis* (Killick-Kendrick *et al.*, 1973) and refined biochemical techniques (Chance *et al.*, 1977), the behaviour of the parasite within the invertebrate host and characteristic biochemical features.

A. SEROLOGY

Studies on the serological reactions of lizard leishmanias and their antigenic relationships with human species of *Leishmania* are few; however,

---

FIG. 2. Behaviour of promastigotes of *Leishmania adleri* inoculated into tissue cultures of hamster peritoneal exudate macrophages, as shown by phase-contrast microscopy. (A) 10 min after inoculation showing promastigotes adhering to macrophages. (B) 30 min after inoculation showing a promastigote attached to a macrophage by its flagellum, and an amastigote (arrowed) within a macrophage. (Photographs by courtesy of Dr P. Scheiber).

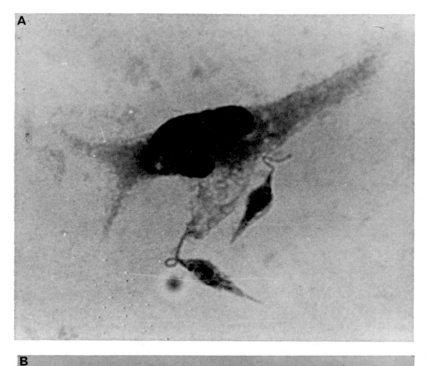

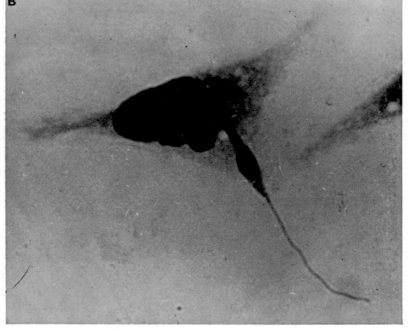

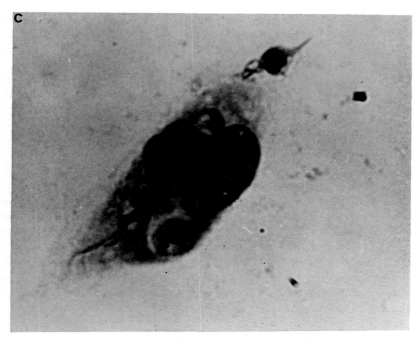

evidence for their serological distinctness from but nevertheless close relationship to, certain human leishmanias has been demonstrated (Aliev *et al.*, 1972; Saf'janova, 1966; Adler, 1964; McMillan, 1965).

Adler (1962a, b, 1964) found that *L. adleri* showed common antigens with *L. donovani*, *L. infantum*, *L. braziliensis* and *L. tropica*. He also showed (McMillan, 1965) that *L. hoogstraali* shared agglutinating antigens with Sudanese, Kenyan and Indian strains of *L. donovani*, *L. infantum*, *L. braziliensis*, *L. mexicana* and *L. adleri*, but was more closely (largest number of common antigens) related to the latter than any other species. However, the antigenic titres of the two lizard species were different, and considerably so in the case of flagellar (as opposed to non-flagellar) antigens.

These antigenic relationships provide further evidence to support the hypothesis that *L. adleri* and probably *L. hoogstraali* and *L. tarentolae*

FIG. 3. Behaviour of promastigotes of *Leishmania adleri* inoculated into monolayer cultures of hamster macrophages on cover-slips, after fixation and staining with Giemsa. (A) 15 min after inoculation showing two promastigotes attached to macrophage. (B) 15 min after inoculation showing promastigote being engulfed by macrophage. (C) 2 h after inoculation, showing a dividing rounded promastigote outside the macrophage, a dividing promastigote within the macrophage, and two amastigotes within the macrophage, with vacuoles forming around them. (Photographs by courtesy of Dr P. Scheiber.)

represent transitional stages in the evolution of *Leishmania* from a purely reptilian to a mammalian parasite.

B. CROSS IMMUNITY BETWEEN THE LEISHMANIAS OF LIZARDS AND MAN

Cross reactivity between different species of *Leishmania* in the vertebrate host has been studied extensively during the past 70 years. For example, as early as 1910, Nicolle and Manceaux demonstrated that in the dog, a cured infection with *L. donovani* protected against subsequent infection with *L. tropica*, whereas dogs cured of *L. tropica* infections were susceptible to infection with *L. donovani*. Since then, numerous attempts have been made to demonstrate cross immunity between human species of *Leishmania*, both in man and in experimental animals. The subject has been fully reviewed, with valuable reference lists, by Adler (1963, 1964), Manson-Bahr (1963a, b), and by Preston and Dumonde (1976).

Cross reactivity in man between lizard and human species of *Leishmania* was first demonstrated by Latyshev and Kryukova (1953). These workers inoculated seven human volunteers subcutaneously with cultures of the gecko flagellate *L. gymnodactyli*; one of the volunteers had been experimentally infected twice in the skin and once intraperitoneally with *L. tropica*, two of the volunteers had recovered from naturally acquired oriental sores; four of the volunteers had never had leishmanial infections. Allergic reactions at the site of infection occurred in the three subjects who had recovered from leishmaniasis, whereas no reactions were produced in the four control subjects. Latyshev and Kryukova concluded that their experiments pointed to the existence of common antigens in *L. tropica* and *L. gymnodactyli*.

Heisch (1958) discovered a new species of lizard *Leishmania* in Kenya, and the parasite *L. adleri* subsequently proved a valuable tool in studying the relationships between human and lizard leishmaniae.

Southgate and Oriedo (1967) found that many people living near a newly-established focus of kala-azar in the Voo location of Kitui district in Kenya had positive leishmanin skin tests although they had never had kala-azar, nor vaccination against it. Southgate and Manson-Bahr (1967) showed that these people were immune to the intradermal and subcutaneous inoculation of cultures of rodent strains of *L. donovani*. It was suggested that their immunity might have resulted from natural skin infections with *L. adleri* caused by the bites of sandflies which normally feed on lizards.

The first suggestion that repeated natural inocula of heterologous non-human species of *Leishmania* could lead to immunity to the specific parasites of man appears to have been made by Berberian (1959), who included lizards in his list of vertebrate hosts of *Leishmania* which could be responsible for this naturally acquired immunity. Manson-Bahr and Southgate (1964) reported that two individuals who had recovered from a transient skin infection with *L. adleri* had positive leishmanin tests two years later, and this observation led Southgate (1967) to carry out more detailed investigations into cross immunity between *L. adleri* and *L. donovani* in man, and into the possible significance of naturally-transmitted *L. adleri* in the epidemiology of human kala-azar in Kenya.

Two of the volunteers inoculated with *L. adleri* two years previously by Manson-Bahr and Heisch (1961) were traced. One of them had yielded a culture from his nodule seven days after inoculation; both of them had shown scanty amastigotes in smears from their nodules, 48 h and 5 days after inoculation. They were given a thorough medical examination and found to be completely healthy; both of them stated that they had been well since the inoculation. They were skin-tested with the following leishmanial and allied antigens: (i) leishmanin made (in the Medical Research Laboratory, Nairobi) from *L. donovani* gerbil strain; Heisch *et al.*, 1959), *L. donovani* (human strain) and *L. adleri*; (ii) Pessoa-type antigen, prepared from *L. braziliensis*, supplied by Professor P. C. C. Garnham, London School of Hygiene and Tropical Medicine; (iii) antigenic fluid prepared from *L. enriettii*, *L. tarentolae* and *Strigomonas oncopelti* by Dr. R. A. Neal, Wellcome Research Laboratories, Beckenham. The method of preparing these antigens and the technique and significance of skin tests were discussed by Manson-Bahr (1961a, b).

Secondly, these two individuals were inoculated intradermally and subcutaneously in their left forearms with five-day cultures of *L. adleri* and seven-day cultures of the ground-squirrel strain of *L. donovani* (Heisch, 1957), both grown at room temperatures on NNN medium. 10^8 flagellates of *L. adleri* were inoculated, and 10^7 of ground squirrel *L. donovani*. The lesions produced were examined one week, two weeks, four weeks and eight weeks after the inoculations. At each examination a smear was made, stained with Leishman's stain and examined for amastigotes; at the same time, fluid aspirated from the lesions was inoculated on to tubes of NNN medium.

Thirdly, three leishmanin-positive volunteers of the Wakamba tribe were inoculated with five-day cultures of *L. adleri*, and the lesions studied in the manner described above. These three persons had acquired their positive leishmanin reactions in different ways: (i) a male aged 45 years from the Voo location of Kitui district was found to be naturally leishmanin-positive, during a medical survey (Southgate and Oriedo, 1967). He had never had kala-azar nor had he been artificially immunized; (ii) a male aged 20 years from the Tseikuru location of Kitui district had had proved kala-azar, which was treated and cured, three years before the study was carried out; (iii) a male aged 19 years from

Kitui was artificially immunized with the ground-squirrel strain of *L. donovani* three years previously, during an experimental vaccination trial (Manson-Bahr and Southgate, 1964).

The results of these experiments are shown in Tables 4, 5 and 6. The results given in Table 4 show that inoculation of leishmanin-negative subjects with cultures of *L. adleri* caused the development of positive leishmanin tests; the greatest reactions occurred with antigens prepared from human and rodent strains of *L. donovani* and from *L. adleri*. The exact epidemiological significance of the leishmanin reaction is not yet fully understood, but there is evidence that it is associated with immunity to experimental inoculations of *L. donovani* (Manson-Bahr, 1959, 1961b; Southgate and Manson-Bahr, 1967) and possibly to natural infection with kala-azar (Southgate and Oriedo, 1967).

Table 5 shows that two years after inoculation with *L. adleri*, two previously susceptible individuals developed Arthus reactions after further inoculations with *L. adleri* and with the ground-squirrel strain of *L. donovani*. The significance of the Arthus reaction in experimental leishmanial infections was discussed by Southgate and Manson-Bahr (1967) and it was concluded that it denoted some degree of immunity to the challenging antigen.

Table 6 shows that a subject with a naturally-acquired positive leishmanin reaction, a patient cured of kala-azar, and an artificially immunized individual, were all immune to challenge with cultures of *L. adleri*.

These results indicated that there was a considerable degree of cross-immunity in humans between *L. adleri* and *L. donovani* (human, ground-squirrel and gerbil strains); there was evidence from leishmanin testing of some degree of cross-immunity between *L. adleri* and *L. braziliensis*, *L. enriettii*, *L. tarentolae* and *S. oncopelti*. The results were in agreement

Table 4. Results of skin testing two human volunteers previously infected with *L. adleri*

Antigen used	Skin reactions	
	Subject No. 1	Subject No. 2
L. donovani (gerbil strain)	+ + +	+ +
L. donovani (human strain)	+ + +	+ +
L. braziliensis	+ +	+
L. enriettii	+ +	+
L. tarentolae	+ + +	+ +
L. adleri	+ + +	+ +
S. oncopelti	+	—

Keys to symbols used: + + + 1·0 to 2·0 cm diameter; + + 0·5 to 1·0 cm diameter; + 0·25 to 0·5 cm diameter; — No reaction.

Table 5. Results of inoculating two human volunteers, previously infected with *L. adleri*, with promastigote cultures of *L. adleri* and *L. donovani*.

Parasite inoculated	Weeks after inoculation	Subject No. 1			Subject No. 2		
		Lesion	Smear	Culture	Lesion	Smear	Culture
L. adleri	1	Arthus reaction	—ve	—ve	Arthus reaction	—ve	—ve
	2	Arthus reaction	—ve	—ve	Arthus reaction	—ve	—ve
	4	Nodule	—ve	—ve	Nodule	—ve	—ve
	8	Nil	—ve	—ve	Nil	—ve	—ve
L. donovani (ground-squirrel strain)	1	Arthus reaction	—ve	—ve	Arthus reaction	—ve	—ve
	2	Arthus reaction	—ve	—ve	Nodule	—ve	—ve
	4	Nil	—ve	—ve	Nil	—ve	—ve
	8	Nil	—ve	—ve	Nil	—ve	—ve

Table 6. Results of inoculating three immune subjects with cultures of *L. adleri*

Subject	Weeks after inoculation	Lesion	Smear	Culture
Leishmanin positive	1	Arthus reaction	—ve	—ve
—naturally acquired	2	Arthus reaction	—ve	—ve
	4	Nil	—ve	—ve
	8	Nil	—ve	—ve
Cured case of kala-azar	1	Arthus reaction	—ve	—ve
	2	Nil	—ve	—ve
	4	Nil	—ve	—ve
	8	Nil	—ve	—ve
Artificially immunized	1	Arthus reaction	—ve	—ve
with *L. donovani*	2	Nil	—ve	—ve
(ground-squirrel strain)	4	Nil	—ve	—ve
	8	Nil	—ve	—ve

with the serological studies of Adler (1962a, b). It is particularly interesting that *L. tarentolae* and *L. adleri* appeared to have common antigens, since *L. tarentolae* produced visceral and cutaneous lesions in the Chinese hamster (Young and Hertig, 1927) and, like *L. adleri*, developed in the anterior station in the sandfly (Adler and Theodor, 1935). It may thus resemble *L. adleri* in representing a transition stage between reptilian and mammalian species of *Leishmania*.

McMillan (1965) reported that a new species of gecko *Leishmania*, *L. hoogstraali* from the Sudan had common antigens with *L. adleri*. Van Peenen and Dietlein (1963) have recorded the finding of unexplained positive leishmanin reactions in the same (Upper Nile) province of the Sudan. It is possible that these reactions have been produced by infection of humans with *L. hoogstraali*.

This study provided supporting evidence for the hypothesis (Southgate and Oriedo, 1967; Southgate and Manson-Bahr, 1967) that naturally-acquired positive leishmanin reactions in Kenya may result from transient infections with sandfly-transmitted *L. adleri* and that these reactions were associated with immunity to kala-azar. These reactions are thus another example of natural zooprophylaxis.

C. LIZARD *LEISHMANIA* AND HUMAN EPIDEMIOLOGY

Since these studies were performed a number of published reports have appeared from areas of endemic cutaneous leishmaniasis, as well as from areas of visceral leishmaniasis, indicating that leishmanin positivity rates are frequently much higher than the known rates of overt, recovered or cured human disease. Thus Lemma *et al.* (1969) found rates of leishmanin positivity in Ethiopia a little more than double the rates for combined active and healed cutaneous lesions, and suggested that the anomaly could be due to "subclinical infection, exposure to non-human *Leishmania* spp., or to some non-specific cause". A series of studies by Cahill and his co-workers (Cahill, 1965, 1971; Cahill *et al.*, 1965a, b, 1966, 1967) in the Sudan, Egypt, Turkey and Somalia have revealed essentially similar findings, as have studies by Imperato and Diakité (1969) and Imperato *et al.* (1970) in Mali.

However, whilst Cahill (1970) regards the heterologous immunity hypothesis as "important to all future studies of the immunity and, hopefully, control of visceral leishmaniasis", it is speculative at present to consider that natural infections of man with non-pathogenic lizard and rodent leishmanias occur often enough to invalidate the leishmanin skin test as an epidemiological tool in kala-azar surveys. Cahill (1970) believes that "subclinical, minimal and cured *L. donovani* infections are the rule rather than the exception in endemic kala-azar areas" and that these infections can explain the differences between observed leishmanin positivity rates and rates of known treated and cured kala-azar cases.

Recently Belova (1971) has written a detailed account of the possible influence of lizard *Leishmania* species on the epidemiology of human leishmaniasis in the Soviet Union, with a full list of references to the Russian literature. She concludes, however, that they play little or no rôle in influencing the distribution of human infections.

VI. Physiology and biochemistry

The metabolism of the lizard leishmanias has been poorly studied when compared with that of the mammalian species and the reader is referred to the review of the physiology and biochemistry of the genus *Leishmania* (Von Brand, 1966). More recent studies on the metabolism of the lizard leishmanias are few and, with one exception (Chance *et al.*, 1977), have employed the use of promastigote cultures of *L. tarentolae* only.

Trager (1969) showed that when cultured in a defined medium, the promastigotes of *L. tarentolae* require, in addition to folic acid, a growth factor in the form of an unconjugated pteridine (biopterin being more active for this parasite than neopterin). He stated that although the metabolic roles of unconjugated pteridine are not yet well-defined, it would appear that they are of importance as co-factors in hydroxylation of phenylalanine, tyrosine, tryptophan and sterols.

Krassner (1969) and Da Cruz and Krassner (1971) studied the sulphur metabolism of *L. tarentolae*. They reported that this parasite was able to grow in a medium free of organic sulphur. The continuous growth of one line, a variant of *L. tarentolae*, was obtained using inorganic ^{35}S-sodium sulphate as the only source of sulphur: the uptake and incorporation of significant amounts of this chemical indicated that the parasite is capable of assimilatory sulphate reduction. This is characteristic of many microorganisms, algae and higher plants, but does not usually take place in protozoan species or higher animals. Krassner and Flory (1971) showed that alanine and aspartate were not essential for the growth of *L. tarentolae*; previous studies on haemoflagellates have revealed that although they require ten essential exogenous amino acids they are also capable of forming other amino acids.

Simpson and Braly (1970) described an interesting investigation into the potential use of the synchronization of DNA synthesis in *L. tarentolae* for the study of certain aspects of mitochondrial biogenesis. They obtained sufficient synchronization of nuclear and kinetoplastic (K) DNA synthesis by hydroxyurea to enable further studies on the regulation of the synthesis of K-DNA.

Recently, exciting biochemical techniques, using enzyme electrophoresis and DNA buoyant density, have been developed to differentiate between species and strains of *Leishmania* (Chance *et al.*, 1974; Gardener *et al.*, 1974; Kilgour *et al.*, 1974).

Certain enzymes which can be used as electrophoretic markers have been found in lizard species. In 1968, Krassner found that promastigotes of *L. tarentolae* contain two types of malate dehydrogenase (MDH) which differ markedly in their physical and kinetic properties; MDH was used as the test enzyme because of its universal distribution and marked variation in animal evolution. Subsequently, Fair and Krassner (1971) found significant activities of ALAT and ASAT* in *L. tarentolae*. This confirmed the importance of a transaminase proline metabolism and the earlier prediction of a proline metabolic pathway requiring aminotransferases (Krassner, 1969).

In 1974, Kilgour *et al.* demonstrated species-characteristic variants of ALAT and ASAT in mammalian species of *Leishmania*; and in 1977, Chance *et al.* examined a number of mammalian and reptilian isolates of *Leishmania* for DNA buoyant density and MDH, isocitrate dehydrogenase (IDH), and glucose-6-phosphate dehydrogenase (G6PDH). They found that the lizard leishmaniae are distinct from mammalian species in terms of DNA buoyant density and, that although there is some similarity of MDH type, the distinction between them is confirmed by their different IDH and G6PDH types. They distinguished four groups of lizard leishmanias: two groups of *L. adleri* (Kenya strain), *L. hoogstraali* (Sudan strain) and *L. tarentolae* (Senegal strain). A fourth lizard parasite, *L. agamae* from the Middle East, has a unique nuclear-DNA buoyant density of 1·720 g/ml.

Undoubtedly, these biochemical methods for the identification and characterization of various species of *Leishmania* have enormous potential for the further clarification of the taxonomy of this group and especially in the epidemiology of lizard and mammalian leishmaniasis.

* ALAT = alanine aminotransferase; ASAT = aspartate aminotransferase.

VII. References

Adler, S. (1962a). The behaviour of a lizard *Leishmania* in hamsters and baby mice. *Revista do Instituto de Medicina Tropical de São Paulo*, **4**, 61–64.

Adler, S. (1962b). Approaches to research in leishmaniasis. *Scientific Reports of the Istituto Superiore di Sanità*, **2**, 143–150.

Adler, S. (1963). Immune phenomena in leishmaniasis. *In:* "Immunity to Protozoa". (P. C. C. Garnham, A. E. Pierce and I. Roitt, eds), Oxford, Blackwell, pp. 235–245.

Adler, S. (1964). *Leishmania. In:* "Advances in Parasitology" (B. Dawes, ed), Vol. 2, Academic Press, New York and London, pp. 35–96.

Adler, S. and Theodor, O. (1929). Observations on *Leishmania ceramodactyli* n sp. *Transactions of the Royal Society of Tropical Medicine and Hygiene*, **22**, 343–356.

Adler, S. and Theodor, O. (1935). Investigations on Mediterranean kala-azar. X. A note on *Trypanosoma platydactyli* and *Leishmania tarentolae*. *Proceedings of the Royal Society of London, Series B*, **116**, 543–544.

Adler, S. and Theodor, O. (1957). Transmission of disease agents by phlebotomine sandflies. *Annual Review of Entomology*, **2**, 203–226.

Akiyama, H. J. and Haight, R. D. (1971). Interaction of *Leishmania donovani* and hamster peritoneal macrophages—a phase microscopical study. *American Journal of Tropical Medicine and Hygiene*, **20**, 539–545.

Aliev, E. I., Saf'janova, V. M., Nadzhafov, H. Y. and Gasanzade, G. B. (1972). Comparative serological study of *Leishmania tropica major* and *Leishmania tropica minor*. *Meditsinskaya parazitologiya: parazitarnÿe bolezni (Moskva)*, **41**, 531–536.

Baker, J. R. (1965). The evolution of parasitic protozoa. *Symposium of the British Society for Parasitology*, **3**, 1–27.

Bayon, H. (1915). Herpetomonidae found in *Scotophaga hottentota* and *Chamaeleon pumilus*. *Transactions of the Royal Society of South Africa*, **5**, 61.

Belova, E. M. (1971). Reptiles and their importance in the epidemiology of leishmaniasis. *Bulletin of the World Health Organization*, **44**, 553–560.

Berberian, D. A. (1959). Relationship of Mediterranean kala-azar to canine kala-azar. *Transactions of the Royal Society of Tropical Medicine and Hygiene*, **53**, 364–365.

Cahill, K. M. (1965). Leishmanin skin testing in Africa and the Middle East. *East African Medical Journal*, **42**, 213–220.

Cahill, K. M. (1970). Field techniques in the diagnosis of kala-azar. *Transactions of the Royal Society of Tropical Medicine and Hygiene*, **64**, 107–110.

Cahill, K. M. (1971). Studies in Somalia. *Transactions of the Royal Society of Tropical Medicine and Hygiene*, **65**, 28–40.

Cahill, K. M., Anderson, G. R. and Türegün, M. (1965a). A leishmanin survey in south-east Turkey. *Bulletin of the World Health Organization*, **32**, 121–123.

Cahill, K. M., Omer, A. H. S. and El-Mubarak, A. R. (1965b). A leishmanin survey in Omdurman, Sudan. *Journal of Tropical Medicine and Hygiene*, **68**, 151–152.

Cahill, K. M., Kordy, M. I., Girgis, N., Atalla, W. and Mofti, A. (1966). Leishmaniasis in Egypt, U.A.R. *Transactions of the Royal Society of Tropical Medicine and Hygiene*, **60**, 79–82.

Cahill, K. M., Mazzoni, P. L. and Aden, H. (1967). A leishmanin survey in Giohar, Somalia. *Transactions of the Royal Society of Tropical Medicine and Hygiene*, **61**, 340–342.

Cameron, T. W. M. (1956). "Parasites and Parasitism", p. 30. London, Methuen and Co. Ltd., p. 30.

Chance, M. L., Peters, W. and Schory, L. (1974). Biochemical taxonomy of *Leishmania*. I. Observations on DNA. *Annals of Tropical Medicine and Parasitology*, **68**, 307–316.

Chance, M. L., Gardener, P. J. and Peters, W. (1977). Biochemical taxonomy of *Leishmania* as an ecological tool. *Colloques Internationaux de Centre National de la Recherche*, **239**, 53–62.

Da Cruz, F. S. and Krassner, S. M. (1971). Assimilatory sulphate reduction by the haemoflagellate *Leishmania tarentolae*. *Journal of Protozoology*, **18**, 718–722.

David, A. (1929a). Note préliminaire sur un *Leishmania* trouvé chez le lézard gris de la région de Tibériade (Basse-Galilée, Palestine). *Annales de Parasitologie Humaine et Comparée*, **7**, 190–192.

David, A. (1929b). Recherche expérimental sur un haematozaire du genre *Leishmania* (*L. agamae* A. David). Doctorate thesis, Faculty of Science, University of Paris. 54 pp.

Dollahon, N. R. and Janovy, J. (1973). *Leishmania adleri*: In vitro phagocytosis by lizard leucocytes and peritoneal exudate cells. *Experimental Parasitology*, **34**, 56–61.

Dollahon, N. R. and Janovy, J. (1974). Experimental infection of New World lizards with Old World lizard *Leishmania* sp. *Experimental Parasitology*, **36**, 253–260.

Edeson, J. F. B. and Himo, J. (1973). *Leishmania* sp. in the blood of a lizard (*Agama stellio*) from Lebanon. *Transactions of the Royal Society of Tropical Medicine and Hygiene*, **67**, 27.

Fair, D. S. and Krassner, S. M. (1971). Alanine aminotransferase and aspartate aminotransferase in *Leishmania tarentolae*. *Journal of Protozoology*, **18**, 441–444.

Fantham, H. B. (1926). Some parasitic Protozoa found in South Africa. IX. *South African Journal of Science*, **23**, 560.

Franchini, G. (1921). Sur les flagellés intestinaux du type *Herpetomonas* du *Chamaeleon vulgaris* et leur culture, et sur les flagellés du type *Herpetomonas* de *Chalcides* (*Gongylus*) *ocellatus* et *Tarentola mauritanica*. *Bulletin de la Société de Pathologie Exotique et de ses Filiales*, **14**, 641.

Gardener, P. J., Chance, M. L. and Peters, W. (1974). Biochemical taxonomy of *Leishmania*. II. Electrophoretic variation of malate dehydrogenase. *Annals of Tropical Medicine and Parasitology*, **68**, 317–325.

Garnham, P. C. C. (1971). The genus *Leishmania*. *Bulletin of the World Health Organization*, **44**, 477–489.

Heisch, R. B. (1957). The isolation of *Leishmania* from a ground-squirrel in Kenya. *East African Medical Journal*, **34**, 183.

Heisch, R. B. (1958). On *Leishmania adleri* (sp. nov.) from lacertid lizards (*Latastia* sp.) in Kenya. *Annals of Tropical Medicine and Parasitology*, **52**, 68–71.

Heisch, R. B., Grainger, W. E. and Harvey, A. E. C. (1959). The isolation of a *Leishmania* from gerbils in Kenya. *Journal of Tropical Medicine and Hygiene*, **62**, 158–159.

Hertig, M., Johnson, P. T. and McConnell, E. (1969). Growth pattern of leishmania in phlebotomine sandflies. *Science*, **165**, 1379–1380.

Hoare, C. A. (1948). The relationship of the haemoflagellates. *Proceedings of the Fourth International Congress of Tropical Medicine and Malaria*, **2**, 1110–1116.

Hoogstraal, H. and Heyneman, D. (1969). Leishmaniasis in the Sudan Republic. 30. Final epidemiologic report. *American Journal of Tropical Medicine and Hygiene*, **18**, 1091–1210.

Imperato, P. J. and Diakité, S. (1969). Leishmaniasis in the Republic of Mali. *Transactions of the Royal Society of Tropical Medicine and Hygiene*, **63**, 236–241.

Imperato, P. J., Coulibaly, B. and Togola, T. (1970). Leishmanin skin sensitivity in north western Mali. *Acta Tropica, Basel*, **27**, 260–265.

Kandelaki, S. P. (1939). Attempts at infecting Radde's hamster with leishmaniases. *In:* "Proceedings of the Third Transcaucasian Congress on the Control of Malaria and other Tropical Diseases", pp. 306–315. Tbilisi.

Khodukin, N. I. and Sofiev, M. S. (1940). Leishmaniae in some Central Asian lizards and their epidemiological significance. *Problemỹ Subtropičeskoj Patologii*, **4**, 218–228.

Kilgour, V., Gardener, P. J., Godfrey, D. G. and Peters, W. (1974). Demonstration of electrophoretic variation of two aminotransferases in *Leishmania*. *Annals of Tropical Medicine and Parasitology*, **68**, 245–246.

Killick-Kendrick, R., Leaney, A. J. and Ready, P. D. (1973). A laboratory culture of *Lutzomyia longipalpis*. *Transactions of the Royal Society of Tropical Medicine and Hygiene*, **67**, 434.

Krassner, S. M. (1968). Isoenzymes in the culture forms of *Leishmania tarentolae*. *Journal of Protozoology*, **15**, 523–528.

Krassner, S. M. (1969). Sulphur metabolism in *Leishmania*. Progress in Protozoology, Third International Congress of Protozoology, Leningrad. Amsterdam, Swets and Zeitlinger.

Krassner, S. M. (1969). Proline metabolism in *Leishmania tarentolae*. *Experimental Parasitology*, **24**, 348–363.

Krassner, S. M. and Flory, B. (1971). Essential amino acids in the culture of *Leishmania tarentolae*. *Journal of Parasitology*, **57**, 917–920.

Lainson, R. and Shaw, J. J. (1972). Leishmaniasis of the New World: Taxonomic problems. *British Medical Bulletin*, **28**, 44–48.

Lainson, R., Ward, R. D. and Shaw, J. J. (1977). *Leishmania* in phlebotomid sandflies. VI. Importance of hindgut development in distinguishing between parasites of the *Leishmania mexicana* and *L. braziliensis* complexes. *Proceedings of the Royal Society. Series B. Biological sciences*, **199**, 309–320.

Latyshev, N. I. and Kryukova, A. P. (1953). The genetic relationship between various species of *Leishmania*. Probl. reg. gen. exp. Parasitol. med. zool. Moscow, **8**, 211–215. (Abstract: *Tropical Disease Bulletin*, 1955, **52**, 22–23.)

Latyshev, N. I. and Pozyvaj, T. T. (1937). Experience in epidemiological investigations in places in Turkmenia where cutaneous leishmaniasis occurs. *In:* "Problemỹ Parazitologii i faunỹ Turkmenii", pp. 163–181.

Laveran, A. (1915). Des lacertiens peuvent-ils etre infectées par des *Leishmania?* *Bulletin de la Société de la Pathologie Exotique et de ses Filiales*, **8**, 104–109.

Lavier, G. (1943). L'évolution de la morphologie dans le genre *Trypanosoma*. *Annales de Parasitologie Humaine et Comparée*, **19**, 168–200.

Léger, M. (1918). Infection sanguine par *Leptomonas* chez un saurien. *Comptes Rendus des Séances de la Société de Biologie et de ses Filiales*, **81**, 772–774.

Lemma, A., Foster, W. A., Gemetchu, T., Preston, P. M., Bryceson, A. and Minter, D. M. (1969). Studies on leishmaniasis in Ethiopia. I. Preliminary investigations into the epidemiology of cutaneous leishmaniasis in the highlands. *Annals of Tropical Medicine and Parasitology*, **63**, 455–472.

Lewis, D. H. (1975). Ultrastructural study of *Leishmania* from reptiles. *Journal of Protozoology*, **22**, 344–352.

McMillan, B. (1965). Leishmaniasis in the Sudan Republic. 22. *Leishmania hoogstraali* sp. n. in the gecko. *Journal of Parasitology*, **51**, 336–339.

Mackie, F. P., Gupta, B. M. Das and Swaminath, C. S. (1923). Progress report on kala-azar. *Indian Journal of Medical Research*, **11**, 591–599.

Manson-Bahr, P. E. C. (1959). East African kala-azar with special reference to the pathology, prophylaxis and treatment. *Transactions of the Royal Society of Tropical Medicine and Hygiene*, **53**, 123–137.

Manson-Bahr, P. E. C. (1961a). The leishmanin test and immunity in kala-azar. *East African Medical Journal*, **38**, 165–167.

Manson-Bahr, P. E. C. (1961b). Immunity in kala-azar. *Transactions of the Royal Society of Tropical Medicine and Hygiene*, **55**, 550–555.

Manson-Bahr, P. E. C. (1963a). Active immunization in leishmaniasis. *In:* "Immunity to Protozoa" (P. C. C. Graham, A. E. Pierce and I. Roitt, eds), pp. 246–252. Oxford, Blackwell.

Manson-Bahr, P. E. C. (1963b). Immunity in the prophylaxis of protozoal diseases. *In:* "Clinical Aspects of Immunology" (P. G. H. Gell and R. R. A. Coombs, eds), pp. 759–774. Oxford, Blackwell.

Manson-Bahr, P. E. C. and Heisch, R. B. (1961). Transient infection of man with a *Leishmania* (*L. adleri*) of lizards. *Annals of Tropical Medicine and Parasitology*, **55**, 381–382.

Manson-Bahr, P. E. C. and Southgate, B. A. (1964). Recent research on kala-azar in East Africa. *Journal of Tropical Medicine and Hygiene*, **67**, 79–84.

Medina, R. (1966). Leishmaniasis experimental en animals silvestres. *Separata Dermatologia Venezolana*, **5**, 91–119.

Medina, R. (1968). Leishmaniasis experimental en reptiles. *In:* "Medicina Tropical" (A. Anselmi, ed.), pp. 133–141. Mexico, Editori Fournier.

Mesnil, F. (1918). (Review of a paper by C. Franca entitled "Quelques considérations sur la classification des hématozoaires"). *Bulletin de l'Institut Pasteur, Paris*, **16**, 536.

Miller, H. C. and Twohy, D. W. (1967). Infection of macrophages in culture by leptomonads of *L. donovani*. *Journal of Protozoology*, **14**, 781–789.

Minchin, E. A. (1908). Investigations on the development of trypanosomes in tsetse-flies and other Diptera. *Quarterly Journal of Microscopical Science*, **52**, 159–167.

Minchin, E. A. (1912). See Minchin, E. A. (1922).

Minchin, E. A. (1914). The development of trypanosomes in the invertebrate host. Section of a report by J. H. Ashworth entitled "Zoology at the British Association" in *Nature, London*, **94**, 405.

Minchin, E. A. (1922). An Introduction to the Study of Protozoa. London, Edward Arnold. 2nd impression (1st impression published 1912).

Minter, D. M. and Wijers, D. J. B. (1963). Studies on the vector of kala-azar in Kenya. IV. Experimental evidence. *Annals of Tropical Medicine and Parasitology*, **57**, 24–31.

Mohiuddin, A. (1959). The behaviour of *Leishmania adleri* in various lizards. *East African Medical Journal*, **36**, 171–176.

Nadim, A., Seyedi-Rashti, M. A. and Mesghali, A. (1968). On the nature of leptomonads found in *Sergentomyia sintoni* in Khorasson, Iran and their relation to lizard leishmanias. *Journal of Tropical Medicine and Hygiene*, **71**, 240.

Nicolle, C. and Manceaux, L. (1910). Recherches sur le bouton d'Orient. Cultures reproduction expérimentale, immunisation. *Annales de l'Institut Pasteur*, **24**, 673–720.

Parrot, L. (1935). L'évolution de *Leishmania tarentolae* Wenyon chez *Phlebotomus minutus* Rond. *Bulletin de la Société de Pathologie Exotique et de ses Filiales*, **27**, 839–843.

Popov, P. P. (1941). Cutaneous leishmaniasis in Azerbardzhan. *In:* "Problemy Koznogo Lejšmanioza, Ashkahabad", pp. 107–112.

Preston, P. M. and Dumonde, D. C. (1976). Immunology of clinical and experimental leishmaniasis. *In:* "Immunology of Parasitic Infections" (S. Cohen and E. H. Sadun, eds), pp. 167–202. Oxford, Blackwell.

Reynal, J. H. (1954). Les phlébotomes de France et leur distribution régionale. *Annales de Parasitologie Humaine et Comparée*, **29**, 297.

Rioux, J. A., Knoepfler, L. P. and Martini, A. (1969). Presence en France de *Leishmania tarentolae* Wenyon 1921 parasite du gecko *Tarentola mauritanica* (L. 1758). *Annales de Parasitologie Humaine et Comparée*, **44**, 115–116.

Saf'janova, V. M. (1966). Serological comparisons of leptomonad strains isolated from sandflies with *Leishmania tropica* and leptomonads from reptiles. *Meditsinskaya Parazitologiya i Parazitarnye Bolezni (Moskva)*, **35**, 686–695.

Scheiber, P. (1972). Studies on the relationships between reptilian and mammalian *Leishmania* species. M.Sc. dissertation (Medical Parasitology), University of London.

Sergent, Ed., Sergent, Et., Lemaire, G. and Severnet, G. L. (1914). Insecte transmetteur et réservoir de virus du clou de Biskra. Hypothèse et expériences préliminaires. *Bulletin de la Société de Pathologie Exotique et de ses Filiales*, **7**, 577–579.

Seyedi-Rashti, M. A., Nadim, A. and Naficy, A. (1971). Further report on lizard leishmaniasis in the Northern part of Iran. *Journal of Tropical Medicine and Hygiene*, **74**, 70–71.

Shortt, H. E. and Swaminath, C. S. (1928). Preliminary note on three species of Trypanosomidae. *Indian Journal of Medical Research*, **16**, 241–244.

Simič, T. (1930). Etude comparative de la biologie de *Phlebotomus perniciosus* et *P. paptasi* en Macédoine. *Annales de Parasitologie Humaine et Comparée*, **8**, 179–182.

Simpson, L. (1968). Behaviour of the kinetoplast of *L. tarentolae* upon cell rupture. *Journal of Protozoology*, **15**, 132–136.

Simpson, L. and Braly, P. (1970). Synchronization of *Leishmania tarentolae* by hydroxyurea. *Journal of Protozoology*, **17**, 511–517.

Southgate, B. A. (1967). Studies in the epidemiology of East African leishmaniasis. 5. *Leishmania adleri* and natural immunity. *Journal of Tropical Medicine and Hygiene*, **70**, 33–36.

Southgate, B. A. and Manson-Bahr, P. E. C. (1967). Studies in the epidemiology of East African leishmaniasis. 4. The significance of the positive leishmanin test. *Journal of Tropical Medicine and Hygiene*, **70**, 29–33.

Southgate, B. A. and Oriedo, B. V. E. (1967). Studies in the epidemiology of East African leishmaniasis. 3. Immunity as a determinant of geographical distribution. *Journal of Tropical Medicine and Hygiene*, **70**, 1–4.

Strong, R. P. (1924). Investigations upon flagellate infections. *American Journal of Tropical Medicine*, **4**, 345–385.

Trager, W. (1969). Pteridine requirement of the haemoflagellate *Leishmania tarentolae*. *Journal of Protozoology*, **16**, 372–375.

Trager, W. and Rudzinska, M. A. (1964). The riboflavin requirements and the effects of acriflavin on the fine structure of the kinetoplast of *Leishmania tarentolae*. *Journal of Protozoology*, **11**, 133–145.

Van Peenen, P. F. D. and Dietlien, D. R. (1963). Leishmaniasis in the Sudan Republic. 14. Leishmanin skin testing in Upper Nile Province. *Journal of Tropical Medicine and Hygiene*, **66**, 171–174.

Von Brand, T. (1966). The physiology of *Leishmania*. *Revista de Biologia Tropical*, **14**, 13–25.

Wenyon, C. M. (1921). Observations on the intestinal protozoa of three Egyptian lizards, with a note on a cell-invading fungus. *Parasitology*, **12**, 350–365.

Wenyon, C. M. (1926). Protozoology, Vol. 1, pp. 438–442. London, Baillière, Tindall and Cox.

Young, C. W. and Hertig, M. (1927). Peripheral lesions produced by *L. donovani* and allied leishmaniae. *Proceedings of the Society for Experimental Biology and Medicine, New York*, **25**, 196–197.

Zmeyev, G. Ja. (1936). Haemoparasite fauna of wild vertebrates in some southern areas of Tadzhikistan. *In:* "Trudy Tadzikskoj bazy AN USSR" (Transactions of the Tadzhik base of the Academy of Sciences of the USSR), **6**, 249–266.

6

Biology of the Trypanosomes and Trypanoplasms of Fish

JIŘÍ LOM

*Institute of Parasitology,
Czechoslovak Academy of Sciences, Prague*

I. Introduction 270

II. Cell structure 271
    A. *Trypanosoma* 271
    B. *Trypanoplasma* 275

III. Life cycle 279
    A. Transmission 279
    B. Vector phase of the life cycle 280
    C. Vertebrate phase of the life cycle 285
    D. Course of spontaneous infections in nature . . . 301

IV. *In vitro* culture 303
    A. *Trypanosoma* 303
    B. *Trypanoplasma* 306

V. Taxonomic considerations 307
    A. *Trypanosoma* 307
    B. *Trypanoplasma* 320

VI. Technique of investigation 325

VII. Conclusions 327

VIII. Acknowledgements 327

IX. References 328

I. Introduction

The rather vague term "piscine haemoflagellates" includes leech-transmitted kinetoplastids from the blood of a large variety of host species, which are united more by following a similar way of life in water rather than by forming a taxonomically homogeneous group. Fish trypanosomes occur in hagfish, in elasmobranchs (these are the largest in the genus—*Trypanosoma gargantua* or *T. gigantea* are far longer than 100 μm) and in bony fishes, each host group constituting a different class. Within the two latter groups, they invade hosts as different as sharks or skates, dipnoans, such as sturgeons, and teleosteans. Thus, regarding their hosts, they are a much more heterogeneous group than the trypanosomes of mammals; however, due to the common features in biology of their hosts and vectors, their divergence is not great.

Fish haemoflagellates have a long history of study. What Valentin (1841) found in the blood of trout may have been either a trypanosome or, more probably (Gauthier, 1920), a trypanoplasm; in the following year, Remak (1842) found what seems definitely to have been a trypanosome in the blood of the pike. Since then there is a long list of findings. In 1901, the genus *Trypanoplasma*, which was established by Laveran and Mesnil, entered the scene. The early records of fish blood flagellates are meticulously documented in the book of these French authors (1912 edition). The first great wave of interest in fish haemoflagellates coincided with the era in which the African trypanosomes were discovered to be the agents of fatal diseases of man and large mammals. Later the fish flagellates became less fashionable and interest dwindled so that only a few descriptive papers were published each several years. That is why our knowledge of their biology is very uneven, and why there have been practically no studies of their physiology, biochemistry and immunology. This may be partly due to the technical problems involved in keeping suitable fish for experimental purposes, but it is most regrettable. The study of fish kinetoplastids yields valuable insights into important problems in the study of pathogenic mammalian trypanosomes and into the phylogeny of the whole group; and it may finally solve the problem of the fish diseases which these flagellates cause—or may cause—in today's large-scale fish husbandry.

The only recent reviews of fish haemoflagellates are those by Becker (1970, 1977) which, unfortunately, are limited in extent since both reviews also deal with other types of fish parasites. The present review deals with the genera *Trypanosoma* and *Trypanoplasma*; the few findings of enigmatic monoflagellates (Becker and Holloway, 1968; Fantham and Porter, 1924) are not included.

II. Cell structure

A. *TRYPANOSOMA* GRUBY

The basic cell organization of fish trypanosomes resembles that of congeneric species—see Vickerman (1971, 1974, 1976) and also Vickerman and Preston (1976) in Volume 1 of this treatise. Special structures related to peculiarities in the biology, invasive processes and physiology of fish trypanosomes might be discovered by electron microscopy; however, in addition to observations by Preston (1969), Vickerman and Preston (1970) and Ranque (1973) on cultural forms of the skate species *T. rajae* and *T. boissoni*, respectively, there are the data of Lom *et al.* (1978) and Paulin *et al.* (1978) on *T. danilewskyi*. Most of the features of fish trypanosomes are identical with those of other, well-studied, trypanosomes; however, several structures are worth mentioning:

The *surface coat* on the surface of the bloodstream forms of *T. danilewskyi* (Figs 2, 3) is very thin and of the "fuzzy" type—similar to that existing in stercorarian rather than in salivarian trypanosomes (Vickerman, 1969). In the Thiéry PATSC-Ag method the silver is deposited throughout the membrane and in the substance of the surface coat. Numerous positively stained vesicles originate probably as pinocytotic coated vesicles in the flagellar pocket (Fig. 1).

A *cytostome* has been visualized in the culture forms of all three trypanosome species. Its mouth—permanently open and unable to constrict —is approximately level with the opening of the flagellar pocket (skate species) or shifted out of the pocket anterior to it on the surface of the body (*T. danilewskyi*; Fig. 1). Unlike the condition in the amphibian *T. mega* or in *T. conorhini*, the cytostome in carp trypanosomes leads into a long, tubular, unit-membrane-lined canal—the cytopharynx—surrounded by 5–8 microtubules and curving posteriorly for up to several microns. During cell division, the structure is retained by one and formed anew in the other daughter individual. The phagocytic function of the cytostome was proved by studying the route of ferritin uptake (Preston, 1969); the force propelling the nutrients into the canal is not known; it may be the flagellar beat.

In the bloodstream forms of *T. danilewskyi* there is also a well developed cytostome, slightly curving and terminating near the nucleus. Membrane-bound dense vesicles are found in juxtaposition to the cytopharyngeal tube (pinocytotic activity?) (Lom *et al.*, 1978).

A *contractile vacuole*, a feature of bodonids and "lower" trypanosomatids (see Vickerman, 1977), was noted near the flagellar pocket in the culture forms of *T. rajae*.

Kinetoplast-mitochondrion. The nucleoid is disc- or dish-shaped (Fig.

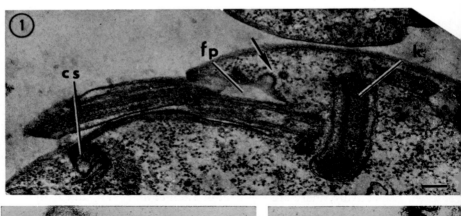

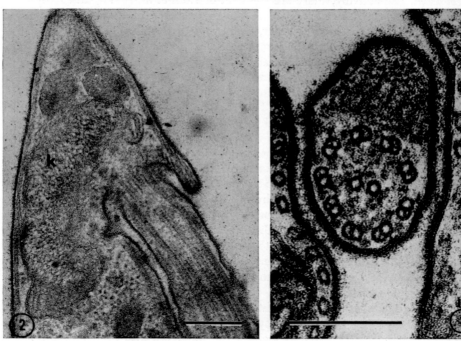

FIGS 1–3.   *Fig. 1*—*Trypanosoma danilewskyi*, cultural form; section through the flagellar pocket (fp) with (?endocytotic) vesicle formation at its walls (arrow). cs—transverse section through the mouth of the cytostomal aperture with surrounding microtubular armature. k = kinetoplast. *Fig. 2*—Longitudinal section through the posterior end of *T. danilewskyi*, bloodstream form: Thiéry (PATSC-Ag) reaction showing polysaccharides in the surface coat. *Fig. 3*—Transverse section through pellicle and flagellum of bloodstream form of *T. danilewskyi* showing the fuzzy surface coat without special staining. The flagellum belongs to the trypanosome body to the left. Scale represents 0·25 μm.

1). In the culture forms of the two skate species, and in both culture and bloodstream forms of *T. danilewskyi*, there are plate-like cristae.

Dyskinetoplasty. In fish trypanosomes, spontaneous occurrences of dyskinetoplastic forms have never been observed. However, preliminary results indicate that with certain strains at least, it is possible to obtain dyskinetoplastic mutants both in bloodstream and culture stages, by certain treatments.

In *T. danilewskyi* strain MA, a single dose of acriflavine (0·01 mg/g body weight administered before the peak of parasitaemia) produced up to 78% dyskinetoplastic trypomastigotes in the bloodstream of the goldfish and also a certain proportion (5%) of flagellates with the kinetoplast reduced in size. The affected populations failed to reproduce in the following syringe passage (Lom, unpublished observations).

In diphasic medium (SNB-9 at +25°C), acriflavin (0·05 mg/ml) induced dyskinetoplasty in 85% of the flagellates when applied in the logarithmic phase of growth of *T. danilewskyi* strain MS. Dyskinetoplastic mutants were able to grow in the presence of the drug for five consecutive passages; finally, the dyskinetoplastic forms amounted to 100%. The dyskinetoplastic forms also changed the general structure of their cells: the long, slender epimastigotes had a conspicuously elongated anterior part, the anterior free flagellum was absent and the undulating membrane was slightly developed. There was no cyclic alternation of epi- and hypermastigotes in dyskinetoplastic cultures, in contrast to untreated cultures (Nohýnková, 1977).

The capacity of dyskinetoplastic forms to grow *in vitro* has not been reported in any other trypanosome. It suggests—along with the observed resistance of these cultures to KCN—that in *T. danilewskyi* culture forms there may be extramitochondrial NADH oxidation, and that the supposedly respiratory granules in their cytoplasm probably endow the dyskinetoplastic forms with this capacity for *in vitro* growth.

The nucleus of *T. rajae* has served as a model for the study of the role of intranuclear microtubules during nuclear division (Vickerman and Preston, 1970). Two groups of these microtubules were described: those converging upon kinetochore-like plaques; and long, interpolar, microtubules occupying the isthmus between dividing nuclei.

Cytoplasmic inclusions. Vesicles with smaller dense bodies are commonly present in both bloodstream and culture forms. In *T. rajae* culture forms, digestive vacuoles with ingested ferritin are present, as well as multivesiculate bodies in the region of the Golgi apparatus.

Cytoplasmic granules are frequent if not universal in fish trypanosome cytoplasm; their conspicuous presence in Giemsa-stained preparations was even used as a differentiating feature in establishing some species (e.g., *T. granulosum*). In *T. danilewskyi* culture and bloodstream forms, microbodies are detectable at the ultrastructural level (Lom and Nohýn-

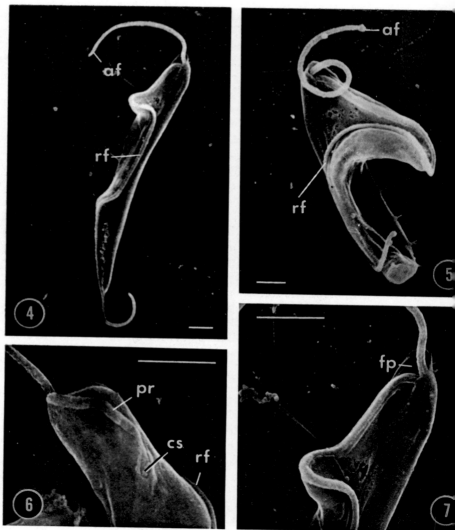

FIGS 4–7.   *Trypanoplasma borelli*, bloodstream phase syringe-passaged in gold-fish. Scanning electron micrograph. *Fig. 4*—Slender form with "slightly wound" undulating membrane. *Fig. 5*—Stout, much contorted form. *Fig. 6*—Ventral face showing preoral ridge (pr) and opening of the cytostome (cs). *Fig. 7*—Enlarged part of Fig. 4 to show apposition of the recurrent flagellum to the body border. af—anterior flagellum. rf—recurrent flagellum. fp—flagellar pocket. The lines equal 1 μm.

ková, unpublished observations). The NADH-oxidoreductase ("dia-
phorase") activity can be demonstrated at the light-microscope level in
numerous granules of various sizes (up to 60 per cell) in both bloodstream and culture forms (Fig. 27). This suggests that at least part of the
microbodies may constitute the extramitochondrial respiratory organelles
of the glycerophosphate oxidase system, as in salivarian trypanosomes
(Ryley, 1966; Bayne et al., 1969).

3. *TRYPANOPLASMA* LAVERAN AND MESNIL

Hardly any progress was made in the knowledge of the cell organization
of trypanoplasms from the time of Minchin (1909), Robertson (1911)
and Breindl (1915) until the first electron micrographs published by
Vickerman and Preston (1970). A detailed study (Lom and Nohýnková,
in press; Brugerolle et al., in press), now available, confirms the close
affinities of trypanoplasms to the *Bodo-Cryptobia* lineage.

The spindle-shaped body (see Figs. 4, 8) of most trypanoplasms,
rounded anteriorly and tapering to the hinder end, can be oriented
according to the location of the cytostome [contrary to Vickerman's
(1977) use in *Cryptobia vaginalis* of the recurrent flagellum to mark the
ventral side]. A crest-like preoral ridge (Figs. 6, 9) emerges from the
flagellar pocket and extends on the ventral surface; it ends in a small
opening—the cytostome—in about one third of the body length. Accordingly, the recurrent flagellum is attached to the body along its left
border (Fig. 7), which—as a largely outstretched fold of the cell—forms
with the flagellum a striking undulating membrane, much more developed than in trypanosomes or in any *Cryptobia* including *C. helicis*.
The outstretched fold extending along the recurrent flagellum delimits a
longitudinal, dorsolateral (left) concavity, detectable in most specimens
in spite of their sometimes incredibly contorted shape. This groove is the
only zone of the cell membrane devoid of and not subtended by longi-
tudinally running microtubules (Figs 8, 12). Similar belts of unsubtended
pellicle are found also in cryptobias and bodonids.

In bloodstream forms, the pellicle is covered by a surface coat of a
"fuzzy" type, up to 200 Å thick (Lom and Nohýnková, 1977a, b). The
Thiéry method reveals the presence of carbohydrates throughout the cell
membrane and in the surface coat, which latter has a granulo-filamentous
appearance (Figs 11, 12). This is at variance with previously reported
findings in trypanosomatids in which there are no records of polysaccharide being detected in both the cell membrane and the surface
coat (Wright and Hales, 1970; Steiger, 1973; Brooker, 1976). Within the
cytoplasm there was regularly a distinct reaction product in the cisternae
of the Golgi apparatus (Fig. 10); this material was similar to that occurring on the cell surface. The variety of positively stained vesicles in the

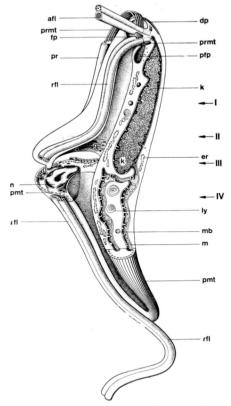

FIG. 8.   Diagram to show cell structure of *Trypanoplasma borelli* bloodstrea
form, as revealed by the electron microscope. Part of the cell is cut off laterally
show the continuity of the kinetoplast (k) with the mitochondrial ribbon (m
Another transverse cutout visualizes the nucleus (n) and the point of the plungir
of the preoral ridge (pr) below the level of the pellicle. At the apex of the cell, t
five microtubules of the preoral ridge (prmt) are laid free. afl—anterior flagellur
rfl—recurrent flagellum, dp—dense plate adhering to the three dorsal micr
tubules, fp—flagellar pocket, g—Golgi apparatus, ly—lysosomes, mb—micr
bodies, pmt—pellicular microtubules, er—endoplasmic reticulum, pfp—posteri
flagellar pocket, I, II, III, IV—levels of transverse sections in Fig. 9 (drawing l
Dr. E. Nohýnková).

cytoplasm may represent the pathway for the movement of cell co
material to the cell surface. No data are available regarding the surfa
coat in the vector and culture stages; if it is not present in these, it m:
well be that the coat of bloodstream forms is an adaptation to blo
parasitism, as it probably is in *Trypanosoma* (Vickerman and Presto
1976).

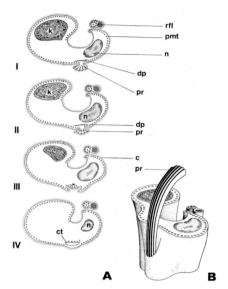

FIG. 9.   *Trypanoplasma borelli*. A: I to IV: diagrams of transverse sections, corresponding to the levels indicated in Fig. 8, to show various profiles of the preoral ridge: an elevated crest in I, it gradually submerges beneath the pellicle in II and III. In IV, a small cytostomal pit is demonstrated. B: Diagram of a section of the cell to show the preoral ridge plunging into the cytostomal cavity. c—cell coat, dp—dense plate beneath the preoral ridge (pr), ct = cytostome; for other abbreviations see Fig. 8 (drawing by Dr. E. Nohýnková).

Bodonid and cryptobiid kinship is well manifested in the fibrillar and membranous structures of *Trypanoplasma*.

The preoral ridge arises near the kinetosome of the recurrent flagellum as a ribbon of five microtubules closely associated with microfibrillar substance on the inner side of the flagellar pocket; it forms, at the opening of the pocket, an elevated crest comparable to the proboscis structure of *Rhynchomonas* (Swale, 1973), or to the rostrum in *Bodo* (Brooker, 1971; Burzell, 1975). The preoral ridge in *C. intestinalis* (Brugerolle *et al.*, in press) and in *C. vaginalis* (Vickerman, 1977) is closely similar; that of *C. helicis* (Brugerolle *et al.*, in press) almost identical.

The cytopharyngeal funnel, less conspicuous and shorter than in other genera, has the same orientation, although it is not reinforced by exactly the same variety of fibrillar structures, as, for example, in *Bodo caudatus*, *C. intestinalis* or *C. helicis* (Brugerolle *et al.*, in press).

The flagellar pocket continues posteriad below the kinetosome level into a postflagellar pocket, as in *C. vaginalis* for example (Vickerman, 1977).

The kinetoplast is single during the whole life cycle, unlike the condi-

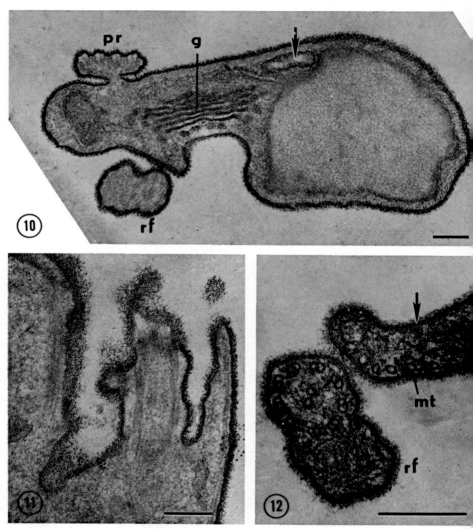

FIGS 10–12. *Trypanoplasma borelli*; bloodstream phase. *Fig. 10*—Transverse section, Thiéry reaction (PATSC-Ag) revealing the presence of polysaccharides on the cell surface, throughout the Golgi apparatus (G) and in cytoplasmic vesicles (arrow). *Fig. 11*—Longitudinal section through the flagellar pocket (Thiéry); the reaction product is deposited throughout the cell membrane and the cell coat. *Fig. 12*—Transverse section of the flagellum associated with the left body margin to form the undulating membrane; the fuzzy cell coat material is visible without special staining. mt—subpellicular microtubules; arrow points at the pellicular zone without microtubules. pr—preoral ridge; rf—recurrent flagellum. Scale represents 0·25 μm.

tion in some other bodonids (Brugerolle *et al.*, in press; Vickerman, 1977); the nucleoid is formed of a fine meshwork of isotropic, homogeneously distributed DNA fibres. The nucleoid extends to the membrane of the mitochondrial tube, which continues posteriorly as an irregularly-branched, continuous network (Fig. 8) containing plate-like cristae. The cytoplasm contains Golgi apparatuses (often in the form of peculiar concentric formations), small digestive vacuoles, and also autophagous vacuoles (vesicles with electron dense bodies), lipoid inclusions, cisternae of the endoplasmic reticulum (Fig. 8) and microbodies. Further research is needed to elucidate the true nature of various cytoplasmic granules, including "black pigment" (*T. guerneyi*; Brumpt, 1906b) and "light-breaking" granules (*T. valentini*; Gauthier, 1920; and *T. salmositica*, Becker and Katz, 1969).

III. Life cycle

A. TRANSMISSION

Leeches were suggested to be vectors for the transmission of fish haemo-flagellates by Doflein (1901), who knew of Leydig's old findings (1857) of flagellates in leeches of the genera *Piscicola* and *Pontobdella*. This suggestion was confirmed in the publications of Hofer (1904), Léger (1904b), Brumpt (1904, 1906a), Keysselitz (1906), Neumann (1909) and Robertson (1907, 1911). In the digestive tract of the leech, the flagellates undergo multiplicative development including a series of morpho-physiological changes; finally, they are transmitted into the fish host by inoculation during the feeding act. There is no evidence of infection taking place by the ingestion of an infected leech by the fish (for latest reference, see Khan, 1976) or of transovarial perpetuation of infection in leeches. Claims that, in crowded salmonid hatcheries, the fishes may become infected without the presence of leeches (Becker and Katz, 1965b, Wales and Wolf, 1955) have not been proven. *Hemiclepsis marginata* and *Piscicola geometra* are known to be vectors of European freshwater trypanosomes and trypanoplasms. *P. salmositica* and *Cystobranchus virginicus* transmit North American trypanoplasms. *Batrochobdella tricarinata* and *Hirudo nipponica* have been recognized as vectors of African and Chinese fish haemoflagellates, respectively. The marine leeches *Calobdella puncta-ta*, *C. vivida*, *Hirudo tractina*, *Platybdella soleae*, *P. muricata*, *P. scorpii*, *Trachelobdella lubricata*, *Branchellion torpedinis*, *Piscicola funduli* and *Johanssonia* sp. transmit marine fish haemoflagellates. To date, there is no evidence that parasitic crustacea (or any other animal) are vectors of piscine haemoflagellates.

B. THE VECTOR PHASE OF THE LIFE CYCLE

1. Development in the leech

Flagellate development has been studied in a few of the known vectors, but especially in the European *Piscicola geometra* and *Hemiclepsis marginata*, which both transmit indiscriminately various flagellate species. In the latter, the flagellates multiply to an incomparably higher number than they do in *Piscicola*; also they seem to persist for a much longer time. Brumpt (1906b) reported *T. granulosum* surviving as epimastigotes at 15°C for up to 9 months in a fasting *Hemiclepsis*. Also, Robertson (1911) reported the trypomastigotes persisting in the proboscis of *H. marginata* for as long as 61 days (without mentioning the temperature). Needham (1969a), however, disclaimed the existence of persistent stages in the leeches and reported the infection in *H. marginata* as lasting only 14 days at +20°C (20 days at +15°C). In *Piscicola geometra*, Brumpt's (1906b) data on trypanosome persistence in the stomach and anterior intestine coincide with those of the writer; the duration of infection of the leech never surpassed 15 days.

The leech becomes infective as soon as the metacyclic trypomastigote forms are produced (and migrate to the proboscis sheath) which takes from 3 (*Trypanosoma granulosum* in *H. marginata*) to 19 days (*Trypanoplasma salmositica* in *Piscicola salmositica*; Becker and Katz 1965b) in hosts in the temperate geographical zone. It is important to note that at some of the European localities, all *H. marginata* or *P. geometra* are infected; both species can transfer infection as young leeches after their first feeding.

Foremost among the many factors which affect the vector phase of development is the ambient temperature. *Trypanosoma murmanensis*, a marine species, takes up to 62 days to complete the cycle within the leech vector *Johanssonia* sp. at 0–2°C in the cold waters of northern Atlantic; when kept at +4–6°C, the cycle takes "only" 42 days (Khan, 1976). The epimastigotes persisted no longer than 90 days in the intestine.

The only worker who studied the preferences of fish haemoflagellates for vector species, or for parts of the vector digestive tract, was Brumpt (1906b). In freshwater trypanoplasms, he found that *T. abramidis* and the flagellate from loaches develop only in *H. marginata*, while *T. guernei*, *T. barbi* and *T. borelli* develop only in *P. geometra*. He also divided trypanosomes from freshwater fish into three groups. In the first group (*Trypanosoma barbi*, *T. percae*, *T. acerinae*, *T. squalii*) the organisms develop only in the stomach (transformation into epimastigotes and then into metacyclic trypanosomes) from whence they are inoculated directly into the blood of the fish. The second group (*T.

granulosum) start to grow as epimastigotes in the leech's stomach, whence the organisms proceed into the anterior digestive part of the intestine; then the flagellates return to the stomach, change into metacyclic trypomastigotes and reach the proboscis sheath; there they await the leech's feeding and inoculation into the blood of the fish host. Trypanosomes of the third group (*T. danilewskyi*, *T. phoxini*) transform in the stomach into epimastigotes, multiply, change into metacyclic trypomastigotes and then invade the proboscis sheath. Among the trypanosomes from osteichthyan marine fish, *T. soleae* and *T. cotti* develop only in the stomach of *Calobdella punctata*; they have not been found in the proboscis sheath. On the other hand, the skate species, *T. scylli* and *T. rajae*, invade also the anterior intestine.

In *H. marginata*, capable of harbouring trypanosomes for a long period, all trypomastigote stages are washed out from the proboscis at each new feeding act. However, a population of sphaeromastigote and epimastigote forms persists in the stomach and this starts a new period of proliferation in the freshly-ingested blood.

Re-examination of these statements, and a detailed study of vector capabilities are most urgently needed.

2. Sequence of stages in the leech

(a) *Trypanosoma*. Ingestion of the trypanosomes in fish blood, by the leech, triggers a series of morpho-physiological changes manifested by a sequence of amastigote, sphaeromastigote, epimastigote and trypomastigote forms, including, possibly (Tanabe, 1924; Baker, 1960; Becker, 1977), promastigotes. It is not known if the vector phase of development can be started indiscriminately by any, or just by some, of the bloodstream forms (young or adult ones in pleomorphic species). Different trypanosome species may differ in the relative abundance (or absence of some) of the above listed forms in the morphological forms in which the main proliferation occurs, and in the presence or frequency of proliferation by multiple division.

In trypanosomes from marine fish—as opposed to freshwater species— a mass of dividing amastigotes (seen already by Brumpt in 1906b in *T. cotti*, *T. soleae*, *T. scylli* and *T. rajae*)—seems to be characteristic for the initial phase of the leech part of the cycle (Fig. 13, A to C). It is not certain if the amastigotes just lack an external flagellum or if they are also devoid of any intracellular axoneme. In *T. rajae*, developing in *Pontobdella muricata* (Robertson, 1907, 1919), there follow actively dividing sphaeromastigote and later epimastigote forms, and six days after feeding there is in the stomach and anterior intestine a series of various intermediate forms leading up to trypomastigotes, which also are able to divide. This is a long lasting phase ending with long slender trypomastigotes returning to the stomach and, finally, to the proboscis. Mutliple

fission seems to be quite common in the sphaeromastigote and epimastigote forms. Neumann (1909), in *T. giganteum* and *T. variabile,* found the
main divisional forms in the same leech species to be sphaeromastigotes.
The extremely slow development of *T. murmanensis* in *Johanssonia* sp.
from the cold Newfoundland waters (taking up to 60 days!) permitted
Khan (1976) to follow the exact time distribution of the individual forms.

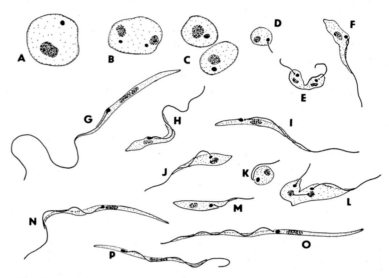

FIG. 13.   Stages of trypanosome development in the leech. A–I, *Trypanosoma
murmanensis*: A, B, C—amastigotes and their division; D—sphaeromastigote;
E—division giving rise to epimastigotes; F—epimastigote; G, H—slender epimastigotes; I—slender metacyclic trypomastigote (after Khan, 1976). J–P—*Trypanosoma danilewskyi*: J, K—epimastigotes and less numerous sphaeromastigotes
found at the start of leech cycle; L—division of epimastigotes with fission product
M; N, O—slender epimastigotes; P—slender metacyclic trypomastigote stage.

The amastigotes were the first to appear (originating from rounded-up
bloodstream trypomastigotes), and they persisted—although in dwindled
numbers—in the leech throughout its infection. Sphaeromastigotes
appeared simultaneously with the epimastigotes but soon vanished
again as they transformed into epimastigotes, which did not themselves
divide. At day 42 after feeding they began to migrate into the proboscis.
Trypomastigotes (resembling midgut forms of Salivaria) arose in the
stomach and also migrated later into the proboscis.

   In the trypanosomes of freshwater fish, the leech phase of the life
cycle (Brumpt, 1906b; Robertson, 1911; Tanabe, 1924; Quadri, 1962b)
has been investigated in only a few species. Detailed data are available
only on *T. danilewskyi* in *Hemiclepsis marginata* (Robertson, 1911;

Quadri, 1962d). Epimastigotes, and, later, trypomastigotes are predominant (Fig. 13, J-P). At the beginning, tadpole-like epimastigotes arise by unequal division of bloodstream trypomastigotes; there are a few sphaeromastigotes. Some of the epimastigotes may have the kinetoplast shifted almost to the anterior end (promastigotes?). The stomach is soon filled by a mass of intermediate stages, which result in the production of long, sometimes even filiform, trypomastigotes (up to 51 μm long) with kinetoplast halfway between nucleus and posterior end; later these prevail and move into the proboscis (starting with day 10, but also as late as several months after feeding). The binary divisions tend to be more or less unequal.

The sequence of forms is always directly correlated to the degree of digestion of the blood meal. As a rule, it is only after the blood has been almost completely digested that the slender trypomastigotes appear—thus their timing depends not only on temperature but also on the amount of blood ingested. If a "late-phase" leech feeds on uninfected blood, the cycle starts in its stomach again, just as after the ingestion of infected blood (Robertson, 1911). The forms which start the cycle are probably the short, "stubby", sometimes almost spherical epimastigotes. These persist in the stomach for a long period of time, while most, if not all proboscis-located trypomastigotes (in any case unable to divide) are washed off into the blood of the newly-attacked host.

The development of other species of trypanosomes of freshwater fish in other leech vectors may follow a modified pattern. For example, Khaybulyayev (1969, 1970) reported the division of an unspecified trypanosome in the form of cyst-like (?) structures, or the origin of epimastigotes from rosettes of hundreds of cells. There may also be leech- and strain-dependent differences. Strain MS of *T. danilewskyi* (Lom, unpublished results) fed to *Piscicola geometra* produces a sequence of epimastigote and trypomastigote forms. Strain Ma, unable to transform in culture (see p. 304), was able to transform in *P. geometra* in the 17th syringe passage (after 2 years of non-cyclical maintenance). In addition to proliferating epimastigotes, it produced sphaeromastigotes as well (Fig. 13, K) which were also capable of division. Amastigote forms also occurred occasionally. Later on, at the 33rd syringe passage, the production of sphaeromastigote forms was inconstant; in some leeches, only very slender epimastigote and trypomastigote forms were produced.

(b) *Trypanoplasma.* The observations of the vector stages in trypanoplasms, although being very uneven, have proved that, similarly to trypanosomes, they undergo a series of morphological changes (existing reports on freshwater species—Léger, 1904b; Keysselitz, 1906; Robertson, 1911; Tanabe, 1924; Putz, 1972a, b; Lom, unpublished observations).

As soon as the flagellates are ingested with the blood meal, they start to divide in the stomach. First, they have a rather "stubby", compact shape, and they exhibit undulatory movements; the flagella seem short compared to the body dimensions. Then there are moderately elongated stages, reminding one of the initial bloodstream forms, which also divide and seem to persist throughout the infection of the leech (Fig. 14F). Beginning on the second day, slender, sometimes even very long, filiform shapes appear (Fig. 14G); in these cells, however, the nucleus is

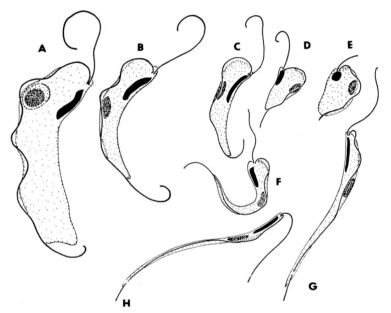

FIG. 14. *Trypanoplasma.* A, B—*T. guerneyorum* bloodstream forms from pike: A—stout adult form, B—young slender form. C–H: *T. borelli,* stages of the leech cycle: C—ingested bloodstream form; transformation into "stubby" (D, E) and slender (F) forms; G—elongated form; H—metacyclic worm-like form. All figures are drawn to the same scale.

some distance behind the end of the kinetoplast, whilst in the bloodstream stages these organelles usually overlap. Then the slender forms start moving into the proboscis of the leech, where they concentrate in large numbers; they are attached to the proboscis wall by means of the anterior flagellum. A similar adherence may be observed also in the stomach and digestive intestine. It is, however, the more compact forms which divide (Fig. 14D, E), evidently giving rise to the "worm-like" stages, in which there is no report of fission.

Near the end of blood digestion, a huge mass of the slender stages (Fig. 14H) may accumulate in the stomach in front of the proboscis. As with trypanosomes, the course of changes affecting the trypanoplasms depends on the degree of digestion of the blood meal. The time for which the leeches remain infected is not exactly known; in *Piscicola geometra*, *T. borelli* is never found later than 15 days after feeding.

C. VERTEBRATE PHASE OF THE LIFE CYCLE

1. Development in the fish

As distinct from salivarian infections in mammals, the course of trypanosome or trypanoplasm infection in fish is discontinuous. It comprises several consecutive periods. Following the bite of an infected leech, or the intraperitoneal introduction of bloodstream trypanosomes or trypanoplasms, there is a first phase in which the flagellates are absent from the peripheral blood. Perhaps this is not just the result of a simple dilution of the inoculum; it is not known where the organisms stay during that phase—no tissue stages have been reported. However, Robertson (1911) mentions the acquisition of infection by a leech which had fed on a goldfish exposed to a *Trypanosoma danilewskyi*-infected leech two days earlier.

The appearance of rather slender forms of flagellates in the peripheral blood starts the second phase—patent and increasing parasitaemia. Division may (or may not) be observed in the peripheral blood; sometimes a heavy parasitaemia is attained. This phase lasts from several days to a few weeks. Heavy infections may result in the death of the host but mostly the infection passes over in the third, chronic, phase. This is characterized by a diminishing number of flagellates in the blood of fish and lasts for a few weeks, or for an indefinite period of time; that is why this phase is the one most often observed. In pleomorphic species of trypanosomes and trypanoplasms, the adult bloodstream forms are typical for this phase. As a rule, no division stages are observed, which has led some (e.g., Khaybulyayev, 1970; Khan, 1976) to conclude that fish trypanosomes multiply only in the vector and not in their vertebrate host.

Finally, the fourth phase is characterized by the complete absence of flagellates in peripheral blood. Although sometimes the flagellates may be found in their preferred sites, the pseudobranchia or the mesonephros of the kidney, mostly the fish appears to be completely devoid of parasites. The disappearance of flagellates is a manifestation of a premunition, of a non-sterile rather than of a sterile immunity: a fish appearing as completely infection free may later suffer a sudden severe relapse. Although this is mostly due to some kind of stress condition (e.g., adverse environmental factors), occasionally it occurs without detectable reasons (Lom, unpublished observations). Various factors may act upon the balance between the parasite and host so that the above mentioned phases two, three and four of infection—or phase three and four—can alternate.

Assuming that during the feeding act the leech pumps most, if not all, the flagellates from its digestive tract into the fish host (Brumpt, 1904, 1905; Keysselitz, 1906; Robertson, 1911), the infecting dose may be anywhere between around several hundreds (in generally weakly infected *Piscicola geometra*) and tens of thousands and more (in heavily infected *Hemiclepsis marginata* or *Piscicola salmositica*). The few reports available on the length of the first, prepatent phase of a leech-vectored infection agree on one week or less; for example, Robertson (1911) recorded 5 days for *Trypanosoma danilewskyi* and 4 days for *Trypanoplasma borelli*; Becker and Katz (1965b, 1966) recorded 5 days for *Trypanoplasma salmositica*; and Khaybulyayev (1970) recorded 5-7 days for unspecified species of both genera.

It is much more informative to follow the course of infection in laboratory experiments under defined environmental conditions, of which the temperature is most important. In goldfish infected with about 500 flagellates per fish via syringe passage and kept at about 20°C (Lom, 1974) several strains of *Trypanosoma danilewskyi* showed an average prepatent period of 7-9 days, with a range of variation between 4 and 35 days. *Trypanoplasma borelli* strains appeared in the blood on the average a little later—13 days after inoculation, with a variation between 4 and 28 days. The variation was due to differences in individual resistance of the goldfish, in the growth phase of the flagellates used for infection and on the number inoculated. As a rule, the length of the prepatent period depends on the infecting dose and is shortest when a large number of organisms (5000 and more per fish) are inoculated. On the other hand, infections which were started with only a few flagellates (two trypanosomes or trypanoplasms injected) took a long time to develop; the longest was 47 days in *Trypanoplasma*. However, the number of flagellates inoculated was not correlated with their number at the peak of parasitaemia; low doses of parasites produced parasitaemias as heavy as very high doses.

The peak of parasitaemia is reached in *T. danilewskyi* strains syringe-passaged in goldfish on average on day 21 post infection, with variation between 11 and 44 days; at the height of parasitaemia, the trypanosome population comprises 10-13% of division stages. The maximum number of trypanosomes counted (which was not necessarily the record number) was 1.6×10^6 per 1 mm^3 (= antilog 9·2 per ml). In *Trypanoplasma borelli*, the peak was reached on average on day 27 after inoculation, within the variation range of 14 to 60 days. The maximum number of trypanoplasms counted was 1.2×10^5 per 1 mm^3 (= antilog 8·1 per ml). The percentage of division stages of *T. borelli* in an acutely infected goldfish never exceeded about 1%; the bulk of the fission stages is probably confined in the internal organs.

Most of the goldfish infected with *Trypanosoma danilewskyi* or *Trypanoplasma borelli* die, usually as they reach the peak of parasitaemia; some perish later, up to 90 days post infection. In a small proportion of goldfish the number of parasites gradually decreases until the fish are completely devoid of infection. A thorough check can reveal no parasites either in blood or in the internal organs. This happens by day 30 to 138 after inoculation; mostly after 2–3 months with *T. danilewskyi* strains (from day 38 to 67), mostly after about two months with *T. borelli* strains. Quite exceptionally, the infection persists at 20°C for what appears an indefinite period of time (Lom and Suchánková, 1974, and unpublished results).

In syringe-infected, aparasitaemic carps (the carp is the natural host of both species tested) of the year, infections with *Trypanosoma danilewskyi* and with *Trypanoplasma borelli* follow a course similar to that occurring in goldfish.

In goldfish surviving infection, aparasitaemic, and kept continuously under the same conditions, no signs of infection could be detected for a period of more than one year. Transfer into another environment, perhaps provoking a stress of adaptation, however, may result in a flare of infection (Lom, unpublished results).

Although in heavy infections the trypanosomes divide in the circulating blood, the site of their reproduction during the prepatent period is not known. The same applies to trypanoplasms in which, moreover, the division index in the blood is disproportionaly low, even during heavy parasitaemias. Both genera are known to invade various body organs, the brain included; to what extent they invade the extravascular space remains to be decided.

2. Effect of temperature

The crucial importance of the ambient temperature in influencing the course of the infection with fish haemoflagellates was reflected in the field observations of the early authors. For instance, Breindl (1912, 1915) noted that the prevalence and intensity of infection by various species of *Trypanosoma* and *Trypanoplasma* of freshwater fish in Czechoslovakia reached a peak in the summer months, while there was a marked drop in the cold season. Much later, Needham (1969a, b) noted the same phenomenon in *Trypanosoma* infections in tenches. However, experimental work has been very scarce. This temperature-dependence may be demonstrated in the course of infection with strains of *Trypanosoma danilewskyi* and *Trypanoplasma borelli* in goldfish (Lom, 1973b). In an ambient temperature of 22° to 25°C, the infection develops very rapidly, the peak of parasitaemia being reached in about 7 to 11 days. If a massive inoculum (100 000 flagellates) is used, the trypanosomes may appear in the blood as early as the second day after inoculation. With an inoculum of about 500 flagellates, the prepatent phase lasts only 2 to 5 days. 22° to 25°C may be taken as optimal for parasite development in this host–parasite system. At temperatures slightly above or below that range, 18° or 28°C, flagellate growth is distinctly slower and, also, their final concentration may be low. At 30°C the parasites are still able to develop. At 10°C and below, the infection develops extremely slowly and never reaches more than 100 000 flagellates per 1 mm³ (= antilog 8·0 per ml). If inoculated goldfish are kept below 10°C, the infection started by an injected inoculum or by leech-feeding may never become patent and it is only after transfer of the fish into the optimal temperature range that the infection proceeds further.

These effects are more the expression of the temperature requirements of the particular species than host-mediated effects, since the optimal temperature for the *in vitro* growth of *T. danilewskyi* is 25°C, although it tolerates 33°C for a short time. In contrast to the finding with anuran trypanosomes (see Bardsley and Harmsen, 1973), the peripheral parasitaemia in fish haemoflagellates does not fluctuate in relation to rapid changes of ambient temperature.

3. Stress factors

Unfavourable conditions generally favour the progress of the infection by prevailing against the host's resistance. Breindl (1915) reported relapses of *Trypanoplasma varium* in loaches starved after the winter period. He also observed a 90% prevalence after spawning in a large sample of female loaches which were all negative before the spawning period. The dramatic increase of infection with *Trypanoplasma salmositica* in salmonid fishes during their laborious upstream migration (Katz and Becker, 1960; Becker and Katz, 1966) is also significant.

However, modelling of a stress situation in a laboratory infection is not so simple (Lom, unpublished observations) although such an investigation might have implications in disease prevention in fish husbandry. Preliminary experiments with cortisone treatment and osmotic shocks did not yield conclusive results in *T. danilewskyi* infections in goldfish. Only in crucian carps infected experimentally with the last cited trypanosome, and exposed to forced motion, was there a slight increase in the infection as compared with controls.

4. Immune reactions

Immune phenomena control the bloodstream phase of fish *Trypanosoma* and *Trypanoplasma* in a way similar to that obtaining in higher vertebrates. The complete disappearance of flagellates in fish surviving a heavy infection can only be interpreted in terms of acquired immunity. Although Brumpt (1906c) and Robertson (1911), on the evidence of rather inconclusive experiments, doubted the ability of fish to acquire a protective immunity following infections with trypanosomes, the experiments summarized by Lom (1974) prove the contrary. Goldfish—but also carp of the year*—surviving heavy infections with various strains of *Trypanosoma danilewskyi* or *Trypanoplasma borelli* (aparasitaemic phase 4 of infection) could not be reinfected with the same strain of flagellates. The resistance to challenges with massive inocula was repeatedly tested. This immunity to superinfection could be seen to last up to 350 days. However, as mentioned above, this is probably no sterile immunity, and it depends on temperature as do all immune phenomena in fish (see review by Avtalion *et al.*, 1973). As noted by Barrow (1954, 1955) in perches, goldfish and tenches, and by Kipp (1968) in tenches, when fish are kept at a low, suboptimal, temperature (0° to 15°C) the infection does not reach phase four and a certain level of parasitaemia is maintained.

Fishes showing a light parasitaemia may be superinfected with the same flagellate species by inoculation or by using a leech and this is said to increase the parasitaemia to a high level (e.g. Brumpt, 1906c; Needham, 1969b). Studies with goldfish (Lom, unpublished results) yielded very inconsistent results; the outcome of infection probably depends on the actual condition of the fish and on the phase of the infection.

The only proof of the existence of trypanocidal antibodies in fish was presented by Barrow (1954, 1955). He observed lytic action of the serum of fish that have recovered from *Trypanosoma* sp. infection at 20°C. This lytic capacity soon diminished; it was lost by three weeks after the disappearance of the parasite from the blood. Fish kept at lower temperatures (5°C), or starving fish, did not produce lytic antibodies; the latter finding is at variance with the statement of Avtalion (1969). Curiously also, the immune phase four of the infection was not reached by fish low in the pecking order in a given aquarium. While the feeding, dominant, fish got rid of the infection, the omega specimens did not feed and kept their parasitaemia. In this instance, some other effects (stress; nutrition) might have been of importance.

Cottrell (1976, 1977) found that plaice infected with *Trypanosoma platessae* had elevated levels of serum immunoglobulins possessing the β-electrophoretic mobility. This might be associated with antibody production. He pointed out the marked seasonal variation of *T. platessae* infections, which could be explained in terms of temperature-controlled immunity to these parasites.

Goldfish surviving a heavy experimental infection with *Trypanosoma danilewskyi* or *Trypanoplasma borelli* were refractory to superinfection, but induction of the same degree of protection by passive immunization, using successive large inocula of thermally-killed haemoflagellates, failed (Lom, unpublished data).

* Means fish less than one year old.

Attempts were made to produce a protective immunity by inoculation of γ-irradiated haemoflagellates—a technique successful with the salivarian trypanosome species, *T. congolense* and *T. rhodesiense*, in laboratory rodents, but less so in dogs and cattle (Duxbury *et al.*, 1972; 1975). Only a partial success was achieved with *Trypanosoma danilewskyi* in goldfish; using massive inocula of flagellates exposed previously to 100 000 rad (lower doses did not prevent division), a challenge inoculum of 1000 flagellates/fish resulted in a very delayed parasitaemia (not appearing before 60–85 days as compared to the normal range of 11–44 days); the infection rate was 60–75%. Using a massive challenge inoculum (500 000 flagellates), no delay of onset of parasitaemia was observed and the decrease in infection rate was inconclusive. Immunization of goldfish with irradiated *Trypanoplasma borelli* had no marked effect on the subsequent infection (Lom, unpublished results).

No data are available on cell mediated immunity to fish haemoflagellates; the observation that trypanosomes may be engulfed by leucocytes (Lom, unpublished results) suggests that cell-mediated immunity may play some role.

5. Pathogenicity

Most haemoflagellate infections in fishes pass without any signs of disease and we largely ignore the changes provoked in the hosts by symptomless infections. Under certain conditions—mostly in cultured hosts and in a less natural environment—the parasites prevail against the defence system of the fish host and the ensuing pathological changes result in a pronounced disease condition and, ultimately, death of the host. Although the symptoms are often very striking, their profound analysis is still lacking; not all of them are due to the flagellates.

(a) *Trypanoplasma*. Species of this genus were reported to cause disease and sometimes heavy losses not only in cultured carps, tenches and crucian carps (Hofer, 1904; Plehn, 1903, 1924; Keyssellitz, 1906; Neresheimer, 1912; Volf, 1934) but also in other hosts, e.g. *Phoxinus phoxinus, Acipenser ruthenus* (Léger, 1904a, b; Breindl, 1915; Ioff *et al.*, 1926). In the textbooks on fish parasitology, the term "sleeping sickness" (Hofer, 1904) of carps and tenches became well-used, derived from the "sleeping" position of moribund, anaemic and ascitic fish lying on their sides beneath the water surface; however, these are symptoms of diseased conditions often of other than flagellate aetiology. More recently, massive infection associated with heavy losses have been reported for various salmonids (see, e.g., Wales and Wolf, 1955; Makeyeva, 1956) and for Chinese grass-carps (Britchuk, 1969; Migala, 1967, 1971). From most of the earlier reports, however, it was not quite certain whether the trypanoplasms were the primary cause of the disease or if their massive occurrence in the host was made possible by the debilitated condition of the fish, preventing its protective immune response. Nowicki (1940) questioned the pathogenic potency of *Trypanoplasma cyprini* on the basis of several experiments with splenectomized carps. The carps failed to develop a disease following injection of *Trypanoplasma*-infected blood, and did not show higher numbers of trypanoplasms in their blood than did controls. He concluded that *T. cyprini* can hardly exert any pathogenic action even in fishes stressed by other infections. Yet, his experiments are not fully unequivocal; the spleen, though the most important organ, is not the only one involved in the immune response; and his carps might have had a previous history of infection.

Putz (1972b) published what seems a decisive proof of the pathogenicity of *Trypanoplasma salmositica*, inoculated intramuscularly into the coho salmon, *Oncorhynchus kisutch*. The first symptom, a slight exophthalmia, appeared on day 6 after inoculation. Within 14 to 18 days all the inoculated fish perished, the blood corpuscle/trypanoplasma ratio reaching 2/3 in some of the specimens.

The syringe-passaged strains of *T. borelli* kill 56 to 80% of their goldfish hosts depending chiefly on the passage level of the inoculum and on the ambient temperature. Young carps reared parasite-free and inoculated intraperitoneally also suffered heavy mortalities. In first year carps (1·3 to 4 cm in length) there was a 40–80% mortality; in their second year, the mortality of young carps only exceptionally reached 40%, thus being considerably lower. This may reflect a resistance increasing with age (Lom, unpublished results).

Thus pathogenicity—at least in certain host–parasite systems—has been fully established. In other such systems, or in specimens which later recover or in which the infection persists at a low level, the state of health may be more or less severely impaired, rendering the hosts more susceptible to various stresses or to other infections. Trypanoplasmosis may well be one of the factors predisposing to haemorrhagic septicaemia of carps (Tesarčík, 1974).

The invariably-occurring symptoms of serious trypanoplasmiasis are: a drastic decrease in the number and in the haemoglobin content of the erythrocytes, resulting in anaemia well apparent on gills and sometimes even visceral organs; lethargic condition; loss of normal reactions; and refusal of food. Very often, and to a different degree in various species of hosts, there is an ample ascites in the body cavity, exophthalmus and haemorrhagic patches on the skin.

Exact analysis of the pathologic changes of trypanoplasmiasis is still not available. Reports on the pathologic changes due to trypanoplasmiasis indicate that, in the blood, the total protein, albumin and haemoglobin values, as well as the erythrocyte number are reduced (Kipp, 1968). Organ changes include haemorrhagic foci, and changes of blood vessels

(Kipp, 1968); capillaries in the gills and suprarenal glands may be plugged by numerous flagellates, kidney glomerula may be oedematous (Putz, 1972b). The latter author deems the mortality to be a result of a general loss of osmoregulation on the evidence of the oedematous and ascitic condition of infected coho salmon. However, the histopathological changes themselves may account for the high fatality of the goldfish heavily infected with *T. borelli* (Dyková and Lom, 1978b). There were many extravascularly located flagellates, numerous vascular lesions and inflammatory infiltrations of tissues. In the kidneys, glomerulitis and tubulonephrosis were observed as well as diffuse degenerative changes and focal necrosis in the livers. Dilated intercellular spaces in the fat tissue were filled with aggregations of trypanoplasmas.

Heavy infections and mortalities are not necessarily limited to young fishes but may affect two- or three-year-old or fully grown fish also.

(b) *Trypanosoma*. It seems, on the evidence obtained from observations of natural infections, that species of this genus live in a more or less balanced state with their host; at most, the sensitivity of the fish to noxious factors may be enhanced by concurrent *Trypanosoma* infection (Kipp, 1968). The old finding of trypanosomes in populations of moribund carps (Doflein, 1901) did not necessarily mean that the flagellates were responsible for the disease. Reports of actual pathological changes produced by naturally-occurring trypanosomiasis are extremely rare. Neumann (1909) observed, in skates (*Raja punctata*) heavily infected with *Trypanosoma variabile*, an inflammation of the brain (which harboured the parasite also), fatty degeneration of body organs, anaemia and eosinophilia. Smirnova (1970) claimed that the presence of *Trypanosoma lotai* in the burbot (*Lota lota*) caused a fall in various blood serum constituents, notably in the serum protein level. Tandon and Joshi (1973) described marked changes in the blood picture in fishes infected with *T. vittati* and *T. maguri*; the peripheral blood contained an increased number of immature or abnormal erythrocytes, the total number of leucocytes reached twice its normal value, while the erythrocyte number and haemoglobin contents decreased. The same authors (1974) noted a marked decrease of the blood glucose level in trypanosome-infected (species not determined) fishes of four Indian species. Cottrell (1977) found, in natural infections of plaice with *T. platessae*, a markedly reduced albumin–globulin ratio in the serum, i.e., an increase of globulins, while the packed cell volume remained unchanged. The trypanosome-induced haematological changes may be age- or size-dependent. Khan (1977b) noted, in *T. murmanensis*-infected cod less than 24 cm in length, parasitaemia to be accompanied by decreased haematocrit and haemoglobin values and an increased erythrocyte sedimentation rate while cod more than 26 cm in length underwent only slight haematological changes. He believes that the infected small cod are more prone to predation or disease.

In heavy *T. danilewskyi* infections in goldfish, Dyková and Lom (1978a) observed the heaviest histopathological changes to be located in the haemopoietic organs—kidneys, spleen and the liver. The spleen turned into a nearly acellular stroma. The changes were evidently irreparable and indicated a fatal prognosis. In contrast to trypanoplasmosis (Dyková and Lom, 1978b) and to mammal trypanosomiases, there was a striking absence of inflammatory reaction.

The mortality caused by syringe-passaged *T. danilewskyi* strains in goldfish varied between 60 to 100%. In some experimental infections at least, *T. danilewskyi* was pathogenic also for carp (Lom and Suchánková, 1974, and unpublished results). Strains MS or Ma introduced intraperitoneally in low doses (500 flagellates per fish), into parasite-free reared carps of the year while still 2 to 4 cm in length, caused a mortality of 10–100% depending on the strain and on the fish-age class used, the average mortality being 46%. In one-year-old carps the mortality averaged no more than 30%, which again may reflect a resistance increasing with the growth of the host (Lom, unpublished results).

These observed mortalities clearly surpass others reported for natural infections. This unheard-of high virulence may be the result of the unfavourable conditions which the carps find in the laboratory tanks and, also, of the injection of bloodstream trypomastigotes, which, not having the need first to readapt to the vertebrate host, may develop a much stronger growth than does a leech-vectored infection. However, it surely shows the pathogenic potential of fish trypanosomes, which—at least in some cases—may escape attention in natural conditions. Careful re-examination of the problem of pathogenicity in large scale experiments in conditions simulating natural settings is needed. This comment applies also to *Trypanoplasma*; although it is known as a pathogen in fish husbandry, the natural infections never seem to be fatal.

6. Virulence of syringe-passaged strains

In the first few passages after the flagellates have become established in goldfish, most of the goldfish develop the infection but there is a fair percentage of survivors. However, this may change with the increasing number of transfers (Lom, unpublished results). *T. danilewskyi* strain Ma, isolated from carp and maintained for more than five years by syringe passage (a total of 100 consecutive transfers) in goldfish, had up to the tenth passage an average infectivity of 96% while there were 28% survivors. Up to the 20th passage, the average values were 95% and 20%, respectively; up to the 40th passage (more than 3 years after isolation), 97% and 14%, respectively. From then on, the infectivity was 100% while the percentage of survivors decreased to 10% in passages

41–60; subsequently there were no survivors. However, in two other *T. danilewskyi** strains, isolated from eels and tenches, G and L respectively, the percentage of survivors increased (instead of diminishing) with the number of passages. Similarly with *Trypanoplasma borelli* strain Ml, isolated from carps; over 41 consecutive passages (which took a total of three and a half years) the infectivity rose from the initial 90% to 99%, and the percentage of survivors rose also from 20% to 44%.

Syringe-passaged strains keep their infectivity for the leech over a considerable period of non-cyclical transmission; *Trypanosoma danilewskyi* strain Ma was able to transform in the leech after 40 syringe-passages.

7. Host specificity

Most early studies on fish haemoflagellates assumed a high degree of the host specificity by assigning species status to populations of trypanosomes and trypanoplasms found in different species of fish host. A different host was often the only considerable distinction for newly erected species (see, e.g., Henry, 1913). Some of the early cross-infection experiments performed in a rather fortuitous way yielded negative results which seemed to corroborate the strict specificity concept (e.g., Breindl, 1915; Ioff *et al.*, 1926). More dependable evidence for strict host specificity is rare; such data were presented by Lebailly (1905) and Cottrell (1977) for *Trypanosoma platessae*; the latter author failed to transmit the infection to taxonomically and biologically related hosts. Bower and Woo (1977b) on the evidence of unsuccessful transmissions of *Trypanoplasma commersoni* to 16 species of taxonomically related or alien hosts claimed a strict host specificity for this trypanoplasma.

Other records of experiments indicate that the haemoflagellates of fish are not species specific, although the results are sometimes ambiguous. Kipp (1968), using inoculation of tench blood infected with *T. borelli*, failed to infect pikes, perches and chubs, but succeeded with carps, breams and crucian carps. Khan (1977a) using leech transmission successfully infected with *Trypanosoma murmanensis* 13 species of marine fish belonging to 4 different orders. Using infection-free leeches, he also transmitted trypanosomes found in four species of perciform and pleuronectiform fish to a total of 6 other taxonomically related and unrelated fish. (He did not, however, work with parasite-free reared fish.) He assumes all the trypanosomes are referable to the single species, *T. murmanensis.*

Barrow (1954), using parasite-free leeches, failed to transmit trypanosomes from eels to goldfish, but succeeded in infecting goldfish with undetermined trypanosomes from nine-spined and blue-spined stickleback, minnow, tench, perch and bullhead; he did not say whether the goldfish used were proved to be parasite-free; unless the innoculated

* See discussion on synonymy of *T. danilewsky* on p. 314.

fish has a parasite-free anamnesis it may prove insusceptible because of superinfection immunity, or the introduction of parasites may cause relapse of a dormant infection. However, Robertson (1911) did use trypanosome-free goldfish; she infected them with leeches carrying trypanosomes from perches and breams. Lom (1973a, and unpublished results), using syringe inoculation to parasite-free reared goldfish, was able to repeatedly, and without failure, infect the goldfish with *T. danilewskyi* from carps, and with populations of trypanosomes from tenches assignable to the same species. He also succeeded with populations of trypanosomes, morphologically identical to *T. danilewskyi* isolated from eel and gudgeon, but failed with *T. anguillae* and *T. elegans* from these same hosts. Inoculations of *T. percae* from perches, *T. acerinae* from *Acerina cernus*, *T. ?remaki* from pikes, and trypanosomes from breams, barbs and roaches gave repeatedly negative results. *Trypanoplasma ?guerneyorum* from pikes also failed to establish itself in the goldfish. On the other hand, *T. danilewskyi* isolated from carps and passaged in goldfish was easily established in parasite-free reared pikes and in *Puntius conchonius*, and also in seemingly uninfected stone perches and crucian carps from the wild. *Trypanoplasma borelli*, isolated from carps and also passaged in goldfish, failed to infect parasite-free reared pikes and *Puntius conchonius*, but did establish itself in minnows, crucian carps, roaches and gudgeons.

Discrepancies between the transfer experiments of Lom (1973a), Barrow (1954) and Robertson (1911) (e.g., in the infection of goldfish with trypanosomes from perches and eels) can be explained, at least in part, by the fact that one fish host may, even if not simultaneously, act as the host of two (or more) di- or poly-xenuous trypanosome species of differing preferences for other hosts. In favour of this assumption are observations on North American trypanoplasms. *T. cataractae* (Putz, 1972a, b) also infects, apart from its principal host, *Rhinichtys cataractae* (prevalence of infection 97%) and four more cyprinid species; intra-peritoneal injection can extend the list to two more hosts, one of which belongs to a different family. *T. salmositica* in addition to its principal host *Oncorhynchus tschawytscha* which is affected by the heaviest infections (Becker and Katz, 1965a–c), infects in the wild a total of 9 species of salmonid fishes, 5 species of cottids, 3 of cyprinids and the three-spined stickleback; the only common feature of the hosts is their cold-water habitat. Inoculation established this species in two more cyprinid hosts. The marine species *Trypanoplasma bullocki* infects in nature four species from two fish families. The case of *Trypanoplasma salmositica* is used by Khaybulyayev (1976) as a part of the evidence for his claim that blood flagellates of fish while having a low specificity for fishes are strictly specific for leeches—which certainly does not hold true for European leeches.

It is obvious—although experimental data are fragmentary and inconsistent—that strict host specificity may be an exception rather than a rule in fish haemoflagellates. The latter may have—in addition to one or more principal hosts (e.g., carp and tench in *Trypanosoma danilewskyi*) which best meet their growth requirements—more hosts which at the same time may serve as principal hosts for other haemoflagellates (e.g., eel—such as *T. granulosum* and *T. danilewskyi*). Thus important commercial fishes such as salmon or carp may contract their leech-vectored infections from sources in "trash" fishes which act in this sense as reservoir hosts.

Sometimes a susceptible host is protected only by an ecological barrier against its potential parasite (e.g., the susceptibility of *Puntius conchonius* (Lom, 1973a) or of *Lebistes reticulatus* (Khaybulyayev, 1976) to *T. danilewskyi*). Interestingly, but similarly to salivarian trypanosomes, fish trypanosome species can thrive in hosts which occupy very different taxonomic positions.

Heterologous sera may exhibit a toxic effect upon trypanosomes and trypanoplasms; for example, trout serum kills carp-derived *Trypanosoma danilewskyi* within 90 minutes (Lom, unpublished observations). *Trypanoplasma catostomi* from *Catostomus commersonii* was found to be sensitive to fresh blood plasma of five heterologous fish hosts, being killed by a 3 hours exposure to plasma diluted to the titre 1 : 16 (in rainbow trout plasma) (Bower and Woo, 1977a). On the evidence of their experiments the authors conclude that the rainbow trout have a natural properdin system activated by the parasite. This is suggested to be one of the mechanisms of natural immunity of fish.

8. Attempts at chemotherapy of fish infections

The only existing report is by Havelka *et al.* (1965) stating that *Trypanoplasma cyprini* (= *T. borelli*) is killed *in vitro* by methylene blue, gentian violet and malachite green in concentrations 1 in 2000 to 1 in 20 000. Exposure of infected carp fingerlings to 1 in 2000 and 1 in 5000 solutions of the above dyes resulted in the disappearance of flagellates from the peripheral blood; in field experiments, the use of these dyes increased the survival rate of heavily infected fish and reduced the parasitaemia. However, using goldfish infected with *T. danilewskyi* or *T. borelli* (Lom, unpublished results), it was found that concentrations tolerated by the goldfish did not in the least affect the flagellates.

9. Pleomorphism in the fish host

In fish blood flagellates, similarly to the condition in trypanosomatids of other host groups (see Lumsden and Evans, 1976), the pleomorphism is understood as a sequential (sometimes overlapping) phenotypic manifestation of one genotype as it appears in the trypanomastigote stage in the vertebrate host. Their appearance is most probably triggered by changes in the host antibody spectrum, as is well known in trypanosomes of mammals and as suggested for amphibian trypanosomes by Barrow (1958). Apart from the numerous fish parasites in which pleomorphism evidently exists, there are fish trypanosomes which seem to be virtually monomorphic. They only display a more or less marked variability in size and/or in length/width ratio. The developmental changes in their vertebrate host, if any, seem in such species to be limited to other than morphologic manifestations. However, as aptly stated by Bardsley and Harmsen (1973), only observation of the parasite in its vertebrate host when it is subjected to a complete variety of naturally-occurring conditions and factors can reveal whether it really is monomorphic. To date, it is only in a few species that such a decision can be reached. One is *Trypanosoma danilewskyi* in which, so far, experimental transfers among various hosts (carps, goldfish, gudgeon, pike, *Barbus conchonius*), varying temperature regimes or study of various stages of infection failed to reveal any true pleomorphism (Lom, unpublished observations).

(a) *Pleomorphism in trypanosomes.* Forms differing conspicuously in their shape and size were designated by the early authors, since Laveran and Mesnil (1901), as "var. *parva*" or "var. *magna*". Sometimes such morphs were even credited with separate taxonomic status by authors who failed to find intermediate stages (Fantham, 1919). However, it soon became clear that these are but extremes in the sequence of forms occurring during the course of infection with one species [e.g. Minchin (1909); Breindl (1915); see also recent papers by Laird (1951), Kahn (1976)]. Out of the large number of piscine trydanosomes, only in a few has the full sequence been established.

The most marked examples of pleomorphism can be drawn from among marine species, e.g. those from skates—*T. giganteum*, *T. rajae*, *T. gargantua* (Fig. 28A–C). The freshwater examples are *T. granulosum* (Fig. 15A–C), *T. percae* (Fig. 23), and *T. remaki*. The pleomorphism is expressed in the following features:

(1) size changes;

(2) changes in length/width ratio, i.e. slender or broad forms;

(3) the number of waves of the undulating membrane, and their width and depth;

(4) the presence or absence of a distinct karyosome in the nucleus by light microscopy;

(5) the presence of subsurface striation ("myonemes") in stained preparations by light microscopy [longitudinal or spirally oriented striations, probably subpellicularly located ribbons of mitochondrial systems—an assumption supported by Paulin's (1975) spatial reconstruction of chondriome in several trypanosomatids];

(6) presence and number of stainable cytoplasmic granules;

(7) distance of the kinetoplast from the posterior end;

(8) length of the free end of the flagellum;

(9) shifts in position of the nucleus in the body.

Separate morphological stages may be defined by the combination of the above characters; marked changes of points 1 to 5 are proper to truly polymorphic species while changes in points 1, 2, 6, 7, 8, 9 may also be found in "monomorphic" species.

In pleomorphic species, the first trypanosomes to appear in the blood of the infected host are the "young" forms—rather small and slender with a few, shallow waves of the undulating membrane (Fig. 15A) and with the nucleus revealing no distinct karyosome. After a certain period,

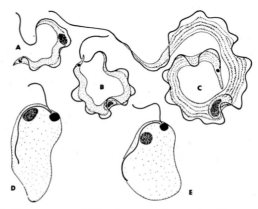

FIG. 15. A–C. Sequences of bloodstream forms in *Trypanosoma granulosum* from eels. A, B—young and intermediate form; C—adult form with subsurface striation (after Minchin, 1909). D–E: *Trypanoplasma* sp. from *Fluta alba* (after Ogawa and Uegaki, 1927).

intermediate forms appear in growing numbers until eventually "adult" forms appear, persisting later during the fourth, chronic, phase of infection. These are large, stout if not very wide, and have mostly a richly spiralling undulating membrane with numerous bends, a nucleus with a prominent karyosome, and subsurface striation. The adult forms tend to have more chromatic granules in their cytoplasm, and a shorter free flagellum, than the young forms. Depending on the phase of infection at which the fish is examined, one can come across young slender or large adult forms only, or a mix of forms in which the intermediate ones prevail. The form that predominates depends on the course of infection, which again in its turn is subject to many factors. Although this time sequence of morphs has been verified in some species only [e.g., *T. variable*, Neumann (1906); *T. barbatulae*, Breindl (1915); *T. murmanensis*,

Kahn (1976)], it most probably holds true for all of the polymorphic species.

Division of cell organelles in the bloodstream forms follows the same pattern as in other congeneric forms (e.g., Noble, 1955). Piscine trypanosomes divide in trypomastigote forms, the fission being mainly unequal, but occasionally equal or almost equal (Laveran and Mesnil, 1902; Lom, unpublished results).

(b) *Pleomorphism in trypanoplasms.* The existence of a sequence of different morphological types of trypanoplasm during the course of infection in carps was firmly established as early as in 1906 by Keysselitz. Although he misinterpreted numerous stages both in the blood and in the leech as gametes, his reproduction of polymorphism is the most complete to be found in existing reports. The sequence of stages was confirmed by Robertson (1911) in goldfish, Breindl (1915) in loaches and Kipp (1968) in tench trypanoplasms. Bower and Woo (1977b) studied *Trypanoplasma catostomi* in parasite-free fingerlings of the host fish and noted a remarkable polymorphism including the size as well as differing body structure coupled with the progress of the infection originally started by the introduction of a single flagellate into the host. Unpublished observations of the writer on organisms affecting goldfish, tenches and pikes concur with these reports. In view of the paucity of information, sequential pleomorphism in blood-stream stages of trypanoplasms may or may not be a generally distributed phenomenon.

Bloodstream forms of the initial stages of infection—which may last only a few days—are always rather small and of a regular shape (young stages have comma-like or crescent-like shapes). In more advanced infections bigger, very irregular forms prevail, reflecting in their shape wave-like undulatory movements of the whole body (Fig. 5). In the chronic, often long lasting, period of infection the number of trypanoplasms is reduced; they assume a large size and an irregular shape, sometimes with numerous large bends of the undulating membrane; they have a nucleus with a conspicuous endosome not seen in young stages. The length of flagellum relative to the body length may also greatly vary during the cycle, as well as the number of stainable granules in the body. There may also be differences in the shape of the kinetoplast, the presence of cytoplasmic vacuoles, but these tend to be more strain- or species-specific.

Given the extreme metaboly of the cell shape, it is difficult to characterize the shape differences in young and advanced infection stages in more precise terms but they are quite conspicuous (Figs. 14A, B; 16–19) as are the differences in size. For example, in *Trypanoplasma* sp. from pikes (*T. ?guerneyorum*) the average size of a young form is 20 by 4 μm, flagella not included, while in the chronic stage form it is 38 by 9 μm.

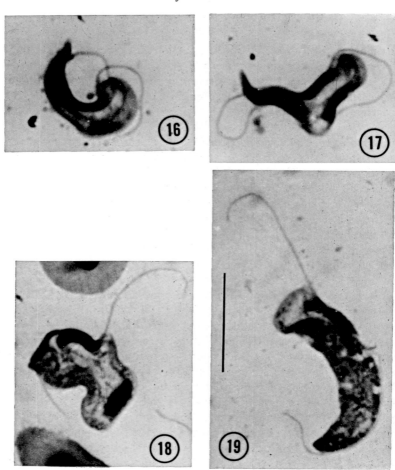

FIGS 16–19. Various forms of *Trypanoplasma borelli* from the blood of the tench. *Figs 16, 17*—Young forms. *Fig. 18*—Contorted form. *Fig. 19*—Large adult form. Methanol-fixed dry films, stained Giemsa. Scale equals 10 μm.

The large forms of trypanosomes and trypanoplasms found in late infection in the circulating blood are considered to be "adult" forms and can be conveniently used as reference stages for taxonomic comparisons. While it seems certain that they are competent to initiate growth in the vector (as proven by Khan, 1978, in *Trypanosoma murmanensis*), there is no evidence as to whether it is this or some cryptic, tissue-inhabiting, persisting, stage which is responsible for relapses of parasitaemia.

Studies of cell division in trypanoplasms are very scarce. Papers by Keysselitz (1906) and Ponselle (1913) made it clear that it follows a pattern found in bodonids in general (Hollande, 1952) and known also in *Cryptobia congeri* (Martin, 1910, 1913). Keysselitz (1906) claimed there were 8 chromosomes discernible in *T. borelli*. While previous authors (Keysselitz, 1906; Ponselle 1913) claimed there was no definite sequence of division of nucleus and kinetoplast, Bower and Woo (1977c) in a more detailed recent paper have proven the contrary. Longitudinally-dividing bloodstream forms of *T. catostomi* start the division in their flagellar apparatus and nucleus, division of kinetoplast following.

D. COURSE OF SPONTANEOUS INFECTIONS IN NATURE

Field observations deal mostly with infection of the economically important cyprinid fish (Plehn, 1903, 1924; Keysselitz, 1906; Breindl, 1912, 1915; Nowicki, 1940; Schäperclaus, 1954; Needham, 1969a, b) or salmonids (Becker and Katz, 1965a, b, c; 1966; McCarthy, 1974). Detailed observations on marine hosts are rather rare (Khan, 1976; Cottrell 1977). Experimental laboratory infections constitute a very helpful model for understanding the course and fluctuations of infections in the wild; perhaps the only significant difference between experimental and natural infections is that the former tend to be much more severe than the latter (see p. 293). Also, natural infections, as far as is known at present, tend to be more long-lasting, infected fish displaying a continuous parasitaemia for long (in terms of years) periods of time [e.g. *Trypanosoma tincae* in tenches (Needham, 1969b), *Trypanoplasma cataractae* in longnose dace (Putz 1972b)].

The haemoflagellate infections of cyprinids in the Middle-European pond systems constitute an example of the fluctuations of the host parasite balance in natural milieu. If not eradicated by special control measures, leeches (*Hemiclepsis, Piscicola*) are present in most bodies of water so that practically all fish of the year are exposed to infection. The findings of Needham (1969a, b) and of the writer prove that tenches and carps of the year in some localities may be 100% infected. Factors in the ecology of the fish host may limit or enhance the role of infection; e.g., fish living near the bottom or in littoral vegetation are more exposed to leeches than pelagic ones; in various seasons the activity of leeches may vary; in fish schools the transmission is more easy than among solitarily living ones.

After an acute phase of infection—there are no exact data on the variety of mortalities in nature—the immune phenomena induce the third, chronic phase of infection which is of variable duration. The immunity is temperature-dependent (like other immune phenomena in fish—see the review by Avtalian *et al.*, 1973). It is not of a sterile type and the host–parasite balance may be upset by environmental factors other than temperature (starvation, oxygen depletion, hibernation stresses, concurrent infections) and, possibly, by reinfections by feeding of infected leeches. Thus various states may ensue from the chronic phase of infection: the fish may stay free from detectable parasites or they may stay chronically infected during their whole life span, or finally, parasitaemic and aparasitaemic periods may alternate.

A seasonal, largely temperature-dependent, fluctuation is well manifested in carp infections with *Trypanosoma danilewskyi* and *Trypano-*

plasma borelli, where serious parasitaemias are commonly found in the early spring, following the hibernation period. This concurs with observations of Barrow (1954) on nine species of European freshwater fish which suffered their highest parasitaemia just after the winter season. Similar phenomena can be met with in the parasite–host system existing in rather cold marine waters; the seasonal incidence of *Trypanosoma platessae* in plaice is consistent with fluctuations of ambient temperature, the highest infection levels coinciding with the lowest sea temperature and *vice versa* (Cottrell, 1977). A decrease of trypanosome numbers in summer has also been noted in other poikilotherms such as Anura (e.g., Bardsley, 1972; Bollinger *et al.*, 1969). However, these seasonal fluctuations of infection in fish are evidently at variance with such regular annual fluctuations of parasitaemia as occur in amphibian trypanosomiasis, which are believed to be hormone-induced (Bardsley and Harmsen, 1973).

Intervention of factors other than temperature may provoke high parasitaemias or a severe relapse during periods when the immunological competence of the host, as far as temperature is concerned, would be unhampered. For example, in warmer seasons of the year the parasitaemia often tends to be much heavier than the light levels reached in the early spring; this happens frequently in one- or two-year-old carps. The mechanism of interplay of all the factors possibly involved has not yet been elucidated.

An intricate interaction of temperature, pre-spawn stress, and increased exposure to infected leeches (*Piscicola salmositica*) acts upon the host–parasite balance in *Trypanoplasma salmositica*-infected salmonids from the U.S. northwest Pacific coast (papers by Becker and Katz, 1965a, b, c, 1966, 1969; also McCarthy 1974). The parasite infects 18 fish species, mostly salmonids, the most susceptible being the pink and coho salmon. Coho salmon (*Oncorhynchus kisutch*) fingerlings, thanks to their infection-preventing ecology, have an average infection rate as low as 5 %. It is not known whether they keep it during the marine period of their life, but adult coho salmon entering the rivers in October have a similarly low prevalence of infection. However, one of the non-salmonid hosts, the torrent sculpin *Cottus rhotheus*, keeps an all-year-round relatively high incidence of trypanoplasms, and may act as a reservoir of the flagellates. In the following fall and winter months, the rate of infection in upstream migrating coho salmon starts soaring, reaching up to 80–100 % in December or January, along with decreasing temperature, constant reinfections and culminating spawning period. Although the intensity of infection is heavy, the infection does not seem to cause any pre-spawn losses in coho salmon. This is of course in contrast to the high or total mortalities produced in coho salmon fingerlings by experimental infections (Putz, 1972b). It is also at variance with claims of Makeyeva (1956) that heavy infections caused by a related species, *T. makeevi* (1·5 parasites to 1 blood cell), cause prespawning mortalities in the pink salmon in the Amur river.

A definite age dependence may be observed in fish haemoflagellate infections which were examined in this respect. As a rule, in older fish there seems to be either a decreasing rate of infection, or the infection is completely absent. However, due probably to ecological factors inhibiting easy transfer of infection, the youngest age class may be the least infected [e.g. *Trypanoplasma salmositica* in the torrent sculpin (Becker and Katz, 1966); *Trypanosoma pacifica* in the English sole (Burreson and Pratt, 1972); *T. platessae* in plaice (Cottrell, 1977)]. Also, in carps of the year and of the second year, parasitaemia more often persists during the whole summer while in older carps the parasitaemic periods are more often limited to early spring periods (Lom, unpublished observations).

No reliable data are available on mixed infections with two trypanosome species in the same host. Concurrent infection with *Trypanoplasma* and *Trypanosoma*, however, are fairly common. In most of the slight haemoflagellate infections of carps both *Trypanosoma danilewskyi* and *Trypanoplasma borelli* are present. In massive infections, one or the other species always prevails. In most of the goldfishes inoculated with a mixed population of the two above-mentioned species, during the subsequent transfers trypanosomes ultimately prevail until the trypanoplasms are completely eliminated (Lom, 1973b).

IV. In vitro culture

A. TRYPANOSOMA

The first reports on *in vitro* culture of fresh water fish trypanosomes date back to the first decade of this century. Various modifications of blood agar media supported the growth of *T. danilewskyi* (Petrie, 1905; Keysselitz, 1906; Thompson, 1908), *T. granulosum* (Brumpt, 1906b; Matthis, 1911; Ponselle, 1913a), *T. scardinii* (Delanoe, 1910), *T. elegans* (Roudsky, 1912) and *T. sp.* from *Misgurnus anguillicaudatus* (Tanabe, 1924). However, none of these authors reported establishment of subcultures, their attempts being limited to the initial primary culture.

As late as 1962, the first really continuous culture with subculturing was achieved by Quadri who maintained *T. striati* from the Indian fish *Ophiocephalus striatus* and *T. winchesiense* (*T. ?danilewskyi*) on Shortt's modification of NNN medium; Peterson (1974) grew *T. percae* on a modified 4N medium. He was more successful in detecting light infection by cultivation than by direct inspection of the perches.

The first to grow trypanosomes from marine fish *in vitro* was Brumpt (1910) who observed *T. rajae* and *T. scyllii* forming colonies of dividing spherical cells giving rise to mastigotes. Continuous cultivation of the former species, using Johnson's (1947) medium at a temperature of 11°C or 20°C, was reported by Preston (1969). Ranque (1973) grew *T. boissoni* on Tobie's and on NNN diphasic media and with much better results on fluid and semi-fluid media (brain-heart-infusion agar with blood, nutrient broth with blood). The latter media also supported abundant growth of *T. triglae senegalensis*. Ranque was unable to grow *T. cephalacanthi* and *T. sphaeroidis* on any of the media.

Trypanosoma danilewskyi from cyprinid fishes, *T. percae* from perches (*Perca fluviatilis*) and *T. ?remaki* from pikes are very easy to cultivate at a temperature of 25°C in diphasic blood agar media with transfers every 10 days (Lom and Suchánková, 1974). *T. danilewskyi* may reach a concentration of more than 5×10^7/ml; there is always a sequence of epimastigote and trypomastigote stages. A short-term stay in culture does not impair the infectivity for goldfish (and carps). After four *in vitro* passages, the infectivity is lowered. However, even after 30 passages the cultural forms may infect the goldfish; in the case observed, the prepatent period of infection took 6 months, compared to 4 to 35 days in syringe-passaged trypanosomes. There was one exception: *T. danilewskyi* strain Ma isolated from goldfish, after 6 consecutive syringe passages which took a period of 1·5 years, grew *in vitro* in the trypomastigote bloodstream stage only. Even after an additional two years of syringe-passaging, it was possible to transfer this strain into a diphasic culture medium. When established in culture, the strain preserved its infectivity for fish even for a considerable number of serial *in vitro* passages. Its unique feature is its conservation of constant biological as well as morphological characters seemingly irrespective of prolonged maintenance *in vitro* or *in vivo*, and can be easily transferred between goldfish and culture, as well as between goldfish and leech, and leech and culture.

T. danilewskyi can also be transferred to fish tissue cultures of the strains FHM and BB (American Type Culture Collection) on Eagle's MEM medium with 10% bovine foetal or calf serum. It can be maintained continuously at the optimal temperature of 25°C (Smolíková *et al.*, 1977a, b). Hemin enrichment (2 mg/100 ml) of the medium considerably promotes the growth. However, hemin-enriched tissue culture medium without the presence of living cells failed to support the trypanosomes continuously. The Ma strain kept its trypomastigote phase in tissue culture, too. The trypanosomes did not penetrate into the cells and showed no cytopathogenic effect.

The abundance of the growth is always temperature dependent; Quadri (1962c) found the growth limits for *T. striati* (its host, *Ophiocephalus striatus*, is a warm-water fish) to be 12° and 32°C.

1. Morphological stages of *in vitro*-grown trypanosomes

Upon transfer into the culture medium, bloodstream stages transform into stages comparable to the forms in the leech vector. As a rule, the occurrence of dividing epimastigotes and later trypomastigotes are typical in all species; the exact structure and shape of these stages varies with species and with conditions of culture. Additional morphological stages were amastigotes, observed in marine species, and promastigotes recorded in freshwater trypanosomes. There is binary, rarely multiple, division in the culture.

In *T. boissoni* from skates, Ranque (1973) observed epimastigotes at the start of the culture growth, and a later differentiation including amastigotes and trypomastigotes; in *T. triglae*, the occurrence of amastigotes was rather exceptional. Preston (1969) observed three main structural types—non-motile "stubby" epimastigotes with a barely emergent flagellum, elongated motile epimastigotes and trypomastigotes.

A little more is known on the morphological diversity of freshwater trypanosomes in culture. The epimastigotes may be extremely variable in shape, the greatest variation recorded being in *T. striati* (from droplike to long filamentous) (Quadri, 1962c). The same author recorded a tendency in *T. winchesiense* (synonym of *T. ?danilewskyi*) to assume broad and globular (?sphaeromastigote) stages. Culture forms divide by binary fission, mostly unequal, sometimes almost equal, and rarely by multiple division (e.g., Thompson, 1908).

The greatest individual variation in morphology may be observed in long lasting cultures, initiated by a small number of individuals, which invariably end with production of bloodstream type trypomastigotes, although the latter may sometimes resemble more a salivarian species than the respective fish trypanosome. In densely growing cultures, passaged at regular, 10 day, intervals at about 25°C, the cyclic alternation of epi- and trypomastigotes is well manifested, while these stages themselves are not that variable (Smolíková *et al.*, 1977). In a diphasic medium (SNB 9) the percentage of trypomastigote stages of the *T. danilewskyi* strain MS decreased on average to 9% on the third day post inoculation, and from then on, it rose to 93% at the tenth day; the reverse applied to epimastigotes.

The dependence of the trypomastigote : epimastigote ratio, as well as of the morphology of the organisms, on conditions of cultivation were evidenced upon transfer of this strain into media of different composition. If cultivated with FHM-cell line in MEM medium, the epimastigote : trypomastigote ratio shifted from 63 : 37 on day 1 after inoculation to 15 : 85 in declining culture, indicating that some trypomastigotes evidently do not transform at all. In the SNB medium the length of the free flagellum in trypomastigotes averaged 2·6 μm, while it was 3·8 μm in the other medium. If this tissue culture medium was enriched by hemin, the epimastigote : trypomastigote ratio shifted from 92 : 8 on the first day to 15 : 85 in the declining culture, while there was almost no change in the trypomastigote free flagellum length (3·2 μm). In the MEM medium without the presence of living tissue cells, while there was a similar shift in epimastigote : trypomastigote ratio (87 : 13 to 7 : 93), there was also a moiety of promastigote stages on day 2 to 4, reaching up to 5 %. The trypomastigote free flagellum length averaged 8·9 μm, and the trypomastigotes were of a typical bloodstream *T. danilewskyi* appearance, while in all former cultures the final trypomastigotes were not exactly like the bloodstream phase (the kinetoplast was more distant from the posterior end, and there was a short free flagellum).

B. TRYPANOPLASMA

Being much less easy to cultivate than fish trypanosomes, the list of successful attempts is very meagre. Ponselle (1913a, b) used his modification of solid blood agar medium for growing *T. varium* in the condensation fluid; he described a successful cloning of the flagellates in subcultures. Tanabe (1924) grew *Trypanoplasma* sp. from *Misgurnus anguillicaudatus* on Ponselle's and NNN medium; he does not mention subcultures. Nowicki (1940) briefly mentioned having cultured *T. cyprini* in Ponselle's medium; he gave no details. Quadri (1962b) established a continuous culture in NNN medium for *T. willoughbyi*. Putz (1972b) was unable to subcultivate *T. cataractae* in three types of diphasic media, tissue culture medium M 199 and in foetal bovine fluid, having achieved only a limited success in the primary culture. In preliminary experiments of the writer, *T. borelli* from carps readily grew in primary culture and for two subcultures (10% of dividing stages) in diluted defibrinated rabbit blood or in SNB and 4N diphasic media; however, continuous culture was not achieved. A short-term stay (one week) in the culture medium did not impair the infectivity for goldfish.

1. Morphological stages of *Trypanoplasma* grown *in vitro*

The paucity of information on this subject corresponds to the rarity of successful cultivation attempts. Ponselle (1913a, b) found, in his culture of *T. varium*, flagellates complying morphologically with bloodstream forms, and failed to find the long slender forms typical of the leech phase. Quadri (1962b) described the primary culture forms as resembling roughly the bloodstream forms, while subcultures contained predominantly slender, elongated stages in which the nucleus was situated far posteriad behind the kinetonucleus or even close to the posterior end of the cell. In addition, there were large stubby forms and small, rounded ones with a rounded kinetoplast. There were both binary and multiple fissions.

V. Taxonomic considerations

A. TRYPANOSOMA

To my knowledge, 153 species of trypanosomes have been described from marine and freshwater hosts. In addition, 33 unnamed records from various hosts exist (there may be more, since they are rather difficult to trace). Since Laveran and Mesnil (1912), numerous descriptions have appeared; some of the papers, though primarily taxonomic, contain also a certain amount of information on life cycles, pleomorphism, ecology and distribution (Yakimoff, 1912; de Fonseca, 1929, 1935; de Fonseca and Vaz, 1929; Nikitin, 1929; Hoare, 1932; Pearse, 1933; Rodhain, 1942; Quadri, 1955, 1962a–d; Chen, 1956; Hawking, 1957; Dogiel and Akhmerov, 1959; Hansan and Qasim, 1962; Becker, 1967; Abolarin, 1970; Vinnichenko *et al.*, 1970; Daly and DeGiusti, 1971; Khaybulyaev, 1971; Misera *et al.*, 1973; Raychaudhuri and Misra, 1973; Mandel, 1975; Lima, 1976).

As a matter of caution, for each species listed below, only the original host and locality are given, since, because of frequently inadequate descriptions, one cannot be sure of later correct identifications.

Trypanosomes from freshwater fishes

1. *Trypanosoma abramis* Laveran and Mesnil, 1904. *Abramis brama*; France.

2. *T. acanthobramae* Warsi and Fattohy, 1976. *Acanthobrama marmid*; Tigris, Iraq.

3. *T. albopunctatus* Fonseca, 1929. *Plecostomus albopunctatus*; Brazil.

4. *T. acerinae* Brumpt, 1906. *Acerina cernua*; France.

5. *T. amurensis* Vinichenko, 1971. *Mesocottus heitei*; Amur river, Asia.

6. *T. andrade-silvae* Dias, 1952. *Clarias gariepinus*; Mozambique, Africa.

7. *T. anguillicola* Johnston and Cleland, 1910. *Anguilla reinhardii, A. mauritans*; Australia.

8. *T. anura* Vinichenko, 1971. *Acipenser schrenki*; Amur river, Asia.

9. *T. aristichthysi* Chen, 1956. *Arystichthys nobilis*; China.

10. *T. armeti* Mandal, 1955. *Mastacembulus armatus*; India.

11. *T. ataevi* Khaibulaev, 1971. *Gobius ratan goebeli, G. kessleri gorlap, G. fluviatilis pallasi, Benthophilus macrocephalus*; Caspian Sea, Asia.

12. *T. bancrofti* Johnston and Cleland, 1910. *Copidoglanis tandanus*; Australia.

13. *T. barbatulae* Léger, 1904. *Noemachailus barbatula*; France (possibly synonym of No. 27; see Breindl 1915).

14. *T. barbi* Brumpt, 1906. *Barbus fluviatilis*; France.

15. *T. batrachi* Quadri, 1961. *Clarias batrachus*; India.

16. *T. batrachocephali* Schapowal, 1954. *Mesogobius batrachocephalus*; Ukrainian SSR, USSR.

17. *T. bliccae* Nikitin, 1929. *Blicca bjoerkna*; European part of the USSR.
18. *T. bourouli* Neiva and Pinto, 1926. *Symbranchus marmoratus*; Brazil.
19. *T. carassi* Mitrofanov, 1883. *Carassius carassius*; European part of the USSR.
20. *T. catostomi* Daly and DeGiusti, 1971. *Catostomus commersonii commersonii*; USA.
21. *T. chagasi* Horta and Machado, 1911. *Plecostomus* sp.; Brazil.
22. *T. cheni* Chen, 1964. *Ophiocephalus argus*; China.
23. *T. chetostomi* Fonseca, 1929. *Chetostomus* sp.; Brazil.
24. *T. choudhuryi* Mandal, 1977. *Tilapia mossambica*; India.
25. *T. clariae* Montel, 1905. *Clarias* (= *Silurus*) *clariae*; Vietnam, Asia.
26. *T. clariae* var. *batrachi* Froilano de Mello and Valles, 1936. *Clarias batrachus*; India.
27. *T. cobitis* Mitrofanov, 1883. *Cobitis fossilis*; European part of the USSR.
28. *T. ctenopharyngodoni* Chen and Hsieh, 1964. *Ctenopharyngodon idellus*; China.
29. *T. danilewskyi* Laveran and Mesnil, 1904. *Cyprinus carpio*; Europe.
30. *T. danilewskyi* var. *saccobranchi* Quadri, 1962. *Saccobranchus fossilis*; India.
31. *T. dogieli* Winichenko, 1971. *Gobio albipinatus tenuicorpus, Chilogobio czerskii*; Amur river, Asia.
32. *T. dorbygnii* Fonseca, 1929. *Rhinodorus dorbigny*; Brazil.
33. *T. elegans* Brumpt, 1906. *Gobio gobio*; France.
34. *T. elongatus* Raychaudhuri and Misra, 1973. *Ophicephalus punctatus*; India.
35. *T. ferreirae* Fonseca, 1929. *Characinidae* sp.; Brazil.
36. *T. francirochai* Fonseca and Vaz, 1928. *Otocinchus francirochai*; Brazil.
37. *T. gachuii* Misra, Chandra and Choudhury, 1973. *Ophiocephalus gachua*; India.
38. *T. gandhei* Rodhain, 1942. *Labeo macrostoma*; Congo river basin, Africa.
39. *T. gasimagomedovi* Khaibulyaev, 1971. *Pungitius platigaster*; Caspian Sea, Asia.
40. *T. gerraroi* Dias, 1955. *Tilapia mossambica*; Africa.
41. *T. granulosum* Laveran and Mesnil, 1909. *Anguilla fluviatilis*; France.
42. *T. hypostomi* Splendore, 1910. *Hypostomus auroguttatus*; Brazil.
43. *T. iheringi* Fonseca, 1935. *Franciscodoras marmoratus*; Brazil.
44. *T. langeroni* Brumpt, 1906. *Cottus gobio*; France.
45. *T. larsi* Fonseca, 1929. *Prochilodus* sp.; Brazil.
46. *T. latinucleata* Vinichenko, 1971. *Parasilurus asotus*; Amur river, Asia.

47. *T. laverani* Breindl, 1912. *Alburnus lucidus*; Czechoslovakia.
48. *T. leucisci* Brumpt, 1906. *Leuciscus* spp.; France.
49. *T. liocassis* Dogiel and Achmerov, 1959. *Liocassis ussuriensis*; Amur river, Asia.
50. *T. loricariae* Fonseca, 1929. *Loricaria* sp.; Brazil.
50a. *T. lotai* Smirnova, 1970. *Lota lota*; European part of the USSR.
51. *T. luciopercae* Nikitin, 1929. *Stizostedion lucioperca*; European part of the USSR.
52. *T. macrodonis* Botelho, 1907. *Macrodon malabaricus*; Brazil.
53. *T. maguri* Tandon and Joshi, 1973. *Clarias batrachus*, *Mystus villatus*; India.
54. *T. malopteruri* Rodhain, 1942. *Malopterurus electricus*; Congo river basin, Africa.
55. *T. margaritiferi* Fonseca, 1929. *Plecostomus margaritifer*; Brazil.
56. *T. markewitschi* Lubinsky in Salewskaja-Schapowal, 1950. *Parasilurus asotus*; Uzbekistan, Asian part of the USSR.
57. *T. marplatensis* Bacigalupo and Delaplaza, 1948. "Las rayas de mar plate"; Brazil.
58. *T. minuta* Chen and Hsieh, 1964. *Erythroculter dabryi*; China.
59. *T. mukasai* Hoare, 1932. *Haplochromis nubilis*, *H. serratus*, *H. cinereus*, *H. humilior*; Lake Victoria, Africa.
60. *T. mukundi* Raychaudhuri and Misra, 1973. *Heteropneustes fossilis*; India.
61. *T. mylopharyngodoni* Chen, 1956. *Mylopharyngodon piceus*; China.
62. *T. napolesi* Dias, 1955. *Tilapia mossambica*; Mozambique, Africa.
62a. *T. neinavana* Fattohy, 1978. *Batbus grypus*; Iraq.
63. *T. nikitini* Schapowal, 1953. *Aspius aspius*; European part of the USSR.
64. *T. occidentalis* Becker, 1967. *Cottus gulosus*, *C. rhotheus*, *Gasterosteus aculeatus*; Washington, USA.
65. *T. ophiocephali* Pearse, 1933. *Ophiocephalus striatus*; Thailand, Asia.
66. *T. orientalis* Chen and Hsieh, 1964. *Hemibarbus maculatus*, *Pseudorasbora parva*; China.
67. *T. pancali* Mandal, 1976. *Mastacembelus pancalas*; India.
68. *T. parasiluri* Chen and Hsieh, 1964. *Parasilurus asotus*; China.
69. *T. pellegrini* Mathia and Léger, 1911. *Macropodus viridi-auratus*; Vietnam, Asia.
70. *T. percae* Brumpt, 1906. *Perca fluviatilis*; France.
71. *T. percae canadensis* Fantham, Porter and Richardson, 1942. *Perca flavescens*; Canada.
72. *T. phoxini* Brumpt, 1906. *Phoxinus laevis*; France.
73. *T. piavae* Fonseca, 1929. Characinidae sp.; Brazil.
74. *T. pingi* Chen and Hsieh, 1964. *Carassius auratus*; China.
75. *T. piracicaboe* Fonseca, 1929. *Loricaria piracicaboe*; Brazil.
76. *T. plecostomi* Fonseca, 1929. *Plecostomus* sp.; Brazil.

77. *T. pseudobagri* Dogiel and Achmerov, 1959. *Pseudobagrus fulvidraco*; Amur river, Asia.

78. *T. punctati* Hasan and Quasim, 1962. *Ophiocephalus punctatus*; India.

79. *T. rebeloi* Dias, 1955. *Tilapia mossambica*; Mozambique, Africa.

80. *T. regani* Fonseca, 1929. *Plecostomus regani*; Brazil.

81. *T. remaki* Laveran and Mesnil, 1901. *Esox lucius*; France.

82. *T. rhamdiae* Botelho, 1907. *Rhamdia quelen*; Brazil.

83. *T. roulei* Mathis and Léger, 1911. *Monopterus javanensis*; Vietnam, Asia.

84. *T. saccobranchi* Castellani and Willey, 1905. *Saccobranchus fossilis*; India.

85. *T. sarcochilichthys* Dogiel and Achmerov, 1959. *Sarcochilichthys sinensis*; Amur river, Asia.

86. *T. scardinii* Brumpt, 1906. *Scardinius erythrophthalmus*; France.

87. *T. schulmani* Khaybulyayev, 1971. *Esox lucius*; Caspian Sea, Asia.

88. *T. serranoi* Dias, 1955. *Tilapia mossambica*; Mozambique, Africa.

89. *T. siluri* Li, in Vinichenko *et al.*, 1971. *Silurus soldatovi, Parasilurus asotus*; Amur river, Asia.

90. *T. simondi* Lebeuf and Ringenbach, 1910. *Anchenoglanis biscutatus*; Africa.

91. *T. siniperca* Chang, 1964. *Siniperca chuatsi*; China.

92. *T. sinipercae* Vinichenko *et al.*, 1971. *Siniperca chua-tsi*; Amur river, Asia.

93. *T. squalii* Brumpt, 1906. *Leuciscus cephalus*; France.

94. *T. striata* Vinichenko *et al.*, 1971. *Liocassis braschnikowi*; Amur River, Asia.

95. *T. striati* Quadri, 1955. *Ophiocephalus striatus*; India.

96. *T. strigaticeps* Fonseca, 1929. *Plecostomus strigaticeps*; Brazil.

97. *T. synodontis* Lebeuf and Ringenbach, 1910. *Synodontis notatus*; Africa.

98. *T. tchangi* Chen and Hsieh, 1964. *Siniperca knerii, Ochetobius elongatus*; China.

99. *T. tincae* Laveran and Mesnil, 1904. *Tinca vulgaris*; France.

100. *T. tobeyi* Dias, 1952. *Clarias angolensis*; Congo river basin, Africa.

101. *T. toddi* Bouet, 1909. *Clarias anguillaris*; Africa.

102. *T. trichogasterae* Pearse, 1933. *Trichogaster trichopterus*; Thailand, Asia.

103. *T. vittati* Tandon and Joshi, 1973. *Clarias batrachus, Mystus vittatus*; India.

104. *T. wangi* Chen and Hsieh, 1964. *Sarcocheilichthys nigripinnis*; China.

105. *T. wincheniense* Quadri, 1962. *Cyprinus carpio*; England.

106. *T. zillii* Léger, 1914. *Tilapia lata*; Africa.

107. *T. zungaroi* Fonseca, 1929. *Pseudopimelodus zungaro*; Brazil.

Trypanosoma sp. Chen and Hsieh, 1964. *Culter bravicauda*; China.

Trypanosoma sp. 1 Dogiel and Achmerov, 1959. *Siniperca chua-tsi*; Amur river, Asia.

Trypanosoma sp. 2 Dogiel and Achmerov, 1959. *Pseudaspius leptocephalus*; Amur River, Asia.

Trypanosoma sp. Fantham and Porter, 1947. *Salvelinus fontinalis*; Canada.

Trypanosoma sp. Hawkings, 1957. *Phoxinus phoxinus, Cottus gobio*; England.

Trypanosoma sp. Kairova, 1970. *Perca schrenki*; Kazahstan, USSR.

Trypanosoma sp. Lingard, 1904. *Ophiocephalus striatus*; India.

Trypanosoma sp. Lingard, 1904. *Trichogaster fasciatus, Macrones seenghala*; India.

Trypanosoma sp. Mathis and Léger, 1911. *Anabas scandens*; Vietnam, Asia.

Trypanosoma sp. Mathis and Léger, 1911. *Ophiocephalus striatus*; Vietnam, Asia.

Trypanosoma sp. Mathis and Léger, 1911. *Ophiocephalus maculatus*; Vietnam, Asia.

Trypanosoma sp. Naeve, 1906. *Bagrus bayad*; Sudan, Africa.

Trypanosoma sp. Naeve, 1906. *Mugil* sp.; Sudan, Africa.

Trypanosoma sp. Naeve, 1906. *Polypterus* sp.; Sudan, Africa.

Trypanosoma sp. Naeve, 1906. *Syndontis schall*; Sudan, Africa.

Trypanosoma sp. Ogawa and Uegaki, 1927. *Anguila mauritiana*; Taiwan, Asia.

Trypanosoma sp. Ogawa and Uegaki, 1927. *Clarias fuscus*; Taiwan, Asia.

Trypanosoma sp. Ogawa and Uegaki, 1927. *Fluta alba*; Taiwan, Asia.

Trypanosoma sp. Ogawa and Uegaki, 1927. *Fulvidraco* sp.; Taiwan, Asia.

Trypanosoma sp. Ogawa and Uegaki, 1927. *Ophiocephalus maculatus*; Taiwan, Asia.

Trypanosoma sp. Rodhain, 1907. *Labeo macrostoma*; Congo river basin, Africa.

Trypanosoma sp. Rodhain, 1907. *Labeo zalzifer*; Congo river basin, Africa.

Trypanosoma sp. Rodhain, 1907. *Malopterus electricus*; Congo river basin, Africa.

Trypanosoma sp. Schapowal, 1953. *Chondrostoma schmidti*; European part of the USSR.

Trypanosoma sp. Wenyon, 1908. *Chrysichthys auratii*; Sudan, Africa.

Trypanosoma sp. Wenyon, 1908. *Ophiocephalus obscurus*; Sudan, Africa.

Trypanosoma sp. Wenyon, 1908. *Tilapia zillii*; Sudan, Africa.

Trypanosoma sp. Zupitza, 1909. *Periophthalmus koelreuteri, Clarias* spp.; Africa.

Trypanosomes from marine fishes

108. *Trypanosoma aulopi* Mackerras and Mackerras, 1925. *Aulopus purpurissatus*; Australian coast.

109. *T. balistes* Saunders, 1959. *Balistes carpiscus*; Atlantic coast of Florida, USA.
110. *T. bleniclini* Fantham, 1930. *Blennius cornutus, Clinus anguillaris*; coast of South Africa.
111. *T. boissoni* Ranque, 1967. *Zanobatus atlanticus*; Senegal coast, Africa.
112. *T. bothi* Lebailly, 1905. *Scophtalmus rhombus*; Atlantic coast of France.
113. *T. callionymi* Brumpt and Lebailly, 1904. *Callionymus dracunculus*; Atlantic coast of France.
114. *T. capigobii* Fantham, 1919. *Gobius nudiceps*; coast of South Africa.
115. *T. carchariasi* Laveran, 1908. *Carcharias* sp.; Australian coast.
116. *T. cataphracti* Henry, 1913. *Agonus cataphractus*; English coast at Plymouth (the only reference found is in Schäperclaus, 1954).
117. *T. caulopsettae* Laird, 1951. *Caulopsetta scapha, Rhombosolea plebeia*; New Zealand coast.
118. *T. cephalacanthi* Ranque, 1967. *Cephalacanthus volitans*; Senegal coast, Africa.
119. *T. coelorhynchi* Laird, 1951. *Coelorhynchus australis*; *Physiculus bachus*; New Zealand coast.
120. *T. congiopodi* Laird, 1951. *Congiopodus leucopaecilus*; New Zealand.
121. *T. cotti* Brumpt and Lebailly, 1904. *Cottus bubalis*; Atlantic coast of France.
122. *T. delagei* Brumpt and Lebailly, 1904. *Blennius pholis*; Atlantic coast of France.
123. *T. dohrni* Yakimoff, 1911. *Solea monochir*; Mediterranean Sea off Naples, Italy.
124. *T. flesi* Lebailly, 1904. *Pleuronectes flesus*; Atlantic coast of France.
125. *T. froesi* Lima, 1976. *Mugil brasilensis*; Atlantic coast of Brazil.
126. *T. gargantua* Laird, 1951. *Raja nasuta*; New Zealand coast.
127. *T. giganteum* Neumann, 1909. *Raja oxyrhynchus*; Mediterranean Sea off Naples, Italy.
128. *T. gobii* Brumpt and Lebailly, 1904. *Gobius niger*; Atlantic coast of France.
129. *T. heptatreti* Laird, 1948. *Heptatetrus cirrhatus*; New Zealand coast.
130. *T. laternae* Lebailly, 1904. *Arnoglossus laterna*; Atlantic coast of France.
131. *T. limandae* Brumpt and Lebailly, 1904. *Limanda limanda*; Atlantic coast of France.
132. *T. murmanensis* Nikitin, 1927. *Gadus callarias*; Arctic Ocean.
133. *T. myoxocephali* Fantham, Porter and Richardson, 1942. *Myoxocephalus octodecemspinosus*; Atlantic coast of Nova Scotia.
134. *T. nudigobii* Fantham, 1919. *Gobius*(?) sp.; South African coast (original paper not seen).

135. *T. pacifica* Burreson and Pratt, 1972. *Parophrys vetulus*; Pacific coast of Oregon, USA.
136. *T. parapercis* Laird, 1951. *Parapercis colias*; New Zealand coast.
137. *T. platessae* Lebailly, 1904. *Pleuronectes platessa*; Atlantic coast of France.
138. *T. pulchra* Mackerras and Mackerras, 1925. *Ellerkeldia semicincta*; Australian coast.
139. *T. rajae* Laveran and Mesnil, 1902. *Raja punctata, R. mosaica, R. macrorhynchus* and *R. clavata*; Atlantic coast of France.
140. *T. scorpaenae* Neumann, 1909. *Scorpaena ustulata*; Mediterranean Sea off Naples, Italy.
141. *T. scyllii* Laveran and Mesnil, 1902. *Scyllium stellare*; Atlantic coast of France.
142. *T. soleae* Laveran and Mesnil, 1901. *Solea vulgaris*; Atlantic coast of France.
143. *T. sphaeroidis* Ranque, 1968. *Sphaeroides spengleri*; Senegal coast, Africa.
144. *T. torpedinis* Sabrazes and Muratet, 1908. *Torpedo marmorata*; French coast.
145. *T. triglae* Neumann, 1909. *Trigla corax*; Mediterranean Sea off Naples, Italy.
146. *T. triglae senegalensis* Ranque, 1967. *Trigla lineata*; Senegal coast, Africa.
147. *T. tripterygium* Laird, 1951. *Tripterygion varium, T. medium*; New Zealand coast.
148. *T. variabile* Neumann, 1909. *Raja punctata*; Mediterranean Sea off Naples, Italy.
149. *T. yakimovi* Wladimiroff, 1910. *Syngnathus acus*; Mediterranean Sea off Naples, Italy.
Trypanosoma sp. Baker and Brown, 1971. *Mugil cephalus*; Atlantic coast of Florida, USA.
Trypanosoma sp. Fantham, 1919. *Raja capensis*; South African coast.
Trypanosoma sp. So, 1972 .*Glyptocephalus cynoglossus*; Newfoundland coast.
Trypanosoma Wurtz and Thiroux, 1909. *Thalassina columna*; Senegal coast, Africa.
Trypanosoma sp. Yakimoff, 1910. *Syngnathus acus*; Black Sea.
Not listed are species established without any description, i.e., *nomina nuda*:
   Trypanosoma zeugopteri Henry, 1910, from *Zeugopterus punctatus* at the British coast. Marine.
   Trypanosoma aeglefini Henry, 1913, from *Melanogrammus aeglefinus* at the British coast. Marine.
   Trypanosoma ezenami Khaybulyayev, 1970, from *Salmo trutta ezenami*, Dagestan, USSR. Freshwater.

Undoubtedly many of the above listed species are either not valid or are synonyms. It is unfortunate that many authors have protected themselves in the "publish or perish" struggle by publishing papers increasing the taxonomic confusion; let us quote a sequence from a recent paper: ". . . it resembles *T. danilewskyi* but is described as new because trypanosomes have not previously been reported from this list or from this or neighbouring countries." This practice has created a lot of synonyms, of which only the most striking will be quoted.

Four separate species were described from *Clarias batrachus* from India (species Nos. 15, 26, 52 and 103); there is another one from *Clarias clarias* from Vietnam (species No. 25). Two separate species from *Siniperca chua-tsi* from China (species Nos. 91 and 92). Three species were recorded in *Parasilurus asotus* from China (species Nos. 45, 67 and 89). From closely related species, *Gobio gobio* and *Gobio albipinnatus*, were described two different species (Nos. 33 and 31). From the Asian *Ophiocephalus striatus* were described two different species (Nos. 64 and 95) while three more hosts of the genus *Ophiocephalus* seem to harbour three different trypanosomes (Nos. 22, 37 and 78; the latter, *T. punctati* may, however, be a valid species if it really has such a huge kinetoplast as described). There is a question of pleomorphic trypanosomes described from skates of the genus *Raja*; for example, Minchin and Woodcock (1910) suggest that *T. variabile* may well be synonymous with *T. rajae*. It may prove to be necessary to reduce these and possibly other species to synonymy, as Baker (1960) did with species described from Africa, limiting the number of valid ones to three (Nos. 58, 100 and 101). An important problem of synonymy concerns *T. danilewskyi*. Its identity with *T. carassii* (Mitrophanow, 1883) from crucian carps seems most probable (as suggested already by Laveran and Mesnil, 1912) because of no contrasting features in morphology and relatively easy transfers of trypanosome populations from carps to crucian carps and *vice versa*. Although in many papers, including those of experimental nature, trypanosome populations from carps are dealt with under this name, it would probably have to be replaced by *T. carassii*. *T. pingi* and *T. winchesiense* (species No. 73 and 105) are its evident junior synonyma, too. Many other species described from fish hosts on the Eurasian continent also seem to be closely related in their morphology (Nos 17, 31, 34, 66 and 67). The problem could be a model one for the study of speciation, if morphologically almost identical species would reveal restrictive adaptations to certain hosts. A question could thus be asked similar to that raised by Hommel and Miltgen (1974) in the *Herpetosoma*-complex; is it a complex of closely related species or one species adapted for a life in different hosts? To solve the problem of species will make us understand host specificity and many important aspects of the host–parasite relationship. However, a meticulous light-microscope study may not be enough. The similarity in structure and the variability of characters in each of the freshwater trypanosomes he studied led Breindl (1915) to assume it would be better to deal with them as biological races of a single species, *T. piscium*. A long-term study of life cycle, cross infection experiments and, possibly, also biochemical and immunological methods will be required. According to existing data, however fragmentary and uneven it is, piscine trypanosomes can be assembled into two large groupings, comprising pleomorphic and monomorphic (with the reservations stated on p. 297) species:

(A) Pleomorphic species: the sequence of forms in the vertebrate host shows changes in body size and structure (see p. 297).
 (1) Species from marine hosts (including Agnatha, Chondreichthyes and Osteichthyes). Kinetoplast not terminal, mostly far from the posterior end. Posterior end of the cell pointed; adult morphs often very large and broad with subsurface striation present. Development in the leech starts with production of amastigotes.

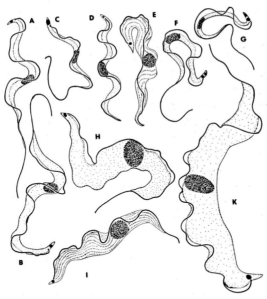

FIG. 20. Trypanosomes of freshwater fish, various morphological types. Redrawn to the same scale from original sources. A—*T. mylopharyngodoni* (from Chen, 1956). B—*T. siluri* (from Vinnitchenko *et al.*, 1971). C—*T. punctati* (from Hasan and Qasim, 1962). D—*T. anura*, E—*T. amurensis* (both from Vinnitchenko *et al.*, 1971). F—*T. ctenopharyngodoni*, G—*T. minuta* (both from Chen and Hsieh, 1964). H—*T. latinucleata*, I—*T. striata* (both from Vinnitchenko *et al.*, 1971). K—*T. striati* (from Qadri, 1955).

(a) Young and adult morphs without or with an extremely short free flagellum and a marked striation. Adult morphs huge and broad: e.g., *T. gargantua* (Fig. 28C), *T. boissoni.*

(b) Free flagellum well developed: e.g., *T. heptatreti* (Fig. 28D), *T. tripterygium, T. variabile, T. caulopsettae, T. giganteum, T. murmanensis* (species with marked striation); *T. coelorhynchi* (Fig. 28F—species with a faintly visible striation); *T. rajae* (Fig. 28G—striation undetected).

(2) Species from freshwater Osteichthyes. Kinetoplast in young morphs almost subterminal, in adults often quite far from the hind end; adult forms not so large as in marine species. Development in the leech starts with production of epimastigotes (and ?sphaero-mastigotes). They can be further subdivided:

(a) Species in which only morphs (evidently adult ones) without a free flagellum were described: e.g., *T. amurensis* (Fig. 20E).

(b) The same as (a), but with a free flagellum: e.g., *T. striata* (Fig. 20I)—with distinct striation, *T. latinucleata* (Fig. 20H)—without distinct striation.

(c) Species in which the sequence of morphs is known; adult forms with striation: e.g., *T. percae* (Fig. 23), *T. granulosum* (Fig. 15C), *T. occidentalis.*

(d) The same as (c), but adult morphs described without striation: e.g., *T. striati* (Fig. 20K), *T. mukasai, T. gandei, T. leucisci.*

(B) Monomorphic species (as defined on p. 297)

(1) Freshwater species

(a) Trypanosomes with a long, slender body, kinetoplast terminal or subterminal, a long free flagellum. Development in the leech starts with the production of epimastigotes (and some sphaero-mastigotes), e.g., *T. danilewskyi* (Figs 21, 22), *T. mylopharyngodoni* (Fig. 20A), *T. tchangi, T. catostomi, T. dogieli, T. vittati, T. sinipercae.*

(b) The same as (a), but with an unusually large kinetoplast: e.g., *T. punctati* (Fig. 20C).

(c) The same as (a), but without a free flagellum: e.g., *T. anura* (Fig. 20D).

(d) The same as (a), but with two kinetoplasts: e.g., *T. ctenopharyn-*

FIGS 21–27. *Figs 21, 22—Trypanosoma danilewskyi* isolated from tench and maintained *in vivo* in goldfish (figures all at the same magnification). *Fig. 23—* Adult form of *T. percae* from perch. *Fig. 24*—Adult form of *T. elegans* from gudgeon. *Fig. 25—T. remaki* from pike. *Fig. 26*—Adult form of *T. acerinae* from ruff. *Fig. 27—T. danilewskyi* from carp. Cultural form with granules with heavy formazan deposits showing $NADH_2$-tetrazolium reductase activity. Scales equal 10 μm.

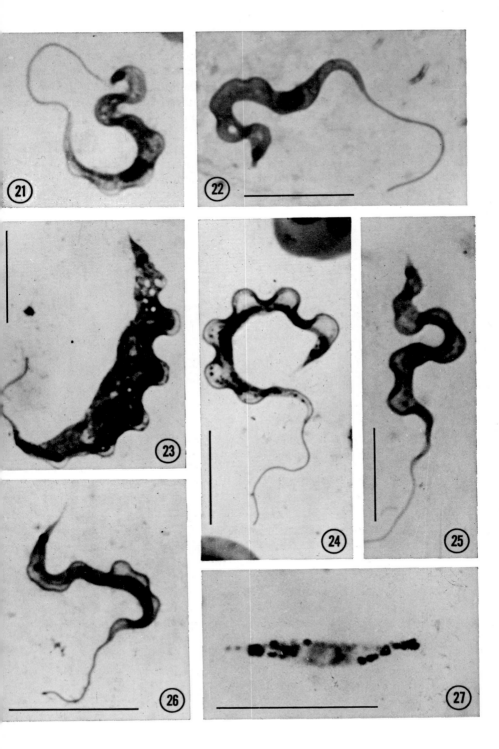

godoni, T. minuta (Figs 20F, G). If the existence of two kinetoplasts is confirmed, this category should constitute a new genus.

(2) Marine species. Similar in appearance to freshwater trypanosomes
but probably differing in the developmental sequence in the leech,
starting with amastigotes. Kinetoplast terminal or subterminal, free
flagellum developed: e.g., *T. cephalacanthi* (Fig. 28E), *T. solae, T.
sphaeroides, T. triglae senegalensis.*

If the criteria in the above scheme seem rather inconsistent, it is also
because of the exasperating unevenness of our knowledge. Differences in
migration routes in the digestive tract of the leech and in the main sites
of reproduction were not listed; so far the data are very scanty.

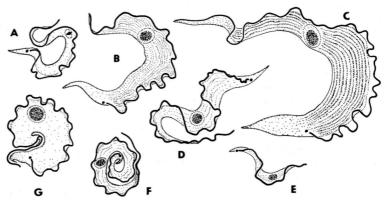

FIG. 28.   Marine fish trypanosomes, redrawn from original sources to the same
scale. A, B, C—young, intermediate and adult forms of *T. gargantua* (from Laird,
1951). D—*T. heptatreti* (from Laird, 1951). E—*T. cephalacanthi* (from Ranque,
1973). F—*T. coelorhynchi* (from Laird, 1951). G—*T. rajae* (from Laird and
Bullock, 1968).

The categories of "piscine" trypanosomes cannot be grouped according to taxonomic position of the hosts: there is no essential difference
either between pleomorphic species from marine hagfish, Chondrich-
thyes and Osteichthyes, or between monomorphic species from marine
elasmobranches and bony fishes. However, the incontestable differences
in the above scheme amount to a level permitting establishment in the
near future (as soon as the salient features are better known in more
species) of supra-specific categories like those erected by Hoare (1964)
for mammalian trypanosomes (for a recent review see Vickerman, 1977).
There may be subgenera, if the divergence between the categories is
deemed profound, as suggested by Lumsden (1974) for Hoare's subgenera, and even genera.

Many piscine trypanosomes reveal a great resemblance of their "adult" morphs to corresponding stages of some of the amphibian, reptilian, avian and, to a certain extent, mammalian species. In the two latter groups, similarities may extend beyond the morphological level as, for example, the fact of division of trypomastigotes in circulating blood brings them close to salivarian trypanosomes; however, the different modes of transmission and adaptation to homoiothermy preclude further comparison. Among reptilian trypanosomes, the leech-vectored species from chelonians reveal considerable resemblances in morphology and developmental stages. Some of the leech-vectored amphibian species differ from all piscine ones in the structure of the adult morphs (*T. rotatorium*), or in other characters (e.g. presence of polysaccharide reserves or the low infectivity of stages from the circulating blood for another host; Bardsley and Harmsen, 1973). However, some are more akin morphologically and biologically (division of trypomastigotes in the blood in *T. grylli*; Nigrelli, 1945).

Thus it may be possible that the subgeneric categories, unlike the guiding principle in Hoare's classification, will not consist in grouping the species of a given high-order taxonomic unit of hosts, but rather within the whole assemblage of leech-vectored trypanosomes. This would be in agreement with possible common phylogenetical lineage of leech-transmitted trypanosomes, as quite plausibly proposed by Baker (1974). The subgenera may thus reach across the piscine–amphibian–reptilian borders as they in fact do across the Agnatha–Chondreichthyes–Osteichthyes boundaries.

These future subgeneric categories would hardly fit into any of Hoare's subgenera or the subgenus *Trypanomorpha* Woodcock resurrected by Baker (1976) for large bird species, nor could they be accommodated by the nominate subgenus *Trypanosoma* comprising *T. rotatorium* complex, differing in their morphology and biology. Yet, the name *Haematomonas* Mitrophanow 1883, as Hoare (1964) pointed out, is available for the use of . . . "those who decide that these (fish) trypanosomes are subgenerically distinct". As one of Mitrophanow's specific names indicates (*H. carassii*) this subgenus could be redefined to include the species of Section B,1 of the above scheme (p. 316). The subgenus *Haematomonas* Mitrophanow 1883 would thus comprise apparently monomorphic species of trypanosomes invading freshwater fish, with a long, slender body, terminal or subterminal kinetoplast and a long free flagellum and with development in the leech predominantly in epimastigote stages, while the proportion of sphaeromastigotes is low. The second species described originally by Mitrophanow, *T. cobitis*, is insufficiently known to be selected as the type species. Nicoli and Quillici (1964) quote *T. cobitis* as belonging to the "genus" *Haematomonas* in a not quite precise position (". . . espèce princeps", not "espèce type"). Type species *T.*

carassi Mitrophanow (synonyms see Nos. 73, 105, possibly 29); other species see Nos. 20, 31, 60, 92, 103.

It would be premature to introduce further taxons now, but an equal rank should be attributed at least to sections A,2, A,1, and B,2. This might be possible in the near future.

B. TRYPANOPLASMA

The original description of the genus (Laveran and Mesnil, 1901) did not go into great detail and it was rather on the evidence of a completely new environment than on the analysis of morphological differences from the existing genus of endoparasitic biflagellates of the genus *Cryptobia* Leidy, 1846, that the French authors established the species they found in blood of the rudd as a new genus. Their lead was soon followed by others who correctly used the name *Trypanoplasma* for flagellates found in fish blood, but also for cryptobiids in the digestive tract of marine fishes (Léger, 1905; Keysselitz, 1906) and on their surface (Swezy, 1919), and even, paradoxically, for snail cryptobiids (Friedrich, 1909; Iollos, 1911). This threatened to end in a general confusion. Alexeieff (1909) pointed out the great resemblance between *Cryptobia* and *Trypanoplasma*; however, he did not expressly synonymize them. Crawley (1909), who studied *Cryptobia* from the North American snail *Polygyra albolabria* and compared them with drawings and descriptions of *Trypanoplasma borelli* from the literature, failed to find salient differences and proposed that the two organisms be considered congeneric. Laveran and Mesnil (1912) agreed that there was a great morphological resemblance between the snail and fish blood parasites; however, they justified the existence of the genus *Trypanoplasma* by its biological distinction manifested by the life in blood and transmission by a vector, as compared to *Cryptobia* which inhabited the organ cavities and was transmitted directly.

Since then, however, the life cycle differences have not been considered sufficient enough to support the genus *Trypanoplasma*, and an increasing number of authors treated fish blood flagellates as *Cryptobia* (e.g., Hollande, 1952; Shulman, 1962; Strout, 1965; Kudo, 1966; Hoffman, 1967; Noble, 1968; Kipp, 1968; Putz, 1972a, b). Some authors recognized the presence of a well-functioning undulating membrane in trypanoplasms and its general absence in cryptobias as a sufficient justification to retain *Trypanoplasma* (e.g.; Plehn, 1924, Doflein and Reichenow, 1952, Reichenbach-Klinke and Elkan, 1965). More recently, Pokorny *et al.* (1975) were in favour of recognizing the contrasting features of *Cryptobia* and *Trypanoplasma*, and Becker (1977) stressed the importance of biological and physiological attributes as aids in establishing taxonomic categories among the parasitic protozoa and endorsed the validity of the genus *Trypanoplasma*.

In the evolutionary sequence *Bodo*–ectozoic *Cryptobia*–endozoic *Cryptobia* of fish and leeches–*C. helicis*, as reflected in ultrastructural patterns, *Trypanoplasma* may be considered the last step following *C. helicis*. While there are distinct differences from *C. vaginalis* as described by Vickerman (1977), the ultrastructural differences from *C. helicis* (Brugerolle *et al.*, in press; Lom, unpublished observations) probably relate to a specific rather than a generic level; for example, in *Trypanoplasma* the kinetoplast is a fine, homogenous isotropic meshwork of DNA fibres, while in *C. helicis* there are distinct knots of DNA fibres surrounded by "empty" spaces; the preoral ridge in *Trypanoplasma* is much more distinctly formed while the cytopharynx is shorter, reinforced by just a few microtubules as contrasted with periodic fibres present in *C. helicis*; the latter has a mitochondrial branch closely adhering to the dorsoventral belt of pellicle unsupported by microtubules and this is not the case in *Trypanoplasma*.

Thus it seems, at the present state of knowledge, difficult to find a distinct morphological boundary between bloodstream forms of *Trypanoplasma* and *Cryptobia*, as it is almost impossible to use ultrastructural data to draw a sharp line between *Bodo* and *Cryptobia*. However, the validity of the genus *Trypanoplasma* is supported by a complex of taxonomically important characters such as the profound physiological adaptations needed to cope with change of hosts (vector⇌vertebrate) plus living media (leech digestive tract⇌fish blood system and tissues) which are reflected in cyclical polymorphism both in the fish and in the leech. The morphological changes (in body shape and respective position of, for example, nucleus and kinetoplast) are quite pronounced, though unlike trypanosomids, shifts of the basal bodies along the body length, due to elaborate fibrillar armature at the anterior end, are impossible. Also, there is an analogy in trypanosomatid genera *Phytomonas* and *Endotrypanum*, distinguished because of their life cycle habits rather than other morphological differences.

To my knowledge, 34 species have been described, only two of them from marine fishes; an additional 9 species have been reported without being assigned a specific status. From authors whose papers are worth mention not only from the taxonomical point of view, several can be quoted: Bullock (1953), Chen and Hsieh (1964), Kairova (1970), Katz (1951), Ogawa and Uegaki (1927), Putz (1972a) and Quadri (1962a–d). The list below gives hosts and geographical areas only as stated in the original description since later identifications may not have all been correct.

*Trypanoplasma from fresh water fishes**
1. *Trypanoplasma abramidis* Brumpt, 1906. *Abramis brama*; France.

* Author's name and date in parentheses indicate that the species was originally described as a *Cryptobia*; this is an emendation.

2. *T. acipenseris* Joff, Lewaschow and Boschenko, 1926. *Acipenser ruthenus*; European part of the USSR.
3. *T. barbi* Brumpt, 1906. *Barbus fluviatilis*; France.
4. *T. borelli* Laveran and Mesnil, 1902. *Leuciscus erythrophthalmus*; France.
5. *T. capoetobramae* (Osmanov, 1963). *Capoetobrama kuschakewitschi*; Uzbekistan, USSSR.
6. *T. carassii* (Kaschkovsky, 1974). *Carassius auratus*; Siberia.
7. *T. cataractae* (Putz, 1972). *Rhinichtys cataractae, R. atratulus, Exoglossum maxilingua, Campostoma anomalum*; Virginia, USA.
7a. *T. catostomi* (Bower and Woo, 1977). *Catostomus commersoni*, USA.
8. *T. clariae* Matthis and Léger, 1911. *Clarias macrocephalus*; Vietnam.
9. *T. cyprini* Plehn, 1903. *Cyprinus carpio*; Germany.
10. *T. erythroculteri* (Chen and Hsieh, 1964) *Erythroculter dabryi*; China.
11. *T. gandei* Rodhain, 1942. *Labeo macrostoma*; Africa.
12. *T. guernei* Brumpt, 1906. *Cottus gobio*; France.
13. *T. guerneyorum* Minchin, 1909. *Esox lucius*; England.
14. *T. keysselitzi* Minchin, 1909. *Tinca vulgaris*; England.
15. *T. lomakini* (Khaybulyaev, 1971). *Gobius melanostomus affinis, G. kessleri gorlap, G. fluviatilis pallasi, Benthophilus macrocephalus*; Caspian Sea.
16. *T. makeevi* (Achmerov, 1959). *Oncorhynchus gorbuscha*; *O. keta*; Amur river, East Asia.
17. *T. markewitschi* Schapowal, 1953. *Anguilla anguilla*; European part of the USSR.
18. *T. megalobrami* (Chen and Hsieh, 1964). *Megalobrama amblycephala*; China.
19. *T. mirabilis* (Dzhalilov, 1965). *Varicorhinus heratensis steindachneri*; Tadzhikistan, USSR.
20. *T. misgurni* (Chen, 1964). *Misgurnus anguillicaudatus*; China.
21. *T. ninae kohl-yakimovi* Yakimov and Schocher, 1917. *Silurus* sp.; Turkestan, USSR.
22. *T. pseudobagri* (Chang, 1964). *Pseudobagrus fulvidraco*; China.
23. *T. pseudocaphirhynchi* (Ostroumov, 1949). *Psuedocaphirhynchus kaufmanni*; Uzbekistan, USSR.
24. *T. rutili* (Osmanov, 1963). *Rutilus rutilus caspicus*; Uzbekistan, USSR.
25. *T. salmositica* (Katz, 1951). *Oncorhynchus kisutch*; US Pacific coast.
26. *T. sarcocheilichthysi* (Chen and Hsieh, 1964). *Sarchocheilichthys nigripinnis*, China.
27. *T. tincae* Schäperclaus, 1954. *Tinca tinca*; Germany.
28. *T. truttae* Brumpt, 1906. *Salmo trutta fario*; France.
29. *T. valentini* Gauthier, 1920. *Salmo trutta fario*; France.

30. *T. varium* Léger, 1904. *Noemacheilus barbatula*; France (syn. *T. magnum* Breindl, 1912).
31. *T. willoughbii* Quadri, 1962. *Salvelinus willoughbii*; England.
Trypanoplasma sp. (Kairova, 1970). *Abramis brama*; Kazakhstan, USSR.
Trypanoplasma sp. (Kairova, 1970). *Schizothorax argentatus*; Kazakhstan, USSR.
Trypanoplasma sp. Nikitin, 1929. *Aspius aspius*; European part of the USSR.
Trypanoplasma sp. Ogawa and Uegaki, 1927. *Fluta alba*; Taiwan.
Trypanoplasma sp. Ogawa and Uegaki, 1927. *Anguilla mauritiana*; Taiwan.
Trypanoplasma sp. (Putz and Hoffman, 1965). *Exoglossum maxilingua, Rhinichthys* spp., *Semotilus corporalis*; USA.
Trypanoplasma sp. (Wolf, 1960). *Dorosoma petenense*; USA.
  Trypanoplasma from marine fishes
32. *T. bullocki* (Strout, 1965). *Pseudopleuronectes americanus, Liopsetta putnami, Fundulus heteroclitus, F. majalis*; US Atlantic coast.
33. *T. parmae* Mackerras and Mackerras, 1925. *Parma microlepis;* Australia.
Trypanoplasma sp. Nigrelli, Pokorny and Ruggieri, 1975. *Opsanus tau*; Long Island Sound, USA.
Trypanoplasma sp. (Zajka, 1966). *Odontogadus merlangus euxinus*; Black Sea.
Not listed as a valid species is *T. flesi* Nowicki 1940; *nomen nudum*, probably misquoted instead of *Trypanosoma flesi* Lebailly.

   As in *Trypanosoma*, the validity of many, if not most, species of *Trypanoplasma* can be questioned. Curiously enough, although the cell of trypanoplasms is much more complicated than in trypanosomes, there is a lack of sufficiently contrasting diagnostic features. This is due to the great uniformity of alleged species and to the extreme metaboly of their cells. The two exceptions are *Trypanoplasma* sp. Ogawa and Uegaki 1927 from freshwater (Fig. 15D, E) and *T. parmae*, both with oval body and a subspherical kinetoplast; the former has also a very short recurrent flagellum. However, the latter may be a gut-dwelling cryptobiid which contaminated the smears during preparation (Mackerras and Mackerras, 1961).

   Keysselitz (1906) who studied *Trypanoplasma* populations from a total of 14 species from European fish claimed that they all constitute but one species, *T. borelli*; his view was more recently upheld by Hollande (1952). This viewpoint seems to be an extreme one as indicated by some failures in experimental transfers (see p. 295) and by differences discernible under close scrutiny of an experienced observer. However, the first objection may be somehow mitigated by the fact that trypanosomatids living for a certain time in a different host may also develop changed sensitivity to original sera (discussed by Targett and Wilson, 1973).

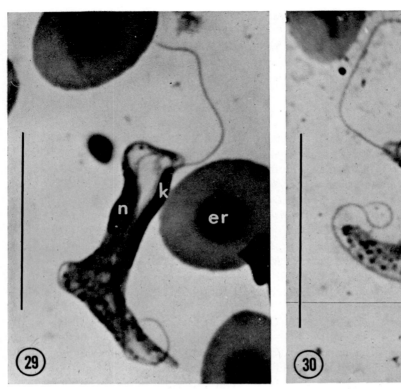

FIGS 29–30. *Fig. 29—Trypanoplasma borelli* from carp. *Fig. 30—Trypanoplasma cataractae* from *Rhinichthys cataractae*. Methanol-fixed dry smears, stained Giemsa. k—kinetoplast, n—nucleus, er—host erythrocyte. Scales equal 10 μm.

The cross-infection experiments of the writer and the lack of sufficient morphological differences suggest that the trypanoplasms found in carps, goldfish and crucian carps are all identical with the type species *T. borelli* and that the species described from those hosts as separate taxons (species No. 5 and 9) are more probably junior synonyms. That is why the name *T. borelli* was used for carp-derived trypanoplasms in the preceding chapters. Minchin (1909) supposed that *T. cyprini* and *keysselitzi* were identical. Similarly, Kipp (1968) has reduced to synonymy with *T. borelli*, trypanoplasms from tenches—the two evidently synonymous species *T. keysselitzi* and *T. tincae*. However, the appearance of young blood stages of tench trypanoplasms seem sometimes rather characteristic (Fig. 16) and different from carp and crucian carp trypanoplasms, and the transfer of *T. borelli* from carps to tenches failed (Lom, unpublished observations). This illustrates the necessity of a thorough study to solve problems of specific taxonomy of trypanoplasms.

Although Becker and Katz (1965a, b) thought it different, *T. salmositica* from North America salmonids may well be identical with the insufficiently-described *T. makeevi* from the Amur salmonids; its relation to *T. truttae* (No. 29) and its possible synonymum, *T. valentini* (No. 30), both from French trouts, as well as to the species found by Conroy and McCarthy (1972) in England also remains to be elucidated. *T. guerneyorum* from pike (Fig. 14) and *T. cataractae* (Fig. 30) from North American cyprinids (No. 7) seem positively different from *T. borelli* because of their morphology as well because of cross-infection restrictions.

VI. Technique of investigation

Only several selected procedures will be mentioned, which have not been common practice in the research on fish, or other congeneric, trypanosomes.

(*a*) *Detection in the host.* There is a method of choice (Lom, unpublished observations) which can be used even for slight infection and for very small fish (e.g., small fingerlings or larger fry) and can be used repeatedly on the same living specimen without any risk to its life. It consists in clipping off a very small piece of gill tissue (tips of the filaments), mincing them in a drop of saline and examining them under low power objective for easily discernible moving flagellates.

In larger fish specimens, gentle cardial puncture or other methods applicable in live fish can be used. If this fails to reveal any parasitaemia, flagellates may still be detected in pieces of minced tissue of pseudobranchia or kidney ("kidney stroke" done by scalpel; Putz, 1972a, b) suspended in saline. Also, spinning down several ml of serum from a suspected fish after the separation of the clotted bloodcake may reveal flagellates in the sediment even if the parasitaemia is extremely slight. This is a modification of the method by Strout (1962) who originally used just a small clot of blood from which the flagellates escaped into the serum, without later centrifugation. However, failure to detect any flagellates does not mean that there is no subpatent chronic infection.

(*b*) *Preparation of smears with trypanoplasms.* As noted already by Minchin (1909), Breindl (1915) and others, a brief fixation of blood smears— while still wet—first with osmic acid vapour prevents undesirable distortion of the trypanoplasms, though it reduces the contrast between the nucleus and cytoplasm in stained preparations.

(*c*) *Separation of blood flagellates from the blood corpuscles.* In citrated, heparinized or otherwise treated blood, it can be done by two step

centrifugation; a low speed spinning removes most of the blood corpuscles (and some flagellates) while the following high speed (2000 g)
centrifugation of the supernatant sediments the flagellates. Cottrell (1977)
used centrifugation of heparinized blood in haematocrit tubes, which
after spinning were broken at the erythrocyte–leucocyte interface and the
buffy layer of white cells examined for live trypanosomes.

DEAE-cellulose column method was successfully employed by Godfrey *et al.* (1970) to separate *T. percae* from the perch's blood. The
buffer of high ionic strength required to elute this highly negatively
charged trypanosome (the negative charge was second only to *T. cruzi*,
Lanham, 1971) also eluted some erythrocytes.

(*d*) *Cryopreservation.* This method enables one to preserve for further
use in unchanged conditions stabilates of the heavier spontaneous infections in feral fish, initial passages of flagellates freshly isolated in goldfish
as well as samples of *in vivo*- or *in vitro*-maintained haemoflagellate
strains. Putz (1972b) kept two strains of *Trypanoplasma* at $-80°$C using
10% v/v glycerol as a cryoprotectant. Ranque (1973) stored cultural
forms of *Trypanosoma boissoni* and *T. triglae* in liquid nitrogen. The
method currently used by the writer (Lom and Suchánková, 1974) for
long-term preservation of strains is to use in the sample a final concentration of 10% v/v of dimethylsulfoxide, to allow some 30 minutes for equi-
libration time and to cool the sample under controlled conditions at a
rate of one centigrade per minute to below $-30°$C. This is followed by
the transfer into a storage tank with liquid nitrogen. However, a method
of Dar *et al.* (1972) using glass capillary tubes is also suitable.

(*e*) *Syringe-passage of laboratory strains.* To avoid the difficulties encountered in procuring a constant supply of uninfected leeches for
laboratory maintenance of strains, syringe passage is the method of
choice. It was introduced as early as 1902 by Laveran and Mesnil for
tentative transmission of *Trypanosoma remaki, T. granulosum* and *Trypanoplasma borelli.* Intramuscular, intracardial, or, most conveniently,
intraperitoneal injection of saline-diluted infected blood (Lom, 1973a) or
flagellate-containing saline extract from kidneys (Putz, 1972b) permits
the introduction of the desired number of flagellates into a laboratory-
bred, uninfected host. In feral fish, the method fails in a large percentage
of animals inoculated or may yield only slight infections [e.g., Plehn's
(1903) transfer of *Trypanoplasma* between carps; Marullaz and Roudsky
in Laveran and Mesnil (1912)—the transfer of *Trypanoplasma* from
carps to goldfish; Cottrell (1977) in infection of plaice with *Trypanosoma
platessae*] since there is no guarantee that the fish used were free of
previous contact with the flagellate. Putz (1972b) used syringe passage to
maintain *Trypanoplasma cataractae* in its laboratory-bred natural host,

Rhinichthys atratulus, and kept another species, *T. salmositica*, for 13 months in its natural hosts.

The goldfish *Carassius auratus auratus* L., which is very easy to keep and to breed in a specific-pathogen-free state, is very susceptible to blood flagellates from several species of cyprinid fish, unlike its feral relative, *Carassius carassius*. It is well suited for their isolation and maintenance, developing a much more severe (usually fatal) infection than the fish species from which the flagellates were isolated (Lom, 1973a; Lom and Suchánková, 1974).

VII. Conclusions

Rather than merely to deplore deficiencies in our knowledge of fish haemoflagellates, we find it more stimulating to set urgent research goals to improve the situation. Such studies may not be just a matter of academic interest—with respect to the pathogenicity of some species for economically interesting fish.

There is an urgent need to investigate, under exactly controlled conditions, the extent of the pathogenicity which some of the trypanosomes may have for youngest age classes of their hosts, and the conditions under which *Trypanoplasma* becomes pathogenic for older fish. Such a study should be followed by investigation into suitable chemotherapeutic measures. Immunological studies, virtually nonexistent, may contribute to the preceding question as well as to immunology of kinetoplastids in general. Experimental transfers of defined strains—easily stored in a cryopreserved state—to heterologous infection-free hosts should help to resolve the question of species-specificity. Since most trypanosomes may prove to be easily grown, modern biochemical methods, too, may be applied for investigations of relations between the real and alleged species. Finally, a very intriguing research of life cycles both in the fish and leech vector, combined with careful morphological examination, may throw light on the problem of supraspecific taxonomy. These are the several points; to answer them, even if partially, would advance our knowledge and, at the same time, it would certainly prove beneficial to applied fish parasitology and to the knowledge needed for complete eradication of mammal trypanosomiases.

VIII. Acknowledgements

I wish to thank Mr. D. Eremiáš for his skilled technical assistance throughout all my previous work with fish haemoflagellates.

IX. References

Abolarin, M. O. (1970). A note on the trypanosomes from the African freshwater fish and some comments on the possible relationships between taxonomy and pathology in trypanosomes. *Bulletin of Epizootic Diseases of Africa, Kenya*, **8**, 221–228.

Alexeieff, A. (1909). Formes de passage entre le genre *Bodo* Ehrenberg et le genre *Trypanoplasma* Laveran et Mesnil. *Comptes rendus de la Société de Biologie, Paris*, **67**, 649–651.

Avtalion, R. A. (1969). Temperature effect on antibody production and immunological memory in carp (*Cyprinus carpio*) immunized against bovine serum albumin (BSA). *Immunology*, **17**, 927–931.

Avtalion, R. A., Duczyminer, M., Malik, Z., Shahrabani, R. and Wojdani, A. (1973). Influence of environmental temperature on the immune response in fish. *Current Topics in Microbiology and Immunology*, **61**, 1–35.

Baker, J. R. (1960). Trypanosomes and dactylosomes from the blood of freshwater fish in East Africa. *Parasitology*, **50**, 515–526.

Baker, J. R. (1974). The evolutionary origin and speciation of the genus *Trypanosoma* (presented at the 24th symposium of the Society for General Microbiology, "Evolution in the Microbiologic World", held at Imperial College London, April 1974. *Symposium of the Society for General Microbiology*, **24**, 343–366.

Baker, J. R. (1976). Biology of the trypanosomes of birds. *In:* "Biology of the Kinetoplastida" (W. H. R. Lumsden and D. A. Evans, eds), Vol. 1, pp. 131–174. Academic Press, London and New York.

Bardsley, J. E. (1972). An investigation of the endocrine control system regulating the distribution of trypanosomes in the bullfrog. Doctoral thesis, Queen's University, Kingston, Canada.

Bardsley, J. E. and Harmsen, R. (1973). The trypanosomes of Anura. *Advances in Parasitology*, **11**, 1–73.

Barrow, J. H. (1954). Observations of some host-specificity and immunological reactions of trypanosomes infections in some freshwater fish of Europe. *Anatomical Record*, **120**, 750–751.

Barrow, J. H. (1955). Social behavior in freshwater fish and its effect on resistance to trypanosomes. *Proceedings of the National Academy of Sciences of the United States of America*, **41**, 676–679.

Barrow, J. H. (1958). The biology of *Trypanosoma diemyctyli* Tobey. III. Factors influencing the cycle of *Trypanosoma diemyctyli* in the vertebrate host *Triturus v. viridescens*. *Journal of Protozoology*, **5**, 161–170.

Bayne, R. A., Muse, K. E. and Roberts, J. F. (1969). Isolation of bodies containing the cyanide-insensitive glycerophosphate oxidase system of *Trypanosoma equiperdum*. *Comparative Biochemistry and Physiology*, **30**, 1049–1054.

Becker, C. D. (1967). *Trypanosoma occidentalis* sp. n. from freshwater teleosts in Washington State. *Journal of Protozoology*, **14**, 153–156.

Becker, C. D. (1970). Haematozoa of fishes, with emphasis on North American records (S. F. Sniezsko, ed), A Symposium on Diseases of Fishes and Shellfishes. Special Publication No. 5, 82–100. American Fisheries Society, Washington.

Becker, C. D. (1977). Flagellate parasites of fish. *In:* "Parasitic Protozoa" (Kreier, ed), Vol. 1, pp. 357–416. New York; Academic Press.

Becker, C. D. and Holloway, H. L. (1968). A survey for haematozoa in antarctic vertebrates. *Transactions of the American Microscopical Society*, **87**, 354–360.

Becker, C. D. and Katz, M. (1965a). Transmission of the hemoflagellate, *Cryptobia salmositica* Katz, 1951, by a rhynchobdellid vector. *Journal of Parasitology*, **51**, 95–99.

Becker, C. D. and Katz, M. (1965b). Distribution, ecology and biology of the salmonid leech, *Piscicola salmositica* (Rhynchobdellae: Piscicolidae). *Journal of the Fisheries Research Board of Canada*, **22**, 1175–1195.

Becker, C. D. and Katz, M. (1965c). Infections of the hemoflagellate, *Cryptobia salmositica* Katz, 1951, in freshwater teleosts of the Pacific Coast. *Transactions of the American Fisheries Society*, **94**, 327–333.

Becker, C. D. and Katz, M. (1966). Host relationships of *Cryptobia salmositica* (Protozoa: Mastigophora) in a western Washington hatchery stream. *Transactions of the American Fisheries Society*, **95**, 196–202.

Becker, C. D. and Katz, M. (1969). Refractive granules in *Cryptobia salmositica*, a hemoflagellate of freshwater teleosts. *Transactions of the American Fisheries Society*, **88**, 300–304.

Bollinger, R. R., Gam, A. A. and Seed, J. R. (1969). Studies on frog trypanosomiasis. II. Seasonal variations in the parasitemia levels of *Trypanosoma rotatorium* in *Rana clamitans* from Louisiana. *Tulane Studies in Botany and Zoology*, **15**, 64–69.

Bower, S. M. and Woo, P. T. K. (1977a). *Cryptobia catostomi*: incubation in plasma of susceptible and refractory fishes. *Experimental Parasitology*, **43**, 63–68.

Bower, S. M. and Woo, P. T. K. (1977b). Morphology and host specifity of *Cryptobia catostomi* n. sp. (Protozoa: Kinetoplastida) from white sucker (*Catostomus commersoni*) in southern Ontario. *Canadian Journal of Zoology*, **55**, 1082–1092.

Bower, S. M. and Woo, P. T. K. (1977c). Division and morphogenesis of *Cryptobia catostomi* (Protozoa: Kinetoplastida) in the blood of white sucker (*Catostomus commersonii*). *Canadian Journal of Zoology*, **55**, 1093–1099.

Breindl, V. (1912). Trypanosomes and trypanoplasms of some fish from Bohemia. *Věstník Král. české společnosti nauk v Praze*, pp. 1–34.

Breindl, V. (1915). Study on the blood parasites of freshwater fishes. *Rozpravy České Akademie Císaře Františka Josefa pro vědy, slovesnost a umění*, **18**, 1–29.

Britchuk, P. F. (1969). *Cryptobia cyprini* Plehn, 1903 (Flagellata, Bodonidae) as a cause of mortality of *Ctenopharyngodon idella* Val. *Parazitologiya*, **3**, 574–576.

Brooker, B. E. (1971). The fine structure of *Bodo saltans* and *Bodo caudatus* (Zoomastigophora: Protozoa) and their affinities with the Trypanosomatidae. *Bulletin of the British Museum (Natural History) Biology*, **23**, 87–102.

Brooker, B. E. (1976). The cell coat of *Crithidia fasciculata*. *Parasitology*, **22**, 259–267.

Brumpt, E. (1904). Contribution a l'étude de l'évolution des hémogragarines et des trypanosomes. *Comptes rendus de la Société de Biologie, Paris*, **57**, 165–167.

Brumpt, E. (1905). Trypanosomes et trypanosomosis. *Revue Scientifique*, **4**, 321–322.

Brumpt, E. (1906a). Sur quelques éspèces nouvelles de trypanosomes parasites des poissons d'eau douce; leur mode d'évolution. *Comptes rendus de la Société de Biologie, Paris*, **60**, 160–162.

Brumpt, E. (1960b). Mode de transmission et évolution des trypanosomes des poissons. Description de quelques espèces de trypanoplasmes des poissons d'eau douce. Trypanosome d'un crapaud africain. *Comptes rendus de la Société de Biologie, Paris*, **60**, 162–164.

Brumpt, E. (1960c). Expériences relatives au mode de transmission des trypanosomes et des trypanoplasmes par les hirundinées. *Comptes rendus de la Société de Biologie, Paris*, **60**, 77–79.

Bullock, W. L. (1953). An interesting blood parasite of a New Hampshire fish. Proceedings of the New Hampshire Academy of Sciences, **2**, 7–8.

Burreson, E. M. and Pratt, I. (1972). *Trypanosoma pacifica* sp. n. from the English sole *Parophrys vetulus* Girard from Oregon. *Journal of Protozoology*, **19**, 555–556.

Burzell, L. A. (1975). Fine structure of *Bodo curvifilus* Griessmann (Kinetoplastida: Bodonidae). *Journal of Protozoology*, **22**, 35–39.

Chen, C. L. (1956). The protozoan parasites from four species of Chinese pond fishes: *Ctenopharyngodon idellus*, *Mylopharyngodon piceus*, *Aristhictys nobillis* and *Hypophthalmichthys molithrix*. II. The protozoan parasites of *Mylopharyngodon piceus*. *Acta Hydrobiologica Sinica*, **1**, 19–42.

Chen, C. L. and Hsieh, S. R. (1964). Parasitic flagellates of fishes from Hwa-ma Lake. *Acta Hydrobiologica Sinica*, **5**, 37–55.

Conroy, D. A. and McCarthy, D. H. (1972). Haematozoa in the Atlantic salmon (*Salmo salar* L.). *Rivista Italiana di Piscicultura e Ittiopatologia*, **7**, 15–16.

Cottrell, B. J. (1976). The immune response of plaice, *Pleuronectes platessa*, to tissue parasites. *Parasitology*, **24**, 74.

Cottrell, B. J. (1977). A trypanosome from the plaice, *Pleuronectes platessa* L. *Journal of Fish Biology*, **11**, 35–47.

Crawley, H. (1909). The priority of *Cryptobia* Leidy, 1846, over *Trypanoplasma* Laveran and Mesnil, 1901. *Bulletin of the U.S. Bureau of Animal Industry*, **119**, 16–20.

Daly, J. J. and de Giusti, D. L. (1971). *Trypanosoma catostomi* sp. n. from the white suckers *Catostomus c. commersoni* (Lacépède). *Journal of Protozoology*, **18**, 414–417.

Dar, F. K., Ligthart, G. S. and Wilson, A. J. (1972). Cryopreservation of pathogenic African trypanosomes in situ: metacyclic and bloodstream forms. *Journal of Protozoology*, **19**, 494–497.

Delanoe, P. (1910). Reference in Laveran and Mesnil, 1912, p. 886.

Doflein, F. (1901). Reference in Laveran and Mesnil, 1912, p. 916.

Doflein, F. and Riechenow, E. (1952). "Lehrbuch der Protozoenkunde", Part II. 6 Auflage. G. Fischer, Jena.

Dogiel, B. A. and Akhmerov, A. X. (1959). New species of parasitic protozoa of the fishes from the Amur River (In Russian). *Československá parasitologie*, **6**, 15–25.

Duxbury, R. E., Anderson, J. S., Muriithi, I. E., Sadun, E. H. and Wellde, B. T. (1972). *Trypanosoma congolense*: immunization of mice, dogs and cattle with gamma-irradiated parasites. *Experimental Parasitology*, **32**, 527–533.

Duxbury, R. E., Sadun, E. H. and West, J. E. (1975). Relative effectiveness of neutron and gamma radiation of trypanosomes for immunizing mice against African trypanosomiasis. *Transactions of the Royal Society of Tropical Medicine and Hygiene*, **69**, 484–485.

Dyková, I. and Lom, J. (1978a). Histopathological changes in *Trypanosoma danilewskyi* infection in goldfish. *Journal of Protozoology*, **25**. In press.

Dyková, I. and Lom, J. (1978b). Histopathological changes in *Trypanoplasma borelli* infections in goldfish. *Journal of Protozoology*, **25**. In press.

Fantham, H. B. (1919). Some parasitic protozoa found in South Africa. II. *South African Journal of Science*, **16**, 185–191.

Fantham, H. B. and Porter, A. (1924). On *Herpetomonas denticis*, a parasitic flagellate found in the blood of the silver-fish *Dentex argytozona*. *Transactions of the Royal Society of South Africa*, **12**, 15–21.

da Fonseca, F. (1929). Novas especies de peixes Brasileiros de aqua doce. *Boletín Biologico Laboratorio Parasitología*, **15**, 36–41.

da Fonseca, F. (1935). Trypanosomas de peixes brazileiros. Descripcao da una nova especie. *Memoarios de l'Instituto Butantan*, **2**, 149–184.

da Fonseca, F. and Vaz, Z. (1929). Novas especies de trypanosomas de peixes brasilieiros de aqua doce. *Boletín Biologico Laboratorio de Parasitología*, **15**, 36–41.

Friedrich, L. (1909). Ueber Bau und Naturgeschichte des *Trypanoplasma helicis* Leidy. *Archiv für Protistenkunde*, **14**, 363–395.

Gauthier, M. (1920). Sur le "trypanosome" de la truite. *Comptes rendus de l'Académie des Sciences, Paris*, **170**, 69–70.

Godfrey, D. G., Lanham, S. M. and Taylor, A. E. R. (1970). Studies on the biology of trypanosomes with special references to their surface properties. *Transactions of the Royal Society of Tropical Medicine and Hygiene*, **64**, 182–183.

Hasan, R. and Qasim, S. Z. (1962). *Trypanosoma punctati* sp. n. from the fish *Ophicephalus punctatus* Bloch, common freshwater murrel of India. *Zeitschrift für Parasitenkunde*, **22**, 118–122.

Havelka, J. Tesarčik, J. and Volf, F. (1965). Research of antiparasitic and antifungal control measurements. I. Investigation of the action of new antiparasitic medicaments on *Cryptobia cyprini* Plehn, 1903 (syn.: *Trypanoplasma cyprini* Plehn, 1903). (In Czech). Papers of the *Výzkumný ústav rybářský a hydrobiologický, Vodňany*, **5**, 67–87.

Hawking, F. (1957). Trypanosomes of English freshwater fish. *Transactions of the Royal Society of Tropical Medicine and Hygiene*, **51**, 375–376.

Henry, H. (1913a). A new Haemosporidian parasite from *Scomber scomber*, the common mackerel. *Journal of Pathology and Bacteriology*, **18**, 228–231.

Henry, H. (1913b). A summary of the blood parasites of British sea-fish. *Journal of Pathology and Bacteriology*, **18**, 218–223.

Hitchen, E. T. (1974). The fine structure of the colonial kinetoplastid flagellate *Cephalothamnium cyclopum* Stein. *Journal of Protozoology*, **21**, 221–232.

Hoare, C. A. (1932). On protozoal blood parasites collected in Uganda. *Parasitology*, **24**, 210–224.

Hoare, C. A. (1964). Morphological and taxonomic studies on mammalian trypanosomes. X. Revision of the systematics. *Journal of Protozoology*, **11**, 206–207.

Hofer, B. (1904). Handbuch der Fischkrankheiten. Allegemeine Fischerei-Zeitung Verlag, 384 pp. Munchen.

Hoffman, G. L. (1967). "Parasites of North American freshwater fishes". University of California Press, Berkeley, Los Angeles.

Hollande, A. (1952). Ordre des Bodonides (Bodonidea ord. nov.). *In:* "Traité de Zoologie" (P. P. Grassé, ed), Vol. I, Fasc. I, 1071 pp. Masson, Paris.

Hommel, M. and Miltgen, F. (1974). Adaptation de deux espèces d'*Herpetosoma* (Trypanosomidae) à un hôte hétérologue, la souris. *Protistologica*, **10**, 17–20.

Ioff, I. G., Bozhenko, V. B. and Levashev, M. M. (1926). *Trypanoplasma acipenseris* sp. n.—a new parasite of sterlet blood. (In Russian). *Russkhyi Gidrobiologhicheskyi Zhurnal*, **5**, 225–233.

Iollos, V. (1911). Bau und Vermehrung von *Trypanoplasma helicis*. *Archiv für Protistenkunde*, **21**, 103–110.

Johnston, E. M. (1947). The cultivation of *Trypanosoma conorrhini*. *Journal of Parasitology*, **33**, 85.

Kairova, N. (1970). On the research of fish blood parasites in the Balkash-Ilyi basin. (In Russian). *In:* "Rybnye resursy vodoimemov Kazakhstana i ikh ispolzovaniya", Vol. 6, 269–275. Kazakh Research Institute of Fish Husbandry.

Katz, M. (1951). Two new hemoflagellates (genus *Cryptobia*) from some western Washington teleosts. *Journal of Parasitology*, **3**, 245–250.

Katz, M. and Becker, C. D. (1960). *Cryptobia salmositica*, a hemoflagellate parasite of Coho salmon. Proceedings of the Eleventh Annual Northwest Fish Culture Conference Olympia, Washington, 38–40.

Keysselitz, G. (1906). Generations und Wirtwechsel von *Trypanoplasma borreli*, Laveran und Mesnil. *Archiv für Protistenkunde*, **7**, 1–74.

Khan, R. A. (1972). On a trypanosome from the Atlantic cod, *Gadus morhua* L. *Canadian Journal of Zoology*, **50**, 1051–1054.

Khan, R. A. (1976). The life cycle of *Trypanosoma murmanensis* Nikitin. *Canadian Journal of Zoology*, **54**, 1840–1849.

Khan, R. A. (1977a). Susceptibility of marine fish to trypanosomes. *Canadian Journal of Zoology*, **55**, 1235–1241.

Khan, R. A. (1977b). Blood changes in Atlantic cod, *Gadus morhua* L. infected with *Trypanosoma murmanensis* Nikitin: a preliminary study. *Journal of the Fisheries Research Board of Canada*, **55**. 34, 2193–2196.

Khan, R. A. (1978). Infectivity of *Trypanosoma murmanensis* to leeches (Johanssonia sp.). In press.

Khaybulyayev, K. Kh. (1969). The role of blood-sucking leeches in the life cycle of blood parasites of fishes. *In:* "Progress in Protozoology" (Abstract of papers read at the 3rd International Congress on Protozoology, Leningrad 2–10.7.1969), p. 302. Nauka, Leningrad.

Khaybulyayev, K. Kh. (1970). On the role of leeches in developmental cycle of blood parasites of fishes. (In Russian). *Parazitologiya*, **4**, 13–17.

Khaybulyayev, K. Kh. (1971). New species of trypanosomes in the blood of fishes from the Caspian Sea. (In Russian). *Parazitologiya*, **5**, 551–556.

Khaybulyayev, K. Kh. (1976). On the specifity of trypanosomes and cryptobiids from the blood of fishes. (In Russian). *Proceedings of the II. All-Union Congress of Soviet Protozoologists*, **1**, 143–144. Naukova Dumka, Kiev.

Kipp, H. (1968). Untersuchungen zum Vorkommen, zur Artsspezifität und Pathogenität der Cryptobien und Trypanosomen bei der Schleie (*Tinca tinca* L.). Inaugural-Dissertation, Tierärztliche Fakultät der Ludwig-Maxmilians-Universität, 115 pp. Munchen.

Kozloff, E. N. (1948). The morphology of *Cryptobia helicis* Leidy, with an account of the fate of the extranuclear organelles in division. *Journal of Morphology*, **83**, 253–273.

Kudo, R. R. (1966). *Protozoology*. 5th edn. Thomas, Springfield, Illinois.

Laird, M. (1951). Studies on the trypanosomes of New Zealand fish. *Proceedings of the Zoological Society of London*, **121**, 285–309.

Laird, M. and Bullock, W. (1968). Marine fish haematozoa from New Brunswick and New England. *Journal of the Fisheries Research Board of Canada*, **26**, 1075–1102.

Lanham, S. M. (1971). The separation of stercorarian trypanosomes from infected blood using DEAE-cellulose. *Transactions of the Royal Society of Tropical Medicine and Hygiene*, **65**, 248–249.

Laveran, A. and Mesnil, F. (1901). Sur les flagellés à membrane ondulante des poissons (genres *Trypanosoma* Gruby et *Trypanoplasma* n. gen.). *Comptes Rendus de l'Académie des Sciences, Paris*, **133**, 670–675.

Laveran, A. and Mesnil, F. (1902). Des Trypanosomes des poissons. *Archiv für Protistenkunde*, **1**, 475–498.

Laveran, A. and Mesnil, F. (1912). Trypanosomes et Trypanosomiases. 2nd edn. Masson, Paris.

Lebailly, C. (1905). Recherches sur les hématozoaires parasites des téléostéens marins. *Archives de Parasitologie*, **10**, 348–404.

Léger, L. (1904a). Sur la structure et les affinités des Trypanoplasmes. *Comptes Rendus de l'Académie des Sciences, Paris*, **138**, 856–859.

Léger, L. (1904b). Sur les hemoflagelles du *Cobitis barbatula* L. *Comptes Rendus de la Société de Biologie*, **57**, 344–345.

Léger, L. (1905). Sur la présence d'un *Trypanoplasma* intestinal chez les poissons. *Comptes Rendus de la Société de Biologie*, **58**, 511–513.

Leydig, J. (1857). Reference in Laveran and Mesnil, 1912. p. 916.

Lima, D. F. (1976). Uma espécie nova de tripanossoma na tainha (*Mugil brasiliensis* Agassiz, 1829) (Pisces, Mugilidae). *Revista Brasileira de Biología*, **36**, 167–169.

Lom, J. (1973a). Experimental infection of goldfish with blood flagellates. *In:* Progress in Protozoology (4th International Congress on Protozoology, Clermont-Ferrand 1973), Université de Clermont, p. 255.

Lom, J. (1973b). Experimental infections of freshwater fishes with blood flagellates. *Journal of Protozoology*, **20**, Supplement, 537.

Lom, J. and Nohýnková, E. (1977). Surface coat of the bloodstream phase of *Trypanoplasma borelli*. *Journal of Protozoology*, **24**, 52A.

Lom, J. and Suchánková, E. (1974). Comments on the life cycle of *Trypanosoma danilewskyi*. Proceedings of the III. International Congress on Parasitology, Vol. I, pp. 66–67. Facta Publication, Munich.

Lom, J., Paulin, J. J. and Nohýnková, E. (1978). Ultrastructural features of *Trypanosoma danilewskyi* with emphasis on the cytopharyngeal complex. *Journal of Protozoology*, **25**. In press.

Lumsden, W. H. R. (1974). Leishmaniasis and trypanosomiasis: the causative organisms compared and contrasted. *In:* Trypanosomiasis and Leishmaniasis, CIBA Foundation Symposium 20, pp. 3–21. Elsevier-Excerpta Medica, North Holland, Amsterdam.

Lumsden, W. H. R. and Evans, D. A. (Eds) (1976). "Biology and Kinetoplastida", Vol. 1. Academic Press, London and New York.

Mackerras, M. J. and Mackerras, I. M. (1961). The haematozoa of Australian frogs and fish. *Australian Journal of Zoology*, **9**, 123–139.

Makeyeva, A. P. (1956). On one of the factors of prespawning mortality of pink salmon in rivers. *In:* "Pacific Salmon", pp. 18–21. Izrael Program Scientific Translation, Jerusalem.

Mandel, A. K. (1975). Two new trypanosomes from Indian freshwater fishes. *Angewandte Parasitologie*, **16**, 487–493.

Martin, C. (1910). Observations on *Trypanoplasma congeri*. Part I. The division of the active form. *Quarterly Journal of Microscopical Science*, **55**, 485–496.

Martin, C. (1913). Further observations on the intestinal trypanoplasm of fishes, with a note on the division on *Trypanoplasma cyprini* in the crop of a leech. *Quarterly Journal of Microscopical Science*, **59**, 175–195.

Matthis, C. (1911). Culture de *Leishmania infantum* et *L. tropica* sur milieu au sang chauffé. *Comptes Rendus de la Société de Biologie, Paris*, **72**, 538–539.

McCarthy, D. H. (1974). Occurrence of hematozoa in Atlantic salmon (*Salmo salar*) smolts and adults in an English river. *Journal of the Fisheries Research Board of Canada*, **31**, 1790–1792.

Migala, K. (1967). A *Cryptobia* (*Trypanoplasma*) infection in the blood of Ctenopharyngodon idella Val. bred in the carp farm ponds (in Polish). *Wiadomosci Parazytologiczne*, **13**, 275–278.

Migala, K. (1971). Observations on the infection by protozoa from the genus *Cryptobia* (*Trypanoplasma*) in the blood-vascular system of grasscarp (*Cteno-*

pharyngodon idella Val.) bred in carp ponds (in Polish). *Roczniki nauk rolniczych*, **93**, 65–73.

Minchin, E. A. (1909). Observations on the flagellates parasitic in the blood of freshwater fishes. *Proceedings of the Zoological Society of London*, **2**, 30.

Minchin, E. A. and Woodcock, H. M. (1910). Observation on certain blood parasites of fishes occurring at Rovigno. *Quarterly Journal of Microscopical Science*, **55**, 113–154.

Misra, K. K., Chandra, A. K. and Choudhury, A. (1973). *Trypanosoma gachuii* sp. n. from a freshwater teleost fish *Ophicephalus gachua* Ham. *Archiv für Protistenkunde*, **115**, 18–21.

Mitrophanow, P. (1883). Beiträge zur Kenntniss der Hämatozoen. *Biologisches Zentralblatt*, **3**, 35–44.

Needham, E. A. (1969a). Ecology of *Trypanosoma tincae* in the tench (*Tinca tinca*) and the leech (*Hemiclepsis marginata*). Progress in Protozoology. III. International Congress on Protozoa, Leningrad, Supplement, p. 23.

Needham, E. A. (1969b). *Trypanosoma tincae*: some ecological aspects. *Parasitology*, **59**, 8.

Neresheimer, E. (1912). Die Gattung *Trypanoplasma*. Prowazek's Handbuch der pathogenen Protozoen, **1**, 101.

Neumann, R. O. (1909). Studien über protozoische Parasiten im Blut von Meeresfischen. *Zeitschrift für Hygiene und Infectionskrankheiten*, **64**, 1–112.

Nicoli, R. M. and Quilici, M. (1964). Phylogénèse et systématique: essai sur l'arbre phylétique des Trypanosomatida (Zoomastigina). *Bulletin de la Société Zoologique de France*, **89**, 702–716.

Nikitin, S. A. (1929). Trypanosomes and trypanoplasms of the Volgo-Caspian fishes. (In Russian). *Raboty volzhskoy biologhicheskoy stancii*, **10**, 127–146.

Nigrelli, R. F. (1945). Trypanosomes from North American amphibians, with a description of *Trypanosoma grylli* Nigrelli (1944) from *Acris gryllus* (Le Conte). *Zoologica*, **30**, 47–57.

Nigrelli, R. F., Pokorny, K. S. and Ruggieri, G. D. (1975). Studies on parasitic kinetoplastids. II. Occurrence of a biflagellate kinetoplastid in the blood of *Opsanus tau* (toadfish) transmitted by the leech (*Piscicola funduli*). *Journal of Protozoology*, **22**, Supplement, 43A.

Noble, E. R. (1955). The morphology and life cycles of trypanosomes. *Quarterly Review of Biology*, **30**, 1–28.

Noble, E. R. (1968). The flagellate *Cryptobia* in two species of deepsea fishes from the eastern Pacific. *Journal of Parasitology*, **54**, 720–724.

Nohýnková, E. (1977). *Trypanosoma danilewskyi*—*in vitro* culture of dyskinetoplastic forms, *Journal of Protozoology*, **24**, 52A.

Nowicki, E. (1940). Zur Pathogenität der *Trypanoplasma cyprini*. *Zeitschrift für Parasitenkunde* **11**, 468–473.

Ogawa, M. and Uegaki, J. (1927). Beobachtungen über die Blutprotozoen bei Tieren Formosas. *Archiv. für Protistenkunde*, **57**, 14–30.

Paulin, J. J. (1975). The chondriome of selected trypanosomatids. A three dimensional study based on serial thick sections and high voltage electron microscopy. *Journal of Cell Biology*, **66**, 404–413.

Paulin, J. J., Lom, J. and Nohýnková, E. (1978). Observation on the surface coat of *Trypanosoma danilewskyi*. *Journal of Protozoology*, **25**. In press.

Pearse, A. S. (1933). Parasites of Siamese fishes and crustaceans. *Journal of the Siamese Society of Natural History*, Supplement, **9**, 179–191.

Peterson, A. C. (1974). Evaluation of a method for bleeding life perch (*Perca fluviatilis* L.) for the isolation and *in vitro* cultivation of parasites. Unpublished manuscript.

Petrie, G. F. (1905). Observations relating to the structure and geographical distribution of certain trypanosomes. *Journal of Hygiene*, **5**, 191.

Plehn, M. (1903). *Trypanosoma cyprini* sp. n. *Archiv für Protistenkunde*, **3**, 175–180.

Plehn, M. (1924). "Praktikum der Fischkrankheiten". E. Schweizerbartische Verlagsbuchhandlung, Stuttgart.

Pokorny, K. S., Nigrelli, R. F. and Ruggieri, G. D. (1975). Studies on parasitic kinetoplastides. I. Fine structure observations of a biflagellate kinetoplastid parasitic in the gut of the North Atlantic fish *Cyclopterus lumpus* L. (lumpfish), with a revision of the order Kinetoplastida. Honigberg, 1963. *Journal of Protozoology*, **22**, Supplement 10A.

Ponselle, A. (1913a). Recherches sur la culture *in vitro* du trypanosome de l'anguille (*Trypanosoma granulosum* Laveran et Mesnil, 1902). Une nouvelle modification au milieu de Novy et McNeal. *Comptes Rendus de la Société de Biologie*, **74**, 339–341.

Ponselle, A. (1913b). Culture *in vitro* du *Trypanoplasma varium* Leger. *Comptes Rendus de la Société de Biologie*, **74**, 685–688.

Preston, T. M. (1966). *In vitro* cultivation of *Trypanosoma rajae*. *Transactions of the Royal Society of Tropical Medicine and Hygiene*, **60**, 10.

Preston, T. M. (1969). The form and function of the cytostome-cytopharynx of the culture forms of the elasmobranch haemoflagellate *Trypanosoma raiae* Laveran and Mesnil. *Journal of Protozoology*, **16**, 320–333.

Putz, R. E. (1972a). *Cryptobia cataractae* sp. n. (Kinetoplastida: Cryptobiidae) a hemoflagellate of some cyprinid fishes of West Virginia. *Proceedings of the Helminthological Society of Washington*, **39**, 18–22.

Putz, R. E. (1972b). Biological studies on the hemoflagellates *Cryptobia cataractae* and *Cryptobia salmositica*. *Technical papers of the Bureau of Sport Fisheries and Wildlife*, **63**, 3–25.

Qadri, S. S. (1955). The morphology of *Trypanosoma striati* sp. n. from an Indian freshwater fish. *Parasitology*, **45**, 79–85.

Qadri, S. S. (1962a). On three new trypanosomes from freshwater fishes. *Parasitology*, **52**, 221–228.

Qadri, S. S. (1962b). *Trypanoplasma willoughbii* sp. n. from British freshwater fish, *Salvelinus willoughbii*. *Rivista di Parassitologia*, **23**, 1–9.

Qadri, S. S. (1962c). The development in culture of *Trypanosoma striati* from an Indian Fish. *Parasitology*, **52**, 229–235.

Qadri, S. S. (1962d). An experimental study of the life cycle of *Trypanosoma danilewskyi* in the leech, *Hemiclepsis marginata*. *Journal of Protozoology*, **9**, 254–258.

Ranque, P. (1973). "Etudes morphologique et biologique de quelques trypanosomides récoltés au Senegal". Thèse. Université d'Aix-Marseilles, Publication de CNRS A. O. 8223.

Raychaudhuri, S. and Misra, K. K. (1973). Two new fish trypanosomes from India. *Archiv für Protistenkunde*, **115**, 10–17.

Reichenbach-Klinke, H. and Elkan, E. (1965). "The Principal Diseases of Lower Vertebrates". Academic Press, London and New York.

Remak (1842). Reference in Laveran and Mesnil, 1912, p. 881.

Robertson, M. (1907). Studies on a trypanosome found in the alimentary canal of *Pontobdella muricata*. *Proceedings of the Royal Physical Society of Edinburgh*, **17**, 83–108.

Robertson, M. (1909). Further notes on a trypanosome found in the alimentary tract of *Pontobdella muricata*. *Quarterly Journal of Microscopical Science*, **54**, 119–139.

Robertson, M. (1911). Transmission of flagellates living in the blood of freshwater fishes. *Philosophical Transactions of the Royal Society of London B*, **202**, 29–50.

Rodhain, J. (1942). A propos de trypanosomes de poissons du bassin du fleuve Congo. *Revue de Zoologique et de Botanique Africaines*, **36**, 411–416.

Roudsky, D. (1912). Reference in Laveran and Mesnil, 1912, p. 886.

Schäperclaus, W. (1954). "Handbuch der Fishkrankheiten" (3rd edn). Akademie Verlag, Berlin.

Shulman, S. S. (1962). Protozoa. *In:* "Key to the parasites of freshwater fish of the USSR" (B. E. Bykhovsky, ed.), pp. 7–197. Publishing House of the USSR Academy of Sciences, Moscow-Leningrad.

Smirnova, T. L. (1970). Trypanosoma in the blood of *Lota lota* L.—T. lotai n. sp. *Parasitologyia*, **4**, 296–297.

Smolíková, V., Lom, J., Suchánková, E. (1977). Growth of the carp trypanosome *T. danilowskyi* in fish tissue culture. *Journal of Protozoology*, **24**, 54A.

Steiger, R. F. (1973). On the ultrastructure of *Trypanosoma (Trypanozoon) brucei* in the course of its life cycle and some related aspects. *Acta Tropica*, **30**, 64–168.

Strout, R. G. (1962). A method for concentrating hemoflagellates. *Journal of Parasitology*, **48**, 100.

Strout, R. G. (1965). A new hemoflagellate (genus *Cryptobia*) from marine fishes of northern New England. *Journal of Parasitology*, **51**, 654–659.

Swale, E. M. F. (1973). A study of the colourless flagellate *Rhynchomonas nasuta* (Stokes) Klebs. *Biological Journal of the Linnaean Society*, **5**, 255–264.

Swezy, O. (1919). The occurrence of *Trypanoplasma* as an ectoparasite. *Transactions of the American Microscopical Society*, **38**, 20–24.

Tanabe, M. (1924). Studies on the hemoflagellata of the loach, *Misgurnus anguillicaudatus*. *Kitasato Archives of Experimental Medicine*, **6**, 121–138.

Tandon, R. S. and Chandra, S. (1977). Studies on ecophysiology of fish parasites: effect of trypanosome infection on the serum cholesterol levels of fishes. *Zeitschrift für Parasitenkunde*, **52**, 199–202.

Tandon, R. S. and Joshi, B. D. (1973). Studies on the physiopathology of blood of freshwater fishes infected with two new forms of trypanosomes. *Zeitschrift für Wissenschaftliche Zoologie*, **185**, 207–221.

Targett, G. A. T. and Wilson, V. C. L. C. (1973). The blood incubation infectivity test as a means of distinguishing between *Trypanosoma brucei brucei* and *T. brucei rhodesiense*. *International Journal of Parasitology*, **3**, 5–11.

Tesarčík, J. (1974). Parasitofauna of pond fishes accompanying spring viremia and erythodermatitis. (In Czech). *Bulletin of the VÚRH Vodňany*, No. 3–4, 18–23.

Thompson, J. D. (1908). Cultivation of trypanosome found in the blood of the goldfish. *Journal of Hygiene*, **8**, 75–82.

Valentin, G. G. (1841). Über ein Entozoon im Blute von *Salmo fario*. *Archiv für Anatomie, Physiologie und Wissenschaftliche Medicine*, **5**, 435–436.

Vickerman, K. (1969). On the surface coat and flagellar adhesion in trypanosomes. *Journal of Cell Science*, **5**, 163–177.

Vickerman, K. (1971). Morphological and physiological considerations of extracellular blood protozoa. *In: Ecology and Physiology of Parasites* (A. M. Fallis ed.), pp. 57–91. *University of Toronto Press*.

Vickerman, K. (1974). The ultrastructure of pathogenic flagellates. *In:* Trypanosomiasis and leishmaniasis. Ciba Foundation Symposium, 20, pp. 171–190. Elsevier-Excerpta Medica North Holland, Amsterdam.

Vickerman, K. (1977). DNA throughout the single mitochondrion of a kineto-plastid flagellate: observations of the ultrastructure of *Cryptobia vaginalis* (Hesse, 1910). *Journal of Protozoology*, **24**, 221–233.

Vickerman, K. and Preston, T. M. (1970). Spindle microtubules in the dividing nuclei of trypanosomes. *Journal of Cell Science*, **6**, 365–383.

Vickerman, K. and Preston, T. M. (1976). Comparative cell biology of the kineto-plastid flagellates. *In: Biology of the Kinetoplastida* (W. H. R. Lumsden and D. A. Evans, eds), pp. 35–130. Academic Press; London and New York.

Vinnichenko, L. N., Shtein, G. A., Shulman, S. S., Timofeyev, V. A. and Zaika, V. E. (1971). Parasitic protozoa of fishes from the Amur River Basin. (In Russian). *Parazitologhicheskyi sbornik*, **25**, 10–40.

Volf, F. (1934). Sleeping sickness in fish. (In Czech). *Československý rybář*, 1–4.

Wales, J. H. and Wolf, H. (1955). Three protozoan diseases of trout in California. *California Fish and Game*, **41**, 183–187.

Wright, K. A. and Hales, H. (1970). Cytochemistry of the pellicle of bloodstream forms of *Trypanosoma (Trypanozoon) brucei*. *Journal of Parasitology*, **56**, 671–683.

Yakimoff, W. (1912). Trypanosomes parasites du sang des poissons marins. *Archiv für Protistenkunde*, **27**, 1–8.

7

Development of *Trypanosoma brucei* in the Mammalian Host

W. E. ORMEROD

London School of Hygiene and Tropical Medicine,
London, England

I.	Introduction	340
	A. Taxonomy of *Trypanosoma brucei*	341
II.	The significance of pleomorphic stages in the blood	342
	A. Variability of blood trypomastigotes	342
	B. Methods of examination	342
	C. Hypotheses to account for the variability of blood forms	345
	D. Filaments of trypomastigotes	352
	E. A view of the significance of pleomorphism	353
III.	The significance of "aberrant" forms in the blood	354
	A. Spherical forms and "tadpole" forms	354
	B. Filtration of infective blood and tissues	355
	C. Multinucleate forms	356
IV.	The significance of culture forms	357
V.	Remission, relapse and the relation between parasitaemia and pathological lesion	358
	A. Experimental production of remissions	359
VI.	Metabolic and fine structural difference between different stages and their implications for the life cycle	360
	A. The chondriome	360
	B. Differences in lipid metabolism	361
	C. The autophagosome	362

VII.   Tissue stages of *T. brucei*   363
       A.   The chancre   363
       B.   Lymphatic spread   364
       C.   Absence of trypanosomes from the blood   364
       D.   Plasmodial and other multinuclear forms   365
       E.   Spherical forms and "latent" bodies   365
       F.   The attitude of English-speaking workers   371
       G.   The attitude of Italian workers   372
       H.   The rediscovery of tissue forms   373

VIII. Hypothetical life cycles of *T. brucei*   375
       A.   Sexual dimorphism of blood forms   375
       B.   The classical hypothesis   376
       C.   The persistence of latent bodies   377
       D.   The "two cycle hypothesis"   379
       E.   The multinucleate hypothesis   381

IX.   Conclusion   383

X.   Acknowledgements   384

XI.   References   384

I. Introduction

The course of development of *Trypanosoma brucei*, both in its vertebrate and its invertebrate hosts, remains uncertain despite its importance to much of Africa. *T. brucei* is the causative organism of sleeping sickness in man, of a disease in horses which has prevented their use for transport, and of a disease in cattle which would probably be considered important were it not overshadowed by those of greater economic importance caused by *Trypanosoma congolense* and *Trypanosoma vivax*.

One would normally expect a biological problem of this magnitude, which has been studied intensively for 80 years, to be approaching solution or at least consensus; but it is a measure of its complexity that we are probably no nearer a consensus now than we were in 1910.

This chapter deals with the life cycle of *T. brucei* in its vertebrate host; such a review is desirable at the present time because many old theories of its life cycle are being revived and discussed in relation to recent findings. These findings tend not to support the "classical" hypothesis, accepted with little question for many years, that reproduction occurs through binary fission in the blood (Hoare, 1949) and that any method of reproduction other than binary fission, if it occurs at all, is likely to be of no importance.

Yet, in reviewing old work, it is important to draw the distinction between observations which have been made and the inferences that have been drawn from them. If there is a lesson that can today be learned from our past mistakes in interpreting the life cycle of *T. brucei* it is that, when an inference has been rejected as being unrealistic or as being out of accord with current theory, the observations on which the inference was based should not necessarily be rejected as well. There are a number of instances in the history of investigation into the life cycle of *T. brucei* where, on the one hand, valid observations have been made but mis-interpreted and, on the other, inadequate observations have been accepted because they happened to support a theory which was then in vogue. I shall attempt in this review to indicate which lines of thought are likely to be fruitful and which are likely to lead to dead ends; but I shall do so with some caution for if I am mistaken I shall be in distinguished company.

A. TAXONOMY OF *TRYPANOSOMA BRUCEI*

The name *Trypanosoma brucei* Plimmer and Bradford, 1899 was given to trypanosomes derived from a dog which had been infected by Bruce in Zululand and sent to England. For the purposes of this chapter the name *T. brucei* is applied also to the sleeping sickness trypanosomes previously called *Trypanosoma gambiense* and *Trypanosoma rhodesiense* following the recommendation of Ormerod (1967).

Hoare (1972) has pointed out that, while this procedure is justifiable on theoretical grounds since these trypanosomes cannot be separated mor-phologically, it is important from the medical and veterinary point of view to distinguish them taxonomically. Trypanosomes that are patho-genic to man should, he states, be called *Trypanosoma (Trypanozoon) brucei gambiense* (gambian and rhodesian forms of the disease being con-sidered as nosodemes), whereas the animal trypanosomes which will not infect man should be called *T. (T.) brucei brucei.*

Recently, Robertson and Pickens (1975) have shown that a clone, which had been established in most of its variants as sensitive to human serum and therefore by presumption unable to infect man, could never-theless produce a single variant which did infect man and was shown subsequently to be resistant to the action of human serum. Since infec-tivity to man now appears to be a matter of degree rather than an absolute difference, it seems convenient as well as logical to use the name *Trypanosoma (Trypanozoon) brucei (T. brucei* for short) without sub-species designation. It is important, however, to bear in mind that there are at least two types of gradation in the variability of strains of this species:

(1) in the degree of pathogenicity to man; so that on the one hand man may readily become infected and on the other only animals may become infected (the *rhodesiense-brucei* gradation);

(2) in the degree of parasitaemia produced; thus some strains give a high parasitaemia while others give such a low, or absence of, parasitaemia, that the infection may be inapparent (the *rhodesiense-gambiense* gradation). That this gradation may apply not only to strains which infect man but also to animal strains is a contingency which is not covered by the classification of Hoare (1972).

The term "strain" is used in this review with latitude to include stocks, isolates, clones and the organisms giving rise to an infection where closer definition of how the population may, or may not, have been selected is not required.

Hoare (1972) has pointed out that *T. evansi* is closely related to *T. brucei* in its morphology and behaviour, and differs from *T. brucei* only in its failure to pass through a cycle of development in the tsetse. Indeed, *T. brucei* is also difficult to transmit through cyclical development in the tsetse so that failure to transmit may not be a very useful taxonomic indication. Moreover, Mathur (1971) claims to have transmitted *T. evansi* by cyclical development in the tsetse; however, this work still lacks confirmation under conditions that leave no doubt as to the provenance of the strains transmitted. There is little doubt that *Trypanosoma* (*Trypanozoon*) *evansi* is closely related to *T.* (*T.*) *brucei* and, since this close relationship is generally accepted, evidence relating to stages of the life cycle of *T. evansi* will, in this chapter, be introduced into the argument which, however, mainly concerns *T. brucei*.

II. The significance of pleomorphic stages in the blood

A. VARIABILITY OF BLOOD TRYPOMASTIGOTES

Infections with *T. brucei* show a marked variability in the size and shape of trypomastigotes circulating in the blood, and Fig. 1 shows something of the range of forms observed. Similar types are also observed in *T. evansi* although the variability tends to be less extreme. While trypomastigotes of other species, such as *T. vivax* or *T. congolense*, produce wide variation in length, there is generally no important difference in shape. *T. brucei* (and to a lesser extent *T. evansi*), are exceptional not so much in their differences in size but in the wide differences in actual shape of the forms that are seen in the blood. In this section of the review, discussion is limited to the types shown in Fig. 1. Other types, frequently regarded as abnormal and/or degenerate, will be considered below.

B. METHODS OF EXAMINATION

Before considering individual hypotheses put forward to account for this

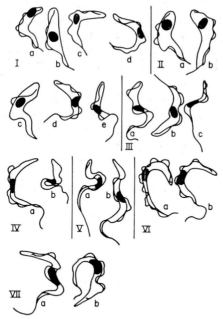

FIG. 1. "Pleomorphism". The different shapes of trypomastigotes as seen in the blood by Swellengrebel (1912) who attempted to divide the forms into different categories other than on the basis of length. Although the forms shown are excellent representations, the grouping seems to have little relevance today. Note IIIc and Va which Ormerod and Venkatesan (1971a) call the "long-narrow" in contradiction to the "long-flat" form (i.e. IVa and b, Vb, VIa and b, VIIa). Dividing forms, which are not shown, are all classified as long-flat.

variability it is necessary to discuss the methods that have been used to investigate it. This is necessary for the following reasons:

(1) The two main methods of assessing variability, namely measuring the trypanosome and counting its granules, represent fundamentally different approaches to the same phenomenon: the terminologies of the two methods are therefore different and need to be reconciled if the results of both are to be introduced into the argument.

(2) In the absence of direct, unassailable evidence for the existence of a tissue phase of development of *T. brucei* the main evidence for the existence of such a phase must rest on interpretation of the sequence of phases which are seen in the blood.

It is, consequently, important to understand the relationship of the different forms to one another and the role that they play in the life cycle.

The classical method (Bruce *et al.*, 1910) for studying variability of trypanosomes has been to make a drawing of the organism by *camera lucida* and to measure its length with dividers or with a mapping wheel.

This method works well for helminths because of their size, but the errors involved in measuring trypomastigotes, many of the dimensions of which are near the limits of microscopic resolution, tend to be large: for this reason measurement of the length only is not a sufficiently reliable parameter and it gives little weight to the differences in shape which are an essential part of the variability of forms of *T. brucei* in the blood. To overcome this difficulty Swellengrebel (1912), in addition to measurements, divided the trypomastigotes into types (Fig. 1); this method was further elaborated by Wijers (1959) who took as his types the drawings of Lady Bruce (Bruce *et al.*, 1912): trypomastigotes which did not conform to her "type" drawings of "slender", "intermediate" and "stumpy" were classified either as "long-intermediate" or "short-intermediate", but in the final percentages of the categories "slender", "intermediate" and "stumpy" half the long-intermediates were counted as slender and half as intermediate, similarly the short intermediates were divided among intermediate and stumpy forms. While this method has been useful both to its originator Wijers (1959), to Luckins (1972) and to Balber (1972) in relieving much of the tedium of drawing and measuring, it involves the possible danger of "creating" an intermediate stage which might otherwise not exist other than in representing the transition between slender and stumpy forms.

In the method of Ormerod (1958) living trypomastigotes are observed on agar by phase contrast microscopy. Trypomastigotes of uniform refractility which first appear in the blood are regarded as slender forms. At about 100 h from inoculation, trypomastigotes begin to acquire dense lipid granules and these are counted up to an arbitrary maximum of ten, although a lower figure may be appropriate for certain strains. This method has certain advantages: firstly, greater speed is achieved so that in a given time many more trypomastigotes can be counted; secondly, the trypomastigotes are alive and motile so that their refractility indicates clearly whether they are normal or degenerate; thirdly, no measurement near the limits of microscopical resolution is involved; and fourthly, the intermediate form is differentiated clearly from the slender form by its acquisition of granules; the identification of the stumpy form, however, remains arbitrary since its production appears to be part of a continuous process. While it is useful to think of slender and stumpy forms as having the same general significance in the classical and in the agar method, it must be appreciated that in the two methods the identification of these forms is not the same, and this dissimilarity is of particular importance (as will be noted below) in identification of the stumpy form for subsequent electron microscopy.

C. HYPOTHESES TO ACCOUNT FOR THE VARIABILITY OF BLOOD FORMS

The difficulty of developing a satisfactory hypothesis to account for the extreme variability of *T. brucei* in the blood of its vertebrate host is probably the main reason why so little progress has been achieved in determining the life cycle of this parasite. It seems, therefore, appropriate to discuss in some detail such hypotheses as have been put forward. They are grouped under the following headings:

(1) The different shape of individual trypomastigotes reflects their different genetic constitution.
(2) The different forms represent a sexual dimorphism.
(3) The different forms represent different stages in the life cycle.
(4) The gradation of forms is due to progressive degeneration.
(5) A combination of two or more of factors 1 to 4 may be in operation.

In addition, a tentative hypothesis was proposed by Robertson (1912a) that division gave rise to two trypomastigotes of unequal size, but since no evidence was brought forward in its support this hypothesis will not be discussed further.

1. Variable genetic constitution (pleomorphism and polymorphism)

The most likely cause for the variability of forms in the blood seemed at first sight to be due to circulation of individuals of differing genetic constitution. This hypothesis seemed all the more reasonable in that some strains, such as the original strain of *T. brucei* (Plimmer and Bradford, 1899), showed no variability, whereas others (Bruce *et al.*, 1910) showed the characteristic variability. Karl Pearson (Pearson, 1914) explained the characteristic variability of some strains in terms of the presence of two components "*T. minus*" and "*T. majus*". Although he considered that these components might merely represent a dimorphism of a uniform strain, he considered that the most likely explanation was that two distinct "strains" (genetic types) were involved.

Fortunately, von Prowazek (1913), Oehler (1913, 1914) and Bruce *et al.* (1914) showed that the variability persisted when the host had been injected with a single trypanosome, thus demonstrating experimentally that the variability had no genetic basis and that Pearson's concept of individual variation as the basic cause of variability of trypanosomes in the blood could only be tenable if the divergent forms represented the dimorphism of a uniform strain.

It has been traditional to refer to the variation in shape of *T. brucei* in the blood as monomorphic, dimorphic, trimorphic or polymorphic. While most of these terms are appropriate and self-explanatory, the term "polymorphism" has since acquired, in biology, the additional meaning of variation occurring as a result of genetic difference; a condition which, as demonstrated above, is not appropriate to *T. brucei*. Vickerman (1965) first introduced the term "pleomorphism" to describe the changes which occur in the flagellates of *T. brucei*. Some will say that this change is unnecessary since Blackwelder (1967) has stated that polymorphism may be either genetic or developmental in origin; nevertheless, since both genetic and developmental polymorphism can occur in *T. brucei*, the term "pleomorphism" is used in this chapter, for the sake of clarity, to describe the normal morphological variation of trypomastigotes in a strain of *T. brucei* in the blood as opposed to other types of variation occurring from one strain to another.

2. Sexual dimorphism

Von Prowazek (1905) seems to have first considered the possibility that slender and stumpy forms of *T. brucei* represented male and female gametes and that the forms of intermediate length were sexually indifferent. Minchin *et al.* (1906) also discussed this possibility, but no satisfactory evidence was put forward. Nevertheless, Ottolenghi (1910) interpreted the multinucleate forms, the probable significance of which will be discussed below (see Fig. 4, and page 370), as dividing into macrogametes in order to produce the sexual forms that von Prowazek and Minchin had postulated. Ottolenghi does not specifically state that he also regards the spherical form as a microgametocyte; nevertheless this is the inference that his paper seems to convey. More recently Fairbairn and Culwick (1946) proposed a sexual process based not on morphology but on the existence of positive and negative charges that trypanosomes had been found to possess (Broom *et al.*, 1936). The evidence that Fairbairn and Culwick put forward consisted of a series of pictures of trypanosomes undergoing what they describe as "syngamy". Indeed it is possible to interpret them either in this way or as fission of dividing forms and, since the latter is known to occur, it would seem a more probable interpretation. Little further attention has been given to the hypothesis that sexual differentiation or syngamy of *T. brucei* might occur in the vertebrate host and it seems unlikely that this hypothesis will bear fruit in the future. The sexual cycle proposed by Penso (1934) (see below Fig. 8) cannot be considered a serious contribution and is only of interest in so far as it appears to represent an extreme example of the process, so common in investigation of the life cycle of *T. brucei*, where theory has tended to overshadow the data, on which it is presumably based, so that the two have tended to become separate.

3. Different stages of the life cycle in circulation—two stages with continuous gradation or three stages?

Salvin-Moore and Breinl (1908) and Valerio (1909) considered that a continuous development of *T. brucei* occurred in the blood and that the slender and stumpy forms represented the extremities of such a range. Minchin (1908), on the other hand, pointed out that the "intermediate form" differed to such an extent in its shape from that of the slender and stumpy forms of *T. brucei* that he considered it to represent a distinct stage in the life cycle. This idea was supported by the biometric studies of Hindle (1910b) who showed that lengths of blood forms taken at a single point in the infection were trimodal in distribution.

Bruce (1911) and Bruce *et al.* (1910) also considered that three distinct forms were involved; their measurements of many hundreds of trypanosomes, although suggestive, gave less clear-cut results and trimodal distributions were not obtained; this was probably because their preparations were taken from different animals at different times of infection. Swellengrebel (1912) also pooled the measurements that he had taken on different days; under these circumstances the varying proportions of different forms in their samples may have obscured any tendency to trimodality. Whatever their results, it is difficult to accept that trimodality should of itself constitute evidence that slender, intermediate and stumpy forms necessarily represent three separate stages in the life cycle; continuous gradation from slender to stumpy could as easily show an "intermediate" mode if the rate of transformation were slowed at any particular part of its course thereby causing an accumulation of transformational forms. Such slowing is implicit in the results of Venkatesan and Ormerod (1976) and Venkatesan *et al.* (1977).

Fairbairn and Culwick (1949) accepted, nevertheless, that slender, intermediate and stumpy forms in the blood did represent distinct stages and tried to use the dimensions of each form, considered in isolation from the other two, as the means of establishing differences between strains. This approach cannot, however, be justifiable because it is impossible to determine objectively which are intermediate forms or, indeed, which are slender and stumpy: a selection has to be made subjectively.

Many workers have demonstrated that the proportion of slender and stumpy forms varies at different phases of the infection and that this seems to be related to whether the trypomastigotes are dividing or not. Muriel Robertson (Robertson, 1913) showed that when a high percentage of slender trypomastigotes was in circulation many of these were dividing, but when the percentage of stumpy forms was high only a few showed signs of division; she concluded that division did not take place below a length of 20 μm.

Ogawa (1913, 1914) who studied infections in which the virulence had been exalted by passage, found that dividing forms which occurred at the beginning of the infection were slender whereas, towards the end of the infection when division had ceased, the trypomastigotes became stumpy.

Reichenow (1921) noted a similar phenomenon in patients: when a relapse occurred and trypomastigotes began to appear in the blood and to increase in numbers, only slender forms were present. However, at the peak of parasitaemia, slender trypomastigotes were transformed into stumpy forms and a remission in the infection occurred.

Ashcroft (1957) and Wijers (1959) both demonstrated clearly that in each wave of parasitaemia the slender forms preceded the stumpy and, as the wave subsided, the stumpy forms replaced the slender forms; both concluded that the intermediate form represented merely a transition between the slender and stumpy forms. Ormerod (1958) also demonstrated that agranular (slender) forms occurred at the beginning of the wave; at its crest all trypomastigotes contained granules (intermediate) which increased in size and number (stumpy form) as the wave decreased. There seems to be little doubt that pleomorphism represents the sequential development of forms of *T. brucei* in that the slender form appears first, divides and is converted into the stumpy form. When this transformation is associated with a wave of parasitaemia, the dividing slender (agranular) form is seen at the beginning of the rise, granules begin to accumulate during the rise and are at a maximum, in size and number, from the peak to the trough. When clearcut waves do not occur but only minor fluctuations, a preponderance of slender forms is generally associated with a rising parasitaemia and a preponderance of stumpy forms with a fall.

4. Degeneration

The stumpy form was known from the early decades of the century to be broader and slower-moving than the slender form and to contain many granules which could become as large as the nucleus (Policard, 1910); moreover, this sluggishness and granularity was particularly striking in the case of the posterior nuclear form. It was also accepted that the slender forms divided and transformed into stumpy forms which themselves were not observed to divide (Robertson, 1911). Oehler (1914) regarded the stumpy forms as "remission forms". Under these circumstances it would seem obvious to conclude, as did Beck (1910), that the stumpy forms were degenerate. But the majority of workers at that time did not accept his view: for instance, Swellengrebel (1912) described them as "surviving" (überlebenden) forms and he, as well as Hindle (1910a), noted that they were the forms remaining longest in the blood after chemotherapy, while Thomson and Robertson (1926) found that, in a strain which had become monomorphic, stumpy forms, previously absent, were produced by chemotherapy; thus the view that stumpy forms were generally resistant to adverse conditions became accepted. It is difficult to understand the reluctance of these and other workers to consider the possibility that the stumpy form of *T. brucei* might be degenerate unless the importance which was attached to the views of Muriel Robertson on the transmission of *T. brucei* in the tsetse is also taken into account.

Robertson (1913) argued persuasively that only the stumpy form was infective to the fly. This view, which was accepted almost universally, was apparently confirmed by Wijers and Willett (1960). However, Mshelbwala (1967) infected a single fly by feeding it solely with slender forms, an observation which has been confirmed on several occasions by Elce (unpublished observations): they were able to have reasonable confidence in the absence of stumpy forms for the feed by using a strain which shows only slender forms in the initial wave of infection. It is now possible to conclude that a totally viable stumpy form is not an essential requirement for cyclical transmission and allows one to accept evidence of degeneration of the stumpy form.

But what is the nature of this degeneration? Bevan and MacGregor (1910), who studied in rats a strain which behaved in the typical manner of *T. brucei*, thought that the conversion of slender into stumpy forms might be due to the action of antibodies, and this appeared to be confirmed by Ashcroft (1957) and Petana (1964) who demonstrated that the immunodepressive action of cortisone produced an increase in the proportion of slender at the expense of stumpy forms. This view of the relation between pleomorphism and the production of antibody was the more compelling because it appeared to fit so well with the concept of antigenic variation developed by Ritz (1914, 1916). According to this concept each wave of parasitaemia heralded the production of a new antigenic variant; thus, according to Ashcroft (1957), the slender form, which carried the new variant, did not react immediately with existing antibody, but when antibody to the new variant had been produced the slender forms reacted with it, their reproduction by binary fission was reduced, they were transformed to stumpy forms and removed from the blood.

Ashcroft's hypothesis, despite its attractions, could not be maintained in face of recent results using more effective techniques of immunodepression. Balber (1972) used a pleomorphic strain which gave no remission but only a plateau at about 80 h before a further rise in the total number of trypomastigotes resulted in the death of the animal; immunodepression abolished this plateau but did not affect the sequence of transformation from slender to stumpy forms. Similarly Luckins (1972) used strains which gave a partial remission. The effect of immunodepression was to produce a plateau in the total number of trypomastigotes; the succession of slender by stumpy forms again remained unaffected. Ormerod *et al.* (1974) used a strain that produced a complete remission; that is, all trypomastigotes disappeared temporarily from the blood. After immunodepression the remission remained complete although in some instances the disappearing stumpy (granular) forms overlapped the new wave of slender (agranular) forms. In the results of these three groups of workers, immunodepression in no way changed the sequence of transformation of slender to stumpy forms but it did cause a delay in the disappearance of stumpy forms from the blood. According to Ormerod *et al.* (1974) the stumpy forms in immunodepressed animals became even more sluggish, broader and more heavily loaded with lipid granules, and they concluded that the transformation had nothing to do with the action of antibody but represented an innate process of degeneration in the blood trypomastigote. Venkatesan and Ormerod (1976) have since clarified the nature of this process of degeneration and have shown that lipid, rich in cholesterol, is absorbed from the plasma of the host into phagosomal vacuoles (Venkatesan *et al.*, 1977). These vacuoles

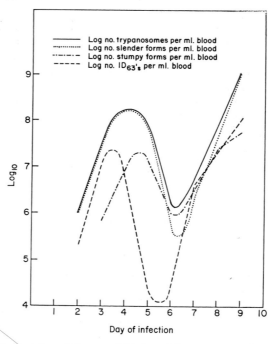

FIG. 2. The infectivity of forms of *T. brucei* in an acute relapsing infection in rats (Cunningham *et al.*, 1963). Note that the minimum infectivity occurs at day 5 when the infection is falling; when slender forms are being transformed to stumpy forms and the latter removed from the blood. It is probable that the method of Ormerod *et al.* (1963) would have indicated that many of the "slender" forms carried granules at day 5, i.e. that degeneration was beginning to occur.

fuse with lysosomes which, in the process of transformation of the trypomastigote from slender to stumpy, liberate hydrolases which destroy the trypomastigote. The process of destruction is, however, a slow one unless the intact immune system is able to remove damaged trypanosomes from the blood.

The degenerate nature of the stumpy form is also shown by its lack of infectivity on transference to a new vertebrate host. This observation has been made by Cunningham *et al.* (1963) (see Fig. 2) and has been confirmed by Venkatesan (unpublished observation).

5. Pleomorphism may be the result of more than one process

Although slender forms are now known to be infective to tsetse, there is no evidence to suggest that stumpy forms are not also infective to tsetse. Such a conclusion, although a reasonable supposition on the evidence to hand, must await the results of direct experiment.

It is possible that a stage of development prior to degeneration may represent the ideal phase for infection of tsetse, and in this connection a process described by Langreth and Balber (1975) and by Venkatesan *et al.* (1977) may be significant; this is the process of "autophagy" or "cellular defaecation" in which a time-expired organelle may be removed from the cell. Such a process, if it removes the phagolysosome after the absorption of lipid and before secretion of hydrolytic enzyme has begun, might reverse the process of progressive degeneration of the cell. Whether or not this process is of significance in the infection of tsetse remains uncertain, but the process is mentioned at this point in the discussion to emphasize that the accumulation of lipid need not necessarily result in the death of the cell; it is possible that it may direct the development of the trypanosome into yet another pathway, namely into the production of tissue forms—this possibility will be discussed later in this review as part of an hypothesis for the development of *T. brucei*.

The first trypomastigotes to appear in the blood are thinner than the normal slender trypomastigote. These forms were first observed by Swellengrebel (1912) (see Fig. 1) who regarded them as typical slender trypomastigotes; also by Wijers (1960) who considered them to be slender forms immediately after division. Ormerod and Venkatesan (1971a) noted that they were the first forms to appear in the blood either at the beginning of the infection or at the relapse, that they had a characteristic movement more like a spirochaete than a trypanosome, and that their refractility suggested that they were circular in cross-section, hence the name "long-narrow" with which they described them to distinguish them from the "long-flat" form, the more familiar dividing form. Long-narrow forms stain differently from long-flat forms (Molloy and Ormerod, 1965) in that there are no Type I granules. There also appears to be a striking difference on electron microscopy (Ellis and Ormerod, un-

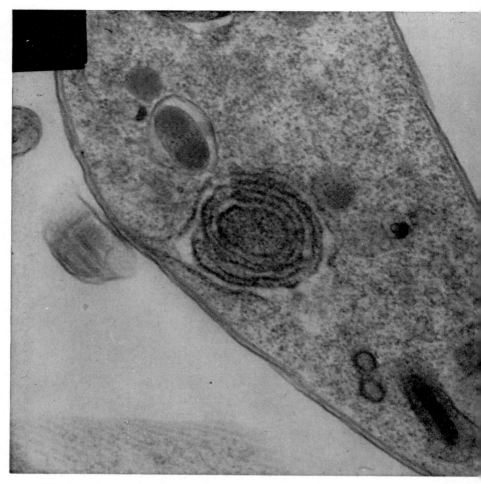

FIG. 3.   Electron micrograph (D. S. Ellis original) of a "long-narrow" form.
Note the whorl shape of the flagellum-associated endoplasmic reticulum.

published) see Fig. 3); the peculiar whorl-shaped endoplasmic reticulum
appears to be an essential characteristic of the long-narrow form.

D. FILAMENTS OF TRYPOMASTIGOTES

Schepilewsky (1912) first noted long thread-like appendages from both
ends of trypomastigotes which appeared to emerge and to be trailed by
them as they swam through the blood. These were first seen by electron
microscopy by Babudieri and Tomasini (1962) and were investigated in
some detail by Ellis et al. (1976). There appear to be two distinct types

of filament. One is associated with the long-narrow and long-flat forms, and is referred to by Ellis *et al.* (1976), using the terminology of Vickerman and Luckins (1969), as the "plasmaneme". It is seen by light in the living trypomastigote and by electron microscopy by means of the negative staining technique. It is absent in any material which has been fixed and sectioned for electron microscopy and there is thus some suggestion that it may appear as a result of artificial manipulation. Clearly, under these circumstances it is not possible to indicate whether it plays any part of significance in the life cycle of *T. brucei*.

The other type of filament is associated with the stumpy trypomastigote. This filament is clearly observed in sections of tissue and of blood viewed by electron microscopy. It appears to emerge from the flagellar pocket and resembles a secretion. It is possible that it is related in some way to the production and liberation of hydrolytic enzymes which were observed in this phase of the parasite by Venkatesan *et al.*(1977): if this interpretation is correct it may be important to the pathogenicity of *T. brucei* but it is still not clear whether it is of any significance to the life cycle.

E. A VIEW OF THE SIGNIFICANCE OF PLEOMORPHISM

Pleomorphism of *T. brucei* in the blood, according to Ormerod and Venkatesan (1971a), appears to represent the successive development of three stages in the life cycle of the parasite: the long-narrow form is the first to appear, it does not divide but transforms into the long-flat form; the long-flat form undergoes binary fission and absorbs lipid which gradually inhibits its division while it becomes transformed into the stumpy form. The forms designated in the older classification, namely slender, intermediate and stumpy, correspond only in part to the new designation given above: the long-narrow form of Ormerod and Venkatesan was previously either ignored or counted in with the slender forms; the long-flat form of Ormerod and Venkatesan can generally be considered to correspond with the slender forms of the older classification. Ormerod and Venkatesan do not recognize "intermediate" as a stage but rather as the early stage of degeneration, and the stumpy form and its extreme posterior–nuclear form they regard as the final stages of degeneration. While it seems likely that the stumpy form continues progressively to degenerate and becomes non-infective for tsetse and mammal alike, the possibility remains that in some instances the lipid phagolysosomes may be removed from its cytoplasm to allow division to be resumed.

Pleomorphism in the blood may therefore be considered to represent the maturation of the long-narrow form into the long-flat form; the long-flat form divides and begins to degenerate; its more degenerate stages are known as stumpy forms. There is no evidence to suggest that the process described above is reversible or that the long-narrow or long-flat forms can ever be generated in the blood from the stumpy form as was suggested by Robertson (1912a) (see Fig. 6). The hypothesis that the long-narrow form is produced from a tissue form will be discussed below.

III. The significance of "aberrant" forms in the blood

While it is generally accepted that the variation of *T. brucei* in the blood includes forms ranging from long-narrow and rapidly moving, to stumpy and relatively sluggish leaf-like forms (also the "posterior–nuclear form" which is the most sluggish of all), a number of other forms have been described which do not fit into this series. These forms are here described as "aberrant", not because they should necessarily be assumed to be abnormal forms but because they do not appear to be part of the usual series characteristic of *T. brucei* parasitaemia. Many workers regard these forms as artefacts or as degenerate forms (Wijers, 1960), however, it is possible that this interpretation may not, in all instances, be justified; for this reason it is important to reconsider the evidence that has been put forward.

A. SPHERICAL FORMS AND "TADPOLE" FORMS

On a number of occasions spherical or "tadpole"-like forms have been observed in the blood. The first observations were by Bradford and Plimmer (1902) and Laveran and Mesnil (1902) who regarded them as "formes d'involution". Holmes (1904) and Lingard (1907) made similar observations on *T. evansi*. The first serious study of their significance was that of Salvin-Moore and Breinl (1908) who regarded the spherical forms as "latent bodies" capable of renewing the infection either by relapse or by passage into another host in the absence of trypomastigotes in the blood. Latent bodies were illustrated as having the structure of a trypanosome nucleus usually surrounded by a small amount of cytoplasm, sometimes with a flagellum which was either partially free or wrapped around the periphery of the organism in the manner of a sphaeromastigote (Brack, 1968). Salvin-Moore and Breinl described the way in which latent bodies were produced as being related to a streak of staining material (usually referred to as the axial filament) which, in their preparations, appeared to form a junction between the nucleus and kinetoplast. Axial filaments, which are only seen occasionally with the staining techniques of today, are probably fixation artefacts in which the stain accumulates in a groove formed in the region of the flagellar pocket.

More detailed studies were carried out by Fantham (1911) who noted in addition the presence of pear-shaped forms, referred to in this chapter as "tadpole forms" (*forme a girino*; Penso, 1934) which Fantham regarded as being an intermediate stage in the development of the latent body into the trypomastigote during the relapse when the parasitaemia was increasing. Fantham made a clear distinction between the tadpole forms which he regarded as an essential part of the cycle of development and degenerating trypomastigotes which he also observed.

At about the same time, Fry (1912), Fry and Ranken (1913) and Balfour (1911) proposed the theory that, when the trypomastigote degenerated, it liberated into the blood a collection of "infective granules", analogous to latent bodies, capable of continuing the infection through a remission period in the absence of trypomastigotes in the blood. Few appeared to accept this theory, and it is likely that the infective granules that were observed being liberated into the blood were in fact the lipid (Type II) granules of Molloy and Ormerod (1965) which Ormerod (1961) also observed being liberated into the blood at the time of the crisis.

Since many circulating trypomastigotes undergo degeneration it is easy to postulate that all unusual forms are the result of degeneration. Thus Hindle (1910b) asserted that all the changes observed were the result of degeneration. Hindle based his conclusions on the effect of an arsenical drug which caused trypomastigotes to swell, burst and liberate their nuclei. Fusco (1908, 1910) studied degeneration of trypomastigotes in dead animals and in culture and, although he concluded that the forms that he observed were a significant part of the life cycle, it is unlikely that either he or Hindle (1910b) were studying any process that can occur during a normal infection; the same criticism also applies to the more recent work of Wijers (1960) who recorded an observation (frequently observed by others) that trypomastigotes tend to round up and become vacuolated *in vitro*.

Tadpole forms frequently occur, especially after immunodepression, in drug-treated infections. This observation was made by von Jancsó (1934) and confirmed by Ormerod (1951). But they also occur in untreated infections (Ormerod and Venkatesan, 1971a) in which they are identical in appearance with those treated with drugs and are active and refractile without the usual appearances of degeneration. Nevertheless Ormerod and Venkatesan (1971b) considered that they were degenerate in the sense that they represented a failure in the maturation process of the long-narrow forms, normally the first stage to appear in the blood.

B. FILTRATION OF INFECTIVE BLOOD AND TISSUES

The most important point in the theory discussed above, *viz.* that *T. brucei* had a stage of development which was small or even ultramicroscopical, depended upon the observation that fluids, passed through a filter with pores that were too small to allow the passage of trypomasti-gotes, would nevertheless generate infection in a new host. Such an observation was first carried out by Salvin-Moore and Breinl (1908) using a technique developed by Novy and McNeal (1907) for the study of *T. lewisi*. Although no details of their technique is given they stated that the filtrate was infective. Bruce and Bateman (1908) carried out a similar experiment with *T. evansi* and found that the filtrate would not infect and neither would filtrate from *T. brucei* (Bruce *et al.*, 1910; Wolbach *et al.*, 1915).

However, extensive experiments by Reich and Beckwith (1922), Reich (1924) and Battaglia (1924) showed that the filtrates, mainly from macerated internal organs of infected animals, were frequently infective in the absence of parasitaemia; both Bruce and Reich controlled their experiments carefully by introducing a marker bacterium so that the discrepancy of their results was not explicable except in terms of some difference between blood and tissue infection. Recently, similar experiments have been carried out by Soltys *et al.* (1969) who showed that an infective filtrate was obtained from a filter with pores of 1·2 μm but not from one of 0·65 μm pore size. The conclusion that these experiments suggest is that infective forms smaller than trypomastigotes (such as infective granules or latent bodies) do not normally occur in the blood but that such forms may occur in the tissues. These conclusions may be valid despite the lack of uniformity of results; I, however, confess myself unconvinced and would prefer to ignore all results obtained by filtration.

C. MULTINUCLEATE FORMS

Forms with more than two nuclei, kinetoplasts or flagella were noted by the early workers (Bradford and Plimmer, 1902; Salvin-Moore and Breinl, 1908; Hindle, 1910a; Robertson, 1912) but no comment about their possible significance was made except by Ottolenghi (1910) who regarded them as macrogametocytes. von Jancsó and von Jancsó (1934) and Ormerod (1951) noted them, together with tadpole forms, as mentioned above, in animals which had been treated with trypanocidal drugs and immunodepressant agents; these "giant" forms are particularly impressive when observed by phase contrast in the living state and resemble, in the way they move, the swimming of a skate. Some of them appear degenerate and contain numerous lipid granules but others show no properties to suggest that they might be degenerate. Moreover, although they had previously attracted most attention in infections which had been influenced by the administration of drugs, Ormerod and Venkatesan (1971a) noted that they were plentiful at some phases in the infection of untreated animals. Thus they considered them to represent part of the normal life cycle in the vertebrate host.

Although the so-called "aberrant" forms have not hitherto received much attention in the literature of *T. brucei* they may nevertheless be of some importance as an indication of processes which may be taking place in less accessible parts of the body and be aberrant only in that they have appeared in the blood. It seems unlikely, on the other hand, that they represent the normal development of *T. brucei* in the tissues.

IV. The significance of culture forms

The relevance of cultured forms of *T. brucei* is marginal to the argument of this review which concerns the nature of the life cycle in the intact vertebrate host. Nevertheless, some useful indications have been given about the possible course of development of certain stages isolated in culture. Three general types of culture method need to be considered:
(1) Development at 28°C (or thereabouts) in blood media has been studied by Thomas and Breinl (1905), Gray and Tulloch (1906), Thomson and Sinton (1912) and latterly by Weinman (1946). These methods bring about development of forms that resemble those that occur in the gut of tsetse. This resemblance was first recognized by Thomson and Sinton (1912).
(2) Development at 25–37°C of specially selected cell lines in defined or semi-defined media by methods of Pittam (1970) or Cross and Manning (1973) where the object is to grow an homogeneous population of organisms for use as a biochemical model of the blood stage. In practice the forms bear so little resemblance to those of a natural parasitaemia that inferences drawn from their development (and probably also their biochemical properties) are not likely to be of much value.
(3) Development of organisms, derived from strains that have recently been isolated, at 37°C in blood media or in the presence of other living cells.

The following discussion is based solely on the third type of culture. Although in some instances growth may be minimal, some indication may be given of the course of development of blood forms or of their subsequent fate.

Erdmann (1915a, b) took trypanosomes from a rat infected 84 h previously and inoculated them into plasma at 37°C. After 24 h multiple division occurred, one organism producing 4 or 8 daughter cells. After 4 days rounded forms, which resembled the latent bodies of Salvin-Moore and Breinl (1908), appeared. Although Erdmann's account of her findings is not very clear, she distinguished the forms which appeared at 37°C from those which appeared at 16–18°C which were rounded and "crithidia-like" and underwent binary fission.

Many workers have successfully grown *T. brucei* and *T. evansi* in hen eggs; this work has been reviewed by Pipkin (1960) but none succeeded in obtaining a cycle of development resembling that in mammals until

Goedbloed and her co-workers (Goedbloed and Southgate, 1969; Goedbloed and Kinyanjui, 1970) showed that recently isolated strains of *T. brucei* would produce the typical cycle of pleomorphism in the chicken embryo. Although culture in eggs cannot strictly be referred to as "*in vitro*" culture, the inability of the chicken embryo to mount an antibody response gives it some of the characteristics of an inert medium. The appearance of pleomorphic trypomastigotes in the blood system and chorioallantoic membranes of eggs indicated clearly (some years before experiments were carried out in immunodepressed mammals) that the presence of antibodies was not essential to the transformation of slender to stumpy trypomastigotes or to the fluctuation in parasitaemia.

Similar pleomorphic development occurs in the cultures of Hirumi *et al.* (1977). This recent work which makes use of cultures of a cell line of bovine fibroblasts not only gives heavy yields of slender and stumpy forms (which may prove useful as biochemical models) but also a small number of multiple-division forms. Further information on the use of this interesting new method is awaited with impatience.

V. Remission, relapse and the relation between parasitaemia and pathological lesion

T. brucei infection, with a strain which has not previously been passaged many times by syringe, usually gives a fluctuating parasitaemia. On the one hand parasitaemias may fluctuate in short waves, as in the strain isolated from the original case of rhodesian sleeping sickness studied by Ross and Thomson (1910) where the peaks were only a few days apart and a constantly fluctuating parasitaemia was always present: on the other hand, in the gambian type of disease, waves may be so long that there are prolonged periods when there is no parasitaemia. Such phases may be protracted, continuing for a number of years as in the cases reviewed by Todd (1911). Similar waves or periods without parasitaemia occur when the strains are isolated in laboratory animals; thus Thomson and Robertson (1926) showed that in rats and guinea-pigs, the parasites of gambian strains were frequently absent from the blood, whereas rhodesian strains gave a continuous fluctuating parasitaemia. This state of affairs tended to persist in both types of strain until increasing virulence of the parasite, the result of frequent consecutive passage, caused the host's death during the first wave of parasitaemia which frequently overwhelmed it.

Laveran (1911) infected a goat with a gambian strain, and over the course of two years he was seldom able to find parasites in the blood. Nevertheless, dogs, which were subinoculated from it became parasitaemic, and the goat, which died two years after the original inoculation, showed the typical lesions of sleeping sickness in the brain and meninges.

A gambian (the Yaoundé) strain studied by Stefanopoulo and his colleagues (Roubaud *et al.*, 1944; Stefanopoulo *et al.*, 1945) showed over a number of years only occasional parasites in the blood of rats and rabbits, yet at post-mortem the animals showed severe lesions in the brain resembling the typical perivascular cuffing of sleeping sickness associated with massive numbers of parasites in the brain substance and in the meninges. On the other hand, Frazer and Duke (1912), who infected a bushbuck with a gambian strain, were able, 315 days later, to demonstrate a very low parasitaemia sufficient to infect 2 out of 59 tsetse flies, yet at *post mortem* they detected no perceptible lesion. Thus, although there seems to be no clear relationship between the extent of the parasitaemia and the severity of the lesion, there is a greater tendency for gambian sleeping sickness to show more intense perivascular cuffing than the rhodesian disease (Ormerod, 1970). This may either be because the gambian disease lasts for longer or because it has the particular propensity suggested by Ormerod and Venkatesan (1971a) for developing in the tissues rather than in the blood.

The nature of the remissions in sleeping sickness has for long appeared incompatible with the established view that binary fission in the blood was the main if not the only method of reproduction of *T. brucei* in the mammalian host: this apparent incompatibility led Gallais *et al.* (1953) to review the possible mechanisms that could give rise to remissions, and they concluded that the existence of an as yet undiscovered cycle of development in the tissues should not be discounted.

A. EXPERIMENTAL PRODUCTION OF REMISSIONS

Various authors have observed that lower infections occur if the animal is kept in the cold. Blanchard (1903) observed that virulent *T. brucei* developed more rapidly in the marmot (*Marmota* sp.) at room temperature than in hibernating animals. Brumpt (1908) showed that dormice (*Eliomis* sp.) did not develop any significant infection when kept in a cellar at 6°C whereas control animals at 15–20°C developed virulent infections. Similarly Van den Branden (1939) showed that infected rats kept at 4–5°C survived for 5–7 days longer than controls at 10–20°C. On the other hand Ross and Williams (1910) obtained equivocal results, and Kligler (1927), working with a strain of *T. evansi*, negative results, but in both these experiments the temperature differentials were lower and less constantly maintained than by workers who had obtained positive results. Petrů and Vojtěchovská (1955) found that animals maintained under the influence of narcotic drugs in a state of semi-hibernation, also showed lower infections and longer periods of survival. It seems certain that abnormally low temperatures are associated with low parasitaemia.

On the other hand, abnormally high temperatures are also associated with low parasitaemia. Otieno (1972) showed that *T. brucei* and *T. evansi* behaved in the same way as *T. cruzi* in showing a reduction of parasitaemia if the host animal was kept at a raised temperature of 35°C. The effect was particularly well marked when a specially virulent strain was used; under these circumstances, the life of an animal, which would normally have been dead in 10 days, would be prolonged sometimes indefinitely. Immunodepressed animals maintained at 35°C (Otieno, 1973) showed, however, a high parasitaemia which appeared to be less pathogenic than infections at room temperature. A strain which was monomorphic at room temperature became pleomorphic and showed many multinucleate and tadpole forms similar to those observed by von Jancsó and von Jancsó (1934).

The relationship of these experiments to the life cycle of *T. brucei* in the mammalian host is not at the moment clear; there can be little doubt, however, that changes in temperature inhibit one phase in the development of *T. brucei*. There is, however, no evidence as to which phase is inhibited, and it is possible that the actions of heat and cold take effect on different parts of the cycle of development. The experiments involving changes of temperature have been included in this review because it is likely that similar procedures will be useful in future investigation of the life cycle of *T. brucei* in the mammalian host.

VI. Metabolic and fine structural differences between different stages and their implications for the life cycle

A. THE CHONDRIOME

Vickerman (1965, 1970) has discussed in detail the changes which occur in the mitochondrion of *T. brucei* during its development from the slender to the stumpy form. He points out that the mitochondrion of the slender form is a narrow tube from which the normal finger-like cristae (Vickerman, 1962; Mühlpfordt and Bayer, 1965) are almost absent. More cristae were said to be present in the intermediate and stumpy forms and the maximum number was present in the stages which develop in the insect vector and in the culture forms that represent similar stages. Similarly, mitochondrial activity, i.e. the ability of cellular organelles to reduce tetrazolium salts in the presence of nicotinamide adenine dinucleotide, absent in the slender forms of old laboratory strains, was found to be present in intermediate and stumpy forms and especially in culture forms. Vickerman suggested that the stumpy trypomastigote has an advantage in acting as the infective form for the fly because it represents an intermediate stage in the development of the chondriome between the "inactive" chondriome of the slender form and the highly active chondriome of the insect/culture form.

The finding, discussed earlier in this review, that the stumpy trypomastigote is not necessarily the only infective form for the fly suggests that Vickerman's useful and widely accepted concept of the development of the chondriome during pleomorphic development of *T. brucei* should be re-evaluated. In this connection two points need to be considered: (1) The concept of an "inactive" chondriome in the slender form was developed at a time when the only pure source of slender forms was from strains which had been passaged many times in the laboratory: there is no doubt that the mitochondrion of such strains is lacking in cristae. However, suspensions of slender forms which can now be obtained from some recently isolated strains (Venkatesan *et al.* 1977) are not conspicuously lacking in mitochondrial cristae even although the mitochondrial tube is significantly narrower in the slender than in the stumpy form (Böhringer and Hecker, 1975).
(2) It is likely, as has been pointed out above, that there is no absolute distinction between slender, intermediate and stumpy forms. Thus one group of workers may call one morphological form "intermediate" (Ormerod, 1976) and another stumpy (Langreth and Balber, 1975). This tendency is exacerbated in electron microscopy in which tradition dictates that a worker should discount degenerate cells thus degenerate stumpy forms tend—some will say *sui generis*—to be rejected from further consideration. This problem does not, however, arise if the blood stage is identified by some less subjective means, e.g. presence or absence of lipid granules (Ormerod *et al.*, 1974) or, ideally, by the total volume of the organism by morphometric analysis on electron microscopy (Böhringer and Hecker, 1974, 1975).

Böhringer and Hecker (1975) have pointed out that the cristae in the mitochondrion of trypomastigotes undergoing development in the fly are plate-like and do not resemble the cristae of blood forms which are finger-like. Similarly Balber and Ward (1972) have shown that culture forms and flagellates from infected tsetse do not reduce tetrazolium salts until growth has been established for several weeks; thus the evidence suggests that development of the slender into the stumpy trypomastigote does not constitute part of the development of the vertebrate stage into the invertebrate stage but rather that it has some different significance related, perhaps, to the cycle in the vertebrate host.

B. DIFFERENCES IN LIPID METABOLISM

The lack of any metabolic gradation from blood forms to culture forms is also shown by the work of Williamson and his colleagues (Dixon and Williamson, 1970; Dixon *et al.*, 1971, 1972) who showed that there is a complete change in lipid metabolism between blood and culture forms in the composition of fatty acids, sterols and phospholipids.

There is also a difference in the lipid metabolism of slender and stumpy forms of *T. brucei* (Venkatesan and Ormerod, 1976). The slender form has 4- to 5-fold more phosphatidylinositol than the stumpy form and this appears to indicate that the slender form is actively engaged in the synthesis of membranes (i.e., mitochondrion, endoplasmic reticulum) which require large amounts of this phospholipid; the stumpy form appears in this respect to be metabolically inert. The stumpy form, on the other hand, contains 6 times as much cholesterol as the slender form. Venkatesan and Ormerod (1976) argue that the trypomastigote has probably taken up the cholesterol in the process of development in the blood by absorption of plasma lipoprotein. The evidence on which they base this argument consists partly in the extent of the esterified cholesterol present —it is inherently unlikely that it has been synthesized in this form by the trypanosomes—and partly as a result of dietary experiments in which abnormal fatty acids (to which cholesterol is in part esterified) appeared in the host's plasma; in these circumstances the abnormal fatty acids are also found in the lipid of the stumpy trypomastigote indicating that at least this part of the lipoprotein complex has been absorbed from the plasma.

Venkatesan *et al.* (1977) further investigated the uptake of lipid by electron microscopy in association with histochemical localization of acid phosphatase activity. Vacuoles of absorbed lipid were found in association with lysosomal enzymes (acid phosphatase) which appeared to be liberated within the cytoplasm of the stumpy trypomastigote. They consider that the absorption of lipid and its activation of hydrolytic enzymes within the cell is the mechanism by which stumpy forms in a pleomorphic infection become degenerate and die. They conclude (Ormerod *et al.*, 1974) that the stumpy forms are indeed degenerate and are removed from the blood without the necessity of any intervention on the part of the host's immune system.

C. THE AUTOPHAGOSOME

The trypomastigote has been observed by Langreth and Balber (1975) and by Venkatesan *et al.* (1977) to contain a mechanism possessed by many other types of cell by which time-expired organelles may be removed. This mechanism may play an important role in cells which are undergoing metamorphosis from one stage to another, such as the removal of the endoplasmic reticular whorl that appears in the long-narrow form but not in the subsequent long-flat form or any succeeding stage in the blood. This mechanism is called variously the autophagosome or the autophagic vacuole, and Langreth and Balber (1975) state that it is a method of "cellular defaecation" in which unwanted organelles may be eliminated from the cell by extrusion on the surface probably within the flagellar pocket. Venkatesan *et al.* (1977) indicate that the "phagolyso-some", that is to say the combined vacuole (which in this instance has absorbed lipid) and the lysosome with which it has fused, may be en-gulfed in an autophagosome, and in this way its damaging effect on the cell may be reversed. It is difficult to see how important this mechanism may be in the life cycle of *T. brucei* in the mammalian host, yet if blood forms are not to be eliminated entirely from the animal, some such mechanism is necessary for ensuring the continued existence of the organism within the vertebrate body. The possible significance of the autophagosome in the life cycle of *T. brucei* in the vertebrate will be considered in the final section of this review.

VII. Tissue stages of T. brucei

A. THE CHANCRE

The discovery of the pre-erythrocytic stage of the malaria parasite by Shortt and Garnham (1948) concentrated attention, in studies of other parasitic protozoa, on the possibility that a cryptic stage might exist at the beginning of the infection, and in the case of *T. brucei* a possible locus for such a stage seemed to be the site of local reaction which fre-quently precedes an infection. Gordon *et al.* (1956) had shown that, when a tsetse deposits metacyclic trypomastigotes in the tissues, some remain *in situ* while others enter the blood stream directly. Gordon and Willett (1957) showed that the site of inoculation of metacyclic trypo-mastigotes, when excised, macerated and re-inoculated into clean animals, carried much the same degree of infectivity as the blood of the animal and of the local lymph glands. After several days, however, local multipli-cation of slender trypomastigotes occurred, and these generally resembled the forms that were multiplying concurrently in the blood. Fairbairn and Godfrey (1957, 1958) showed that metacyclic forms developed into slender trypomastigotes within and below the dermis in man. These results indicate that a cryptic stage in *T. brucei* infection is unlikely to occur during the prepatent period between the time of inoculation and the time when trypomastigotes first appear in the blood, or if it does occur it is not intrinsically different since tissue forms of the parasite found at this stage seem to be exactly the same as those seen in the blood. The significance of the prepatent period seems generally to depend more on the paucity of trypomastigotes which have not yet had time to re-produce and produce sufficient numbers to be found in the blood than on the existence of a cryptic phase of development that precedes evolution in the blood.

B. LYMPHATIC SPREAD

Nevertheless, development in the blood is not necessarily the only or even the main site of reproduction of trypanosomes in the early stages of the infection. Swollen glands have long been recognized as an early sign of chronic gambian disease (Macfie, 1913). They are also seen in some cases of the more acute rhodesian form but may cease to be a feature (Kunert, 1939) at other epidemic phases of the disease. The importance of lymphatic spread of *T. brucei* was noted by Schuberg and Böing (1913), who compared it with syphilis in its ability to spread through the tissues without involving the blood, and by Reichenow (1921). Recently, Ssenyonga and Adam (1975) have shown that more stumpy forms are to be found in the blood than in the thoracic duct. While the interpretation of this experiment is not yet clear it appears to indicate that forms in the blood are more mature than those which have developed extravascularly in peritoneal fluid and are taken up by the thoracic duct. Further study of the development of *T. brucei* in peritoneal and other body fluids appears to be necessary.

C. ABSENCE OF TRYPANOSOMES FROM THE BLOOD

The remissions that occur in sleeping sickness and *T. brucei* infections of animals, which may be short in duration or prolonged to periods of months or years, focus attention on the possibility that there may be an occult phase of development in the tissues in which the infection is suspended without development of the usual parasitaemia. Arguments in favour of such a phase have been developed by Gallais *et al.* (1953) who believed that such sequestration was a necessary part of the phenomenon of remission in gambian disease; also by Walker (1964), who pointed out the extent of the evidence suggesting that the cycle of development of *T. brucei* was not confined to the blood but that multiplication in tissues might occur either within blood vessels, as with erythrocytic schizogony in *P. falciparium*, or extravascularly. The tissue phase forms may be similar to those of the blood phase as demonstrated by Stevenson (1917, 1922), Stefanopoulo *et al.* (1945) and Gordon and Willett (1957) or may be "plasmodial", cystic or multinuclear (see below) and of these possibilities by far the most likely seemed to be the existence of amastigote forms which had been familiar for many years as the tissue phase of *T. cruzi*. Deane (1969) has suggested that an amastigote phase, which has now been identified in most trypanosomes infecting vertebrates, will ultimately be found to be a part of the cycle of development in all.

D. PLASMODIAL AND OTHER MULTINUCLEAR FORMS

Several early workers described "plasmodial" stages that might represent a tissue stage. Bradford and Plimmer (1902) noted such a stage in the original strain of *T. brucei* and Walker (1912) described a multinucleate form of *T. evansi* which, he believed, underwent schizogony. More recently, a similar plasmodial stage was observed by Gallais *et al.* (1953). Spectacular multiple division forms were observed by Ottolenghi (1910) who infected animals with *T. brucei* and *T. evansi* by inoculating heart blood from a donor animal. 0·25–1·0 ml was injected, depending on the size of the recipient, into the peritoneal cavity: after 24 h the exudate contained numerous large flagellates often with many nuclei and flagella (Fig. 4). The tendency of the large forms to be joined at the posterior end with smaller forms led him to propose a process of gametogamy. The conjunction of forms at the posterior end is frequently seen to occur in trypomastigotes *in vitro* and it does not seem reasonable to attribute any special significance to its occurrence when one organism involved is a "giant" multinuclear form. What, however, cannot fail to impress the reader is the frequency, size and multiplicity of organelles of these forms which Ottolenghi demonstrated in a series of micrographs; some are reproduced in Fig. 4.

Philiptshenko (1929) observed multinucleate forms in the blood and related them to clusters of bodies resembling amastigotes which he also saw in the lungs of infected animals. Similar bodies were also seen in smears of liver and spleen by Soltys and Woo (1969, 1970), by Soltys *et al.* (1969) and by Ormerod and Venkatesan (1971b) who also found clusters similar to the bodies noted by Philiptschenko (1929). These were, however, found in the choroid plexus of the brain.

E. SPHERICAL FORMS AND "LATENT" BODIES

The latent bodies noted in spleen and lung by Salvin-Moore and Breinl (1908), were observed in these and other organs by several early authors. These include Fantham (1911), Laveran (1911), Buchanan (1911), Mott and Stewart (1907), Vianna (1911) and Sant'ana (1913) who found them with considerable frequency in animals infected with a strain of human origin from Mozambique. Many of these observers (e.g., Laveran, Sant'ana) considered that these and other spherical forms that they observed were degenerate, others (Salvin-Moore and Breinl, Fantham), that they represented resistant forms which were able to survive the remission and produce new parasitaemias on relapse. Some of the forms seen, such as those of Buchanan (1911) in wild rodents which had been inoculated in the laboratory, may have been other parasites such as

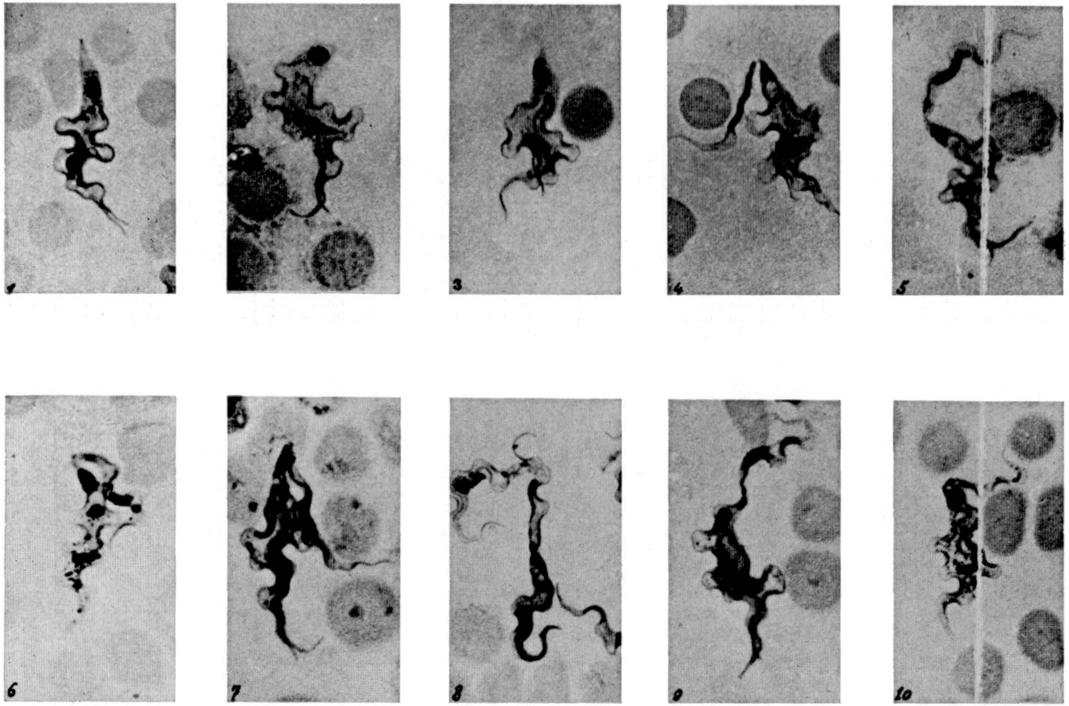

FIG. 4 (see page 370 for legend).

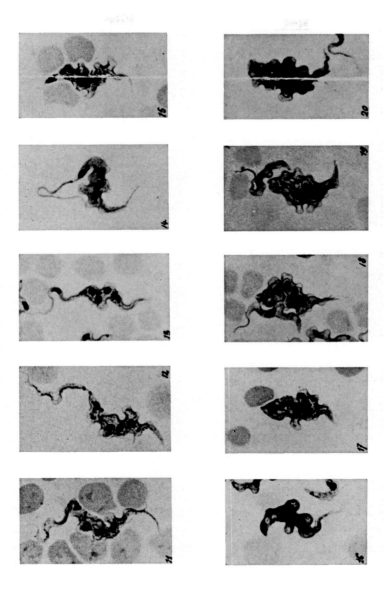

FIG. 4 (see page 370 for legend).

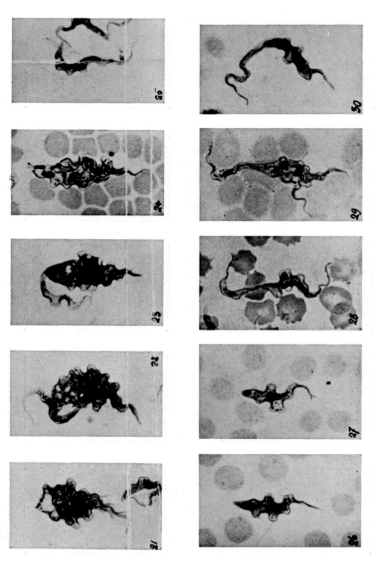

FIG. 4 (see page 370 for legend).

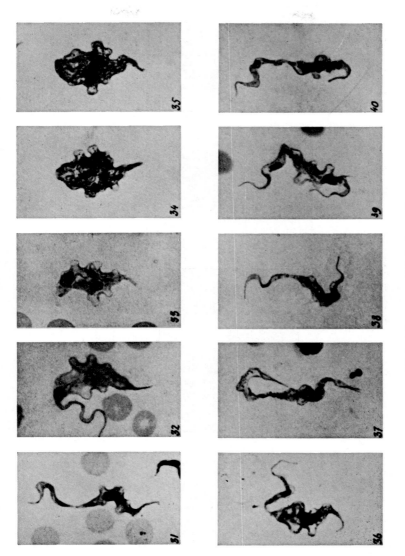

FIG. 4 (see page 370 for legend).

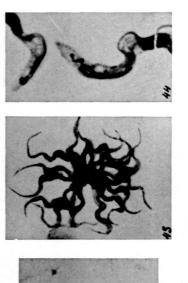

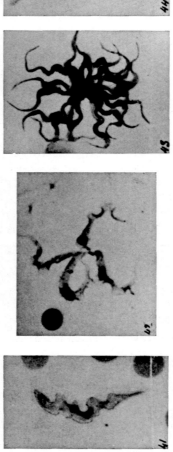

FIG. 4. Multiple division forms found by Ottolenghi (1910) in the peritoneal fluid and interpreted by him as macrogametocytes.

Clossiella or *Pneumocystis*, and it is practically certain that Vianna (1911) observed animals that had been inoculated erroneously with *T. cruzi*, so clearly does his description (a preliminary note only) resemble this parasite. Nevertheless, a body of support for the existence of these spherical forms does appear to have been established.

The subsequent history seems to have depended to a large extent on the divergence of views of certain authorities whose followers were either English-speaking or Italian. German workers on trypanosomiasis had largely withdrawn from the more academic aspects of the field after the 1914–1918 War, although much of the work of the Italian groups was published in German.

F. THE ATTITUDE OF ENGLISH-SPEAKING WORKERS

The work of Salvin-Moore and Breinl (1908) and others who studied the significance of the latent bodies, came under criticism from Robertson (1912a) and Hindle (1910a). Wenyon (1926), in reporting the argument, maintained a scrupulously open view of the subject and indicated that the evidence was conclusive neither in favour of the existence of resistant forms nor against it: nevertheless, the clear importance of binary fission in the blood as the only certain means of reproduction of *T. brucei* tended to overshadow the importance of other possible methods of reproduction.

A characteristically confused account of the life cycle of *T. brucei* (called *Castellanella rhodesiense* in the 3rd Edition) is given by Castellani and Chalmers (1910, 1913, 1919) emphasizing the importance of spherical forms which Castellani claimed to have discovered (see below). Spherical forms were mentioned by Manson (1914) but reference to them was omitted in subsequent editions of his textbook (Manson, 1919). Thomson and Robertson (1929) ignored the problem of tissue multiplication, as did Hoare (1949), and it is probable that the content of these two important textbooks determined the attitude of workers to such an extent that a generation of English-speaking protozoologists has grown up in the belief that *T. brucei* multiplied solely by binary fission in the blood. Nevertheless, Noble (1955) in reviewing earlier literature reached the conclusion, see below, which was at the time much at variance with current attitudes, that an amastigote phase occurred in the development of *T. brucei* in the vertebrate host; his conclusion was also noted by Levine (1961); Hoare (1972), on the other hand, does not refer to the earlier work other than to state that, in the past, tissue forms were regarded as degenerate; he refers however to the recent work of Soltys and Woo (1969, 1970) and to that of Ormerod and Venkatesan (1970).

G. THE ATTITUDE OF ITALIAN WORKERS

Castellani (1904) observed rounded and oval forms of *T. brucei*, which in this paper is called *Trypanosoma castellani*, in the cerebrospinal fluid of sleeping sickness patients. Sceptics may consider that these rounded forms correspond to the *Streptococcus* that he first observed (Castellani, 1903) and believed, initially, to be the causative organism of sleeping sickness. The spherical forms that he described do, however, generally correspond to the "latent" forms of Salvin-Moore and Breinl (1908) so that it is now difficult to dispute his claim to have been the first to observe them in man and to recognize their similarity to the "plasmodial" forms of Bradford and Plimmer (1902). Lumsden (1974) has given an account of the acrimony between the different individuals involved in discovery of the cause of sleeping sickness in Uganda and the writer recalls vividly the animosity with which Sir Philip Manson-Bahr, a man noted for his friendly disposition, spoke of Castellani: it is possible that persistent ill-feeling against Castellani may have had some bearing on the subsequent divergence of views and have unwittingly prejudiced British workers against accepting a view which had been espoused by Castellani. Be that as it may, in a period when no British paper mentions the possibility of a visceral stage of *T. brucei*, Italian workers continued for several decades to describe spherical and oval forms from blood and viscera.

Reference has already been made to the work of Ottolenghi (1910), who described not only spherical and oval forms but also frequent multinuclear stages, and to the work of Fusco (1908, 1910), which, although concerned with oval forms, deals with them in culture and in the dead animal and is therefore unlikely to be significant. Battaglia (1924) described similar forms which passed filters and he attributed the properties of cysts to them. Peruzzi (1928) mentioned the presence of amastigotes in internal organs, particularly in the heart. Penso (1934) developed a complicated life cycle based on the appearance of spherical and oval forms and their relationship to multinuclear forms. This was further discussed by Peruzzi (1935). Castellani and Jacono (1937) further described spherical and oval forms in cerebrospinal fluid; this paper was criticized by Wenyon (1938) as follows: "some of the figures in the coloured plates appear to the reviewer to depict organisms which resemble flagellates from contaminated distilled water rather than trypanosomes". Abnormal blood forms were also mentioned by Guidetti (1937). During this period similar work was also carried out in other countries, for example, by Hoeppli and Regendanz (1930) in Hamburg; they, like Peruzzi (1928), had found amastigotes in various internal organs. Philiptschenko (1929) in Leningrad, as mentioned earlier, found multinucleate forms in blood and in the lungs. The only relevant publication from an English-speaking worker during this period is that of Reich (1924) from Berkeley, California.

H. THE REDISCOVERY OF TISSUE FORMS

There is, however, another possible cause for the disappearance of tissue forms from the British literature. After the first World War, highly virulent strains of *T. brucei*, producing acute rhodesian sleeping sickness, began to spread north from the Zambesi Basin and involved the British Protectorate of Tanganyika and subsequently Uganda and Kenya (Ormerod, 1961). These strains gave a high mortality in man and, when injected into laboratory animals, gave a rapidly developing parasitaemia. Not only was there official pressure for workers to study these strains (e.g. the setting up of the Tinde and Shinyanga Laboratories in Tanzania and the Tororo Laboratory in Uganda) but they also produced high and reliable parasitaemias and were thus attractive to work with. On the other hand, these virulent strains of sleeping sickness trypanosomes did not produce the characteristic lesion (perivascular cuffing) in animals and very little of it in man. There was little tendency for remission, and such tendency as remained disappeared entirely after a few passages; the only strains used in laboratories outside Africa were virulent "rhodesiense" strains which had been passaged many times, and their almost universal use in parasitological research may to some extent account for the failure of English-speaking workers to find visceral forms.

Soltys and Woo (1969, 1970) who found multinucleate and spherical forms in the smears of liver and spleen were concerned mainly with trypanosomes of animals, and it seems possible that they were working with strains which were less exalted in virulence and had retained their tendency to relapse. Ormerod and Venkatesan (1971a) used strains from Botswana which had been collected (Apted *et al.*, 1963) because of their striking difference (Ormerod, 1958, 1963) from strains obtainable in Uganda. One of these differences lay in the reliability with which the Botswana strains underwent a short remission of the infection.

Soltys and Woo (1969, 1970) were apparently unaware of the earlier work which had been done on visceral forms of *T. brucei*. Similarly, Ormerod and Venkatesan (1971a, b) were unaware of all previous work but that of Soltys and Woo; indeed they, like most other British protozoologists, treated Soltys and Woo's results with polite disbelief. The attitude of Ormerod and Venkatesan changed, however, as soon as Venkatesan had pointed out that the first form to appear in the blood, which they subsequently called the "long-narrow" form, did not divide until, after about 12 h, it had transformed into the dividing "long-flat" form. Previous to their transformation, long-narrow forms, which are not themselves dividing, tend to accumulate in the blood in increasing numbers and this seems to indicate that division must be occurring elsewhere, namely in the internal organs.

Ormerod and Venkatesan therefore began to search for particular sites for the development of a visceral phase and were led to the choroid plexus of the brain by the earlier ideas of LePort (1935), who considered that cerebral hypertension, a possible cause of the severe headache of sleeping sickness, might be the result of inflammation and swelling of the choroid plexus which might effectively plug the foramina of the lateral ventricles and inhibit the circulation of cerebrospinal fluid. The finding of a visceral stage of the sleeping sickness trypanosome in the choroid plexus would not only have solved the problem of the tissue phase but also would have indicated the cause of the specific headache which occurs early in the disease with such regularity.

Another factor which led Ormerod and Venkatesan to the choroid plexus was the similarity of its vascular structure to that of the *vasa recta* of the kidney in which developing multinucleate stages of *T. lewisi* had been found (Ormerod and Killick-Kendrick, 1956). The vessels of both structures present a series of alternative pathways so that if one or more become blocked others are available for circulation. Thus they considered that the multinucleate stages of these two species of *Trypanosoma* might be analogous. In the event, they found a body in the lumen of a choroid plexus vessel; on serial section it contained "amastigotes"; sphaeromastigotes and other spherical forms were seen in tissue smears.

While it appeared at first that the choroid plexus might be the specific, or at least the most important site for the formation of visceral stages, subsequent work showed that this was unlikely. Work on the pathophysiology of the choroid plexus in infected rabbits indicated that, although disturbance in the flow of cerebrospinal fluid did occur (Ormerod and Segal, 1973), this could be explained rather better by a general inflammation of the leptomeninges than by specific blockage of the foramina. Moreover, further observations by electron microscopy (Ellis and Ormerod, 1973) indicated that a variety of different stages could be found throughout the leptomeninges and that these stages tended to be diffusely distributed and not arranged in a "body", as had been suggested by Ormerod and Venkatesan (1971b). Moreover, they were not usually found within the lumen of the vessels but more frequently around the periphery of vessels as had been demonstrated by Goodwin (1971) in his study of the vessels of the ear in rabbits infected with trypanosomiasis.

Multinucleate forms were seen by Ellis and Ormerod (1973) in studies of choroid plexus and meninges by electron microscopy. A small number of organisms resembling sphaeromastigotes were seen, but amastigotes, although they had previously been seen by light microscopy, were not observed. This work is being repeated.

Mattern *et al.* (1972) studied the choroid plexus in the brain of mice infected for 150 days with a strain of *T. brucei* isolated from a patient suffering from the gambian type of disease; as in man, long remissions occurred in this infection of the mouse. In this instance "amastigote" forms appeared to be present in great profusion both in and around the vessels of the choroid plexus. This appearance led them to suggest that this type of development might be characteristic of long-standing infections. Similar collections of amastigotes had also been noted in the choroid plexus of cats infected with *T. evansi* by Choudbury and Misra (1973).

Among the unusual shaped forms seen by Ormerod and Venkatesan was the "succession of forms in the process of unrolling" that they considered to represent the transition between sphaeromastigotes and "long-narrow" forms. Similar forms had previously been seen by Sant'ana (1913) who attributed much the same significance to them as did Ormerod and Venkatesan. Penso (1934) and Peruzzi (1935) also saw these forms but thought that they were inside red cells, representing an endoglobular phase resembling *Endotrypanum*.

VIII. Hypothetical life cycles of T. brucei

Today there seems to be little doubt that a tissue phase exists in the life cycle of *T. brucei* but its significance is uncertain, as is its exact nature and distribution in the body of the vertebrate host. The final section of this review will therefore consist of an account of the different hypotheses that have been put forward to explain the facts as they were seen at the time. Most are, today, only of historical interest and there is still sufficient doubt about the real nature of the life cycle in the vertebrate and, for that matter, in the invertebrate host, for new approaches may yet be made as well as the revival of old ones.

A. SEXUAL DIMORPHISM OF BLOOD FORMS

Based on the work of von Prowazek (1905), Minchin *et al.* (1906), Ottolenghi (1910) and Fairbairn and Culwick (1946), this hypothesis may be put in the following terms. The multinucleate stage (macrogametocyte) divides to produce the long-thin female form which fuses with the stumpy male, which may have developed from the small spherical microgametocyte. No views have been expressed as to what happens after fertilization. However, it might be envisaged that the "oocyst" develops in the tissues to produce the blood stages—this seems most unlikely. A less unlikely (but nevertheless unsupported) view that the gametes meet in the tsetse fly cannot be totally rejected until more is known about the life cycle in the fly (a tentative diagram of such a cycle

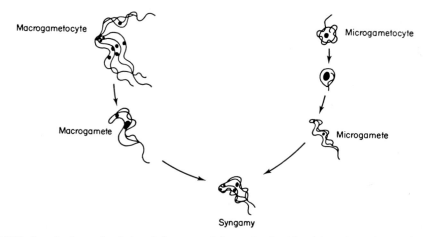

FIG. 5.   An hypothesis involving sexual forms in the blood based on the work of various authors (see text). This method of development seems highly improbable but cannot be totally rejected until syngamy in the tsetse has been excluded.

is shown in Fig. 5). The last word on sexuality in trypanosomes has probably not yet been said. No thorough search for sexual stages in the tsetse has yet been made and until this has been done the possibility that sexual forms may occur in the blood of the vertebrate host must still be entertained. Nevertheless, there is no evidence that any sexual dimorphism occurs and if it does it seems to correspond in no way to the variation in form which has hitherto been observed.

B. THE CLASSICAL HYPOTHESIS

The classical hypothesis that *T. brucei* divides solely in the blood by binary fission is derived mainly from Robertson (1912, 1913) (Fig. 6). In this hypothesis the stumpy form alone is infective for the tsetse (Wijers and Willett, 1960) and its production is the basis of pleomorphic development in the blood. In Robertson's original hypothesis the intermediate form is derived from the stumpy, and presumably the slender form is similarly derived from the intermediate. The experimental evidence with which she supported this hypothesis has been strongly criticized by Walker (1964) as being "based on one monkey, too few trypanosomes, no accurate counting method and was only demonstrated in two of the three cycles given". Few workers today accept that the slender form is developed from the stumpy via the intermediate; most would follow Ashcroft (1957) and Wijers (1959) in believing that the intermediate form occurs in transition from the dividing slender forms and the non-dividing stumpy forms. Nevertheless, many people believe

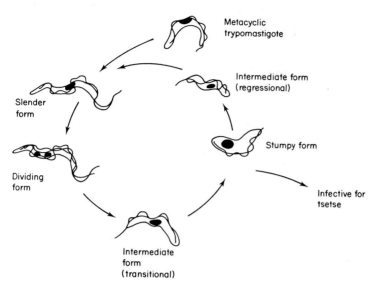

FIG. 6. The "classical hypothesis" (Robertson, 1912) involves reversible transformation between slender, intermediate and stumpy forms, with division occurring in the slender and possibly in the intermediate form. Only the stumpy form is regarded as infective for tsetse.

that the slender form is derived from stumpy forms that have transformed in the blood. One of the implications of this transformation is that the stumpy form must change its antigenic structure and presumably its surface coat (Cross, 1975). Another is that in gambian strains the stumpy form must be sequestered in some part of the circulation for months or possibly years before it transforms to the dividing slender form to give a parasitaemia. This hypothesis is certainly acceptable when heavy parasitaemias and negligible remissions are involved, but when parasitaemias are occasional and scanty, and the tissues contain many parasites, some resembling blood forms, others spherical, oval or multinucleate, it becomes somewhat unrealistic.

C. THE PERSISTENCE OF LATENT BODIES

Salvin-Moore and Breinl (1908) recognized that spherical forms of *T. brucei* occurred in the internal organs of rats during a prolonged latent period when the animal was without parasitaemia. They considered that latent bodies were formed by contraction of the trypomastigote when the kinetoplast moved into proximity with the nucleus along the "axial filament". Fantham (1911) claimed to have seen the rounding off process occur in the space of 30 minutes, with the flagellum and part of the

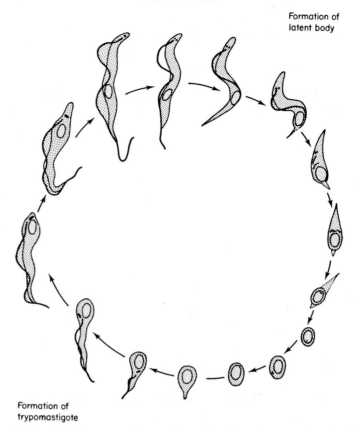

Formation of
latent body

Formation of
trypomastigote

FIG. 7. The development and transformation into trypomastigotes of "latent bodies" according to Fantham (1911).

cytoplasm actively discarded (Fig. 7). He also claimed to have observed the gradual elongation of the latent body into a pseudopodium, development of a flagellum and gradual assumption of all the characteristics of the trypomastigote. Most workers agree with Hindle (1910a), Robertson (1912) and Wijers (1960) that the process of formation of the latent body is one of degeneration. Certainly the disintegration of trypomastigotes leaving only the nucleus (as described by Fantham) is similar to the process that most workers with trypanosomes have observed from time to time; however, the individual stages observed by Fantham can all be seen in a healthy, refractile and (except for the aflagellated bodies) active state, so that there is little doubt that they can occur as a result of some process other than one involving degeneration.

Today, there is not much relevance in the latent body hypothesis. It explains remissions and long incubation periods; it partially explains pleomorphism, but not in a way which would account for the pleomorphic forms that are actually seen in the blood.

D. THE "TWO CYCLE HYPOTHESIS"

The "two cycle" hypothesis of Penso (1934) has a peculiar fascination since it appears to include all the stages that have ever been seen in any

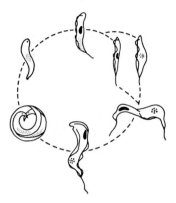

FIG. 8.   The sexual cycle of *T. brucei* according to Penso (1934). Note that syngamy involves the formation of a "pushmi-pulyu" and an oocyst resembling *Endotrypanum*.

known species of *Trypanosoma*. Basically, he proposed two cycles: a sexual cycle (Fig. 8) which involves "double ended" forms resembling a fabulous beast, the "Pushmi-Pulyu" (Lofting, 1925). Such forms have been described by Ottolenghi (1910) and by Thomson and Sinton (1912) and are frequently seen in culture (Fig. 9). It also involves an *"endotrypanum"* stage. The asexual cycle (Fig. 10) is even more complicated and involves all other stages then known to occur in trypanosomes. While it is difficult to state that the hypothesis of Penso (1934) is wrong in any major respect, it is of little value as a scientific hypothesis because it excludes nothing and therefore cannot be tested by experiment.

A more modest hypothesis along similar lines is that of Noble (1955) (Fig. 11). It seems to have been an attempt to reconcile the views expressed in earlier literature with the established findings of other species of *Trypanosoma*. While it was probably of value in reminding English readers that the "classical hypothesis" was not entirely satisfactory, it did not take enough account of established facts to suggest new experiments and it seems to have been little noticed.

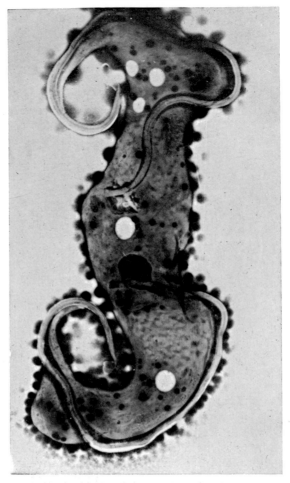

FIG. 9. Electron micrograph of a culture form viewed by negative staining
(D. A. Evans, D. S. Ellis original) representing the double ended "pushmi-pulyu"
form mentioned in the text.

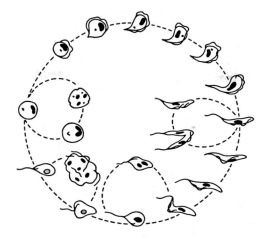

FIG. 10. The asexual cycle of Penso (1934). The cycles involve tissue forms which appear more characteristic of *Trypanosoma lewisi* than of *T. brucei*.

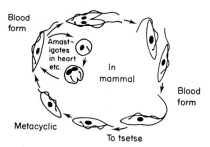

FIG. 11. A more modest hypothesis for the development of *T. brucei* based on the work of earlier authors by Noble (1955).

E. THE MULTINUCLEATE HYPOTHESIS

This hypothesis was proposed by Ormerod and Venkatesan (1971a) and Fig. 12 is the figure which appeared in their paper, modified by removal of the amastigote form. Thus the multinucleate form divides only into sphaeromastigotes which initiate the flush of long-narrow forms into the blood. Since 1971 it has been recognized that stumpy forms are unnecessary as the sole infective stage of the tsetse: it is still not known whether they are, or are not, infective for the fly; however, long-narrow and/or long-flat forms can by themselves infect the fly; more information is also available about the formation of stumpy forms. Ormerod *et al.* (1974), Venkatesan and Ormerod (1976) and Venkatesan *et al.* (1977) have demonstrated a lethal process associated with the uptake of lipid into the cytoplasm (see above). This process, in its early stages, may

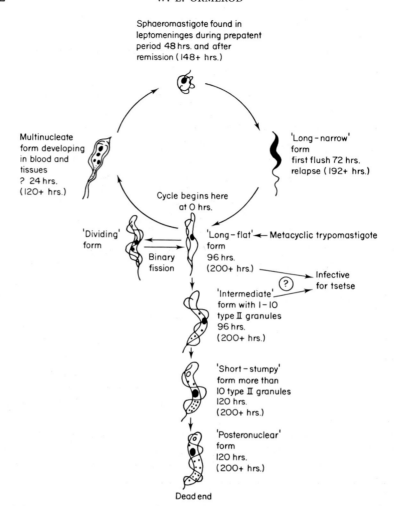

FIG. 12. The multinucleate hypothesis adapted from Ormerod and Venkatesan (1971a). An important addition to the original hypothesis consists in the removal of lipid granules from the multinucleate form, by means of the autophagosome, so that it is not destroyed in the manner of a stumpy form but is allowed to continue its development.

result in failure of the cytoplasm to divide, with consequent accumulation of nuclei and other organelles in the multinucleate form. Many multinucleate forms contain lipid granules, and the presence of these granules probably indicates that the cell will die without reproducing itself. However, the autophagosome may under certain circumstances be able to remove the lipid granules and their associated lysosomes from the cell. It is thus proposed as part of the "multinucleate hypothesis" that the multinucleate cell is formed by accumulation of small amounts of lipid and its division subsequently permitted to continue by removal of the lipid phagolysosome by means of the autophagosome. Trypomastigotes, on the other hand, which have absorbed more lipid become stumpy forms and die without further division. The possibility remains that a proportion of granular trypomastigotes may "defaecate" their lipid by means of the autophagosome and resume division once they have passed into the fly, into culture, or into the tissues of the host.

IX. Conclusion

The enigma which surrounds the history of investigation of the life cycle of *T. brucei* concerns the elimination of most information about the tissue stages of this parasite from the English literature between 1912 and 1969. It is true that much of the work done on tissue forms was inadequate, incomplete, badly written and highly speculative, but much the same can be said of work supporting the rival theories which nevertheless appeared to prevail. It is suggested that an important factor may have been in Castellani having first seen these forms in man and that the problem of the life cycle of *T. brucei* may, unwittingly, have become linked to the bitter contention which surrounded the discovery of the cause of sleeping sickness. This seems a fruitful subject for future historical research. Another factor may have been the increasing virulence of rhodesian strains and their popularity with British workers. Yet another factor may be the great eminence of the authorities Sir David Bruce, Sir Patrick Manson, Muriel Robertson, Edward Hindle, Wenyon and others. These were the people who, between 1910 and 1930, are likely to have been consulted by editors on the publication of results by British workers. It is likely, also, that they would not have agreed to the publication of work which they regarded as based on an outmoded hypothesis.

Reference must be made to the sheer complexity of the problem of unravelling the life cycle of *T. brucei* which has both entranced and daunted research workers, but has led to as much error as truth. But, for the future, I must express my confidence that the existence of a tissue phase of development of *T. brucei* will eventually be proved. Although its exact nature is at present in doubt, it seems likely that it will be found distributed among the fibrous tissues in the immediate periphery of the smaller blood vessels of the brain and meninges and probably also throughout the body, that it will divide by multiple fission, and that by so doing it will initiate the course of development, division and degeneration in the blood that we recognize as "pleomorphism". It also seems likely that the change, from one antigenic variant to the next in sequence (Gray, 1975), occurs during the sojourn of the trypanosome in the tissues, and that the "long-narrow" form, emerging from the tissues, carries into the blood a surface coat (Vickerman and Luckins, 1969) specific to the new variant. It is unlikely that sexual forms are involved, but this problem must await closer investigation of the development of *T. brucei* in the tsetse.

The dangers of accepting any hypothesis which attempts to explain the life cycle of *T. brucei* are illustrated in the above review, and many cautious scientists have avoided these dangers by not committing themselves. Yet little progress in such a difficult subject seems possible, unless one is prepared to commit oneself to an hypothesis and to run the risk, if necessary, of having it destroyed beneath one.

X. Acknowledgements

I wish to acknowledge the help of my colleagues, Dr. R. G. Bird, Dr. D. S. Ellis, Dr. D. A. Evans, Mr. C. B. Hill, Professor W. H. R. Lumsden, Mr. J. O. Molloy, Dr. A. S. Mshelbwala and Dr. S. Venkatesan, who have worked with me in this field in various ways, and of Dr. F. Hawking who first introduced me to "aberrant" trypanosomes. This work has been supported for 23 years by the Ministry of Overseas Development and its predecessors.

XI. References

Apted, F. I. C., Ormerod, W. E., Smyly, D. P., Stronach, B. W. and Szlamp, E. L. (1963). A comparative study of the epidemiology of endemic Rhodesian sleeping sickness in different parts of Africa. *Journal of Tropical Medicine and Hygiene*, **66**, 1–16.

Ashcroft, M. T. (1957). The polymorphism of *Trypanosoma brucei* and *T. rhodesiense*, its relation to relapse and remission of infections in white rats and the effect of cortisone. *Annals of Tropical Medicine and Parasitology*, **51**, 301–312.

Babudieri, B. and Tomasini, N. (1962). Fine struttura dei trypanosomi. *Parasitologia*, **4**, 89–95.

Balber, A. E. (1972). *Trypanosoma brucei*: fluxes of the morphological variants in intact and X-irradiated mice. *Experimental Parasitology*, **31**, 307–319.

Balber, A. E. and Ward, R. A. (1972). Diaminobenzidine staining of the mitochondrion of *Trypanosoma brucei*. *Journal of Parasitology*, **58**, 1004–1005.

Balfour, A. (1911). The role of the infective granule in certain protozoal diseases. *Journal of Tropical Medicine and Hygiene*, **14**, 263–264.

Battaglia, M. (1924). Uber Infektion mit einiger menchlichen und tierischen Protozoen. *Zentralblatt Zur Bakteriologie, Parasitenkunde und Infektionskrankheiten*, **92**, 540–542.

Beck, M. (1910). Experimentelle Beiträge zur Infektion mit *Trypanosoma gambiense* und zur Heilung der menschlicher Trypanosomiasis. *Arbeiten aus dem Kaiserlichen Gesundheitsamate*, **34**, 318.

Bevan, L. E. W. and MacGregor, M. E. (1910). Notes on trypanosomes of the *dimorphon* group. *The Veterinary Journal*, July, 386–390.

Blackwelder, R. E. (1967). *In:* "Taxonomy—A Text and Reference Book", p. 115. New York: Wiley.

Blanchard, R. (1903). Expériences et observations sur la marmotte en hibernation. V. Réceptivité à l'égard de trypanosomes. *Comptes Rendus de la Société de Biologie*, **55**, 1122–1124.

Böhringer, S. and Hecker, H. (1974). Quantitative ultrastructural differences between strains of *Trypanosoma brucei* subgroup during transformation in blood. *Journal of Protozoology*, **21**, 694–698.

Böhringer, S. and Hecker, H. (1975). Quantitative ultrastructural investigation of the life cycle of *Trypanosoma brucei*: a morphometric analysis. *Journal of Protozoology*, **22**, 463–467.

Brack, C. (1968). Elektronenmikroscopische untersuchungen zum Lebenszyklus von *Trypanosoma cruzi* unter besonderen Berücksichtigung der Entwicklungsformen im Überträger *Rhodnius prolixus*. *Acta Tropica*, **25**, 289–356.

Bradford, J. R. and Plimmer, H. G. (1902). The *Trypanosoma brucii* (sic) the organism found in Nagana, or tsetse fly disease. *Quarterly Journal of Microscopical Science*, **45**, 449–472.

Broom, J. C., Brown, H. C. and Hoare, C. A. (1936). Studies in microelectrophoresis. The electric charge of haemoflagellates. *Transactions of the Royal Society of Tropical Medicine and Hygiene*, **30**, 87–100.

Bruce, D. (1911). The morphology of *Trypanosoma gambiense* Dutton. *Proceedings of the Royal Society*, Series B, **84**, 327–332.

Bruce, D. and Bateman, H. R. (1908). Have trypanosomes an ultramicroscopical stage in their life-history? *Proceedings of the Royal Society*, Series B, **80**, 394–398.

Bruce, D., Hamerton, A. E., Bateman, H. R. and Mackie, F. P. (1910). Trypanosome diseases of domestic animals in Uganda. II. *Trypanosoma brucei* (Plimmer and Bradford). *Proceedings of the Royal Society*, Series B, **83**, 1–14.

Bruce, D., Harvey, D., Hamerton, A. E., Davy, J. B. and Bruce, M. E. (1912). The morphology of the trypanosome causing disease in man in Nyasaland. *Proceedings of the Royal Society*, Series B, **85**, 423–433.

Bruce, D., Hamerton, A. E., Watson, D. P. and Bruce, M. E. (1914). Morphology of various strains of the trypanosome causing disease in man in Nyasaland. *Proceedings of the Royal Society*, Series B, **88**, 190–205.

Brumpt, E. (1908). Guérison de la maladie du sommeil chez le lérot vulgaire en hibernation. Action du froid sur le *Trypanosoma inopinatum in vivo*. *Comptes Rendus de la Societé de Biologie*, **64**, 1147–1149.

Buchanan, G. (1911). Notes on developmental forms of *Trypanosoma brucei* (*pecaudi*) in the internal organs, axillary glands and bone marrow of the gerbil (*Gerbillus pygargus*). *Proceedings of the Royal Society*, Series B, **84**, 161–164.

Castellani, A. (1903). The etiology of sleeping sickness: preliminary note. *Lancet*, **1**, 723–725.

Castellani, A. (1904). Die Aetiologie der Schlafkrankheit der Neger. *Zentralblatt für Bakteriologie, Parasitenkunde und Infektionskrankheiten*, **35**, 62–67.

Castellani, A. and Chalmers, A. J. (1910, 1913, 1919). Manual of Tropical Medicine. Baillière, Tindall and Cox, London, England.

Castellani, A. and Jacono, J. (1937). Richerche sperimentali sul poliomorfismo della *Castellanella gambiensis*. *Rivista di Parasitologia*, **1**, 211–220.

Choudhury, A. and Misra, K. K. (1973). Occurrence of amastigote and sphaeromastigote stages of *T. evansi* in the brain tissue of the cat. *Transactions of the Royal Society of Tropical Medicine and Hygiene*, **67**, 609.

Cross, G. A. M. (1975). Identification, purification and properties of clone-specific glycoproteins and antigens constituting the surface coat of *Trypanosoma brucei*. *Parasitology*, **71**, 393–417.

Cross, G. A. M. and Manning, J. C. (1973). Cultivation of *Trypanosoma brucei* sspp. in semi-defined and defined media. *Parasitology*, **67**, 315–331.

Cunningham, M. P., Van Hoeve, K. and Lumsden, W. H. R. (1963). Variable infectivity of organisms of the *T. brucei* subgroup during acute relapsing infections in rats, related to parasitaemia, morphology and antibody response. *Annual Report of East African Trypanosomiasis Research Organization*, 1962–63, p. 21.

Deane, M. P. (1969). On the life cycle of trypanosomes of the *lewisi* group and their relationship to other mammalian trypanosomes. *Revista do Instituto de Medicina Tropical do São Paulo*, **11**, 34–43.

Dixon, H. and Williamson, J. (1970). The lipid composition of blood and culture forms of *Trypanosoma lewisi* and *T. rhodesiense* compared with that of their environment. *Comparative Biochemistry and Physiology*, **33B**, 111–128.

Dixon, H., Ginger, C. D. and Williamson, J. (1971). The lipid metabolism of blood and culture forms of *Trypanosoma lewisi* and *T. rhodesiense*. *Comparative Biochemistry and Physiology*, **39B**, 247–266.

Dixon, H., Ginger, C. D. and Williamson, J. (1972). Trypanosome sterols and their metabolic origins. *Comparative Biochemistry and Physiology*, **41B**, 1–18.

Ellis, D. S. and Ormerod, W. E. (1973). Electron microscopy of the occult visceral forms of *Trypanosoma brucei*. Short note. *Transactions of the Royal Society of Tropical Medicine and Hygiene*, **67**, 276.

Ellis, D. S., Ormerod, W. E. and Lumsden, W. H. R. (1976). Filaments of *Trypanosoma brucei*: some notes on differences in origin and structure in two strains of *Trypanosoma* (*Trypanozoon*) *brucei rhodesiense*. *Acta Tropica*, **33**, 151–168.

Erdmann, R. (1915a). The life cycle of *Trypanosoma brucei* in the rat and in rat plasma. *Proceedings of the National Academy of Sciences*, **1**, 504–512.

Erdmann, R. (1915). Formveränderungen von *Trypanosoma brucei* in Plasmamedium. *Berliner Klinische Wochenschrift*, **52**, 812.

Fairbairn, H. and Culwick, A. T. (1946). A new approach to trypanosomiasis. *Annals of Tropical Medicine and Parasitology*, **43**, 421–452.

Fairbairn, H. and Culwick, A. T. (1949). The differentiation of the polymorphic trypanosomes. *Annals of Tropical Medicine and Parasitology*, **43**, 90–95.

Fairbairn, H. and Godfrey, D. G. (1957). The local reaction in man at the site of infection with *Trypanosoma rhodesiense*. *Annals of Tropical Medicine and Parasitology*, **51**, 464–470.

Fairbairn, H. and Godfrey, D. G. (1958). Sections cut through a chancre developing in a human volunteer previously exposed to the bite of an infected tsetse (laboratory demonstration). *Transactions of the Royal Society of Tropical Medicine*, **52**, 21.

Fantham, H. B. (1911). The life-history of *Trypanosoma gambiense* and *Trypanosoma rhodesiense* as seen in rats and guinea-pigs. *Proceedings of the Royal Society*, Series B, **83**, 212–227. *Annals of Tropical Medicine and Parasitology*, **4**, 465–485.

Frazer, A. D. and Duke, H. L. (1912). Antelope infected with *Trypanosoma gambiense*. *Proceedings of the Royal Society*, Series B, **84**, 484–492.

Fry, W. B. (1912). The infective granule. *Reports of the sleeping sickness Commission of the Royal Society*, **12**, 25.

Fry, W. B. and Ranken, H. S. (1913). Further research on the extrusion of granules by trypanosomes and their further development. *Proceedings of the Royal Society*, Series B, **86**, 377–393.

Fusco, G. (1908). Osservazioni sulle forme involutive et sulla cultura del *Trypanosoma brucei*. *Riforma Medica*, **24**.

Fusco, G. (1910). Dove s'indovano i tripanosomi nel periodo di latenza dell' infezione sperimentale. *Riforma Medica*, **26**, 539–542.

Gallais, P., Cros, R. and Arquié (1953). Contribution a l'étude des périodes de latence clinique et parasitologique de la trypanosomiase humaine Africaine. *Médecine Tropicale*, **13**, 844–856.

Goedbloed, E. and Southgate, B. A. (1969). *Trypanosoma rhodesiense* and *T. brucei*: absence of antibodies in chicken embryos. *Experimental Parasitology*, **26**, 282–289.

Goedbloed, E. and Kinyanjui, H. (1970). Development of African pathogenic trypanosomes in chicken embryos. *Experimental Parasitology*, **27**, 464–478.

Goodwin, L. G. (1971). Pathological effects of *Trypanosoma brucei* on small blood vessels in rabbit ear-chambers. *Transactions of the Royal Society of Tropical Medicine and Hygiene*, **65**, 82–88.

Gordon, R. M. and Willett, K. C. (1957). Studies on the deposition, migration and development to the blood forms of trypanosomes belonging to the *Trypanosoma brucei* group. II. An account of the migration of the trypanosomes from the site of their deposition in the rodent host to their appearance in the general circulation, with some observations on their probable routes of migration in the human host. *Annals of Tropical Medicine and Parasitology*, **51**, 471–492.

Gordon, R. M., Crewe, W. and Willett, K. C. (1956). Studies on the deposition, migration and development to the blood forms of trypanosomes belonging to the *Trypanosoma brucei* group. I. An account of the process of feeding adopted by the tsetse fly when obtaining a bloodmeal from the mammalian host, with special reference to the ejection of saliva and the relationship of the feeding process to the deposition of the metacyclic trypanosomes. *Annals of Tropical Medicine and Parasitology*, **50**, 426–437.

Gray, A. C. H. and Tulloch, F. M. G. (1906). An experiment on the cultivation of *T. gambiense*. *Proceedings of the Royal Society, Series B*, **78**, 253–254.

Gray, A. R. (1975). A pattern in the development of agglutinogenic antigens of cyclically transmitted isolates of *Trypanosoma gambiense*. *Transactions of the Royal Society of Tropical Medicine and Hygiene*, **69**, 131–138.

Guidetti, C. (1937). Ulteriore contributo alla conoscenza della morfologia delle *Castellanelle brucei*. *Giornale Italiano di Clinica Tropicale*, **15**, 227–234.

Hindle, E. (1910a). Degeneration phenomena of *Trypanosoma gambiense*. *Parasitology*, **3**, 423–435.

Hindle, E. (1910b). A biometric study of *Trypanosoma gambiense*. *Parasitology*, **3**, 455–458.

Hirumi, H., Doyle, J. J. and Hirumi, K. (1977). African trypanosomes: cultivation of animal-infective *Trypanosoma brucei in vitro*. *Science*, **196**, 992–994.

Hoare, C. A. (1949). Handbook of medical protozoology: for medical men, parasitologists and zoologists. Baillière, Tindall and Cox, London.

Hoare, C. A. (1972). The trypanosomes of mammals: a zoological monograph. Blackwell, Oxford, England.

Hoeppli, R. and Regendanz, P. (1930). Beiträge zur Pathogenese und Histopathologie der Trypanosomen infektionen der Tiere. *Archiv für Schiffs- und Tropenhygien*, **34**, 67–99.

Holmes, J. D. E. (1904). Evolution of the *Trypanosoma evansi*. *Journal of Comparative Pathology and Therapeutics*, **17**, 210–214.

von Jancsó, N. and von Jancsó, H. (1934). Mikrogiologische Grundlagen der chemotherapeutischen Wirkung: I. Wirkungsmechanismus des Germanins (Bayer 205) bie Trypanosomen. *Zentralblatt für Bakteriologie, Parasitenkunde und Infektionskrankheiten*, **132**, 257–292.

Kligler, I. J. (1927). Relation of temperature to susceptibility of host to disease. *Proceedings of the Society for Experimental Biology and Medicine*, 25, 20–21.

Kunert, H. (1939). Veränderungen im klinischen Bild der ostafrikanischen Schlafkrankheit. *Archiv für Schiffs- und Tropenhygien*, 43, 205–209.

Langreth, S. G. and Balber, A. E. (1975). Protein uptake and digestion in bloodstream and culture forms of Trypanosoma brucei. *Journal of Protozoology*, 22, 40–53.

Laveran, A. (1911). Des infection expérimentales par *T. gambiense* chez les moutons et chez les chèvres. *Bulletin de la Société de Pathologie Exotique*, 4, 619.

Laveran, A. (1911). Les trypanosomes ont-il des formes latentes chez leurs hôtes vertèbres? *Comptes rendus de l'Academie de Science (Paris)*, 15, 649–652.

Laveran, A. and Mesnil, E. (1902). Recherches morphologique et expérimentales sur le trypanosome du Nagana ou maladie de la mouche tsétsé. *Annales de l'Institute Pasteur*, 16, 1–55.

LePort, L.-R. (1935). Les plexo-choroïdites rhomboïdiennes au début de la maladie du sommeil. *Bulletin Médical du Katanga*, 12, 41–55.

Levine, N. D. (1961). Protozoan parasites of domestic animals and man. 1st Edition. Burgess, Minneapolis.

Lingard, A. (1907). Different species of trypanosomata observed in India. *Journal of Tropical Veterinary Science*, 2, 4–50.

Lofting, H. (1925). Doctor Dolittle's circus. Cape, London.

Luckins, A. G. (1972). Effects of X-irradiation and cortisone treatment of albino rats on infections with *brucei*-complex trypanosomes. *Transactions of the Royal Society of Tropical Medicine and Hygiene*, 66, 130–139.

Lumsden, W. H. R. (1974). Some episodes in the history of African trypanosomiasis. *Proceedings of the Royal Society of Medicine*, 67, 789–796.

Macfie, J. S. (1913). On the morphology of the trypanosome (*T. nigeriense* n. sp.) from a case of sleeping sickness from Eket, Southern Nigeria. *Annals of Tropical Medicine and Parasitology*, 7, 339–358.

Manson, P. (1914, 1919). Tropical Diseases: a manual of diseases of warm climates. Cassell, London.

Mathur, S. C. (1971). Cultivation of a pleomorphic variant of Trypanosoma (*Trypanozoon*) *evansi* and its transmission by *Glossina morsitans* (laboratory demonstration). *Transactions of the Royal Society of Tropical Medicine and Hygiene*, 65, 427–428.

Mattern, P., Mayer, G. and Felici, M. (1972). Existence de formes amastigotes de Trypanosoma gambiense dans le tissues choroïdien de la souris infectée experimentalement. *Comptes rendus des séances de l'Academie des Sciences*, 274, 1513–1515.

Minchin, E. A. (1908). Note on the polymorphism of *Trypanosoma gambiense*. *Parasitology*, 1, 236–237.

Minchin, E. A., Gray, A. C. H. and Tulloch, F. M. G. (1906). Glossina palpalis in its relation to *Trypanosoma gambiense* and other trypanosomes (preliminary report). *Proceedings of the Royal Society, Series B*, 78, 242–258.

Molloy, J. O. and Ormerod, W. E. (1965). Two types of cytoplasmic granule in Trypanosoma rhodesiense. *Experimental Parasitology*, 17, 57–64.

Mott, F. W. and Stewart, H. G. (1907). Some further observations on the cell changes in dourine and sleeping sickness. *British Medical Journal*, 2, 1327–1330.

Mshelbwala, A. S. (1967). Infectivity of Trypanosoma rhodesiense to tsetse flies fed through animal membranes. *Nature, London*, 215, 441.

Mühlpfordt, H. and Bayer, M. (1961). Elektronenmikroskopische Untersuchungen an Protozoen (*Trypanosoma gambiense*). *Zeitschrift für Tropenmedizin und Parasitologie*, **12**, 334–346.

Nobl, E. R. (1955). The morphology and life cycle of trypanosomes. *Quarterly Review of Biology*, **30**, 1–28.

Novy, F. G. and McNeal, W. J. (1907). On filtration of trypanosomes. *Studies from the Rockefeller Institute for Medical Research*, **6**, 375.

Oehler, R. (1913). Zur Gewinnung, reiner Trypanosomastamme. *Zentralblatt für Bakteriologie, Parasitenkunde une Infektionskrankheiten*, **70**, 110–111.

Oehler, R. (1914). Den Dimorphismus des *Trypanosoma brucei* bei experimentellen Behanlung. *Zeitschrift für Hygiene und Infektionskrankheit*, **78**, 188–191.

Ogawa, M. (1913). Quelques observations sur le dimorphism de *Trypanosoma pecaudi*. *Zentralblatt für Bakteriologie, Parasitenkunde und Infektionskrankheiten*, **68**, 332–334.

Ogawa, M. (1914). Etude morphologique et biologique sur *Trypanosoma pecaudi*. *Annals del'Institut Pasteur*, **28**, 667.

Ormerod, W. E. (1951). The mode of action of Antrycide. *British Journal of Pharmacology and Chemotherapy*, **6**, 325–333.

Ormerod, W. E. (1958). A comparative study of cytoplasmic inclusions (volutin granules) in different species of trypanosomes. *Journal of General Microbiology*, **19**, 271–288.

Ormerod, W. E. (1961a). The study of volutin granules in trypanosomes. *Transactions of the Royal Society of Tropical Medicine and Hygiene*, **55**, 313–332.

Ormerod, W. E. (1961b). The epidemic spread of Rhodesian sleeping sickness 1908–1960. *Transactions of the Royal Society of Tropical Medicine and Hygiene*, **55**, 525–538.

Ormerod, W. E. (1963). A comparative study of the growth and morphology of strains of *Trypanosoma rhodesiense*. *Experimental Parasitology*, **13**, 374–385.

Ormerod, W. E. (1967). Taxonomy of the sleeping sickness trypanosomes. *Journal of Parasitology*, **53**, 824–830.

Ormerod, W. E. (1970). Pathogenesis and pathology of trypanosomiasis in man. *In:* "The African trypanosomiases" (H. W. Mulligan and W. H. Potts, eds), pp. 587–601. London, England: Allen and Unwin.

Ormerod, W. E. (1976). Comment on paper by Langreth and Balber (1975). *Tropical Diseases Bulletin*, **73**, 318.

Ormerod, W. E. and Killick-Kendrick, R. (1956). Developmental forms of *Trypanosoma lewisi* in the vasa recta of the kidney. Laboratory demonstration. *Transactions of the Royal Society of Tropical Medicine and Hygiene*, **50**, 4.

Ormerod, W. E. and Segal, M. B. (1973). The function of the choroid plexus in the brain of rabbits infected with the sleeping sickness trypanosome. *Journal of Tropical Medicine and Hygiene*, **76**, 121–125.

Ormerod, W. E. and Venkatesan, S. (1970). The choroid plexus and African sleeping sickness. *Lancet*, **2**, 777.

Ormerod, W. E. and Venkatesan, A. (1971a). The occult visceral phase of mammalian trypanosomes with special reference to the life cycle of *Trypanosoma (Trypanozoon) brucei*. *Transactions of the Royal Society of Tropical Medicine and Hygiene*, **65**, 722–735.

Ormerod, W. E. and Venkatesan, S. (1971b). An amastigote phase of the sleeping sickness trypanosome. *Transactions of the Royal Society of Tropical Medicine and Hygiene*, **65**, 736–741.

Ormerod, W. E., Healey, P. and Armitage, P. (1963). A method of counting trypanosomes allowing simultaneous study of their morphology. *Experimental Parasitology*, **13**, 386–394.

Ormerod, W. E., Venkatesan, S. and Carpenter, R. G. (1974). The effect of immune inhibition on pleomorphism in *Trypanosoma brucei rhodesiense*. *Parasitology*, **68**, 355–367.

Otieno, L. H. (1972). Influence of ambient temperature on the course of experimental trypanosomiasis in mice. *Annals of Tropical Medicine and Parasitology*, **66**, 15–24.

Otieno, L. H. (1973). Effects of immunosuppressive agents on the course of *Trypanosoma* (*Trypanozoon*) *brucei* infections in heat-stressed mice. *Transactions of the Royal Society of Tropical Medicine and Hygiene*, **67**, 856–869.

Ottolenghi, D. (1910). Studien über die Entwicklung einiger pathogener Trypanosomen im Säugetierorganismus. *Archiv für Protistenkunde*, **18**, 48–82.

Pearson, K. (1914). On the probability that two independent distributions of frequency are really samples of the same population, with special reference to recent work on the identity of trypanosome strains. *Biometrica*, **10**, 85–143.

Penso, G. (1934). Sul ciclo di sviluppo del "*Trypanosoma gambiense*" negli ospiti vertebrati. *Annali di Medicina navale e coloniale*, (40th Year), **1**, 25–77.

Peruzzi, M. (1928). Pathological-anatomical and serological observations on the trypanosomiases. Final Report of the League of Nations International Commission on Human Trypanosomiasis, Geneva (1928), 245–324.

Peruzzi, M. (1935). Poliomorfismo e transformazioni globulari de alcuni tripanosomi africani nei loro rapporti con la patologia. *Pathologia*, **27**, 577–586.

Petana, W. B. (1964). Effects of cortisone upon the course of infection of *Trypanosoma gambiense*, *T. rhodesiense*, *T. brucei* and *T. congolense* in albino rats. *Annals of Tropical Medicine and Parasitology*, **58**, 192–198.

Petrů, M. and Vojtěchovská, M. (1955). Průběh experimentální trypanosomiase v barbiturátové narkose. *Československa Parasitologie*, **2**, 105–156. Abstract: Tropical Diseases Bulletin (1956), **53**, 1320.

Philiptschenko, A. (1929). Zur Frage über den Ertwicklungszyklus von Trypanosomen im Säugetierorganismus. *Zentralblatt für Bakteriologie, Parasitenkunde und Infektionskrankheit*, **111**, 125–138.

Pipkin, A. C. (1960). Avian embryos and tissue culture in the study of parasitic protozoa. II. Protozoa other than *Plasmodium*. *Experimental Parasitology*, **9**, 167–203.

Pittam, M. D. (1970). Medium for *in vitro* cultivation of *Trypanosoma rhodesiense* and *T. brucei*. *Comparative Biochemistry and Physiology*, **33**, 127–128.

Plimmer, H. G. and Bradford, J. R. (1899). A preliminary note on the morphology and distribution of the organism found in the tsetse-fly disease. *Proceedings of the Royal Society, Series B*, **65**, 274–281.

Policard, A. (1910). Sur la coloration vitale des trypanosomes. *Comptes Rendus de la Société de Biologie*, **68**, 505–507.

von Prowazek, S. (1905). Studien über Säugetientrypanosomen. *Arbeiten aus dem Kaiserlichen Gesundheitsamte*, **22**, 1.

von Prowazek, S. (1913). Über reine Trypanosomenstämme. *Zentralblatt für Bakteriologie, Parasitenkunde und Infektionskrenkheiten*, **68**, 498–501.

Reich, W. W. (1924). *Trypanosoma brucei* as a filterable virus: studies on the site of origin of the filter-passing bodies. *Journal of Parasitology*, **10**, 171–181.

Reich, W. W. and Beckwith, T. D. (1922). *Trypanosoma brucei* as a filterable virus —a preliminary note. *Journal of Parasitology*, **9**, 93–98.

Reichenow, E. (1921). Untersuchungen über das Verhalten von *Trypanosoma gambiense* in menschlichen Körper. *Zeitschrift für Hygiene und Infektionskrankheiten*, **94**, 266–385.

Ritz, H. (1914). Über Rezidive bei experimenteller trypanosomiasis. I. *Deutsche medizinisches Wochenschrift*, **40**, 1355.

Ritz, H. (1916). Über Rezidive bei experimenteller trypanosomiasis. II. *Archiv für Schiffs- und Tropenhygiene*, **20**, 397–420.

Robertson, M. (1912a). Notes on the polymorphism of *Trypanosoma gambiense* and its relation to the exogenous cycle in *Glossina palpalis. Proceedings of the Royal Society, Series B*, **85**, 527–539.

Robertson, M. (1912b). Notes on the life history of *Trypanosoma gambiense. Proceedings of the Royal Society, Series B*, **85**, 66–71.

Robertson, M. (1913). Notes on the behaviour of a polymorphic trypanosome in the bloodstream of the mammalian host. *Report of The Sleeping Sickness Commission of the Royal Society*, **13**, 111–119.

Robertson, D. H. H. and Pickens, S. (1975). Accidental laboratory infection with *Trypanosoma brucei rhodesiense*. A case report. *Communicable diseases in Scotland*, No. 32, iii–vi.

Ross, R. and Thomson, D. (1910). A case of sleeping sickness studied by precise enumerative methods; regular periodic increase of the parasites disclosed. *Proceedings of the Royal Society, Series B*, **82**, 411–415.

Ross, R. and Williams, C. L. (1910). Preliminary experiments on the effect of cold on various diseases in small animals. *Annals of Tropical Medicine and Parasitology*, **4**, 225–232.

Roubard, E., Stefanopoulo, G. J. and Duvolon, S. (1944). Etude chez le rat blanc d'une souche neurotrope de *Trypanosoma gambiense. Bulletin de la Société de Pathologie Exotique*, **37**, 292–300.

Salvin-Moore, J. E. and Breinl, A. (1908). The cytology of trypanosomes. I. *Annals of Tropical Medicine and Parasitology*, **1**, 441–489.

Sant'ana, J. F. (1913). Observações sobre as formas não flagelados do *Trypanosoma rhodesiense* nos animais de experiéncia e em especial no rato. *Arquivos de Higiene e Parasitologia Exoticos*, **4**, 77–105.

Schepilewsky, E. (1912). Fadenförmige Anhängsel bei den Trypanosomen. *Zentralblatt für Bakteriologie, Parasitenkunde und Infektionskrankheiten*, **65**, 79–83.

Schuberg, A. and Böing, W. (1913). Über der Weg der Infektion bei Trypanosomen- und Spirochätenerkrankungen. *Deutsche medizinische Wochenschrift*, **39**, 877.

Shortt, H. E. and Garnham, P. C. C. (1948). The pre-erythrocytic development of *Plasmodium cynomolgi* and *Plasmodium vivax. Transactions of the Royal Society of Tropical Medicine and Hygiene*, **41**, 785–795.

Soltys, M. A. and Woo, P. (1969). Multiplication of *Trypanosoma brucei* and *Trypanosoma congolense* in vertebrate hosts. *Transactions of the Royal Society of Tropical Medicine and Hygiene*, **63**, 490–694.

Soltys, M. A. and Woo, P. (1970). Further studies on tissue forms of *Trypanosoma brucei* in a vertebrate host. *Transactions of the Royal Society of Tropical Medicine and Hygiene*, **64**, 692–694.

Soltys, M. A., Woo, P. and Gillick, A. C. (1969). A preliminary note on the separation and infectivity of tissue forms of *Trypanosoma brucei. Transactions of the Royal Society of Tropical Medicine and Hygiene*, **63**, 495–496.

Ssenyonga, G. S. Z. and Adam, K. M. G. (1975). The number and morphology of trypanosomes in the blood and lymph of rats infected with *Trypanosoma brucei* and *T. congolense. Parasitology*, **70**, 255–261.

Stefanopoulo, G. J., Caubet, P. and Duvolon, S. (1945). Méningocéphalite a *Trypanosoma gambiense* (souche neurotrope) observée chez le lapin. *Bulletin de la Société de Pathologie Exotique*, **38**, 271–275.

Stevenson, A. C. (1917). Trypanosomes in the brain tissue of an experimental guinea-pig (laboratory demonstration). *Transactions of the Royal Society of Tropical Medicine and Hygiene*, **11**, 104.

Stevenson, A. C. (1922). Demonstration of sections showing *Trypanosoma gambiense* in the brain substance of a case of sleeping sickness. *Transactions of the Royal Society of Tropical Medicine and Hygiene*, **16**, 135.

Swellengrebel, N. H. (1912). Zur Kenntnis des Dimorphismus von *Trypanosoma gambiense* (var. *rhodesiense*). *Zentralblatt für Bakteriologie, Parasitenkunde und Infektionskrankheiten*, **61**, 193–206.

Thomas, H. W. and Breinl, A. (1905). Report on trypanosomes, trypanosomiasis and sleeping sickness: the cultivation of trypanosomes. *Liverpool School of Tropical Medicine Memoirs*, **16**, 43–48.

Thomson, J. G. and Robertson, A. (1926). Variations in the virulence and in the morphology of certain laboratory strains of *Trypanosoma gambiense* and *Trypanosoma rhodesiense* isolated from human cases. *Journal of Tropical Medicine and Hygiene*, **29**, 403–410.

Thomson, J. G. and Robertson, A. (1929). Protozoology—a manual for medical men. Baillière, Tindall and Cox, London.

Thomson, J. G. and Sinton, J. A. (1912). The morphology of *Trypanosoma gambiense* and *Trypanosoma rhodesiense* in cultures: and a comparison with the developmental forms described in *Glossina palpalis*. *Annals of Tropical Medicine and Parasitology*, **6**, 331–356.

Todd, J. L. (1911). The duration of trypanosome infections. *Archives of Internal Medicine*, **7**, 500–505.

Valerio, F. (1909). Sulla riproduzione del *Trypanosoma brucei*. *Riforma Medica*, **23**, 617–618.

Van den Branden (1939). Influence du froid sur l'évolution de la trypanosomiase expérimentale du rat blanc infecté de *Trypanosoma brucei*. *Annales de la Société Belge de Médecine Tropicale*, **19**, 243–244.

Venkatesan, S. and Ormerod, W. E. (1976). Lipid content of the slender and stumpy forms of *Trypanosoma brucei rhodesiense*: a comparative study. *Comparative Biochemistry and Physiology*, **53B**, 481–487.

Venkatesan, S., Bird, R. G. and Ormerod, W. E. (1977). Intracellular enzymes and their localization in slender and stumpy forms of *Trypanosoma brucei rhodesiense*. *International Journal for Parasitology*, **7**, 139–147.

Vianna, G. (1911). Algumas notas sobre o cyclo evolutivo do *Trypanosoma gambiense*. *Brasil Medico*, **25**, 61.

Vickerman, K. (1962). The mechanism of cyclical development in trypanosomes of the *Trypanosoma brucei* sub-group: an hypothesis based on ultrastructural observations. *Transactions of the Royal Society of Tropical Medicine and Hygiene*, **56**, 487–495.

Vickerman, K. (1965). Polymorphism and mitochondrial activity in sleeping sickness trypanosomes. *Nature, London*, **208**, 762–766.

Vickerman, K. (1970). Morphological and physiological considerations of extracellular blood protozoa. *In:* "Ecology and physiology of parasites: a symposium held at the University of Toronto" (A. M. Fallis, ed.). Toronto: University of Toronto Press.

Vickerman, K. and Luckins, A. G. (1969). Location of variable antigens in the surface coat of *Trypanosoma brucei*. *Nature, London*, **244**, 1125–1126.

Walker, E. L. (1912). The schizogony of *Trypanosoma evansi* in the spleen of the vertebrate host. *Philippine Journal of Tropical Medicine*, **7**, 53–63.

Walker, P. J. (1964). Reproduction and heredity in trypanosomes: a critical review dealing mainly with the African species in the mammalian host. *International Review of Cytology*, **17**, 51–98.

Weinman, D. (1946). Cultivation of African sleeping sickness trypanosomes on improved, simple, cell-free medium. *Proceedings of the Society of Experimental Biology and Medicine*, **63**, 451–458.

Wenyon, C. M. (1926). *Protozoology*. Baillière, Tindall and Cox, London, England.

Wenyon, C. M. (1938). Tropical Diseases Bulletin, **35**, 327–328.

Wijers, D. J. B. (1959). Polymorphism in *Trypanosoma gambiense* and *Trypanosoma rhodesiense*, and the significance of the intermediate forms. *Annals of Tropical Medicine and Parasitology*, **53**, 59–68.

Wijers, D. J. B. (1960). Studies on the behaviour of trypanosomes belonging to the *brucei* sub-group in the mammalian host. Thesis, University of Amsterdam.

Wijers, D. J. B. and Willett, K. C. (1960). Factors that may influence the infection rates of *Glossina palpalis* with *Trypanosoma gambiense*. II. The number and morphology of the trypanosomes present in the blood of the host at the time of the infected feed. *Annals of Tropical Medicine and Parasitology*, **54**, 341–350.

Wolbach, S. B., Chapman, W. H. and Stevens, H. W. (1915). Concerning the filterability of trypanosomes. *Journal of Medical Research*, **33**, 107–117.

8

Biology of *Leishmania* in phlebotomine sandflies

R. KILLICK-KENDRICK

Medical Research Council External Staff,
Department of Zoology and Applied Entomology,
Imperial College, London, England

I. Introduction 396

II. Life cycles in the sandfly 398
    A. Mammalian leishmanias 400
    B. Saurian leishmanias 423

III. Pathogenicity of leishmanias to sandflies 428

IV. Factors affecting development in the sandfly 429
    A. Intrinsic insusceptibility of some sandflies . . . 430
    B. Number of parasites ingested 433
    C. Time, temperature and humidity 435
    D. The infecting meal and digestion 437
    E. Sugars 438
    F. Attachment to chitin and invasion of head . . . 441
    G. Concomitant infections 442

V. Physiology and behaviour of sandflies 443

VI. Summary and conclusions 447

VII. Acknowledgements 449

VIII. References 449

En fait, les recherches sur les leishmanioses humaines sont liées à l'etude des phlébotomes........ (Adler, 1933).

I. Introduction

At one time or another, almost every anthropophilic haematophagous arthropod has been suspected of transmitting leishmaniasis to man (Wenyon, 1932). Even today there are still occasional speculations, without experimental evidence, that there are vectors other than phlebotomine sandflies. If this is so, it has yet to be satisfactorily demonstrated and, except for rare infections acquired by blood transfusions (references in Bruce-Chwatt, 1972) or bizarre venereal transmission (Symmers, 1960), the weight of evidence is that the way man normally becomes infected with *Leishmania* is by the bite of a sandfly infected at a previous bloodmeal.

Although it has seldom been found possible predictably to transmit the parasite experimentally by the bite of sandflies, a number of workers have obtained laboratory transmissions of 3 species of *Leishmania* (Table 1). There are unsolved problems in obtaining the complete life cycle in experimentally maintained sandflies, and it has proved difficult to keep many species of flies alive at oviposition and to persuade them to feed more than once. Nevertheless, there is ample proof that sandflies transmit *Leishmania* by bite, but no experimental evidence that any other haematophagous arthropod can do the same except by noncyclical transmissions at interrupted feeds (Lainson and Southgate, 1965).

Remarkably little is known of the biology of *Leishmania* in its invertebrate host. Complete life cycles in the vector have seldom been seen and, because many strains of *Leishmania* are readily cultured *in vitro* in the form seen in the invertebrate, it is usually assumed that observations on cultured promastigotes can be applied to morphologically similar forms in the alimentary tract of the vector. This may be misleading. Nearly fifty years ago, Adler and Theodor (1931b) reported that *L. infantum* had a life cycle in *Phlebotomus perniciosus* "in which fairly definite morphological forms follow in regular order". In a review of the life cycle of *L. donovani* in *P. argentipes*, Shortt (1928) noted that "certain types [of the parasite] have a selective affinity for certain situations in the gut". From recent studies on the ultrastructure of *L. m. amazonensis* in different parts of the sandfly, it is clear that this parasite also displays a sequence of morphological forms related to the parts of the gut in which development takes place (Killick-Kendrick *et al.*, 1974, 1977c; Molyneux *et al.*, 1975). These changes, which are not readily demonstrable in cultures, are presumably in response to differing physiological conditions in the various microhabitats within the alimentary tract of the sandfly; it can be assumed, moreover, that these conditions change during the process of digestion of blood and, possibly, the utilization of sugars obtained in nature by the sandfly directly or indirectly from plants (see Section

Table 1. Laboratory transmissions of *Leishmania* species by the bite of experimentally-infected sandflies.

Parasite	Sandfly	Vertebrate infected by bite	References
L. donovani	*P. argentipes*	Chinese hamsters	Shortt *et al.* (1931), Napier *et al.* (1933), Smith *et al.* (1936, 1940)
L. donovani	*P. argentipes*	Golden hamsters	Smith *et al.* (1941)
L. donovani	*P. argentipes*	White mice	Smith *et al.* (1940)
L. donovani	*P. argentipes*	Man	Swaminath *et al.* (1942)
L. donovani	*P. chinensis*	Chinese hamsters	Feng and Chung (1941), Ho *et al.* (1943), Chung *et al.* (1951)
L. donovani	*Lu. longipalpis*	Golden hamsters	Lainson *et al.* (1977b)
L. tropica	*P. papatasi*	Man	Adler and Ber (1941)
L. tropica	*P. papatasi*	Gerbils	Kryukova (1941)
L. m. mexicana	*Lu. panamensis* (?)[a]	Man	Strangways-Dixon and Lainson (1962, 1966)
L. m. mexicana	*Lu. longipalpis*	Golden hamsters	Coelho and Falcão (1962)
L. m. mexicana	*Lu. renei*	Golden hamsters	Coelho and Falcão (1962)
L. m. mexicana	*Lu. cruciata*	Man	Williams (1966)
L. m. amazonensis	*Lu. longipalpis*	Golden hamsters	Killick-Kendrick *et al.* (1977c)
L. m. amazonensis	*Lu. flaviscutellata*	Golden hamsters	Ward *et al.* (1977)

[a] The identity of this experimental vector is in doubt (Williams, 1966; 1970).

IV E). Unfortunately, the physiology of sandflies is so inadequately studied that it is not possible to match changes in form and metabolism of the parasite with the conditions in the various parts of the alimentary tract of the fly, except by extrapolating from that which is known of other haematophagous flies, particularly mosquitoes.

An understanding of the biology of leishmanias is complicated by the multiplicity of vector species. It is not known to what degree the life cycle of a species of *Leishmania* may vary according to the species of the vector. It has been suggested that the virulence of leishmanias might be influenced by the species of sandfly (Barnett and Suyemoto, 1961), but there is no supporting experimental evidence.

In the present review, I have drawn on unpublished observations on *L. braziliensis braziliensis* in *Lutzomyia wellcomei** and *L. b. guyanensis* in *Lu. umbratilis* made in Brazil in collaboration with Dr. R. Lainson, Dr. R. D. Ward and Dr. J. J. Shaw, on *L. infantum* in *P. ariasi* made by an Anglo-French team headed by Prof. J. A. Rioux in southern France, and on *L. mexicana amazonensis* in *Lu. longipalpis* made by Mr. A. J. Leaney in my laboratory. I am greatly indebted to these colleagues for permission to quote this work.

II. Life cycles in the sandfly

There is no single life cycle of all species of *Leishmania*. The development of some is restricted to parts of the alimentary tract anterior to the pylorus (e.g. *L. mexicana*, *L. infantum*, *L. tropica*), that of others to parts of the gut posterior to the stomodaeal valve, including the ileum and rectum (some saurian *Leishmania*); in yet others, initial establishment of infection is in the pylorus and ileum followed by an anterior migration (the *braziliensis* group) (see Fig. 1). In current work, other less prominent differences such as in the sites of division or in the morphological forms of promastigotes are being revealed, and further work is likely to disclose other variations. Observations on a species or subspecies of *Leishmania* in a sandfly other than *the actual population* of a fly transmitting the isolate in nature must, however, be interpreted with some caution.

As with other trypanosomatids, there is no evidence in *Leishmania* of any genetic recombination. If it occurs, however, it is more likely to take place in the invertebrate than the vertebrate host. Although it may seem like heresy or iconoclasm, it can be argued that the generally accepted case for the absence of conjugation in the family Trypanosomatidae is unproven but, from ultrastructural studies of trypanosomes (Deane and Milder, 1966; Brener, 1972; Ellis and Evans, 1977) it now seems, as

---

* Forattini (1971, 1973) raised the subgenus *Psychodopygus* in which *Lu. wellcomei* lies to full generic status, a move approved by Fraiha *et al.* (1971). Cogent arguments for not recognizing *Psychodopygus* as a genus are given by Lewis *et al.* (1977).

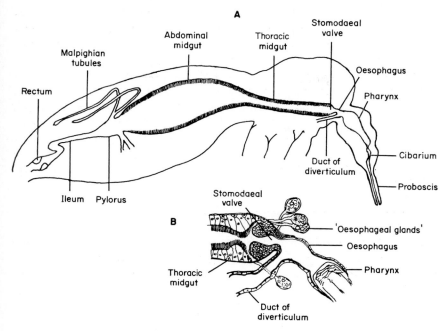

FIG. 1.   Alimentary tract of a sandfly. A. Sites of development of leishmanias (modified from Johnson and Hertig, 1970). B. The stomodaeal valve and adjacent parts (after Adler and Theodor, 1926a).

suggested by Trager (1974b), that the possibility should be re-assessed. The search for conjugation has been made with trypanosomes (e.g. Fairbairn and Culwick, 1946; Amrein, 1965), but it can be assumed that what applies to *Trypanosoma* will also apply to *Leishmania*. However, the "desperate attempts to find a sex life for trypanosomes" (Baker, 1974) may have been mistakenly directed. With a notable exception (Wallace, 1966), there is general agreement that trypanosomatids arose in invertebrates; relatively few have evolved with life cycles involving vertebrates. Even the non-cyclically transmitted species of salivarian trypanosomes now restricted to development in vertebrates (*T. evansi* sspp. and *T. equinum*) have an accepted origin from a tsetse-borne species (*T. brucei*) (Hoare, 1972). It follows, therefore, that if conjugation takes place in Trypanosomatidae, it is more likely to be found in invertebrates than vertebrates. Yet the evidence for the lack of conjugation in the family comes from studies on trypanosomes in vertebrates.

Recently devised methods of demonstrating the isoenzymes of try-panosomatids (e.g. Godfrey, 1976; Chance *et al.*, 1978) provide, for the first time, firm genetic markers which are essential in a search for re-combination, and the stage is now set for a new appraisal of the possibility of the exchange of genetic material in *Leishmania, Trypanosoma* and other trypanosomatids. The search has been in the wrong part of the life cycle before suitable genetic markers were demonstrable. Although there are slight indications in studies on the ultrastructure of trypanosomes, cited above, of forms which could perhaps be the products of conjugation, no such forms have yet been seen in similar studies on *Leishmania* in the sandfly. If, however, conjugation is a rare event and not obligatory as, for example, in the life cycle of malaria parasites, the chances of demonstrating pairing parasites would be small and their product may be morphologically unrecognizable. A surer approach would be, as with bacteria, to search for recombinants in a mixed population, cultured from a sandfly, by means of genetic markers.

A. MAMMALIAN LEISHMANIAS

1. Forms in the sandfly

It is usually assumed that the only morphological form of *Leishmania* in the fly other than the amastigote ingested with the bloodmeal is the promastigote. It now seems, however, that leishmanias have three morphological forms in the fly, namely, amastigotes, promastigotes and paramastigotes.

The amastigote stage is restricted to the first part of the life-cycle; there is evidence that the amastigotes taken in with a bloodmeal divide at least once before changing into promastigotes (see Section II, A, 2). This early development has been examined in only a few species of *Leishmania*.

The dominant morphological form is the promastigote, two different types of which are seen in the life cycle of *L. m. amazonensis* and possibly some other leishmanias (Fig. 4). One type, for which the term nectomonad was resurrected (Killick-Kendrick *et al.*, 1974; Molyneux *et al.*, 1975), is characteristically found in the abdominal midgut of the sandfly. In electronmicrographs it is a slender, elongate, electron-dense promastigote; without the flagellum its length is $> 12 \mu m$; its mitochondrion is a straight antero-postero ramus; it has 76–91 subpellicular microtubules; and, since its flagellum is not modified for attachment to chitin, it does not adhere by means of hemidesmosomes.

As promastigotes of *L. m. amazonensis* move forward to colonize the thoracic midgut (= cardia of some authors), their shape and appearance change to a morphological type for which the term haptomonad was revived (Killick-Kendrick *et al.*, 1974). Intermediate forms between nectomonads and haptomonads have not been seen, and the transition is, therefore, presumably rapid. In electronmicrographs, the haptomonad is a short, broad, electron-lucid promastigote; without the free flagellum its length is $< 12 \mu m$; its mitochondrion winds through the body; it has

115–138 subpellicular microtubules the diameter and distance apart of which are the same as in the nectomonad; and its flagellum is swollen and able to attach to chitin by means of hemidesmosomes formed within the flagellar sheath (Fig. 9).

The change from nectomonad to haptomonad is a modification associated with the establishment of infection in a different part of the gut which represents a change in habitat. It appears to be associated with the indispensable step of forming hemidesmosomes and attaching to the chitinized parts of the stomodaeal valve (see Section II, A, 4). In species other than *L. m. amazonensis* seen with the electron-microscope, the separation of promastigotes in the midgut into the two types is not always clear, and the terms nectomonad and haptomonad may not be applicable to all species of *Leishmania* (Fig. 4).

The commonest morphological form in the foregut and hindgut of the sandfly is a paramastigote (Figs. 2, 3). This term was employed by Janovy *et al.* (1974) to describe transitional forms between promastigotes and opisthomastigotes in the genus *Herpetomonas*. Wallace (1977) found it an acceptable and useful word to describe such forms although he noted two difficulties pointed out to him by Hoare. One is the original use of the word to describe trypanosomatids with two recurrent flagella (Minchin, 1912), and the other the etymological imprecision of the prefix para, which means both beside and near.

When I and my colleagues realized that the forms of *L. m. amazonensis* in the pharynx of the sandfly could not rightly be called promastigotes because the kinetoplast was level with or posterior to the nucleus, not anterior to it, we at first described them from electron-micrographs as opisthomastigotes (Molyneux *et al.*, 1975). We were reluctant to coin a new word if a suitable one were available,* but made the mistake of basing our interpretation solely on electron-micrographs. Since then, I have seen stained smears of pharynges infected with *L. b. braziliensis*, *L. b. guyanensis* and *L. infantum* and believe that we misinterpreted the morphology of the sectioned parasites seen with the electron-microscope. The objections to the word paramastigote seem of less importance than the wrong use of the term promastigote for forms which cannot rightly be considered as such without the definition of this now well accepted word being changed. Janovy's resurrected term, paramastigote, describes round or oval parasites with the kinetoplast lying beside or slightly posterior to the nucleus, and bearing a free flagellum. These forms have

---

* Hoare and Wallace (1966) proposed six names for the morphological forms of trypanosomatids which are now internationally accepted. To these was added the sphaeromastigote (not spheromastigote) of Brack (1968), a term which is now also in common use (Hoare, 1972). In an epidemic of "mastigotes", seven other terms have been proposed or resurrected almost all of which appear to be unnecessary or confusing (see Wallace, 1977). There is much to be said for using existing terms if possible or, failing that, resurrecting and re-defining a suitable forgotten word. Only as a last resort, should a new term be coined.

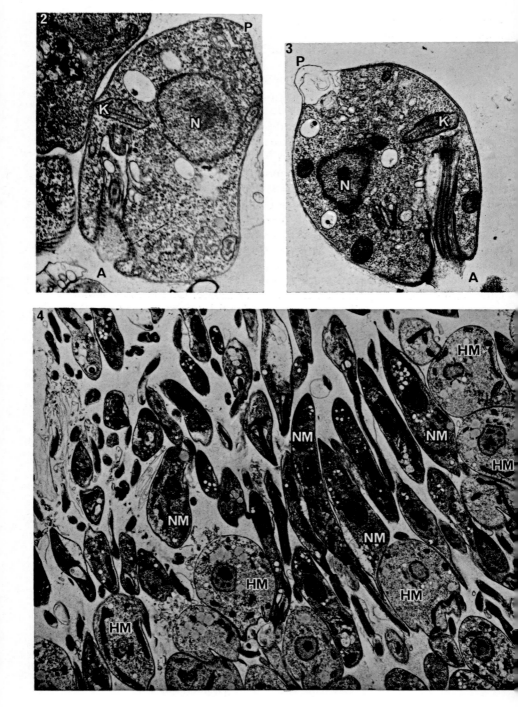

been seen in the pharynx of sandflies infected with *L. m. amazonensis*, *L. braziliensis* and *L. infantum*, and in the pylorus and ileum of flies infected with *L. b. braziliensis*; they have a deep, voluminous flagellar reservoir and are broadly intermediate between the promastigote and the opisthomastigote (Figs. 2, 3) (the latter form is at present known only in the genus *Herpetomonas*).

It is generally assumed that promastigotes in the gut of sandflies are invariably infective to a susceptible vertebrate (Adler, 1964), and many isolates of dermatropic species of *Leishmania* have been made from wild-caught sandflies by inoculating parasites into the skin of hamsters. Similarly, human volunteers have been infected with *L. tropica* by the inoculation of material from sandflies (Wenyon, 1926). There is, however, evidence suggesting that leishmanias in sandflies, perhaps at particular stages of the life cycle, are not necessarily infective to normally susceptible vertebrates. Parrot and Donatien (1927) failed to infect four mice inoculated intradermally with promastigotes from the midguts of *P. papatasi* with 34–48 h old infections of *L. tropica*. The flies were heavily infected, and the method used—inoculating the skin of the tails of mice— was routinely successful with cultured promastigotes. Feng and Chung (1941) inoculated 28 hamsters with *L. donovani* from the guts of experimentally infected sandflies. Of 20 given material from *P. chinensis* (the natural vector of the strain), only six became infected; and of eight given material from *P. mongolensis* (a poor host), two became infected. Earlier, Hindle (1931) had failed to infect six hamsters by inoculating them with material from *P. mongolensis*. The infectivity of paramastigotes of the pharynx has not been examined.

2. Development in the bloodmeal

Sandflies are considered to be pool feeders and take blood from a minute haemorrhage in the skin made by the mouthparts (Shortt and Swaminath, 1928; Lewis, 1975). The number of amastigotes ingested is remarkably low, and even when a fly has engorged on a histiocytoma of *L. mexicana* on the nose of an experimentally infected hamster, which is a solid mass of infected macrophages, it is difficult to find parasites in a stained smear of the bloodmeal. Although the lumen of the mouthparts of the sandfly is remarkably narrow (Lewis, 1975), smears of fresh blood-meals of sandflies show normal numbers of white cells. Infected macro-

---

FIGS 2–4. Morphology of flagellated forms of *Leishmania* in the sandfly. *Figs 2 and 3*—Electronmicrographs of paramastigotes (*L. b. braziliensis*) in the pylorus of *Lu. longipalpis* ($\times$ 15 000). N = nucleus; k = kinetoplast; A = anterior end; P = posterior end (Killick-Kendrick *et al.*, 1977d). *Fig. 4*—Electronmicrograph of promastigotes (*L. m. amazonensis*) in the thoracic midgut of *Lu. longipalpis* ($\times$ 5000). NM = nectomonad; HM = haptomonad (Killick-Kendrick *et al.*, 1974).

phages, however, are distorted and swollen and may not be taken intact in a bloodmeal. The few amastigotes ingested are probably the ones released when host-cells are ruptured as a sandfly probes or begins to suck blood, or which are broken by the cibarial teeth (Lewis, 1975).

Engorgement is quickly followed by the production of a peritrophic membrane which is secreted by the epithelial cells lining the midgut (Gemetchu, 1974). The membrane encloses the bloodmeal and, where intact, appears to be impenetrable by promastigotes a few of which become embedded in it (Killick-Kendrick et al., 1974). In sectioned sandflies, the encased bloodmeal is seen to lie wholly in the distended abdominal midgut and, as suggested by Lewis (1965), it is probable that the cells lining the narrower thoracic midgut play no part in the formation of the peritrophic membrane (see Section V).

Most sandflies engorge only once in each gonotrophic cycle, and the bloodmeal remains encased in the peritrophic membrane until digestion in the midgut is well advanced and the then crumpled or broken sac of digested blood is passed through the pylorus into the ileum. After defaecation, the female lays eggs and seeks a second bloodmeal. In flies which engorge again before digestion of a bloodmeal is complete, the partially digested sac containing the earlier bloodmeal becomes encased with the new bloodmeal in a second peritrophic membrane (Dolmatova, 1942; Gemetchu, 1974).

Ingested amastigotes of some, if not all, species of Leishmania undergo division before transformation into promastigotes. This part of the life cycle has been little studied, but Shortt (1928), in an account of the life cycle of L. donovani in P. argentipes, mentioned that division stages "representing multiplication before the flagellate condition" were present 24 h after an infective bloodmeal, and Strangways-Dixon and Lainson (1966) described and figured an enlargement of amastigotes of L. m. mexicana in the bloodmeal of sandflies, apparently followed in the first 24 h by at least one division of that form before transformation into the promastigote. There appear to be no similar observations on other species of Leishmania, presumably because of the difficulty of finding parasites in fresh bloodmeals.*

Within the bloodmeal, promastigotes of L. m. amazonensis, and probably other species of Leishmania, lie in nests of actively dividing parasites (Leaney, 1977). Some become free from the enclosing peritrophic membrane, perhaps through an open anterior end (Feng, 1951) or, in some species of flies, as the membrane breaks up towards the end of digestion (Gemetchu, 1974). These promastigotes, or others which may escape as the digested meal passes through the pylorus into the ileum, initiate the establishment of infection in the midgut or, in the braziliensis group, in

---

* In fresh preparations, leishmanias early in the infection are immotile, and stained preparations are indispensable in studies of the first stages in the bloodmeal (Shortt, 1928).

the hindgut. The old bloodmeal may be broken by an armature in the pylorus (Christensen *et al.*, 1971), or its peristalsis may break up a still intact meal which then passes to the ileum in disconnected fragments.

The rate of digestion, and in consequence the period of this initial part of the life cycle in the sandfly, is dependent on temperature and the size of the bloodmeal. At 25°C, a typical 0·55 mg bloodmeal of *Lutzomyia longipalpis* (Killick-Kendrick *et al.*, 1977b) is digested and passes into the hindgut on the third day. Smaller bloodmeals are more quickly digested, and higher temperatures increase, and lower temperatures reduce, the rate of digestion. In addition to temperature and size of bloodmeal, a third factor is an intrinsic variation in the rate of digestion between species of sandflies, a characteristic which possibly influences the susceptibility of a sandfly to a given parasite (see Section V).

3. Initial establishment of infection

The development of leishmanias in the bloodmeal of a sandfly cannot be considered as a true establishment of infection. This preliminary part of the life cycle can take place in the bloodmeal of many different haemato-phagous arthropods (Wenyon, 1926) but, as in a sandfly which is an unsuitable host, the parasites are later destroyed or passed out with the faeces (see Patton and Hindle, 1927). In mammalian leishmanias other than the *braziliensis* group, the next development is in the abdominal midgut. In *L. braziliensis* and related parasites, infections become established in the pylorus and ileum. There are differences in the morphology of the parasites in these two sites of development which are, therefore, considered separately.

(a) *In the abdominal midgut.* After the peritrophic membrane is produced, the epithelial cells lining the midgut are shed and pass, with the digested blood, into the hindgut (Killick-Kendrick *et al.*, 1974). The cells bear long microvilli (a "brush border") which increase the surface area of the lining of the gut and presumably play a part in digestion.* As digestion proceeds, the epithelial cells rapidly regenerate and by the time pro-mastigotes are free from the bloodmeal, the midgut is again lined with microvilli to which the promastigotes become attached by inserting their flagella (Fig. 6). In places where the microvilli have not attained their full length, the flagella of promastigotes may be pushed into the cyto-plasm of the cells below the microvilli and their close proximity to the *muscularis* led Molyneux *et al.* (1977) to postulate that parasites could possibly pass through into the coelomic cavity (see Section III). As men-tioned above, promastigotes of *L. m. amazonensis* in the abdominal mid-

---

* The epithelial cells of the abdominal midgut of *P. papatasi* and *P. orientalis* (but not the thoracic midgut) are said to lack microvilli (Adler and Theodor, 1926a; Davis, 1967); this requires confirmation.

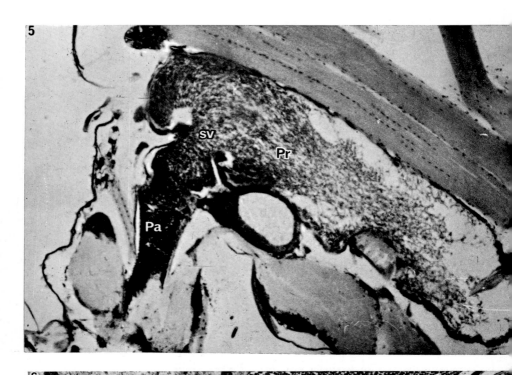

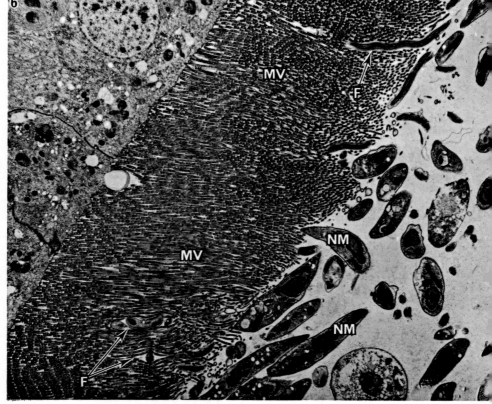

gut have been termed nectomonads (Section II, A, 1) to distinguish them from the morphologically different promastigotes, haptomonads, which are found in the thoracic midgut (Killick-Kendrick *et al.*, 1974; Molyneux *et al.*, 1975). This sharp distinction of two types of promastigotes is not, however, typical of all species; for example, we have not seen these differences between the promastigotes of *L. infantum* or *L. braziliensis* in the two different parts of the gut.

Promastigotes in the abdominal midgut rapidly multiply until the whole gut is swollen with parasites. The sequence of division of organelles leading to binary fission appears generally to be the same for all species. Before division, promastigotes increase in size and the bodies of the two daughter parasites will be little more than half the length of that of the parent. This explains the wide range of sizes of promastigotes in the midgut. At the beginning of division, three changes take place simultaneously. A daughter flagellum, which throughout division remains shorter than that of the parent, arises from a second basal body which is probably the so-called barren basal body seen in electron-micrographs (Molyneux *et al.*, 1975). The kinetoplast enlarges, becomes diffuse and stains less densely with Giemsa's stain than that of forms not in division; presumably replication of kDNA is taking place. At the same time, the nucleus becomes larger.

Unlike many other trypanosomatids, the nucleus of the promastigote in the sandfly divides completely before the kinetoplast. The two recently divided nuclei generally lie side by side across the body of the parasite, although they are occasionally seen in tandem. The rod-shaped kinetoplast lies across the anterior part of the body, and the first signs of its division are a change to a dumb-bell shape. After division, the two kinetoplasts are small, compact and stain densely; they lie just anterior to the nuclei. The body of the promastigote divides into two equal parts by a cleft which arises between the two flagella and progressively continues posteriorly leaving one nucleus and one kinetoplast in each daughter individual. The products of division are identical except that one has the smaller of the two flagella.

In cultures of *Leishmania*, the order of division of the nucleus and kinetoplast may be reversed (Christophers *et al.*, 1926) or either organelle may divide before the other (Killick-Kendrick, personal observation). According to Adler (1964), division of the kinetoplast (of cultured pro-

---

FIGS 5–6. *Fig. 5*—Sagittal section of *P. ariasi* infected with *L. infantum* (× 380). Pr = promastigotes in the thoracic midgut; Pa = paramastigotes in the pharynx; SV = stomodaeal valve. *Fig. 6*—Electronmicrograph of promastigotes (nectomonads of *L. m. amazonensis*) in the abdominal midgut of *Lu. longipalpis*; flagella (F) of the nectomonads (NM) are inserted between the microvilli (MV) of the gut (× 4300). (Killick-Kendrick *et al.*, 1974).

mastigotes) begins when the nucleus is in prophase, continues during metaphase and is completed during anaphase (i.e. before division of the nucleus is complete). The development of the second flagellum was thought probably to begin when the nucleus was in early anaphase. In the sandfly, however, it is only rarely that the kinetoplast divides before the nucleus (see Figure 1 (33) of Parrot and Donatien, 1927) and the second flagellum is formed before changes in the nucleus are demonstrable. In infections of *L. tropica* in *P. papatasi*, Adler and Theodor (1926b) state that the "blepharoplast" divides before the nucleus; in their figures, however, they show two dividing parasites (Fig. nos 36 and 37) the nuclei of which have divided before the kinetoplasts. They also described multinucleate dividing forms similar to stages seen in cultures in the presence of homologous immune serum. In other accounts, multinucleate forms have not been reported in the sandfly, and it is not known if they are a normal part of the life cycle of *L. tropica*.

(b) *In the pylorus and ileum.* The initial establishment of infection in the sandfly of species and subspecies of the *braziliensis* group (*sensu* Lainson and Shaw, 1972) is in the pylorus (= "hind-triangle") and the ileum of the fly. This development was first described by workers in Panama in studies on the life cycle of *L. b. panamensis* (Johnson *et al.*, 1963; Hertig and McConnell, 1963; Johnson and Hertig, 1970). More recently, Killick-Kendrick *et al.* (1977d) have described the ultrastructure of *L. b. braziliensis* in the pylorus and ileum of experimentally infected *Lu. longipalpis*, and Lainson *et al.* (1977c) have confirmed that development of mammalian leishmanias in these unusual sites is characteristic of only the *braziliensis* group. The latter workers emphasize the evolutionary and taxonomic significance of the difference between the life cycle of this group and that of other mammalian leishmanias.

In the ultrastructural studies in the writer's laboratory, attachment by *L. b. braziliensis* to the microvilli of the abdominal midgut of experimentally infected *Lu. longipalpis* or naturally infected *Lu. wellcomei* (a natural vector; Lainson *et al.*, 1973) has never been seen, although free promastigotes, usually few in number, are present in that part of the gut. By the 3rd day after an infective meal, however, infections of rounded paramastigotes of this parasite (Figs 2, 3, 7, 8) are established in the pylorus and, to lesser degree, in the ileum of the sandfly.

These parts of the gut, like the parts anterior to the stomodaeal valve, are ectodermal in origin and, in contrast to the midgut, are lined with a cuticular intima (Fig. 8). Trypanosomatids other than those of the subgenus *Trypanozoon* become attached to cuticular parts of the alimentary tract of their vectors by means of junctional complexes, termed hemidesmosomes, formed within the flagellar sheath (see the review by Molyneux, 1977). Attachment is presumed to be essential for the

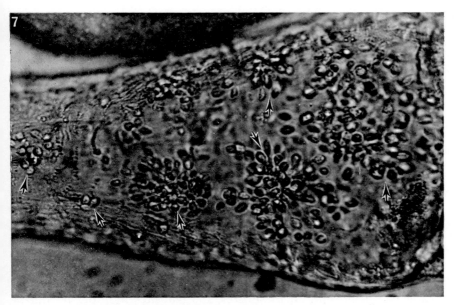

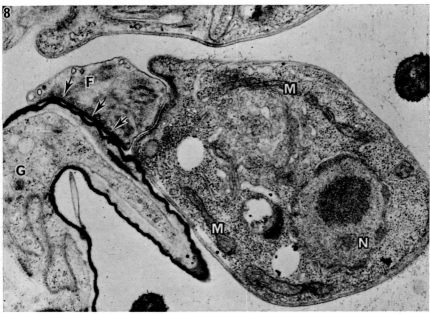

FIGS 7–8.   Paramastigotes of the *braziliensis* complex in the hindgut of the sand-fly. *Fig. 7*—Paramastigotes (arrowed) of *L. b. braziliensis* in the pylorus of *Lu. longipalpis*; fresh preparation, phase contrast illumination (× 630). (Lainson *et al.*, 1977c). *Fig. 8*—Electronmicrograph of a paramastigote (*L. b. braziliensis*) in the pylorus of naturally-infected *Lu. wellcomei* (× 25 500).   N = nucleus; F = flagellum; arrows point to hemidesmosomal attachment to the cuticular intima of the gut (G). (Material collected in 1976 at Serra dos Carajás, Pará, Brazil in collaboration with R. Lainson, R. D. Ward and J. J. Shaw; prepared by A. J. Leaney).

parasites to maintain their position in selected parts of the gut (Brooker, 1971). Predictably, therefore, paramastigotes of *L. b. braziliensis* were found to be attached to the intima of the pylorus and ileum of the sandfly by hemidesmosomes (Fig. 8). The flagella of the parasites are grossly enlarged and, in parts of the pylorus where the intima is thrown into deep folds, attachment is additionally by the insertion of the expanded flagella into the folds (Killick-Kendrick *et al.*, 1977d).

The sequence of development of parasites of the *braziliensis* group leading to the establishment of infection posterior to the midgut is imperfectly known. Promastigotes in the bloodmeal are presumably freed from the digested bloodmeal as it passes through the pylorus. They must then transform into paramastigotes and become attached to the cuticular lining after modification of their flagella without which it is unlikely that hemidesmosomes can be formed. (All leishmanias which form hemidesmosomes have grossly swollen flagella.) While attached in the pylorus and ileum, the paramastigotes, as seen in fresh preparations (Fig. 7), are almost immotile and little movement is seen except for an occasional twitch of a flagellum. In these sites, the parasites multiply by binary fission. Presumably active forms with the configuration of promastigotes are then produced and it is these parasites which migrate forwards to the thoracic midgut.

4. Migration to the stomodaeal valve

The initial establishment of infection of mammalian and some saurian leishmanias, whether in the midgut attached to microvilli or in the hindgut attached to the intima by hemidesmosomes, is followed by an anterior migration to the thoracic midgut. Although, like the abdominal midgut, this part of the alimentary tract is lined with epithelial cells bearing microvilli, most species of *Leishmania* appear not to attach here by the insertion of flagella. An exception, which requires confirmation, is *L. tropica* in *P. papatasi* (see Adler and Theodor, 1926a). In infections of *L. m. amazonensis*, the forward movement is accompanied by a transformation of promastigotes from nectomonads to haptomonads, presumably in response to a changed microhabitat and in preparation for the modifications to the flagellum associated with the production of hemidesmosomes. The change of form is remarkably quick; in the anterior part of the abdominal midgut, infections are a mixture of nectomonads and haptomonads with no signs of intermediate forms (Fig. 4). Further forward, all promastigotes of *L. m. amazonensis* are haptomonads, none of which appears to divide (Killick-Kendrick *et al.*, 1974).

In infections of all species of mammalian leishmanias examined with the electron microscope, promastigotes in the anterior part of the thoracic midgut have been found to be attached to chitinous parts of the stomodaeal valve (= oesophageal valve) by means of hemidesmosomes (Figs 9,

10). Like paramastigotes of *L. b. braziliensis* in the hindgut, the flagella of promastigotes attached to the valve are swollen. Hemidesmosomes form in the inner surface of the flagellar membrane at points not more than 30 nm from the cuticle. No hemidesmosomal attachment has been seen between flagella of different individuals (Killick-Kendrick *et al.*, 1974).

While the general pattern of anterior migration and attachment to the valve seems to be common to all mammalian leishmanias, there are some differences between species. *L. m. amazonensis* divides in the abdominal midgut of *Lu. longipalpis* and forms in the thoracic midgut are never in division (Molyneux *et al.*, 1975). Lainson *et al.* (1977b) showed that promastigotes of "*L. chagasi*" (= *L. donovani*; see Gardener, 1977) divided in the thoracic as well as the abdominal midgut of *Lu. longipalpis*, a natural vector of this parasite. Adler and Theodor (1926a) found that the principal site of division of *L. tropica* in *P. papatasi* was the thoracic midgut, and not the abdominal midgut. Similarly, in preliminary unpublished studies on the ultrastructure of *L. infantum* in *P. ariasi*, one of the natural vectors of this parasite, Prof. D. H. Molyneux and the writer have seen parasites attached to the valve in division; furthermore, unlike *L. m. amazonensis*, no clear separation of promastigotes into nectomonads and haptomonads was discernible. In an ultrastructural study of a parasite believed to be *L. b. braziliensis* in two wild-caught, naturally infected specimens of *Lu. wellcomei* (a known vector), Killick-Kendrick *et al.* (1977a) found nectomonads beneath the cuticular intima of the stomodaeal valve and inside epithelial cells of the unlined part of the valve. As more species of *Leishmania* are examined in their vectors with the electron microscope, other differences will doubtless be found.

In fresh preparations of heavily infected midguts the numbers of promastigotes packed in the thoracic midgut and attached to the valve is so great that this normally narrow part of the midgut is much swollen; such infected material can be readily recognized even under the dissecting microscope. Heavily parasitized valves everted by pressure of a coverslip are covered in actively moving attached parasites (Fig. 10), thus demonstrating the strength of attachment of the hemidesmosomal junction.

The mass of parasites attached to the valve appears to be embedded in a gel-like substance. This is well shown in a photograph of *L. infantum* broken free from the valve of *P. ariasi* published by Rioux *et al.* (1972). The origin of the gel is unknown. In cultures of *L. donovani*, Christophers *et al.* (1926) noted a gel-like "matrix" which, like the gel in the valve, stained pink with Giemsa's stain; they thought it may have been excreted from the anterior end of the parasites. It is possible, therefore, that the gel surrounding the parasites in the valve (and pharynx) is of parasitic origin. It has not been demonstrated in studies with the electron-microscope, but it may have been removed during processing.

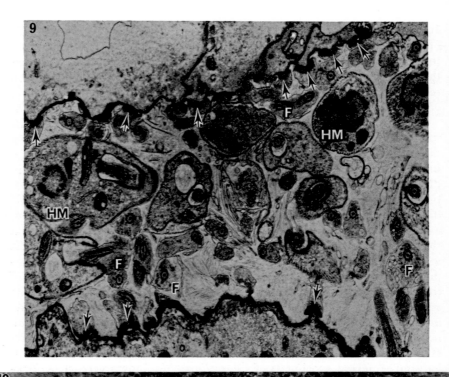

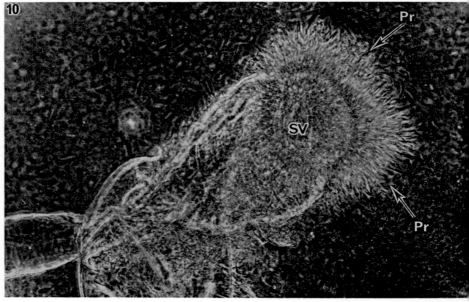

5. Invasion of the head

The stomodaeal valve in the thorax of the sandfly is linked to the pharynx, a pear-shaped pumping organ which lies in the head, by a short oesophagus. The duct of a diverticulum (= crop) opens into the oesophagus (not into the pharynx as stated by Davis (1967); see Fig. 1B); the opening of the duct is controlled by sphincter muscles (Adler and Theodor, 1926a). Although parasites are sometimes seen in the diverticulum (Gemetchu, 1976), infections in this site are generally assumed to be aberrant and not to be a normal part of the life cycle of the parasite. Gemetchu (1974), however, suggests that infections in the anterior midgut may arise from parasites in the diverticulum being moved back into the gut.

The diverticulum of the sandfly plays no direct part in the digestion of the bloodmeal but acts as a receptacle for sugars taken by the sandfly (Section IV, E); it may also play a rôle in osmoregulation (see Section V). Infections of the diverticulum may arise in two ways: during the act of feeding, infected blood may leak into the diverticulum (Adler and Theodor, 1926a; Gemetchu, 1976), or parasites in the oesophagus could perhaps be swept into the diverticulum as the fly takes solutions of sugars.

In the normal development of mammalian leishmanias in the sandfly, the infection in the stomodaeal valve spreads forwards into the oesophagus and pharynx (Fig. 5). As in the stomodaeal valve, a few nectomonads of *L. b. braziliensis* may be found beneath the cuticular lining of the oesophagus (Killick-Kendrick *et al.*, 1977a). Since the intima is unlikely to be penetrable, these parasites presumably move forward to this position having first entered the cells of the unlined part of the valve. The forward movement in the lumen of the oesophagus to the pharynx is typically accompanied by a reduction in the size of the parasites which change from elongate promastigotes (Fig. 10) to round or oval paramastigotes (Figs 11, 12). There is, however, a possibility that this morphological change may not take place in all mammalian leishmanias. In a small number of *Lu. longpalpis* experimentally infected with "*L. chagasi*", Lainson *et al.* (1977b) describe forms in the pharynx as short active promastigotes (see Section II, A, 7). Like the promastigotes in the valve, paramastigotes in the oesophagus and pharynx attach to the cuticular lining by means of hemidesmosomes formed in the flagellar sheath.

FIGS 9–10.   Attachment of *Leishmania* to the stomodaeal valve of the sandfly. *Fig. 9*—Electronmicrograph of promastigotes (haptomonads of *L. m. amazonensis*) in a fold of the stomodaeal valve of *Lu. longipalpis* (× 15 000). HM = haptomonads; F = flagellum; arrows point to hemidesmosomal attachment to the cuticular intima of part of the valve. (Killick-Kendrick *et al.*, 1974). *Fig. 10*—Promastigotes (Pr) (*L. infantum*) attached to everted stomodaeal valve (SV) of *P. ariasi*; (× 250) fresh preparation, phase contrast illumination.

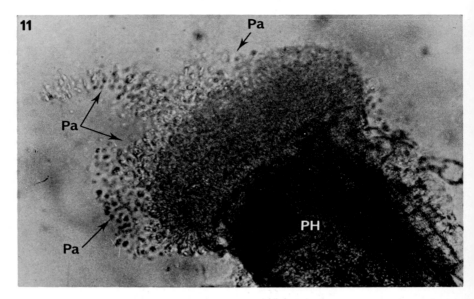

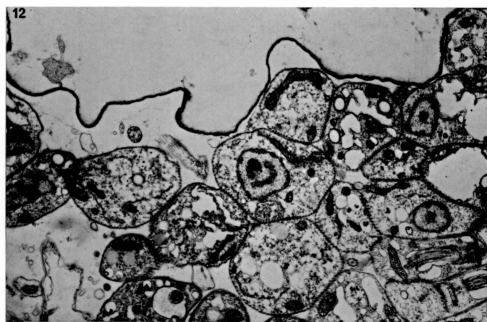

FIGS 11–12. Paramastigotes of *Leishmania* in the pharynx of the sandfly. *Fig. 11*—Paramastigotes (Pa) (*L. infantum*) pressed out of the pharynx (PH) of *P. ariasi*; (× 375) fresh preparation, phase contrast illumination. *Fig. 12*—Electronmicrograph of paramastigotes (*L. infantum*) in the pharynx of *P. ariasi* (× 13 000) (prepared by A. J. Leaney).

They are sessile forms which have never been seen to multiply (Molyneux *et al.* 1975; Killick-Kendrick *et al.*, 1977c).

As in the valve, the mass of parasites in the pharynx appears to be imbedded in a gel which is not apparent in uninfected pharynges. The life of the paramastigote in the pharynx is short. In photomicrographs of *L. m. amazonensis* in the pharynx of *Lu. longipalpis*, Killick-Kendrick *et al.* (1977c) found dead and disintegrating parasites in some pharynges, but healthy paramastigotes in others. This observation must be cautiously interpreted because the fly is not a natural vector of this parasite (although three transmissions by bite were obtained). It does, however, suggest that the infection in this organ may be maintained by a continual migration of parasites from the valve.

The reduction in size of the parasites as the infection spreads forwards, the lack of division and motility, and the suspected short life of the paramastigotes imply that the pharynx represents a more barren environment than the midgut (see Section V). In experimentally infected sandflies, this part of the life cycle is difficult to demonstrate; some of the factors thought probably to affect the spread of infection forward from the stomodaeal valve are discussed in Section IV.

From the pharynx, the infection may spread forwards to the cibarium (= buccal cavity) where paramastigotes indistinguishable from those of the pharynx become attached mainly to the roof of the cibarium which is formed by the junction of two lateral plates. Infections in this site may be considered as simply an overflow from the pharynx rather than as an indispensable step.

The forward movement from the valve is presumably accompanied by detachment and re-attachment of parasites. The hemidesmosomal attachment is remarkably secure when attached parasites are seen in fresh preparations, but there must be some mechanism whereby parasites can become detached and move their position. Hemidesmosomes of trypanosomatids may be considered as biological magnets which, it has been suggested (Killick-Kendrick *et al.*, 1974), act by a difference in charge between the gut lining and the flagellum. If this is so, detachment must be by a change in charge of either the parasite or, under some unknown stimulus, of the insect tissue. In a study of *Crithidia fasciculata*, a monoxenous trypanosomatid of mosquitoes, Brooker (1971) demonstrated that haptomonads detached in response to lowered tonicity, and in sandflies it is possible that detachment and re-attachment of leishmanias in the foregut of sandflies are related to changes in the gut as the insect imbibes sugar solutions or water (see Section IV, E). Hommel and Robertson (1976) demonstrated hemidesmosomal attachment of cultured *Trypanosoma blanchardi* to plastic, and with such a model it should be possible further to determine the factors influencing attachment and detachment.

6. Proboscis forms

The number of parasites deposited in the skin, their morphological form, biochemistry and antigenic composition are of particular interest in studies on vaccination or chemoprophylaxis; it is against infection by these parasites—not amastigotes or cultured promastigotes—that man should ideally be protected.

There is no universally accepted opinion on the form of *Leishmania* which is deposited in the skin when an infected fly bites (see Section II, A, 7). Adler had no doubt: in his view, man became infected by the short proboscis forms he and Theodor demonstrated in the prosboces of Mediterranean sandflies infected with *L. infantum* and *L. tropica*. In infections of the former parasite in a natural vector, *P. perniciosus*, Adler and Theodor (1931b) described the forms in the proboscis (Fig. 13),

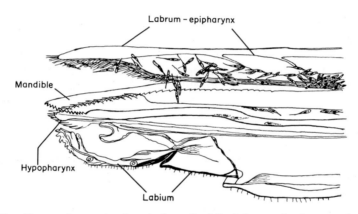

FIG. 13. Promastigotes (proboscis forms) of *L. infantum* in the mouthparts of *P. perniciosus* (from a drawing by Wenyon (1932) of a preparation made by Adler and Theodor in Catania, Italy).

typical only of late infections, as "very short flagellates from 4·7 to 10 μm in length and up to 1 μm broad. The flagellum is usually longer than the body." Measurements of proboscis forms of *L. tropica* seen in fluid seeping from a puncture in the skin of a volunteer just bitten by an infected specimen of *P. papatasi* were: body length, 6·5–13·0 μm; flagellum, 12–24 μm (Adler and Ber, 1941). Adler and Theodor (1931b) considered the short forms as "the end point of this cycle in the sandfly, and under natural conditions these are the most likely to enter the vertebrate host". Similarly, Shortt *et al.* (1926; 1928) described the most anteriorly positioned flagellates in the cibarium of *P. argentipes* infected with *L. donovani* as "elongate free forms" and "small elongated forms with well-developed flagellum". Although Shortt appeared to attach less importance to these forms than Adler, he at first believed that they were "the most likely to be transferred to the wound and so lead to infection of the vertebrate host" (Shortt *et al.*, 1926). [Later, Shortt gave support to the idea of transmission by regurgitation of a plug of parasites from the cibarium or pharynx of the fly (Shortt and Swaminath (1928); see Section II, A, 7.]

Small active promastigotes have been seen in the proboscis in other combinations of parasite and fly including *L. tropica* in *P. sergenti; L. infantum* in *P. major* (Adler *et al.*, 1938); *L. donovani* in *P. chinensis* (Feng and Chung, 1939); *L. donovani* in *Lu. longipalpis* (references in Deane and Deane, 1962; see also: Sherlock and Sherlock, 1961; Lainson *et al.*, 1977b); *L. b. panamensis* in *Lu. sanguinaria* (Hertig and McConnell, 1963); *L. m. mexicana* in *Lu. ylephiletor* (Strangways-Dixon and Lainson, 1966); and *L. braziliensis* in *Lu. longipalpis* and *Lu. renei* (Coelho *et al.*, 1967a).

In current work, the writer and colleagues have seen similar forms of three different parasites in the probosces of sandflies, all natural vectors (*L. b. braziliensis* in *Lu. wellcomei*, *L. b. guyanensis* in *Lu. umbratilis* and *L. infantum* in *P. ariasi*). No other morphological form has been seen in the proboscis and, on present evidence, the description by Adler and Theodor can be assumed to apply to all mammalian leishmanias (see Fig. 13).

Little is known of the numbers of parasites in the proboscis and, therefore, the probable infective dose. In the writer's experience, there are seldom more than ten parasites in even a well-infected fly. Occasionally, however, several hundred may be present (Adler and Theodor, 1931b; 1935).

It is uncertain which parasites are the precursors of the proboscis forms. It is plausible to think of the pharynx as a "base camp" and the proboscis as a "summit". The sequence of events would then be: multiplication in the midgut or hindgut; migration forward and attachment of promastigotes to the stomodaeal valve; cessation of division and migration to the pharynx accompanied by a morphological change to sessile paramastigotes; metamorphosis of a few paramastigotes to highly motile proboscis forms; and a final anterior migration to the mouthparts. Like paramastigotes in the pharynx, the proboscis forms do not divide in the fly, and the numbers of parasites anterior to the stomodaeal valve must be augmented by a constant trickle of parasites from the thoracic midgut. Some of these may already have changed to proboscis forms. Adler and Theodor (1931b) stated that proboscis forms of *L. infantum* in *P. perniciosus* first appeared in the thoracic midgut. In our studies on the same parasite in *P. ariasi*, we have not seen them in this part of the gut but find them, rarely, among the paramastigotes in the pharynx. Similarly,

Lainson *et al.* (1977b) figured proboscis forms of *L. donovani* in pharyngeal smears of *Lu. longipalpis*.

The proboscis, like the pharynx and cibarium, is a comparatively barren niche for the parasite (Adler and Theodor, 1926a). Although proboscis forms are apparently capable of division (as promastigotes) in cultures (Adler and Theodor, 1929a), they have never been seen to divide in the proboscis. Parts of degenerate parasites have been seen in the proboscis of *Lu. longipalpis* infected with *L. m. amazonensis* (Killick-Kendrick *et al.*, 1977c) and Adler and Theodor (1931b) noted that some proboscis forms of *L. infantum*, recovered from the proboscis of *P. perniciosus* with a Hertig apparatus (a capillary tube slipped over the proboscis of an infected fly), were uncharacteristically sluggish in movement and, it would seem, possibly moribund. Adler and Ber (1941) saw promastigotes of *L. tropica* in fluid from a puncture in the skin of a volunteer just bitten by an infected sandfly, and noted that the majority of the parasites were obviously dead. The life of proboscis forms seems, therefore, to be short and their presence in the mouthparts is dependent upon continual replacement as first suggested by Adler and Theodor (1926b).

It is remarkable that workers have often neglected to examine the proboscis and pharynx of flies with infections in the midgut, and much valuable information has thus been lost. The presence of parasites in the proboscis may be unrelated to the density of infection in the midgut, and the head and proboscis of any infected wild-caught sandfly, even with only a light infection of flagellates in the gut, should routinely be dissected and examined.

7. Transmission by bite

So little is known of the mechanism of transmission by bite that this has been considered as "the most important gap in our knowledge" of the leishmaniases (Bray, 1974). Lewis (1978) pointed out that this lack is the main obstacle to forging a mathematical model of the epidemiology of leishmaniasis for which it is necessary to predict the likelihood of the deposition of parasites into the skin when an infected fly takes blood.

In all well-studied life cycles of *Leishmania* spp. of mammals in the sandfly, migration to the stomodaeal valve has been seen to be followed, in at least a proportion of flies, by invasion of the oesophagus, pharynx, cibarium and, usually rarely, the proboscis of the fly. In spite of this, the suggestion persists that this complete development is not necessary for transmission by bite and that, in the act of biting, parasites from the stomodaeal valve or apparently blocking the pharynx or oesophagus may be forced forwards and deposited in the skin (Parrot and Donatien, 1952; Bray, 1974; Molyneux, 1977; Lainson *et al.*, 1977b). This idea was suggested by Shortt and Swaminath (1928) and supported by Napier

(1946) presumably because of similarities between the transmission of plague by "blocked" fleas and transmission of *Leishmania* by the bite of "blocked" sandflies.

Adler and Theodor (1935) strongly opposed the blockage theory on the grounds that the strong dilator muscles activating the cibarium and pharynx would widen the lumen sufficiently for blood to pass without difficulty at a calculated velocity of 2300 μm per second; the blockage seen in sectioned flies, with the organs at rest, could therefore be considered more apparent than real. Molyneux (1977) recommended a re-examination of the theory because, although he accepted Adler and Theodor's explanation that the pharynx was unlikely to be blocked, he believed that blockage of the oesophagus or stomodaeal valve, which are not pumping organs, might impede the passage of blood. He did not, however, explain how this would lead to parasites from these sites being deposited in the skin. Molyneux pointed out that there are several examples of experimental transmissions by infected flies which appear to have had difficulty in taking blood. Killick-Kendrick *et al.* (1977c) discussed this behaviour of flies at potentially infecting bloodmeals and suggested an explanation of the apparent difficulty. The cibarial sensilla probably control engorgement but, if covered by attached parasites, would cease to function. External distal labral sensilla (Lewis, 1975) would continue to stimulate attempts to engorge, but the infected fly would presumably have difficulty and would probe many times. This would increase the chances of parasites in the proboscis being deposited and left in the skin (Adler and Theodor, 1926b), and such altered behaviour of an infected fly could have a selective advantage in the evolution of a life cycle culminating in transmission by bite.

There is no experimental evidence wholly disproving the blockage theory and it is hard to see how it could be put to the test. The extreme difficulty often experienced in experimentally transmitting *Leishmania* by bite compared to the ease with which massive infections of the stomodaeal valve can be obtained, is one reason against accepting Molyneux's suggestion that the parasites deposited in the skin may be from the valve; if they were, transmission should be easy. It is also unlikely that they are from the oesophagus since this is a highly expansible part of the gut which becomes much distended during the act of feeding (Shortt and Swaminath, 1928). Furthermore, efficient transmission by bite without the migration of parasites to the pharynx and proboscis could be considered as an absence of selective pressure for the evolution of the highly characteristic forms seen in the mouthparts.

In spite of the unlikely deposition in the skin of parasites from the stomodaeal valve, the experimental transmissions of neotropical *L. donovani* recently achieved by Lainson *et al.* (1977b) by the bite of experimentally infected *Lu. longipalpis* once again raise the question of transmission arising from pharyngeal parasites. In dissections on days 5–17 of 21 positive flies from a batch with which transmissions to hamster by bite were obtained on days 7, 11, 13, 14 and 15, Lainson *et al.* found no infections in the proboscis until day 14. The first pharyngeal infection was seen on day 7 and it was suggested that, since transmissions took place on this and two later days before the first demonstration of forms in the proboscis, there was a possibility that transmission may have been by a "surge of parasites forward from the pharynx, to the mouthparts, during the feeding process." The morphology of the forms in the pharynx figured by Lainson *et al.* is closer to that of proboscis forms than the sessile paramastigotes seen in the pharynx of flies infected with other species of *Leishmania*. By the light microscope, the pharyngeal parasites were seen to be remarkably active—again in contrast to other species. It thus seems as if the parasite may have produced proboscis forms in the pharynx in the absence of the production of an established infection of paramastigotes in that organ. Two possible explanations are either that the life cycle of the strain studied in *Lu. longipalpis* is different from that of other parasites, or that the experimental conditions in which the flies were kept affected the development of the parasite.

There is no doubt that the conditions in which sandflies are kept in the laboratory can lead to physiological changes, such as incomplete digestion of the bloodmeal (Adler *et al.*, 1938), which could affect the development of leishmanias in the fly, and studies on the life cycles and transmission by bite are greatly hampered by lack of knowledge of the biology, in particular the behaviour, of sandflies in nature. This is well illustrated in a study on the life cycle of *Leishmania* in a natural vector (*P. ariasi*) in marked infected flies released in their habitat and later recaptured and dissected (Rioux *et al.*, in press). Determined attempts to demonstrate the complete life cycle of *L. infantum* in this species of sandfly *in the laboratory* have always failed and, although massive infections of the stomodaeal valve were readily demonstrable (Rioux *et al.*, 1972), development stopped at the valve. In natural conditions, however, the full life-cycle with migration of parasites to the proboscis was readily seen. From observations in the laboratory alone, the erroneous but logical conclusion was that transmission must have been accomplished without the presence of parasites anterior to the stomodaeal valve. This work, discussed in more detail in Section V, highlights the dangers of formulating theories on the transmission by bite solely on results seen in sandflies maintained in the laboratory.

In spite of all opinions to the contrary, experiments by Adler and Theodor (1929a, 1931b, 1935) on the life cycles of *L. tropica* in *P. papatasi* and *L. infantum* in *P. perniciosus* strongly suggest that the transmission of leishmaniasis is by the transfer of short, highly characteristic promastigotes from the tip of the fascicle into the skin. These workers recovered parasites from the proboscis of infected flies both with the aid of a capillary (Hertig's apparatus) and by feeding infected flies through a membrane; they also described their morphology and demonstrated their infectivity to laboratory animals. Adler and Ber (1941) saw proboscis forms of *L. tropica* in fluid oozing from a puncture wound immediately after an infected sandfly (*P. papatasi*) had engorged on the arm of a volunteer. In the face of these observations and elegant experiments, the normal mechanism of transmission of these parasites seems to be proven beyond reasonable doubt.

Adler and Theodor noted that some forms recovered from the proboscis were immotile, but nevertheless suggested that even immotile parasites, if at the tip of the proboscis, would become free in the skin during movements of the mouthparts as the fly probed. The possibility of their being flushed in by saliva is discounted by Davis (1967) on the grounds that the common duct of the salivary glands opens too anteriorly in the hypopharynx for the flow of saliva to be effective. While it is true that most of the parasites in the proboscis would escape the flow of saliva, those at the very tip would easily be carried into the wound. As an alternative, Davis suggested that if the contents of the crop were unloaded as a sandfly began to feed, parasites in the pharynx, cibarium or proboscis would be swept forwards into the skin. Young *et al.* (1978) demonstrated fructose in almost all female *P. ariasi* collected as they alighted to feed on a dog, an observation which suggests that females of at least this species normally have a full crop as they begin to probe. Unfortunately, no comparisons of the presence of fructose in flies arriving to feed and flies which had just taken a bloodmeal have been made; this might show whether or not flies empty the crop before they begin to engorge.

Davis' hypothesis is a plausible explanation for the successful transmissions of *L. donovani* to man and hamsters by the bites of experimentally infected *P. argentipes* [reviewed by Shortt (1945) and summarized by Killick-Kendrick *et al.* (1977c); see Section IV, E]. When infected flies were maintained on blood alone (i.e. with empty diverticula), transmission by bite was exceptional, but when maintained on sugar, given by providing raisins (i.e. with potentially full diverticula), transmissions were accomplished with remarkable ease.

There are two ways other than by bite that a vertebrate may become infected by sandflies. Yuan *et al.* (1943) successfully infected 5 out of 12 Chinese hamsters with *L. donovani* by feeding them 3–6 specimens of *P. chinensis* which had engorged on leishmanial-infected dogs 4–9 days earlier. Since dogs breathe with the mouth open, they suggested that transmission by ingestion should be further investigated.

During collections of *P. ariasi* from eight different dogs in the south of France, the writer and colleagues have observed differences in the behaviour of the dogs when being bitten. On dogs, *P. ariasi* generally engorges on the rim of the black skin of the nose and, in response to their probes, some dogs lick off the flies; others are more tolerant, or cover the nose with their forefeet. When the fly is abundant, a dog may ingest hundreds of flies in a single night and it is likely that dogs commonly become infected by the oral route. Man behaves differently and probably only rarely becomes infected by the accidental ingestion or inhalation of an infected fly.

The second way is by crushing an infected fly on the skin as it bites; it is assumed that infection is then caused by some of the large number of released promastigotes contaminating the wound made by the fly. This recurring idea has been much discussed over the past fifty years (Patton, 1919; Adler and Theodor, 1926b; Adler, 1929; Hu *et al.*, 1929; Southwell and Kirshner, 1938; Strangways-Dixon and Lainson, 1966). Some have considered contamination of the wound as a strong possibility, whereas others have thought it was an occasional alternative to infection by the inoculation of parasites by the proboscis of the fly. Williams and Coelho (1978), however, came to the remarkable conclusion that the majority of leishmanial infections of man are acquired by squashing probing flies on the skin, and not by the bite of infected flies. The chance of occasional transmission to man by contamination in this way cannot be denied, but there are many reasons for rejecting the idea that this is the principal means of transmission. It does not explain transmission to babies (or to animals such as the sloth) which are unable to slap a fly, or to people bitten while sleeping who presumably do not squash the sandflies. It does not take into account the fact that, when conditions are right, transmission by bite takes place with such "ridiculous ease" (Adler and Ber, 1941) that it is inconceivable to believe it is an uncommon mode of transmission. For example, Smith *et al.* (1940) successfully infected 5/5 Chinese hamsters and 2/8 white mice with *L. donovani* by the bites of 6–32 experimentally infected *P. argentipes*. The same workers (1941) similarly infected 5/5 golden hamsters. Adler and Ber (1941) permitted 26 *P. papatasi* experimentally infected with *L. tropica* to bite 45 times on 5 volunteers; 28 of the bites gave rise to lesions. In man-biting catches of wild-caught flies in the Amazon Basin, 6/7 workers exposed to bites became infected (5 with *L. b. guyanensis* and 1 with *L. b. braziliensis*) (Ward, 1977a; Lainson, personal communication); the workers took great care to ensure flies were not squashed on their skin. These and other field and laboratory observations support the view that transmission is normally by bite but do not, of course, exclude the possibility that infection might be acquired if a heavily infected fly were crushed on the skin.

B. SAURIAN LEISHMANIAS

Of eleven named species of *Leishmania* of lizards (Strong, 1924; Adler, 1964; McMillan, 1965), eight are parasites of macrophages of the blood and internal organs, and three are promastigotes in the intestinal tract of the vertebrate. The latter may represent temporary infections of trypanosomatids of invertebrates eaten by the lizard (see Vickerman, 1965), or they may be true parasites of lizards transmitted *via* the faeces. The most likely way of transmission would seem to be by the lizard eating an invertebrate which had ingested parasites from faeces, rather than by lizards eating faeces directly.

Two species of presumed saurian leishmanias, both inadequately known, have been reported in the New World. One, *L. davidi*, was found in the gut of *Cnemidophorus lemniscus* in Central America (Strong, 1924). The other, *L. henrici*, was reported from Martinique and is unusual in that it not only inhabits the cloaca of *Anolis*, but is also occasionally present in the blood; it is thought to represent a step in the evolution of tissue-inhabiting species (Adler, 1964). A third gut-inhabiting species is *L. chamaeleonis* of Old World chameleons. It is not certain that these *Leishmania* spp. of the intestine of lizards are correctly classified in this genus (Dollahon and Janovy, 1974; Vickerman, 1976).

Sandflies are presumed to be the vectors of the eight species of *Leishmania* of the blood of lizards. Since all eight are found only in the Old World, the principal vectors are probably species of the widespread Old World genus *Sergentomyia*, which probably feed mainly or exclusively on reptiles or amphibia.

Some saurian leishmanias migrate anteriorly in the fly and are transmitted by bite, whereas others have a development restricted to the midgut and hindgut and are transmitted by ingestion of an infected fly. The development of most of the parasites, however, has been seen in only a few sandflies which, moreover, were often not natural vectors. Most experiments have been done by feeding sandflies on cultured promastigotes, not amastigotes, and it is possible that infections seen in unnatural vectors fed on promastigotes may not be the same as in natural hosts fed on infected lizards. On critically examining the original accounts, the conclusion is that in no instance is the life cycle of any saurian leishmania fully known and, furthermore, that there is doubt about the means of transmission of five of the eight vector-borne species.

Even with the best studied parasite, *L. tarentolae*, observations on its life cycle in the fly are conflicting. Parrot (1934a, b, 1935) found that Algerian strains of *L. tarentolae* of the gecko, *Tarentola mauritanica*, multiplied massively in the bloodmeal of *S. antennata* (not *S. minuta*, as originally reported; see Parrot, 1942), and that the infections disappeared when the blood was passed after digestion. The flagellates died in the hindgut and rectum, and degenerate parasites were demonstrable in the faeces. Parrot (1934b, 1935) examined a total of 193 sandflies which had fed on naturally-infected geckos. Of 53 flies dissected before the digestion of blood was complete, 35 were infected, whereas of 140 flies dissected after digestion, none was infected. Parrot concluded that transmission of *L. tarentolae* was by geckos eating infected flies which still contained a bloodmeal.

Adler (1933) thought that development of *L. tarentolae* was in the "anterior station" of the sandfly and that transmission was by either bite or ingestion. Adler and Theodor (1929b, 1930b) fed cultured promastigotes of two strains of *L. tarentolae* through a membrane to *P. papatasi* and found that the parasite behaved similarly to *L. tropica* in this fly, i.e. the flagellates multiplied, ascended to the thoracic midgut and pharynx, and occasionally entered the proboscis. Adler and Theodor (1935) fed three *S. minuta* on a gecko with a double infection of *L. tarentolae* and *Trypanosoma platydactyli*. On dissection of the flies on days 4, 10 and 12, both parasites were found in the midguts of the flies and *L. tarentolae* was said to be in the "stomach and anterior part of the cardia".

The differing conclusions of Adler and Parrot can be explained in several ways. Perhaps Parrot's fly was not the natural vector of his parasite. Adler's strains of *L. tarentolae* developed well in *P. papatasi* and, although generally regarded as mammalophilic, it also feeds readily on lizards (Adler and Theodor, 1929b); possibly this fly is the natural vector of the gecko parasite in North Africa. With mammalian leishmanias, the development Parrot described is thought to show that the fly is an unsuitable host (see Section IV, A). Slight doubt is cast on Parrot's conclusion that transmission is solely by ingestion because Sergent *et al.* (1915) were unable to find any trace of sandflies in the stomachs of several hundred geckos and, although geckos will eat engorged sandflies in the laboratory (Adler and Theodor, 1935), they may not in nature.

A second explanation is that Adler was mistaken in believing that the parasites moving forward in the gut of *S. minuta* were *L. tarentolae*. The lizard was also infected with *T. platydactyli* which, in the same work, Adler and Theodor (1935) showed moved forward into the oesophagus. Furthermore, firm conclusions cannot confidently be drawn from observations on only three sandflies, especially since the pharynges and probosces were apparently not examined. Considerable weight must, however, be given to the anterior infections seen in *P. papatasi* fed on cultured promastigotes. A third possibility is that Parrot's parasite (from Algeria) and Adler's strains [one from Tunis and another sent to Adler from the Pasteur Institute, Paris (Adler, 1947)] were not the same species and had different life cycles. It is quite possible that *Tarentola mauritanica* harbours different species of *Leishmania* in some parts of its extensive distribution.

In current work on sandflies and leishmaniasis in the south of France by Prof. J. A. Rioux, the writer and colleagues, five *S. minuta* have been found with natural infections of promastigotes. Four of the five were collected at Banyuls where promastigotes were readily cultured from the blood of geckos (*T. mauritanica*) and where Rioux *et al.* (1969) had earlier seen amastigotes in a blood film from a gecko. The flies were aspirated from drainage holes in stone walls where geckos live in close contact with the flies. The fifth was taken from a similar site in Gard.

All five flies had light, moderate or heavy infections of promastigotes in the Malpighian tubules. In one fly from Banyuls the midgut was packed with promastigotes, a mass of which were attached to the stomodaeal valve. On dissection of the head, the pharynx was found to be heavily infected with paramastigotes. No parasites were seen in the cibarium, proboscis, pylorus or ileum. Two other flies from Banyuls with heavily infected tubules had no parasites in the midgut, but had heavy or moderate infections of apparently healthy promastigotes in the pylorus and ileum. The two remaining flies, one from Banyuls and the other from Gard, had light infections of the tubules, but no parasites elsewhere.

It cannot be said that the parasites in the flies were *L. tarentolae*, but the finding of flagellates in the midgut and pharynx of one fly and the hindguts of others illustrates how experiments on geckos with wild-caught *S. minuta* could give confusing results. No epimastigotes were found, and it is therefore unlikely that the flies were infected with a trypanosome. The promastigotes in the Malpighian tubules may have been part of the life cycle of saurian *Leishmania* or all five flies were perhaps infected with a monoxenous trypanosomatid, such as *Leptomonas*, and the only one with parasites also in the midgut, oesophageal valve and pharynx was coincidentally infected with *Leishmania*. Enzyme typing of promastigotes isolated from both geckos and wild-caught flies will explain the findings.

Adler's work on *L. tarentolae* provides evidence that some (but not all) saurian leishmanias have a life cycle in the sandfly culminating in invasion of the pharynx and proboscis. The evidence cannot be considered conclusive because (1) the main grounds are experiments in a host (*P. papatasi*) which is not a proven natural vector, (2) the three *S. minuta* in which the parasite was seen were also infected with a trypanosome, (3) although anterior migration was reported in these flies, no observations were made anterior to the stomodaeal valve, and (4) the conclusions disagree with the findings of Parrot who, in numerous *S. antennata*, found no evidence of anterior migration.

When closely examined, a similar supposition that *L. adleri* is transmitted by bite is less convincing. Heisch (1958) isolated this parasite by culture from lacertid lizards (*Latastia longicaudata*) in Kenya. In *Sergentomyia clydei* living in close association with the lizards, Heisch (1954) found promastigotes "in the anterior position"; dissections of engorged flies revealed nucleated erythrocytes and it was concluded that there was "little doubt" that the promastigotes were derived from the lizards. On the evidence available this seems unlikely. The flies were shown, by precipitin tests, also to feed on gerbils (Heisch, 1954) from which Heisch (1958) isolated a strain of *Leishmania* different from *L. adleri*. Furthermore, of several trypanosomatids found in *S. clydei*, one was a promastigote "in the posterior station". Since *S. clydei* clearly fed on both lizards and gerbils, it seems probable that the parasite in the "anterior position" was a mammalian *Leishmania*, and that in the "posterior station" was *L. adleri* of the lizards. Heisch's (1958) description of *L. adleri*, in which he noted morphological differences between the promastigotes of *L. donovani* and *L. adleri*, was made on strains cultured from lizards. Unfortunately, no similar observations appear to have been made on parasites isolated from *S. clydei*.

Observations on the life cycle of *L. agamae* in sandflies have been restricted to laboratory experiments with *P. papatasi* fed on cultured promastigotes. According to Adler and Theodor (1930b), the behaviour of the parasite was irregular in that the flagellates usually "confined themselves to the stomach, occasionally they descended into the hindgut and very rarely ascended the cardia and attached themselves to the rhabdorium". Later, Adler and Theodor (1957) stated that when cultured promastigotes of *L. agamae* were fed to *P. papatasi*, heavy infections were produced in which "the flagellates did not progress anteriorly but descended into the hindgut". Adler's conclusions were based on observations by Anna David (1929), a student in his laboratory. Since her work was published in a thesis which is difficult to obtain, the results are worth quoting in detail. David fed a total of 35 laboratory bred *P. papatasi* through a membrane on suspensions of cultured promastigotes of *L. agamae*. The estimated numbers of promastigotes were 500–700/ mm³ of suspension, and the average size of the meal taken was calculated as 0·1 mm³. The flies were kept at 30°C and, to keep them alive, they were given a bloodmeal on day 3 or 4. Omitting flies contaminated by bacteria, 22 out of 25 flies dissected and examined on days 1–5 were infected. Except in a few very heavily infected flies, parasites were confined to the abdominal midgut and hindgut; when infections were intense, parasites were also found in the thoracic midgut. Since flagellates were attached to the cuticular intima of the hindgut by the tip of the flagellum, the infections were truly established in the posterior station and parasites were not simply being passed with the faeces. No infections were found in 4 flies which were dissected 3–5 days after they had engorged on an infected lizard.

Although *P. papatasi* may not be the vector of *L. agamae* in nature, the development seen by David appeared healthy and normal. It is likely, therefore, that this parasite in its natural vector has a life cycle in the posterior parts of the alimentary canal and that transmission is not by bite, but by ingestion.

L. ceramodactyli of the gecko *Ceramodactylus doriae* in Baghdad also develops in the posterior station of the sandfly. Adler and Theodor (1929b) found that 6 out of 17 *P. papatasi* fed on an infected lizard developed heavy infections of the abdominal midgut, hindgut and rectum. The flies were kept at 30°C and were dissected 2–5 days after the potentially infecting bloodmeal. Two of the 6 had a few flagellates in the thoracic midgut, but there were no parasites attached to the stomodaeal valve. In the hindgut, parasites were attached to the cuticular intima from the pylorus down to and, in some flies, including the rectum.

In a series of 10 experiments, Adler and Theodor (1929b) studied the development of *L. ceramodactyli* in *P. papatasi* permitted to engorge, through a membrane, on suspensions of cultured promastigotes (120–1300 promastigotes per mm³). Infections were found in 109 out of 115 flies which had taken a meal without becoming contaminated by bacteria. In dissections of flies kept at 27–30°C, the following observations were made 3–13 days after the infecting meal. (1) The principal sites of infection were the abdominal midgut and the hindgut. (2) Multiplication of the parasites was almost exclusively in the midgut, and division was only rarely seen in the hindgut. (3) Establishment of infection in the hindgut began on day 3 when long, thin promastigotes were first seen attached to the intima just posterior to the pyloric valve; these forms were never present elsewhere and remained throughout the life of the infected fly. (4) The parasites in the ileum and rectum, which were morphologically diverse, were mostly typical elongate promastigotes of medium size, or rounded promastigotes with or without a short flagellum. (5) It appeared as if the infections in the hindgut were constantly replenished from the actively dividing population of the midgut. (6) When infections in the abdominal midgut were intense, the thoracic midgut was also invaded. (7) Parasites were sometimes attached to the stomodaeal valve, but invasion of the pharynx was seen in only one fly. (8) Infections in the thoracic midgut tended to die out after day 6, but infections in the hindgut persisted.

These observations show that *L. ceramodactyli* develops principally in the posterior station of the sandfly with anterior spread only when infections are intense and, moreover, that in *P. papatasi* there is a sequence of development of different morphological forms. The ease with which *P. papatasi* fed on geckos, the high susceptibility of this sandfly and the speed of development of the parasite led Adler and Theodor (1929b) to suggest that *P. papatasi* might be the natural vector of *L. ceramodactyli*, and that transmission must be by the oral route. Adler (1933) assumed that the parasite would probably develop similarly in *S. minuta* and possibly other sandflies found in Iraq, and left open the question of which were the vectors in nature.

L. gymnodactyli of lizards in the USSR develops only in the mid and hindguts of both an experimental host, *P. papatasi*, and the natural vector, *S. murgabiensis* (= *S. sintoni*, = *S. arpaklensis* pro parte; M. M. Artemier and D. J. Lewis, personal communication); transmission of the species seems clearly, therefore, to be by ingestion (Saf'janova and Alekseev, 1967).

The life cycle of *L. hoogstraali* of Sudanese geckos (*Hemidactylus turcicus*) in sandflies is unknown. No development was seen in 38 *P. papatasi* dissected 7 days after engorgement on infected lizards (Mc-Millan, 1965), and only one scanty infection of the midgut and pylorus (with unattached, apparently degenerating parasites) was found in 18 *Lu. longipalpis* fed on cultured promastigotes (Lainson *et al.*, 1977c).

If there are lizard leishmanias which are transmitted by bite, man may sometimes be inoculated with parasites which, although causing no disease, may give rise to a demonstrable immune response (Southgate and Oriedo, 1967; Southgate and Manson-Bahr, 1967). This could be misleading in epidemiological surveys, and it is therefore desirable that the transmission of saurian leishmanias should be re-examined, particularly in flies known to bite both lizards and man. Further work on *Leishmania* of lizards would also be helpful in refining hypotheses on the evolution of the genus (Hoare, 1949).

III. Pathogenicity of leishmanias to sandflies

In field studies on the epidemiology of cutaneous leishmaniasis in Ethiopia, Ashford *et al.* (1973) presented evidence that *L. aethiopica* is pathogenic to *P. longipes*. They found differences in the proportions of infected flies grouped according to their state of engorgement and parousness. The presumed oldest group of flies—parous and with no bloodmeal—had a lower infection rate than other groups judged by the condition of the ovaries and digestion to be younger. It was suggested that the infection caused mortality.

Parousness was recognized by the presence of granules in the accessory glands, a method accepted by Ashford *et al.* to be of "somewhat question-able value" but, they thought, to be sufficiently reliable with *P. longipes* in nature. The conclusion that the parasite was harmful to the fly must be set against increasing doubt of the accuracy of assessing parous states by this method (Chaniotis and Anderson, 1967; Foster *et al.*, 1970; Ward, 1974).

There is, however, other evidence, from laboratory observations, that

Leishmania may be pathogenic to sandflies. In experimental infections, promastigotes of *L. m. amazonensis* are found in the epithelial cells of the midgut of *Lu. longipalpis* (Molyneux *et al.*, 1977). Similarly, in two wild-caught specimens of *Lu. wellcomei* infected with a parasite believed to be *L. b. braziliensis*, Killick-Kendrick *et al.* (1977a) found intracellular promastigotes in damaged epithelial cells near the stomodaeal valve. The assertion by Johnson and Hertig (1970) that the neotropical leishmanias which they studied in *Lu. sanguinaria* and *Lu. gomezi* appeared to have no adverse affect on the longevity of the flies cannot be given much weight because most of the flies, whether infected or not, died at or shortly after oviposition only 3–7 days after their first bloodmeal.

Molyneux (1977) suggested that leishmanias may regularly invade the body cavity of the sandfly. This does indeed happen occasionally, but its effect on the fly is not known. Adler and Theodor (1929a) found promastigotes in the coelomic and muscle spaces throughout the body and appendages of several *P. sergenti* infected with *L. tropica*. They believed this had no significance, and assumed invasion took place just before or during death. In a report on the transmission of *L. tropica* by the bite of *P. papatasi*, Adler and Ber (1941) infer that *L. tropica* also occasionally invades the coelomic cavity of this natural vector when infections of the midgut are intense. In sections of more than 100 specimens of *Lu. longipalpis* infected with *L. m. amazonensis*, Leaney (personal communication) has, however, never seen parasites outside the alimentary tract, and there is no reason yet to suppose that invasion of the body cavity is a regular feature of the life cycle of *Leishmania*, nor that it is a common cause of death of infected flies.

Alekseev *et al.* (1975) found that double infections of two species of *Leishmania*, one mammalian and the other saurian, killed artificially-fed *P. papatasi* and *S. murgabiensis* (= *S. sintoni*); notably, each species of fly seemed most affected by the parasite not normally transmitted by it in nature.

For any mathematical model of the epidemiology of leishmaniasis, it is essential to know the life expectancy of sandflies carrying leishmanias and, for this reason, the pathogenicity of the parasite to the fly should be investigated in controlled experiments. It is clear that the cells of the midgut of flies may be damaged by promastigotes, but it is not known if this is invariable nor if it shortens the life of the fly.

IV. Factors affecting development in the sandfly

The difficulty of transmitting leishmanias by bite in the laboratory has led to much speculation on the factors affecting the development of the parasite in the fly and, in particular, the migration of promastigotes from the midgut into the head. The steps in the life-cycle at which development may stop are readily recognized. Growth in the bloodmeal may be inhibited; parasites may multiply in the meal but be passed into the rectum without infections becoming established in the abdominal midgut or pylorus; forward migration from the abdominal midgut or hindgut to the stomodaeal valve and attachment to the inner chitinous surface may not take place; anterior movement from the valve into the head of the fly is a common point when the life cycle is interrupted; and even when the pharynx and cibarium are invaded, transmission by bite may not be achieved, perhaps because parasites have not entered the proboscis.

With few exceptions, knowledge of the development of *Leishmania* in sandflies is founded on observations on infected flies maintained in the laboratory in conditions which differ in many ways from those experienced by vector species in nature. As Adler *et al.* (1938) pointed out, it is highly likely that transmission in nature is much more efficient than it would seem to be from experiments in the laboratory. In evolutionary terms, *Leishmania* is a successful parasite with a wide distribution and occupying a variety of microniches (in many different species of mammals, lizards and sandflies), and natural transmission is obviously sufficiently effective for survival. Rioux *et al.* (1978) carried out field experiments to investigate the dynamics of transmission in the field and estimated that 60% of sandflies (*P. ariasi*) which lived long enough after an infective bloodmeal (on a dog infected with *L. infantum*) could be expected to become infected in the pharynx; one in ten of the flies with pharyngeal infections would have parasites in the proboscis and might transmit leishmaniasis when next they took a bloodmeal.

These observations were made by marking the freshly engorged flies with fluorescent powders, releasing them and recapturing them up to 29 days after release (Killick-Kendrick *et al.*, 1978). Further similar work with other species of sandflies in suitably uninhabited places would be of interest since the longevity of parasitized flies and the number of ovarian cycles could then be estimated with sufficient accuracy to help in the creation of mathematical models of transmission.

There are a number of conditions which appear to have either adverse or beneficial effects on the development of leishmanias in the vector. Empirically designed experiments have sometimes markedly improved the chances of transmission by bite (even though it has proved difficult to understand the reason), or aspects of the behaviour of sandflies in nature have led to hypotheses suggesting why the full life cycle is often not readily demonstrable in the laboratory. These are considered below.

A. INTRINSIC INSUSCEPTIBILITY OF SOME SANDFLIES

Although the genetics of susceptibility of sandflies to leishmanias have not been studied, it can be assumed that there are genetically controlled differences in susceptibility between individuals of the same population of a species. This is the most likely explanation of why all of a batch of sandflies taking potentially infective bloodmeals do not necessarily become infected and, in those that do, infections are not all of the same intensity. Adler *et al.* (1938) demonstrated differences in the distribution of parasites in two specimens of *P. major* hatched from the same pot. Both were infected with *L. tropica* and, on dissection at 10 days, parasites in one were confined to the midgut but in the other had spread as far as the anterior end of the pharynx. Differences in the susceptibility of individual mosquitoes infected with malaria parasites or filarial worms are well known and have been shown to be genetically determined (Rutledge *et al.*, 1970; Macdonald, 1967). No such investigations have been undertaken with sandflies infected with *Leishmania*.

Of about 600 named species of phlebotomine sandflies, 52 species or subspecies are known or suspected vectors of leishmaniasis of man (Lewis, 1974; Kalra and Lewis, 1975; Killick-Kendrick, 1978). To this total may be added a few more species which transmit *Leishmania* among mammals other than man or among lizards. Some species of sandflies rarely or never engorge on vertebrates which are hosts of *Leishmania* and so have never become part of the "web of causation" (Bray, 1974) within which the parasites have evolved; others appear to be naturally insusceptible to the parasite. The intrinsic resistance to infection of many species of sandflies is presumably because the conditions in the alimentary tract of the majority of species are inimical to the parasite.

Although promastigotes of most species of *Leishmania* may be cultured *in vitro*, it has been shown that, *in vivo*, the parasites of the Old World seem to develop well in only the species of fly by which they are transmitted in nature (Patton and Hindle, 1927; Adler and Theodor, 1930b, 1931b; Hindle, 1931; Adler *et al.*, 1938; Adler, 1947; Heyneman, 1963). This restriction is sometimes said to extend even to geographical populations of a vector which are assumed to be able to support full development only of the strains of a given parasite actually transmitted by them in nature (e.g. Molyneux, 1977). This is one interpretation of the observations of Adler *et al.* (1938) who compared the development in sandflies of two strains of *L. tropica*, one from Crete and the other from Jericho. The parasite from Crete is transmitted in nature by *P. sergenti*, and that from Jericho by *P. papatasi*. In experimental conditions, both parasites developed well in only their natural vectors. Most interestingly, *P. papatasi* from both Crete and Jericho was poorly susceptible to Cretan *L. tropica*. This observation perhaps reveals as much about differences in geographical populations of *L. tropica* as about the relative susceptibilities of two populations of *P. papatasi*. Adler (1929) stressed that isolates of *L. tropica* from different localities in the Mediterranean littoral exhibit many differences notably in their behaviour in mice and infectivity to sandflies. In addition, there is normally no cross immunity between geographically distinct isolates.

Similar differences in the ability to infect different sandflies have been demonstrated between strains of *L. donovani*. Hindle (1931) showed that Chinese isolates of *L. donovani* developed well in the local vector, *P. chinensis*, but Indian isolates of the same parasite, of which *P. argentipes* is the natural vector, failed to become properly established. It thus seems that, in the Old World, the ecology of the parasite, and in particular the species of fly by which it is transmitted in a given place, moulds the parasite in such a way that its characteristics become different from closely related parasites in other ecological situations (Kirk, 1949). It is particularly interesting that a population of an Old World species of sandfly which readily supports development of one parasite is unlikely to be a suitable host of another.

While it is true that in the Old World there is this general pattern of a dominant or sole vector of a parasite in any one area, too little is known of the relative susceptibilities of sympatric species of sandflies in most places for this to be considered as an unbroken rule. In Italy, for example, there is evidence that only *P. perniciosus* transmits *L. infantum*, whereas *P. perfiliewi* is the sole vector of *L. tropica* (Adler and Theodor, 1930c, 1931a; Corradetti, 1936, 1960, 1964). Recent studies, however, suggest that in some parts of Italy *P. perfiliewi* may transmit *L. infantum* (Maroli and Bettini, 1977; Killick-Kendrick *et al.*, 1977e).

In epidemiological investigations, rigid adherence to the assumption that, in the Old World, the rôle of a sandfly as a vector of one particular parasite is immutable may be misleading; in the New World, it is untenable. There is much evidence that some neotropical sandflies have but little intrinsic resistance to many species of *Leishmania* not transmitted by them in nature. An extreme example is the work of Coelho *et al.* (1967b) who found that about 80% of batches of two neotropical sandflies, *Lu. longipalpis* and *Lu. renei*, were susceptible to isolates of *L. tropica* from Israel; invasion of the proboscis was, however, not observed and the parasite did not develop as well as in its natural vector, *P. papatasi*.

Of all the neotropical leishmanias, *L. mexicana* and its subspecies have the widest range of infectivity to sandflies. In nature these parasites are transmitted by flies of the *flaviscutellata* group (Biagi *et al.*, 1965; Williams, 1966, 1970; Disney, 1968; Shaw and Lainson, 1972; Ward *et al.*, 1973, 1977; Tikasingh, 1975). In the laboratory, however, Strangways-Dixon and Lainson (1966) showed that nine species of sandflies of Belize, not in this group, were readily infected with *L. m. mexicana* and parasites moved forwards to the stomodaeal valve in all of these flies; they saw a few promastigotes in the proboscis of one species (*Lu. ylephiletor*) and transmitted the parasite to man by the bite of another (probably *Lu. panamensis*) (Strangways-Dixon and Lainson, 1962, 1966;

see Williams, 1970). The same parasite, the natural vector of which is *Lu. olmeca*, has also been transmitted experimentally by the bite of *Lu. longipalpis*, *Lu. renei* and *Lu. cruciata* (Coelho and Falcão, 1962; Coelho *et al.*, 1967c; Williams, 1966). Similarly, the life cycle of *L. m. amazonensis*, naturally transmitted by *Lu. flaviscutellata*, has been demonstrated in *Lu. longipalpis* (Killick-Kendrick *et al.*, 1974; Molyneux *et al.*, 1975), and the parasite has been transmitted by the bite of the same fly in the laboratory (Killick-Kendrick *et al.*, 1977c).

The range of the susceptibility of neotropical sandflies to the *braziliensis* group is not yet known although, from the isolation of parasites from wild-caught flies, there appear to be at least four species (*Lu. trapidoi*, *Lu. ylephiletor*, *Lu. gomezi* and *Lu. panamensis*) in Panama which naturally transmit *L. b. panamensis*, and at least three (*Lu. wellcomei*, *Lu. pessoai* and *Lu. intermedia*) in Brazil which are vectors of *L. b. braziliensis* (Lainson and Shaw, 1973). Furthermore, Coelho *et al.* (1967a) reported that all of ten species of Brazilian sandflies with which they worked became infected with *L. braziliensis* when fed on experimentally infected hamsters.

The differences in degrees of restriction of leishmanias to particular populations of sandfly species in the Old and New Worlds are thus markedly different. This is of practical importance in the incrimination of vectors. No species of Old World *Leishmania* has been transmitted in the laboratory by the bite of a sandfly which is clearly not a natural vector, and successful transmission is, therefore, strong evidence of the rôle of an Old World sandfly as a vector in nature. In the neotropics, poor development and an inability to transmit in the laboratory may generally be taken as evidence that a sandfly is unlikely to transmit a given parasite in nature, but good development, even with experimental transmission by bite, cannot by itself be considered as proof that the fly is a vector. The bionomics of neotropical sandflies, in particular their host preferences, appear to be more important factors in the limitation of transmission than, as in the Old World, any inherent insusceptibility of a species or, perhaps, of a population of a species (Williams, 1966).

B. NUMBER OF PARASITES INGESTED

Flourishing infections of the midgut of highly susceptible sandflies, readily arise even though very few amastigotes may have been ingested (e.g. Shortt, 1945; Strangways-Dixon and Lainson, 1966). Sandflies which have a low susceptibility to a given strain of *Leishmania* do not normally become infected when they take up only a few parasites, but this natural resistance can be overcome if they ingest artificially high numbers. Although the parasites are then usually confined to the abdominal midgut, in some individuals infections may spread to the head as in a highly susceptible species. Adler and Theodor (1930c, 1931b) fed

P. papatasi through a membrane on amastigotes of *L. infantum* in the bone marrow of a patient. This fly was not the vector of the strain studied. From rough estimates of the numbers of amastigotes, it was found that no females became infected when the parasites were scanty (about one amastigote per 40 microscope fields of a stained smear; 6x ocular, 100x objective) but when the density of parasites was doubled (1 per 20 fields), small numbers became infected. The maximum proportion of *P. papatasi* ever to become infected was 26%; the bone marrow in this experiment was described as heavily infected. With more natural numbers of parasites, the comparative insusceptibility of *P. papatasi* to *L. infantum* was clearly revealed. Thus, when *P. perniciosus* (the natural vector) and *P. papatasi* were fed on the same Chinese hamster infected with an Italian strain of *L. infantum* 15/18 *P. perniciosus* (83%) but only 1/123 *P. papatasi* (0·8%) became infected. In both species of flies, the parasites "adopted an anterior position".

Adler and Theodor (1927, 1939) and Adler (1947) carried out a series of comparative observations on *Leishmania* species fed as cultured promastigotes to *P. papatasi*, the only fly they worked with which would readily feed through a membrane. The results are difficult to interpret because even when a parasite was normally transmitted by *P. papatasi*, the variation in its behaviour in individual flies was considerable. Three observations nevertheless show that the intrinsic insusceptibility of an Old World sandfly to a parasite it does not transmit in nature can be overcome when it ingests much higher numbers of parasites than would be taken up naturally. *P. papatasi* were permitted to engorge through a membrane on suspensions of promastigotes of a strain of *L. infantum* from France where the only known natural vectors of visceral leishmaniasis are *P. perniciosus* and *P. ariasi*. The number of promastigotes was 50 000 to 200 000 per mm³ of suspension. The parasite developed as well as a strain of *L. tropica* transmitted in nature by *P. papatasi*, and in several flies infection spread to the pharynx (Adler and Theodor, 1927).

Adler (1947) fed *P. papatasi* on promastigotes of a Sudanese strain of *L. donovani* which is transmitted in nature by *P. orientalis* (see Heyneman, 1963). Infections died out in flies fed on suspensions containing an estimated 200–1000 promastigotes per 0·1 mm³, but in flies fed on heavier suspensions (about 500 000 promastigotes per 0·1 mm³) infections persisted and parasites moved forward to the cibarium within 3 days.

The quantitative effect of raising the density of promastigotes in the fluid taken up by the sandfly on the proportion of flies becoming infected in the midgut is also shown in a series of experiments in which *P. papatasi* were fed on promastigotes of "*L. chagasi*", the neotropical *L. donovani* transmitted in nature by *Lu. longipalpis* (see Lainson *et al.*, 1977b). Infections were seen in 24% of flies fed on a suspension of 3000 promastigotes per mm³, in 71% fed on suspensions of 10 000–20 000 per mm³ and in 89% fed on suspensions of 20 000 per mm³ (Adler and Theodor, 1939). Clearly the inability of the fly to support development was partially overcome by increasing the numbers of parasites. A possible explanation is that, while in the bloodmeal (of even an unsuitable fly), promastigotes multiply and, if large numbers were to leave the bloodmeal as it passed into the hindgut, parasites dying in an inhospitable midgut would provide a source of nourishment for others. As in cultures of *Leptomonas* (Jadin and Creemers, 1968), parasites in the gut could be expected to cannibalize dead promastigotes. The chances of an infection becoming established in this way would be enhanced if a fly initially ingested large numbers of parasites.

C. TIME, TEMPERATURE AND HUMIDITY

Both the rate at which a sandfly digests a bloodmeal and the speed of development of *Leishmania* in the fly are influenced by temperature. They are fastest at higher temperatures, but the survival of the sandfly is progressively reduced as temperatures increase. At about 10°C or more below the ambient temperature of the habitat of a sandfly, the flies become torpid, digestion is arrested and the development of the parasite stops.

It is probable that each combination of parasite and vector has evolved according to the habitat preferred by the sandfly so that the changes in the fly during digestion of blood are matched by the development of the parasite. Sandflies occupy microniches and, in spite of generally fluctuating temperatures in a habitat, they are thought to select conditions most suitable for digestion and ovarian development. In the extensive studies on *P. argentipes* in India, it was found that temperature was a vital factor in survival at oviposition. Only when engorged flies were maintained at 28 ± 1°C, was it possible for reasonable proportions of flies to survive oviposition, refeed and oviposit again (Shortt *et al.*, 1926). With such a finely tuned response of the host, the optimum temperature for the development of *L. donovani* in *P. argentipes* may be expected to be the same and, although controlled comparisons were not made, it is noteworthy that transmissions by bite were achieved only with flies incubated at 28°C.

Humidity alone has not been shown to affect the life cycle of *Leishmania* in sandflies, although all species of sandflies need comparatively high humidities if they are to live long enough to transmit the parasite. In the microniches occupied by sandflies, temperature and humidity are related, with wetter places being cooled by evaporation. Adler *et al.* (1938) recorded the behaviour of *P. major* in a large enclosed sandfly trap (2 × 1 × 1½ m) in which one end was kept at high humidity (R.H. 100%) by water dripping from porous jars on to earth and stones, whereas elsewhere in the trap the humidity was lower (R.H. 60–80%). Engorged flies which entered the trap at night rested between the stones and jars at high humidity. During the day, they moved out and rested at a lower humidity for varying periods after which they moved back to the stones. Although no measurements of temperature were made, evaporation from the wetter part of the trap would have lowered the temperature by a few degrees Centigrade. Adler *et al.* (1938) postulated that this behaviour of the fly was governed by its physiological state. If the behaviour of sandflies does indeed vary in this way according to stages of digestion or ovarian development, the development of the parasite in the fly may be affected by the temperature changes as the fly moves from place to place.

The only controlled comparisons of the effect of temperature on *Leishmania* in the fly were made by Leaney (1977). Flies (*Lu. longipalpis*) fed on lesions on hamsters infected with *L. m. amazonensis* were randomly divided into 3 groups and incubated at 28°C, 25°C and 22°C. The proportions of flies developing infections of the midgut varied from 30% at 28°C, to 75% at 25°C and 70% at 22°C. At 28°C, infections were generally less heavy than at the lower temperatures and, whereas pharyngeal infections were demonstrable in flies incubated at 25°C and 22°C, invasion of the head in flies at the highest temperature was never seen. These observations show that too high a temperature may not only interfere with the establishment of infection in the midgut, but may also inhibit anterior migration to the pharynx and mouthparts.

Transmissions of *L. m. amazonensis* by bite were obtained with *Lu. longipalpis* incubated at 25°C (Killick-Kendrick *et al.*, 1977c), and from this and the work of Leaney (1977), it seems probable that this temperature is close to the optimal for this combination of fly and parasite. It is not, however, the best temperature for all other pairs. For *L. tropica* in *P. sergenti* it is 30°C (Adler and Ber, 1941) and for *L. donovani* in *P. argentipes* it is 28°C (Shortt, 1945). If the requirements of the fly and parasite do not match, it is unlikely that the fly will be able to transmit the parasite.

The speed of development of leishmanias varies with different species. *L. mexicana* is the most rapid with a minimum time from infecting meal to infective bite of less than 4 days at high ambient temperatures (Strangways-Dixon and Lainson, 1966; Williams, 1966; Ward *et al.*, 1977). *L. infantum* from Italy completes its development in *P. perniciosus* in 6 days (Adler and Theodor, 1931b). These and other parasites have life cycles which fit one ovarian cycle of the vector which, if gonotrophically concordant, transmits the infection at the first bloodmeal after the infecting feed. In contrast, the development of *L. donovani* in *P. argentipes* is not complete by the time the ovarian cycle of the fly is finished and the eggs are laid (Shortt, 1928). Transmission is not therefore possible at the first bloodmeal after the infecting meal. Similarly, the life cycle of *L. infantum* from France west of the Rhône is still unfinished when the natural vector, *P. ariasi*, oviposits, and transmission appears not to be possible until at least the second bloodmeal after the infecting feed. In natural conditions, the life cycle of this parasite in *P. ariasi* is not complete until more than 14 days after the infecting bloodmeal (Rioux *et al.*, 1978).

D. THE INFECTING MEAL AND DIGESTION

There are a few observations suggesting that the development of leishmanias in the sandfly is affected by the nature of the infecting meal. After years of failure (Adler and Theodor, 1929b), Adler and Ber (1941) succeeded in transmitting *L. tropica* by the bite of experimentally-infected *P. papatasi* and attributed the success either to the temperature at which the flies had been incubated (30°C), or to the fact that the salinity of the suspension of promastigotes on which the flies had fed was high. Hertig and McConnell (1963) investigated the influence of salt on the life cycle of *L. b. panamensis* in *Lu. sanguinaria*, *Lu. gomezi* and *Lu. trapidoi*. Flies which fed on suspensions of promastigotes of the same salinity as that used by Adler and Ber (1941) (a final concentration of 2·24%—three times the normal salt concentration of mammalian blood), or slightly lower (2·14%), never lived for more than 4 days. In comparison with control flies, survival was unaffected when the saline concentration was reduced to 1·47%, but no differences were seen in the development of the parasite. The success of Adler and Ber remains unexplained.

The amount of serum in an infecting meal can affect the proportion of flies which become infected. Adler *et al.* (1938) fed *P. papatasi* on suspensions of promastigotes of two strains of *L. tropica*, one from Crete (transmitted in nature by *P. sergenti*) and another from Jericho (transmitted in nature by *P. papatasi*). The Cretan strain was known normally to be poorly infective to *P. papatasi* but when the proportion of serum in the infecting meal was reduced to 10%, 15/16 *P. papatasi* (94%) became infected. When an infecting meal contained 50% serum, only 6/51 flies (12%) became infected with the Cretan strain compared to 13/13 flies (100%) with the strain from Jericho. Thus, a reduction in the amount of serum in the infecting meal in some way led to an increase in the proportion of flies becoming infected by a strain to which the fly was normally insusceptible.

As sandflies engorge, it is common for a small proportion to take up a milky white fluid, presumably lymph, but neither the development of the leishmanias nor the health of the fly are adversely affected. An unusual change in blood taken by some specimens of *P. major*, in which crystals form soon after engorgement, was, however, found to inhibit the development of *L. infantum* (Adler *et al.*, 1938).

The rates at which different species of sandflies digest a bloodmeal differ, even at comparable temperatures, and it is probable that the growth rates of leishmanias have evolved to match the speed of digestion of their vectors. Promastigotes attach to the microvilli of the midgut which are lost when the epithelial cells of the midgut are shed shortly after a bloodmeal is taken. As promastigotes become free from the digested bloodmeal when it passes into the hindgut, the midgut epithelium must have been replaced if the parasites are to have a surface suitable for attachment.

Another aspect of the digestive process which, it has been suggested, may influence the ability of a fly to support development of *Leishmania* is the nature of the peritrophic membrane. In adult sandflies, this is a delamination membrane secreted by cells of the wall of the midgut (Le Berre, 1967). Feng (1951) studied the peritrophic membranes of three species of sandflies and postulated that the explanation of differences in vectorial capacity was that in some (poor hosts of *Leishmania*) the membrane remained intact, enclosing the parasites, whereas in another (a good host of *Leishmania*) the membrane broke up in the midgut and the parasites were freed. It is unlikely that the explanation is as simple as Feng suggested since apparent differences in the peritrophic membranes are only one facet of differences in digestion between species, the influence of which on the parasite is unknown.

E. SUGARS

Like other Nematocera, sandflies feed on sugars (Lewis and Domoney, 1966; Chaniotis, 1974; Young *et al.*, 1978). The frequency with which they are taken and, most importantly, their origin are unknown. The sugars, which are taken into the diverticulum, are doubtless utilized as an easily assimilated source of energy (Chaniotis, 1974) and may play a part in osmoregulation.

It is probable that sugars affect the development of leishmanias in sandflies. The most striking examples are the experimental transmissions of *L. donovani* by the bite of *P. argentipes*. The complete life cycle of Indian strains of this parasite is not completed in a single ovarian cycle of the sandfly, and in the first attempts at transmission by bite flies were kept alive by permitting survivors at oviposition to take more bloodmeals. Eleven volunteers were bitten 11 537 times by specimens of *P. argentipes* which, having engorged on kala azar patients, were refed on blood two or more times to ensure that the flies lived long enough for the parasite to complete its development. None of the volunteers became infected. However, when infected flies were kept alive by giving them raisins, 5/5 volunteers bitten by the flies contracted leishmaniasis (see review by Shortt, 1945). Similarly, in a controlled experiment, Smith *et al.* (1941)

infected 5/5 golden hamsters (*Cricetus a. auratus*) by the bites of *P. argentipes* maintained on raisins, but failed to infect four hamsters bitten by flies maintained on blood alone.

Although it is now general practice to give infected sandflies sugars of some sort, either as raisins or a sucrose solution, transmission by bite in the laboratory remains unpredictable. Some workers in Latin America have, moreover, reported that raisins or glucose had no noticeable effect on the development of leishmanias in neotropical sandflies (Coelho *et al.*, 1967a; Hertig and McConnell, 1963). Comparative trials to determine possible different effects of various sugars, alone or in combination, on the development of leishmanias in sandflies have, however, not been done, and it is possible that optimum growth in any given combination of sandfly and parasite depends upon the actual sugars taken in nature by the wild population of the fly. This would fit the concept of landscape epidemiology of the leishmaniases (Pavlovsky, 1966; Garnham, 1971) and explain, in part, the characteristic focality of this group of diseases.

There is, unfortunately, little information on the sugars taken by sandflies in nature. Fowler (in Kirk and Lewis, 1951) examined the diverticula of 7 *P. papatasi* from the Sudan and found glucose and sucrose in all, and fructose in one. In 18 individually tested crops of 4 species of sandflies in Belize, Lewis and Domoney (1966) demonstrated traces of sugar in all and identified fructose in 16, maltose in 10, glucose in 6, sucrose in 4, raffinose in 4 and melibiose in 2. Using a simple anthrone test for fructose (Van Handel, 1972), Young *et al.* (1978) demonstrated this sugar in almost all female *P. ariasi* in the south of France alighting to engorge on dogs.

Chaniotis (1974) showed that of 11 sugars offered to *Lu. trapidoi* in the laboratory, the ones preferred were sucrose, fructose, maltose, raffinose and D-glucose in descending order of preference. Of these, sucrose and fructose most stimulated flies to take large amounts. Chaniotis inferred that, since these sugars are the principal constituents of nectar, and fructose and glucose are abundant in many wild fruits, sandflies probably obtain sugars in nature from nectar, sweet exudates of plants or ripe fruits. If the source were nectar, it should be easy to find pollen on sand-flies but neither Ashford (personal communication) nor the writer have been able to do so. Ripe fruit is an unlikely source because the gut and crop of sandflies is normally sterile (Adler, 1964) and yeasts and other fungi on fruit would contaminate the flies and lead to death. This commonly happens if sandflies feed on unsterilized raisins.

Ashford (1974) saw 4 species of sandflies in Ethiopia (*P. longipes*, *P. orientalis*, *S. magna* and *S. bedfordi*) apparently probing the leaves and stems of a wide variety of plants and suggested that these were the sources of sugars in the crop of wild-caught flies. However, the mouth-parts of male sandflies seem ill equipped to probe plants, and fluids taken by probing are more likely to be taken into the midgut than the diverticulum (Ready, 1976) (see Section V).

Although it cannot be assumed that all species of sandflies obtain sugars the same way (nor, indeed, that they all take sugar), honeydew seems to be a more probable source than nectar, fruit or plant sap. This is a sugary solution excreted in large quantities from the anus of aphids, coccids and many other plant-sucking insects. It is known to form an important part of the diet of 246 species of insects of 49 families (Auclair, 1963). The kinds of sugars in honeydew and their relative proportions vary, but the commonest are fructose, glucose, sucrose and oligosaccharides (fructomaltose, melizitose, glucosucrose, etc.). The last are thought to be synthesized from sucrose or other simple sugars in the gut of aphids or coccids (Lamb, 1959; Auclair, 1963; Sidhu and Patton, 1970) and form a high proportion of the sugars of many honeydews.

Reasons for supposing honeydew to be a likely source are: (1) it is available in all habitats of sandflies, even in arid places (where scale insects feed on desert plants); (2) it falls to the ground where it is sure to be found by sandflies moving in short flights at ground level as well as by flies living closer to the source; (3) it is passed as tiny droplets which could be taken by sandflies without probing; (4) drops of some honeydews are coated with wax (Lamb, 1959) which protects against contamination and delays evaporation; and (5) the commonest sugars of honeydews (other than the oligosaccharides which no one has looked for) have been demonstrated in the diverticula of sandflies and have been shown to be among the ones preferred in the laboratory.

It has been suggested that natural sugars may provide an essential substrate for leishmanias in the barren environment of the foregut of the sandfly (Sherlock and Sherlock, 1961; Killick-Kendrick et al., 1977c). Honeydews, however, contain not only sugars but also significant amounts of many amino acids including proline (Auclair, 1963) which plays a key rôle in the nutrition of promastigotes (Trager, 1974a). The possibility that the sugars taken by sandflies are from honeydews could be investigated by a search for the characteristic oligosaccharides in the contents of the crop of wild-caught specimens. If evidence of honeydew is found, its influence on the development of leishmanias in the fly should be assessed. As pointed out by Johnson and Hertig (1970), substances available to wild sandflies may contain factors which facilitate the transmission of Leishmania, and information on the fluids taken by the flies in nature may thus provide the key to predictable transmission by bite in the laboratory.

F. ATTACHMENT TO CHITIN AND INVASION OF THE HEAD

For a leishmanial infection to become established in a sandfly, the parasites must become attached to the chitinous intima of the hindgut or foregut. Most saurian leishmanias attach in only the pylorus, ileum or rectum, whereas mammalian species of *Leishmania* except those of the *braziliensis* group attach only to the chitin lining part of the stomodaeal valve, the oesophagus, pharynx and cibarium. *L. braziliensis* and related parasites attach in both the hindgut and the foregut. The differing tropisms for these parts of the gut are probably governed mainly by variations in conditions in different parts of the fly, which must presumably match the requirements of each of the three groups of parasites at particular stages of development, rather than by any special characteristics of the chitin in the two places.

Adler and Ber (1941) suggested that the physiological conditions in the sandfly determine the properties of the inner chitin, and thus the anterior spread of mammalian leishmanias. Promastigotes of *Leishmania* are negatively charged (Adler, 1962; Gunders and Yaari, 1972) and Adler (1962) thought that the establishment of infection in the foreparts of the sandfly must depend upon an appropriate charge of the lining.

Although anterior spread of mammalian leishmanias from the abdominal midgut to the stomodaeal valve is not dependent solely upon numbers of parasites, from unpublished observations by the writer and colleagues it appears as if a massive infection of the thoracic midgut and valve is a prerequisite for invasion of the pharynx. If this is so, one stimulus for the spread of infection from the thorax into the head may be the density of parasites in the anterior part of the midgut. This could be simply overcrowding, but it might be a chemically mediated stimulus perhaps arising from secretions from the parasites or from the heavily infected gut.

It seems probable that the properties of the intima of the gut of different species of sandflies and of individuals of a vector species, perhaps dependent upon the physiological state of the fly, are vital influences on the development of *Leishmania* in its invertebrate host and, in particular, invasion of the head and transmission by bite. The difficulties of experimental transmissions by bite can, once again, be assumed to be related to differences in the physiology of infected female flies maintained in the laboratory compared to that of sandflies in nature (Adler *et al.*, 1938).

G. CONCOMITANT INFECTIONS

Sandflies harbour a wide variety of organisms (see Young and Lewis, 1977) some of which may either shorten the life of the fly or interfere with the development of leishmanias. Some are rarely present and are of little consequence, whereas others may be found in a high proportion of a population of sandflies and could be important factors affecting the transmission of *Leishmania* in nature or, in colonized flies, in the laboratory.

The gut of adult sandflies is normally sterile. Bacterial or fungal infections, unless very light, usually inhibit the development of *Leishmania* and kill the fly (Chung *et al.*, 1951; Adler, 1964). The heavily contaminated guts of sandfly larvae are believed to be a factor in the insusceptibility of larvae to infection by leishmanias (Killick-Kendrick and Ward, 1975).

Among protozoa, the commonest parasites of sandflies are acephaline eugregarines, high prevalences of which are sometimes recorded (e.g. Shortt and Swaminath, 1927; Adler and Mayrink, 1961). The parasites may be pathogenic to the fly (Ayala, 1973) but, since the classical work in India on the transmission of *L. donovani* was done with *P. argentipes* which were commonly infected with a eugregarine, it seems unlikely that these protozoa interfere with the development of *Leishmania*. Schizogregarines, which would be more likely than eugregarines to be pathogenic to sandflies, have only once been recorded (Killick-Kendrick *et al.*, 1976).

Microsporidia, many of which are highly pathogenic to insects (Tanada, 1967) and at least one of which interferes with the development of malaria parasites in mosquitoes (Hulls, 1971; Ward and Savage, 1972), were unknown in sandflies until recently; this is undoubtedly because they had been overlooked. In Brazil, microsporidia of several different genera are now known to be parasitic in a number of species of *Lutzomyia* (Ward and Killick-Kendrick, 1974; Lainson *et al.*, 1976, 1977a), and there are at least two different microsporidia in *P. ariasi* in the south of France west of the Rhône (Killick-Kendrick unpublished observation). In both places, the organs infected are either the midgut or the Malpighian tubules. None of the microsporidia of sandflies has been named, and nothing is known of their pathogenicity to sandflies or possible effect on the development of leishmanias.

Sandflies are vectors of a variety of protozoa of reptiles and amphibia, including trypanosomes, haemogregarines and malaria parasites (see Young and Lewis, 1977). However, since these parasitized flies are species which never or only rarely feed on mammals, the parasites are of no direct importance in the transmission of leishmaniasis to man. It is not known if they interfere with the development of saurian leishmanias.

V. Physiology and behaviour of sandflies

In the previous sections of this review, I have constantly touched upon aspects of the physiology and behaviour of sandflies relevant to the biology of *Leishmania* in its invertebrate host. A number of the comments have been speculative because detailed investigations of many facets of these subjects have not been made, and the information available is generally fragmentary coming, as it does, from scattered observations in the field and laboratory. In the present section, an attempt is made to draw together the little that is known of the physiology and behaviour of sandflies, excluding aspects not directly relevant to the rôle of these insects as hosts of *Leishmania*, and to point the way to new work.

To understand more of the biology of leishmanias in the sandfly, the dynamics of blood digestion must be studied. Only then will it become possible to relate the variations of form and multiplication of different species of *Leishmania* to the different sites of development in the alimentary tract of the vector. Present knowledge on the digestion of blood by sandflies is based mainly on relatively simple observations on *P. papatasi* by Adler and Theodor (1926a) and on a pioneering ultra-structural study of the gut of *P. longipes* by Gemetchu (1974). Adler and Theodor found that complement was rapidly inactivated in the midgut of sandflies and that an anticoagulant was produced in this part of the gut of the fly. Unfortunately, nothing is known of the enzymes involved in the digestion of the bloodmeal and in reviews on the blood digestion of haematophagous insects (e.g. Freyvogel, 1975), it is rare for sandflies to be even mentioned.

As with mosquitoes, it seems probable that there are differences between the functions of the epithelial cells lining the thoracic and abdominal midguts of sandflies. From morphometric and ultrastructural studies of the epithelial lining of the gut of mosquitoes, it is believed that in the thoracic midgut sugars are absorbed and a mucus-like material is formed, but that the main functions of the cells of the abdominal midgut are the formation of the peritrophic membrane, the synthesis of digestive enzymes, and the absorption of the nutrients derived from the digestion of the bloodmeal (Rudin and Hecker, 1976; Hecker, 1977; Bauer *et al.*, 1977). From Gemetchu's (1974) ultrastructural observations on the gut of *P. longipes* similar conclusions can be drawn about sandflies. Gemetchu found that the peritrophic membrane was formed in the abdominal midgut and that there was, as in mosquitoes, a proliferation of rough endoplasmic reticulum in the cells of this part of the gut which is associated with the production of digestive enzymes.

If there are functional differences between the anterior and posterior parts of the midgut of sandflies, it can be postulated that the anterior migration of promastigotes from either the pylorus and ileum, for the *braziliensis* group, or the abdominal midgut, for other mammalian and some saurian leishmanias, is a chemotrophic response to secretions produced by the cells of the anterior part of the midgut (Sherlock and Sherlock, 1961). Adler and Theodor (1926a) described four minute "oesophageal glands" the "ducts" of which were connected to the stomodaeal valve (Fig. 1 B). Perfiliew (1966), however, considered that these bodies were nephrocytes and that the "ducts" had no lumen. Davis (1967) was unable to see the "glands" in sections and dissections of *P. papatasi* and *P. orientalis*; I have often seen them in fresh dissections of midguts of *P. ariasi*. Since these bodies are in a place to which parasites are attracted, it would be interesting to know more of their function; if they produce secretions which are discharged into the fold between the thoracic midgut and the valve, this may be a stimulus for the anterior migration of promastigotes.

There are contradictory accounts of the morphology of the epithelial cells of the abdominal midgut of sandflies which, in most species bear long microvilli (Gemetchu, 1974) to which mammalian species of *Leishmania* other than those of the *braziliensis* group attach by inserting their flagella (Killick-Kendrick *et al.*, 1974); *P. papatasi* and *P. orientalis* are said to lack microvilli in this part of the gut but, like all other sandflies, to have microvilli in the thoracic midgut (Adler and Theodor, 1926a; Davis, 1967). If confirmed, this observation suggests there are major variations in the physiology of blood digestion between some species of sandflies which are of obvious importance in the relationships between parasite and invertebrate host.

Most species of sandflies are gonotrophically concordant and therefore take only one bloodmeal during each ovarian cycle. *P. papatasi* is one exception which, although the females can mature a batch of eggs after only one bloodmeal, frequently feeds again before the first meal is fully digested. This behaviour increases the chances of transmission of *Leishmania* by bite. Multiple feeding is a feature only of the beginning of ovarian development and a female fly with mature eggs, or eggs which are nearly mature, will not feed again until after oviposition (Adler and Theodor, 1926a). When a fly with a partially digested meal feeds a second time, the earlier bloodmeal becomes encased with the later one in a second peritrophic membrane (Dolmatova, 1942; Gemetchu, 1974), and digestive enzymes are presumably secreted anew. The effects of the consequences of multiple meals on the development of leishmanias in the sandfly have not been investigated, but it can be predicted that the parasites transmitted in nature by *P. papatasi* will have evolved in accord with this behaviour.

The life cycles of most species of *Leishmania* are completed during a single ovarian cycle of the fly and, with gonotrophically concordant sandflies, transmission is then possible at the second bloodmeal. There are, however, at least two exceptions. The development of *L. donovani* in *P. argentipes* is not complete by the time the fly has laid eggs and is seeking a second bloodmeal. At 28°C, female *P. argentipes* oviposit and take a second bloodmeal by the fifth day after the infecting feed. At this time, the infection will have spread no further forward than the posterior part of the pharynx. The second bloodmeal has no deleterious effect on development and, as soon as it has been taken, invasion of the anterior end of the pharynx and cibarium proceeds without interruption (Shortt, 1928). The second bloodmeal is not an essential stimulus for the parasite, and the life cycle is completed in flies denied this meal and maintained solely on raisins (Shortt, 1945).

The life cycle of *L. infantum* in *P. ariasi* in the south of France is somewhat similar to that of *L. donovani* in *P. argentipes*. In natural conditions, the thoracic midgut and stomodaeal valve are heavily infected by the time the fly has digested the first bloodmeal and has oviposited six or more days after the infecting bloodmeal. The time depends upon temperature which, in the natural habitat of the fly, varies at different times of the year, and from year to year. There are no parasites present anterior to the valve in flies caught as they seek a second bloodmeal. Immediately after this meal, the infection in the gut appears to diminish slightly, then recovers and spreads forwards to the oesophagus, pharynx and cibarium. Since there are no parasites in the heads of infected flies maintained in the laboratory on sugar solutions for as long as 16 days (at 24°C), it seems likely that the second bloodmeal is indispensable for the complete development of the parasite. It is not possible to confirm this experimentally because *P. ariasi* rarely survives oviposition in the laboratory (Rioux *et al.*, 1978).

The foregut and hindgut of sandflies, like other Diptera, are ectodermal in origin and are lined by a cuticular intima (see Snodgrass, 1935). Leishmanias in both these sites are in the form of paramastigotes, and are attached to the lining by hemidesmosomes. The fore and hind guts are not, however, identical niches; the chitinous lining of the foregut of insects is generally less permeable than that of the hindgut (Richards, 1975) and, whereas parasites in the pylorus and ileum are nourished by the products of the digestion of a bloodmeal and possibly by substances passing through from the body cavity, paramastigotes in the oesophagus, pharynx and cibarium have little to sustain them. This is perhaps why, as parasites move forwards from the stomodaeal valve, they stop dividing and become progressively smaller. Probably their only nourishment is sugar taken by the sandfly into the oesophageal diverticulum which must pass through the proboscis, cibarium, pharynx and oesophagus before being taken into the diverticulum.

It is likely that the diverticulum of sandflies plays a part in osmo-regulation. Haematophagous insects commonly reduce the volume of a bloodmeal by passing clear fluid from the anus as they engorge. Sandflies rarely do this, but appear to conserve all possible moisture; by two days after engorgement, the crop is distended with fluid (Adler and Theodor, 1926a) which must have come from the bloodmeal. In a study of the presence of sugar in wild-caught sandflies, it was shown that almost all female flies contain fructose as they take a bloodmeal (Young et al., 1978). The movement of excess fluid from the bloodmeal in the ab-dominal midgut to the crop may be simply by osmosis into strong solu-tions of sugar taken up by the sandfly before engorgement. Possible sources of these sugars were discussed in Section IV, E. The reason sugars are taken into the crop rather than the midgut is explained by Ready's (1976) observations on sandflies fed on a range of fluids either through a membrane or on cotton wool. Ready found it possible partially to reverse the destinations of fluids, irrespective of their nature, by changing the way in which they were taken by the sandflies. Sugar solutions or plasma taken by probing through a chick skin went pre-dominantly into the midgut, but the same fluids taken from cotton wool normally entered the crop. Ready postulated that the entry of fluids in the midgut was controlled by labral sensilla activated during the act of probing. Without activation, any fluid (even blood) would be largely taken into the diverticulum.

The saliva of sandflies is slightly alkaline and contains an unidentified anticoagulant (Adler and Theodor, 1926a). Like mosquitoes, the fly in-jects saliva as it probes skin immediately before taking blood, and it is likely that at least some of the saliva is taken up into the midgut with the blood. The effect of the saliva on the parasite has not been studied.

Further work is needed on all aspects of the physiology of sandflies and, when considering the rôle of sandflies as vectors of the leishmaniases in the broader sense, also on host-finding behaviour, the natural breeding places and nutrition of larvae, autogeny, diapause, dispersion and, above all, the genetics of sandflies (see Killick-Kendrick, 1978). For much of this work, laboratory colonies are indispensable. In comparison with mosquitoes, tsetse flies or reduviid bugs, work on sandflies has been in-hibited by the generally held view that these insects are difficult or impossible to colonize. This is true of some species, but not of others. Eleven species of sandflies have been bred in good numbers in the laboratory including 7 neotropical species of Lutzomyia (longipalpis, gomezi, sanguinaria, trapidoi, trinidadensis, vespertilionis and flaviscutel-lata) and 4 Old World species of Phlebotomus (argentipes, perniciosus, *longipes* and *papatasi*) (references in Killick-Kendrick *et al.*, 1977b; see also Chaniotis, 1975; Gemetchu, 1976; Ready and Croset, 1977; Ward, 1977b). Of these 11, the least difficult to colonize are 3 species with peridomestic habitats (*Lu. longipalpis, P. argentipes* and *P. papatasi*), all of which are ideal sandflies for laboratory experimentation. With a few notable exceptions, medical entomologists have been slow to accept the challenge of investigating the biology of colonized sandflies, a subject of inestimable value in advances in the epidemiology and transmission of the leishmaniases; this fertile but virtually untouched field is certain to produce results relevant to the biology of *Leishmania* in the sandfly.

VI. Summary and conclusions

In the present review, an attempt has been made to glean all the pertinent facts on the biology of leishmanias in sandflies from the observations scattered through the literature. The picture that emerges is incomplete and, in some instances, contradictory. Some controversial findings have never been confirmed and it is difficult to judge what weight should be given to them. In addition, it is often necessary to assume that observations on one or other well studied combination of parasite and fly are applicable to less well known pairs. If, however, the minor contradictions are ignored and the writer's convictions are allowed free rein, it is possible to summarize, somewhat dogmatically, the present knowledge of *Leishmania* in sandflies.

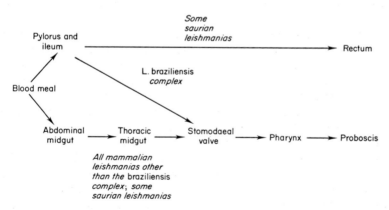

FIG. 14.   Three series of sites of development of *Leishmania* spp. in the sandfly.

Three patterns of development are depicted in Fig. 14, in all of which growth of the parasite begins in the bloodmeal. Infections of most saurian leishmanias and of the parasites of the *L. braziliensis* complex then become established in the pylorus and ileum. Most of the species parasitizing lizards colonize the whole hindgut down to and including the rectum, and are transmitted by the fly being eaten by a susceptible lizard. *L. braziliensis* and related parasites colonize the pylorus and, to a lesser degree, the ileum but do not infect the rectum. From the hindgut, they move forward to the stomodaeal valve to which they attach in large numbers. Anterior movement continues into the pharynx and cibarium where small, active, unattached promastigotes arise which move forwards into the proboscis. Transmission is by bite.

All other mammalian species of *Leishmania* and a few saurian leishmanias develop in a third pattern. The initial site of major multiplication is in the abdominal midgut, and any parasites swept into the hindgut fail to develop and are passed with the faeces. From the abdominal midgut, there is a progressive anterior spread of infection to the thoracic midgut, oesophagus, pharynx and cibarium culminating, as in the *L. braziliensis* complex, in the production of small promastigotes which move into the mouthparts. Transmission is again by bite.

From observations *in vitro*, the stimulus for the transformation of amastigotes to promastigotes is assumed to be the fall in temperature from vertebrate to invertebrate host (e.g. Hommel, 1978). In the sandfly, however, it seems probable that the transformation is preceded by at least one division of the amastigote. *Leishmania* in the blood of lizards is often in the amastigote form and transformation into promastigotes in the gut of the sandfly is presumably not stimulated solely by a change in temperature. The factors governing the morphological changes *in vivo* are clearly more complex than they appear to be from studies on *Leishmania in vitro*.

In the midgut and stomodaeal valve of the sandfly, the dominant morphological form is the promastigote, two kinds of which are present in infections of some mammalian leishmanias—the slender nectomonad in the abdominal midgut and the fatter haptomonad, with its flagellum modified for the production of hemidesmosomes, in the thoracic midgut.

The paramastigote is the typical morphological form in the parts of the alimentary tract which, unlike the midgut, are lined with a cuticular intima. These are round, oval or pear-shaped flagellates with the kinetoplast lying at the side of or slightly posterior to the nucleus. Both in the hindgut and the foregut, paramastigotes are attached to the lining of the gut by means of hemidesmosomes. In the hindgut they divide, but in the foregut they do not. The proboscis forms which arise in the pharynx and cibarium represent a reversion to the promastigote form which, unlike the paramastigote, has a flagellum unmodified for attachment.

Of several theories on the mechanism of transmission by bite, the most plausible is that proboscis promastigotes at the tip of the mouthparts are deposited in the skin as an infected sandfly feeds; promastigotes anterior to the forwardly placed opening of the common salivary duct would be swept into the skin by the flow of saliva. Proboscis forms are probably short-lived, and are replaced by a steady transformation of paramastigotes in the pharynx and cibarium. The generally barren environment in the foregut, reflected in a diminution in size and cessation of division as the parasites move forwards from the thoracic midgut through the stomodaeal valve, results in the paramastigotes having a short life, and infections in the pharynx are maintained by a continual anterior migration. Sugars taken by sandflies in nature may play an indispensable part in the nutrition of parasites in the foregut and the production of proboscis forms.

Some species of sandflies are totally refractory to infection by leishmanias, whereas others are susceptible to either a range of species of *Leishmania*, or to only the parasite transmitted by them in nature. In the Old World, the ecological relationships of the vertebrate and invertebrate hosts appear to have led to a more marked host restriction than in the New World.

Further work is needed on the biochemistry of *Leishmania* in the sandfly, the life cycles of the various species of mammalian and saurian parasites in different sandflies and on the physiology of sandflies and their behaviour in nature. Of particular importance is the study of the mechanism of transmission by bite for which a predictable model is required in the laboratory; this is unlikely to be achieved without a greater understanding of the natural history of sandflies.

VII. Acknowledgements

I wish to thank Prof. T. R. E. Southwood, F.R.S. for providing me with facilities for my work on *Leishmania* and sandflies; Prof. P. C. C. Garnham, F.R.S., Dr. R. Lainson, Dr. D. J. Lewis and Prof. W. Peters for constant encouragement and advice; and Dr. R. Lainson, Dr. R. D. Ward, Dr. J. J. Shaw, Prof. J. A. Rioux and Mr. A. J. Leaney for permitting me to quote collaborative unpublished work. I am especially indebted to Dr. Lewis who critically read a manuscript of this chapter. Mr. Leaney prepared the figures for this review and has given skilled assistance in work both in the field and in the laboratory. I gratefully acknowledge financial support from the Medical Research Council, London; the Wellcome Trust, London; the World Health Organization, Geneva; and I.N.S.E.R.M., Paris.

VIII. References

Adler, S. (1929). An analysis of the *Leishmania* sandfly problem. *Transactions of the Royal Society of Tropical Medicine and Hygiene*, **23**, 289–300.
Adler, S. (1933). Mode de transmission des protozoaires sanguicoles et particulièrement des leishmanioses. *Bulletin de la Société de Pathologie Exotique*, **26**, 207–222.

Adler, S. (1947). The behaviour of a Sudan strain of *Leishmania donovani* in *Phlebotomus papatasii*. A comparison of strains of *Leishmania*. *Transactions of the Royal Society of Tropical Medicine and Hygiene*, **40**, 701–712.

Adler, S. (1962). Approaches to research in leishmaniasis. *Scientific Reports of the Istituto Superiore di Sanità*, **2**, 143–150.

Adler, S. (1964). *Leishmania. Advances in Parasitology*, **2**, 35–96.

Adler, S. and Ber, M. (1941). The transmission of *Leishmania tropica* by the bite of *Phlebotomus papatasii*. *Indian Journal of Medical Research*, **29**, 803–909.

Adler, S. and Mayrink, W. (1961). A gregarine, *Monocystis chagasi* n. sp., of *Phlebotomus longipalpis*. Remarks on the accessory glands of *P. longipalpis*. *Revista do Instituto de Medicina Tropical de São Paulo*, **3**, 230–238.

Adler, S. and Theodor, O. (1926a). The mouthparts, alimentary tract and salivary apparatus of the female in *Phlebotomus papatasii*. *Annals of Tropical Medicine and Parasitology*, **20**, 109–142.

Adler, S. and Theodor, O. (1926b). Further observations on the transmission of cutaneous leishmaniasis to man from *Phlebotomus papatasii*. *Annals of Tropical Medicine and Parasitology*, **20**, 175–194.

Adler, S. and Theodor, O. (1927). The behaviour of cultures of *Leishmania* sp. in *Phlebotomus papatasii*. *Annals of Tropical Medicine and Parasitology*, **21**, 111–134.

Adler, S. and Theodor, O. (1929a). Attempts to transmit *Leishmania tropica* by bite: the transmission of *L. tropica* by *Phlebotomus sergenti*. *Annals of Tropical Medicine and Parasitology*, **23**, 1–16.

Adler, S. and Theodor, O. (1929b). Observations on *Leishmania ceramodactyli* n. sp. *Transactions of the Royal Society of Tropical Medicine and Hygiene*, **22**, 343–356.

Adler, S. and Theodor, O. (1930a). The exit of *Leishmania infantum* from the proboscis of *Phlebotomus perniciosus*. *Nature, London*, **126**, 883.

Adler, S. and Theodor, O. (1930b). The behaviour of insect flagellates and leishmanias in *Phlebotomus papatasii*. *Annals of Tropical Medicine and Parasitology*, **24**, 193–196.

Adler, S. and Theodor, O. (1930c). Infection of *Phlebotomus perniciosus* Newstead with *Leishmania infantum*. *Nature, London*, **126**, 437.

Adler, S. and Theodor, O. (1931a). A study of the sandfly population in endemic foci of infantile kala-azar in Italy. *Bulletin of Entomological Research*, **22**, 105–113.

Adler, S. and Theodor, O. (1931b). Investigations on Mediterranean kala azar. I–V. *Proceedings of the Royal Society, London, Series B*, **108**, 447–502.

Adler, S. and Theodor, O. (1935). Investigations on Mediterranean kala azar. VII–X. *Proceedings of the Royal Society, London, Series B*, **116**, 494–544.

Adler, S. and Theodor, O. (1939). The behaviour of *Leishmania chagasi* in *Phlebotomus papatasii*. *Annals of Tropical Medicine and Parasitology*, **33**, 45–47.

Adler, S. and Theodor, O. (1957). Transmission of disease agents by phlebotomine sandflies. *Annual Review of Entomology*, **2**, 203–226.

Adler, S., Theodor, O. and Witenberg, G. (1938). Investigations on Mediterranean kala azar. XI. A study of leishmaniasis in Canea (Crete). *Proceedings of the Royal Society, London, Series B*, **125**, 491–516.

Alekseev, A. N., Safjanova, V. M. and Karapetian, A. B. (1975). On the viability of sandflies (Diptera, Psychodidae, Phlebotominae) after infection with promastigotes of different species of *Leishmania*. (In Russian). *Parazitologiya*, **9**, 271–277.

Amrein, Y. U. (1965). Evidence against sexuality in *Trypanosoma gambiense*. *Journal of Protozoology*, **4**, 67–68.

Ashford, R. W. (1974). Sandflies (Diptera: Phlebotomidae) from Ethiopia: taxonomic and biological notes. *Journal of Medical Entomology*, **11**, 605–616.

Ashford, R. W., Bray, M. A., Hutchinson, M. P. and Bray, R. S. (1973). The epidemiology of cutaneous leishmaniasis in Ethiopia. *Transactions of the Royal Society of Tropical Medicine and Hygiene*, **67**, 568–601.

Auclair, J. L. (1963). Aphid feeding and nutrition. *Annual Review of Entomology*, **8**, 439–490.

Ayala, S. C. (1973). The phlebotomine sandfly-protozoan parasite community of central California grasslands. *American Midland Naturalist*, **89**, 266–280.

Baker, J. R. (1974). Discussion. *In:* "Trypanosomiasis and Leishmaniasis with Special Reference to Chagas' Disease", p. 248. Ciba Foundation Symposium 20 (new series), Associated Scientific Publishers, Amsterdam.

Barnett, H. C. and Suyemoto, W. (1961). Field studies on sandfly fever and kala-azar in Pakistan, in Iran and in Baltistan (Little Tibet) Kashmir. *Transactions of the New York Academy of Science, Series 2*, **23**, 609–617.

Bauer, P., Rudin, W. and Hecker, H. (1977). Ultrastructural changes in midgut cells of female *Aedes aegypti* L. (Insecta, Diptera) after starvation or sugar diet. *Cell and Tissue Research*, **177**, 215–219.

Biagi, F., Biagi, A. M. and Beltran, F. (1965). *Phlebotomus flaviscutellatus*, transmisor natural de *Leishmania mexicana*. *La Prensa Medica Mexicana*, **30**, 267–272.

Brack, C. (1968). Elekronenmikroskopische Untersuchungen zum Lebenszyklus von *Trypanosoma cruzi*. Unter besonderer Berücksichtigung der Entwicklungsformen im Uebertäger *Rhodnius prolixus*. *Acta tropica*, **25**, 289–356.

Bray, R. S. (1974). Epidemiology of leishmaniasis: some reflections on causation. *In:* "Trypanosomiasis and Leishmaniasis with Special Reference to Chagas' Disease", pp. 87–100. Ciba Foundation Symposium 20 (new series), Associated Scientific Publishers, Amsterdam.

Brener, Z. (1972). A new aspect of *Trypanosoma cruzi* life cycle in the invertebrate host. *Journal of Protozoology*, **19**, 23–27.

Brooker, B. (1971). Flagellar attachment and detachment of *Crithidia fasciculata* to the gut wall of *Anopheles gambiae*. *Protoplasma*, **73**, 191–202.

Bruce-Chwatt, L. J. (1972). Blood transfusion and tropical disease. *Tropical Diseases Bulletin*, **69**, 825–862.

Chance, M. L., Gardener, P. J. and Peters, W. (1978). Biochemical taxonomy of *Leishmania* as an ecological tool. *Colloques Internationaux du C.N.R.S.*, No. 239, Ecologie des Leishmanioses, pp. 53–61.

Chaniotis, B. N. (1974). Sugar-feeding behaviour of *Lutzomyia trapidoi* (Diptera: Psychodidae) under experimental conditions. *Journal of Medical Entomology*, **11**, 73–79.

Chaniotis, B. N. (1975). A new method for rearing *Lutzomyia trapidoi* (Diptera: Psychodidae), with observations on its development and behaviour in the laboratory. *Journal of Medical Entomology*, **12**, 183–188.

Chaniotis, B. N. and Anderson, J. A. (1967). Age structure, population dynamics and vector potential of *Phlebotomus* in Northern California. Part I. Distinguishing parous from nulliparous flies. *Journal of Medical Entomology*, **4**, 251–254.

Christensen, H. A., Herrer, A. and Fairchild, G. B. (1971). Pyloric armature of New World phlebotomine sandflies (Diptera, Psychodidae). *Journal of Medical Entomology*, **8**, 118–119.

Christophers, S. R., Shortt, H. E. and Barraud, P. J. (1926). The morphology and life cycle of the parasite of Indian kala-azar in culture. *Indian Medical Research Memoirs*, No. 4, 19–53.

Chung, H. L., Feng, L. C. and Feng, S. L. (1951). Observations concerning the successful transmission of kala-azar in North China by the bites of naturally infected *Phlebotomus chinensis*. *Peking Natural History Bulletin*, 19, 302–326.

Coelho, M. de V. and Falcão, A. R. (1962). Transmissão experimental de *Leishmania braziliensis*. II. Transmissão de amostra mexicana por picada de *Phlebotomus longipalpis* e de *Phlebotomus renei*. *Revista do Instituto de Medicina Tropical de São Paulo*, 4, 220–224.

Coelho, M. de V., Falcão, A. R. and Falcão, A. L. (1967a). Desenvolvimento de espécies do gênero *Leishmania* em espécies brasileiras de flebótomos do gênero *Lutzomyia* França, 1924. I. Evolução de *L. braziliensis* em flebótomos. *Revista do Instituto de Medicina Tropical de São Paulo*, 9, 177–191.

Coelho, M. de V., Falcão, A. R. and Falcão, A. L. (1967b). Desenvolvimento de espécies do gênero *Leishmania* em espécies brasileiras de flebótomos do gênero *Lutzomyia* França, 1924. II. Cicolo vital de *L. tropica* em *L. longipalpis* e *L. renei*. *Revista do Instituto de Medicina Tropical de Sao Paulo*, 9, 192–196.

Coelho, M. de V., Falcão, A. R., and Falcão, A. L. (1967c). Desenvolvimento de espécies do gênero *Leishmania* em espécies brasileiras de flebótomos do gênero *Lutzomyia* França, 1924. V. Infectividade de leptomonas evoluindo no flebótomo e experiências de transmissão de leishmanioses. *Revista do Instituto de Medicina Tropical de São Paulo*, 9, 367–373.

Corradetti, A. (1936). Ricerche sui flebotomi della zona endemica di Leishmaniosi cutanea in Abruzzo. *Annali d'Igiene*, 46, 13–17.

Corradetti, A. (1960). I focolai Italiani di kala azar e il problema della leishmaniosi nel sud Europa. *Parassitologia*, 2, 95–98.

Corradetti, A. (1964). Mediterranean kala azar. *Parassitologia*, 6, 275–277.

David, A. (1929). *Recherches expérimentales sur un hématozoaire du genre* Leishmania (*L. agamae* A. David). Doctorate thesis, Faculty of Science, University of Paris, 54 pp.

Davis, N. T. (1967). Leishmaniasis in the Sudan Republic. 28. Anatomical studies on *Phlebotomus orientalis* Parrot and *P. papatasi* Scopoli (Diptera: Psychodidae). *Journal of Medical Entomology*, 4, 50–65.

Deane, L. M. and Deane, M. P. (1962). Visceral leishmaniasis in Brazil: geographical distribution and transmission. *Revista do Instituto de Medicina Tropical de São Paulo*, 4, 198–212.

Deane, M. P. and Milder, R. (1966). A process of reproduction of *Trypanosoma conorhini* different from binary or multiple fission. *Journal of Protozoology*, 13, 553–559.

Disney, R. H. L. (1968). Observations on a zoonosis: leishmaniasis in British Honduras. *Journal of Applied Ecology*, 5, 1–59.

Dollahon, N. R. and Janovy, J. (1974). Experimental infection of New World lizards with Old World lizard *Leishmania* species. *Experimental Parasitology*, 36, 253–260.

Dolmatova, A. V. (1942). Life cycle of *Phlebotomus papatasi* (Scopoli). (In Russian). *Medsinskaya Parazitologiya i Parazitarnye Bolezni*, 11, 32–70 (English Translation RTS 9218, British Library, Boston Spa, Yorkshire, England).

Ellis, D. S. and Evans, D. A. (1977). Electron microscope studies of "cyst-like bodies" found in cultures of *Trypanosoma brucei rhodesiense*. *Transactions of the Royal Society of Tropical Medicine and Hygiene*, 71, 385.

Fairbairn, H. and Culwick, A. T. (1946). A new approach to trypanosomiasis. *Annals of Tropical Medicine and Parasitology*, 40, 421–452.

Feng, L. C. (1951). The role of the peritrophic membrane in *Leishmania* and trypanosome infections of sandflies. *Peking Natural History Bulletin*, 19, 327–334.

Feng, L. C. and Chung, H. L. (1939). The development of *Leishmania* in Chinese sandflies fed on dogs with canine leishmaniasis. *Chinese Medical Journal*, **56**, 35–46.

Feng, L. C. and Chung, H. L. (1941). Experiments on the transmission of kala-azar from dogs to hamsters by Chinese sandflies. *Chinese Medical Journal*, **60**, 489–496.

Forattini, A. P. (1971). Sôbre a classificão da subfamilia Phlebotominae nas Americas (Diptera: Psychodidae). *Papéis avulso do Departamento de zoologia. Secretaria de agricultura São Paulo*, **24**, 93–111.

Forattini, A. P. (1973). "Entomólogia Medica. 4. Psychodidae, Phlebotominae. Leishmanioses. Bartonelose". Blucher, Sao Paulo.

Foster, W. A., Tesfa-Yohannes, T. M. and Tesfai Tacle (1970). Studies on leishmaniasis in Ethiopia. II. Laboratory culture and biology of *Phlebotomus longipes* (Diptera: Psychodidae). *Annals of Tropical Medicine and Parasitology*, **64**, 403–409.

Fraiha, H., Shaw, J. J. and Lainson, R. (1971). Phlebotominae brasileiros. II. *Psychodopygus wellcomei*, nova espécie antropófila de flebótomo do grupo *squamiventris*, do sul do estado do Pará, Brasil (Diptera: Psychodidae). *Memórias do Instituto Oswaldo Cruz*, **69**, 489–500.

Freyvogel, T. A. (1975) (Ed.). Blood digestion in haematophagous insects. *Acta tropica*, **32**, 81–124.

Gardener, P. J. (1977). Taxonomy of the genus *Leishmania*: a review of nomenclature and classification. *Tropical Diseases Bulletin*, **74**, 1069–1088.

Garnham, P. C. C. (1971). "Progress in Parasitology". Athlone Press, London.

Geering, K. and Freyvogel, T. A. (1974). The distribution of acetylcholine and unspecific esterases in the midgut of female *Aedes aegypti* L. *Comparative Biochemistry and Physiology*, 49B, 775–784.

Gemetchu, T. (1974). The morphology and fine structure of the midgut and peritrophic membrane of the adult female, *Phlebotomus longipes* Parrot and Martin (Diptera: Psychodidae). *Annals of Tropical Medicine and Parasitology*, **68**, 111–124.

Gemetchu, T. (1976). The biology of a laboratory colony of *Phlebotomus longipes* Parrot and Martin (Diptera: Phlebotomidae). *Journal of Medical Entomology*, **12**, 661–671.

Godfrey, D. G. (1976). Biochemical strain characterization of trypanosomes. *In:* "New Approaches in American Trypanosomiasis Research", pp. 91–97. Washington: P.A.H.O. (Scientific Publication 318).

Gunders, A. E. and Yaari, A. (1972). Mobility of *Leishmania tropica* promastigotes in an electric field: effect of homologous antiserum and rifampicin. *International Journal of Parasitology*, **2**, 113–117.

Hecker, H. (1977). Structure and function of midgut epithelial cells in Culicidae mosquitoes (Insecta, Diptera). *Cell and Tissue Research*, **184**, 321–341.

Heisch, R. B. (1954). Studies in leishmaniasis in East Africa. I. The epidemiology of an outbreak of kala-azar in Kenya. *Transactions of the Royal Society of Tropical Medicine and Hygiene*, **48**, 449–469.

Heisch, R. B. (1958). On *Leishmania adleri* sp. nov. from lacertid lizards (*Latastia* sp.) in Kenya. *Annals of Tropical Medicine and Parasitology*, **52**, 68–71.

Hertig, M. and McConnell, E. (1963). Experimental infection of Panamanian *Phlebotomus* sandflies with *Leishmania*. *Experimental Parasitology*, **14**, 92–106.

Heyneman, D. (1963). Leishmaniasis in the Sudan Republic. 12. Comparison of experimental *Leishmania donovani* infections in *Phlebotomus papatasi* (Diptera: Psychodidae) with natural infections found in man-baited *P. orientalis* captured in a kala-azar endemic region of the Sudan. *American Journal of Tropical Medicine and Hygiene*, 12, 725–740.

Hindle, E. (1931). The development of various strains of *Leishmania* in Chinese sandflies. *Proceedings of the Royal Society, London, Series B*, 108, 366–383.

Ho, E. A., Chu, H. J. and Yuan, I. C. (1943). Transmission of leishmaniasis to the Chinese hamster (*Cricetulus griseus*) by the bite of Chinese sandflies (*Phlebotomus chinensis*). *Chinese Medical Journal*, 62, 207–209.

Hoare, C. A. (1949). The relationships of the haemoflagellates. *Proceedings of the 4th International Congress on Tropical Medicine and Malaria*. Washington, 1948, Vol. 2, 1110–1116.

Hoare, C. A. (1972). "The Trypanosomes of Mammals". Blackwell, Oxford.

Hoare, C. A. and Wallace, F. G. (1966). Developmental stages of trypanosomatid flagellates: a new terminology. *Nature, London*, 212, 1385–1386.

Hommel, M. (1978). The genus *Leishmania*: biology of the parasites and clinical aspects. *Bulletin de l'Institut Pasteur*, 75, 5–102.

Hommel, M. and Robertson, E. (1976). *In vitro* attachment of trypanosomes to plastic. *Experientia*, 32, 464–465.

Hu, C. H., Huie, D. and Lee, C. U. (1929). Slapping as a factor of transmission of kala-azar by sandflies (*Phlebotomus*). *Proceedings of the Society of Experimental Biology and Medicine*, 26, 280–284.

Hulls, R. H. (1971). The adverse effects of a microsporidan on sporogony and infectivity of *Plasmodium berghei*. *Transactions of the Royal Society of Tropical Medicine and Hygiene*, 65, 421–422.

Jadin, J. M. and Creemers, J. (1968). Etude de la pinocytose dans les formes en rosace de *Leptomonas ctenocephali*. *Acta tropica*, 25, 363–366.

Janovy, J., Lee, K. W. and Brumbaugh, J. A. (1974). The differentiation of *Herpetomonas megaseliae*: ulstructural observations. *Journal of Protozoology*, 21, 53–59.

Johnson, P. T. and Hertig, M. (1970). Behaviour of *Leishmania* in Panamanian phlebotomine sandflies fed on infected animals. *Experimental Parasitology*, 27, 281–300.

Johnson, P. T., McConnell, E. and Hertig, M. (1963). Natural infections of leptomonad flagellates in Panamanian *Phlebotomus* sandflies. *Experimental Parasitology*, 14, 107–122.

Kalra, N. L. and Lewis, D. J. (1975). The identity of the probable vector of *Leishmania tropica* among rodents in India. *Transactions of the Royal Society of Tropical Medicine and Hygiene*, 69, 522.

Killick-Kendrick, R. (1978). Recent advances and outstanding problems in the biology of phlebotomine sandflies. A review. *Acta tropica*, 35, 297–313.

Killick-Kendrick, R. and Ward, R. D. (1975). *Leishmania* in phlebotomid sandflies. II. The insusceptibility of sandfly larvae to *Leishmania*. *Proceedings of the Royal Society, London, Series B*, 188, 229–231.

Killick-Kendrick, R., Molyneux, D. H. and Ashford, R. W. (1974). *Leishmania* in phlebotomid sandflies. I. Modifications of the flagellum associated with attachment to the mid-gut and oesophageal valve of the sandfly. *Proceedings of the Royal Society, London, Series B*, 187, 409–419.

Killick-Kendrick, R., Leaney, A. J., Molyneux, D. H. and Rioux, J. A. (1976). Parasites of *Phlebotomus ariasi*. *Transactions of the Royal Society of Tropical Medicine and Hygiene*, 70, 2.

Killick-Kendrick, R., Lainson, R., Leaney, A. J., Ward, R. D. and Shaw, J. J. (1977a). Promastigotes of *L. b. braziliensis* in the gut wall of a natural vector, *Psychodopygus wellcomei*. *Transactions of the Royal Society of Tropical Medicine and Hygiene*, 71, 381.

Killick-Kendrick, R., Leaney, A. J. and Ready, P. D. (1977b). The establishment, maintenance and productivity of a laboratory colony of *Lutzomyia longipalpis* (Diptera: Psychodidae). *Journal of Medical Entomology*, **13**, 429–440.

Killick-Kendrick, R., Leaney, A. J., Ready, P. D. and Molyneux, D. H. (1977c). *Leishmania* in phlebotomid sandflies. IV. The transmission of *Leishmania mexicana amazonensis* to hamsters by the bite of experimentally infected *Lutzomyia longipalpis*. *Proceedings of the Royal Society, London, Series B*, **196**, 105–115.

Killick-Kendrick, R., Molyneux, D. H., Hommel, M., Leaney, A. J. and Robertson, E. S. (1977d). *Leishmania* in phlebotomid sandflies. V. The nature and significance of infections of the pylorus and ileum of the sandfly by leishmaniae of the *braziliensis* complex. *Proceedings of the Royal Society, London, Series B*, **198**, 191–198.

Killick-Kendrick, R., Ready, P. D. and Pampiglione, S. (1977e). Notes on the prevalence and host preferences of *Phlebotomus perfiliewi* in Emilia-Romagna, Italy. *Colloques Internationaux du C.N.R.S.*, No. 239, Ecologie des Leishmanioses, pp. 169–175.

Killick-Kendrick, R., Leaney, A. J., Rioux, J. A., Turner, D. P., Young, C. J. and Lanotte, G. (1978). Marking sandflies with fluorescent powders. *Symposium Proceedings; Medical Entomology Centenary*, November 1977. London: *Royal Society of Tropical Medicine and Hygiene*, p. 132.

Kirk, R. (1949). The differentiation and nomenclature of *Leishmania*. *Parasitology*, **39**, 263–273.

Kirk, R. and Lewis, D. J. (1951). The Phlebotominae of the Ethiopian Region. *Transactions of the Royal Entomological Society, London*, **102**, 383–510.

Kryukova, A. P. (1941). Experimental cutaneous leishmaniasis of wild rodents of Turkmenia. (In Russian). *In:* "Problemy Kozhnogo Leishmanioza", pp. 241–248. Ashkhabad: Turkmengosizdat. (Quoted from Perfiliew, 1966).

Lainson, R. and Shaw, J. J. (1972). Leishmaniasis of the New World: taxonomic problems. *British Medical Bulletin*, **28**, 44–48.

Lainson, R. and Shaw, J. J. (1973). Leishmanias and leishmaniasis of the New World, with particular reference to Brazil. *Bulletin of the Pan American Health Organization*, **7**, 1–19.

Lainson, R. and Southgate, B. (1965). Mechanical transmission of *Leishmania mexicana* by *Stomoxys calcitrans*. *Transactions of the Royal Society of Tropical Medicine and Hygiene*, **59**, 716.

Lainson, R., Shaw, J. J., Ward, R. D. and Fraiha, H. (1973). Leishmaniasis in Brazil. IX. Considerations on the *Leishmania braziliensis* complex: Importance of sandflies of the genus *Psychodopygus* (Mangabeira) in the transmission of *L. braziliensis braziliensis* in North Brazil. *Transactions of the Royal Society of Tropical Medicine and Hygiene*, **67**, 184–196.

Lainson, R., Ward, R. D., Young, D. G., Shaw, J. J. and Fraiha, H. (1976). Preliminary entomological and parasitological studies in Humboldt, Aripuana, Mato Grosso State, Brazil. *Acta Amazonica*, **6** (4) Suppl., 55–60.

Lainson, R., Killick-Kendrick, R., Canning, E. U., Shaw, J. J., Ward, R. D., Leaney, A. J. and Nicholas, J. P. (1977a). Microsporidia of Brazilian sandflies. *Transactions of the Royal Society of Tropical Medicine and Hygiene*, **71**, 381.

Lainson, R., Ward, R. D. and Shaw, J. J. (1977b). Experimental transmission of *Leishmania chagasi*, causative agent of neotropical visceral leishmaniasis by the sandfly, *Lutzomyia longipalpis*. *Nature, London*, **266**, 628–630.

Lainson, R., Ward, R. D. and Shaw, J. J. (1977c). *Leishmania* in phlebotomid sandflies. VI. Importance of hindgut development in distinguishing between parasites of the *Leishmania mexicana* and *L. braziliensis* complexes. *Proceedings of the Royal Society, London, Series B*, **199**, 309–320.

Lamb, K. P. (1959). Composition of the honeydew of the aphid *Brevicorne brassicae* (L.) feeding on swedes (*Brassica napobrassica*) (DC.). *Journal of Insect Physiology*, **3**, 1–13.

Leaney, A. J. (1977). The effect of temperature on *Leishmania* in sandflies. *Parasitology*, **75** (2), xxviii–xxix.

Le Berre, R. (1967). Les membranes péritrophiques chez les arthropodes. Leur rôle dans la digestion et leur intervention dans l'évolution d'organismes parasitaires. *Cahiers O.R.S.T.O.M. serie Entomologie medicale*, **5**, 147–204.

Lewis, D. J. (1965). Internal structures of some Central American phlebotomine sandflies. *Annals of Tropical Medicine and Parasitology*, **59**, 375–385.

Lewis, D. J. (1974). The biology of Phlebotomidae in relation to leishmaniasis. *Annual Review of Entomology*, **19**, 363–384.

Lewis, D. J. (1975). Functional morphology of the mouth parts in New World phlebotomine sandflies (Diptera: Psychodidae). *Transactions of the Royal Entomological Society of London*, **126**, 497–532.

Lewis, D. J. (1978). Phlebotomine sandfly research. *Symposium Proceedings; Medical Entomology Centenary*, pp. 94–99, November 1977, London. Royal Society of Tropical Medicine and Hygiene.

Lewis, D. J. and Domoney, C. R. (1966). Sugar meals in Phlebotominae and Simuliidae. *Proceedings of the Royal Entomological Society, London*, (A), **41**, 175–179.

Lewis, D. J., Young, D. G., Fairchild, G. B. and Minter, D. M. (1977). Proposals for a stable classification of the phlebotomine sandflies (Diptera: Psychodidae). *Systematic Entomology*, **2**, 319–332.

Macdonald, W. W. (1967). The influence of genetic and other factors on vector susceptibility to parasites. *In:* "Genetics of Insect Vectors of Disease (J. W. Wright and R. Pall, eds), pp. 566–584. Elsevier, Amsterdam.

Maroli, M. and Bettini, S. (1977). Leishmaniasis in Tuscany (Italy): (I) An investigation on phlebotomine sandflies in Grosseto Province. *Transactions of the Royal Society of Tropical Medicine and Hygiene*, **71**, 315–321.

McMillan, B. (1965). Leishmaniasis in the Sudan Republic. 22. *Leishmania hoogstraali* sp. n. in the gecko. *Journal of Parasitology*, **51**, 336–339.

Minchin, E. A. (1912). "An Introduction to the Study of the Protozoa". London.

Molyneux, D. H. (1977). Vector relationships in the Trypanosomatidae. *Advances in Parasitology*, **15**, 1–82.

Molyneux, D. H., Killick-Kendrick, R. and Ashford, R. W. (1975). *Leishmania* in phlebotomid sandflies. III. The ultrastructure of *Leishmania mexicana amazonensis* in the midgut and pharynx of *Lutzomyia longipalpis*. *Proceedings of the Royal Society, London, Series B*, **190**, 341–357.

Molyneux, D. H., Lewis, D. H. and Killick-Kendrick, R. (1977). Aspects of the microecology of *Leishmania*. *Colloques Internationaux du C.N.R.S.*, No. 239, Ecologie des Leishmanioses, pp. 31–40.

Napier, L. E. (1946). "Principles and Practice of Tropical Medicine". Macmillan, New York.

Napier, L. E., Smith, R. O. A. and Krishnan, K. V. (1933). The transmission of kala-azar to hamsters by the bite of the sandfly *Phlebotomus argentipes*. *Indian Journal of Medical Research*, **21**, 299–304.

Parrot, L. (1934a). Évolution d'un hématozoaire du gecko (*Leishmania tarentolae*) chez un moucheron piqueur, du group des phlébotomes (*Phlebotomus minutus*). *Comptes rendus des séances de l'Académie des Sciences, Paris*, **199**, 1073–1074.

Parrot, L. (1934b). L'évolution de *Leishmania tarentolae* Wenyon chez *Phlebotomus minutus* Rond. *Bulletin de la Société de Pathologie exotique*, **27**, 839–843.

Parrot, L. (1935). Nouvelles recherches sur l'évolution de *Leishmania tarentolae* chez *Phlebotomus minutus* Rondani. *Bulletin de la Société de Pathologie exotique*, **28**, 958–960.

Parrot, L. (1942). Notes sur les *Phlebotomes*. XXXIX. A propos de deux *Prophlebotomus* d'Algérie: *Phlebotomus minutus* var. *signatipennis* et *Phlebotomus fallax*. *Archives de l'Institut Pasteur d'Algérie*, **20**, 322–335.

Parrot, L. and Donatien, A. (1927). Le parasite du bouton d'Orient chez le phlébotome. Infection naturelle et infection expérimentale de *Phlebotomus papatasi* (Scop.). *Archives de l'Institut Pasteur d'Algérie*, **5**, 9–21.

Parrot, L. and Donatien, A. (1952). Autres observations sur l'infection naturelle des phlébotomes par la leishmaniose générale de l'homme et du chien en Algérie. *Archives de l'Institut Pasteur d'Algérie*, **30**, 146–152.

Patton, W. S. (1919). Note on the etiology of Oriental sore in Mesopotamia. *Bulletin de la Société de Pathologie exotique*, **12**, 500–504.

Patton, W. S. and Hindle, E. (1927). The development of Chinese *Leishmania* in *Phlebotomus major* var. *chinensis* and *P. sergenti* var. *Proceedings of the Royal Society, London, Series B*, **101**, 369–390.

Pavlovsky, E. M. (1966). "Natural nidality of transmissible disease" (N. D. Levine, ed.). University of Illinois Press, Urbana.

Perfiliew, P. P. (1966). *Fauna of the USSR. Diptera, vol III, No 2. Phlebotomidae (sandflies)*. Academy of Sciences of the USSR, new series No. 93. English translation from Russian, Israel Program for Scientific Translations, Jerusalem, 1968.

Ready, P. D. (1976). *Studies on the biology of phlebotomid sandflies*. Ph.D. thesis: University of London.

Ready, P. D. and Croset, H. (1977). Rearing methods for two sandfly species (Diptera: Phlebotomidae) from the "Midi", France. *Transactions of the Royal Society of Tropical Medicine and Hygiene*, **71**, 384.

Richards, A. G. (1975). The ultrastructure of the midgut of haematophagous insects. *Acta tropica*, **32**, 83–95.

Rioux, J. A., Knoepfler, L. P. and Martini, A. (1969). Présence en France de *Leishmania tarentolae* Wenyon, 1921 parasite du gecko *Tarentola mauritanica* (L. 1758). *Annales de Parasitologie humaine et comparée*, **44**, 115–116.

Rioux, J. A., Lanotte, G., Croset, H., Houin, R., Guy, Y. and Dedet, J. P. (1972). Écologie des leishmanioses dans le sud de la France. 3. Receptivité comparée de *Phlebotomus ariasi* Tonnoir, 1921 et *Rhipicephalus turanicus* Pomerancev et Matikasvili, 1940 vis-à-vis de *Leishmania donovani* (Laveran et Mesnil, 1903). *Annales de Parasitologie humaine et comparée*, **47**, 147–157.

Rioux, J. A., Killick-Kendrick, R., Leaney, A. J., Turner, D. P., Young, C. J. and Lanotte, G. (1978). The ecology of leishmaniasis in the south of France. Mark-release-recapture of *Phlebotomus ariasi* infected with *Leishmania donovani*: the biology of the fly and its rôle as a vector. *Annales de Parasitologie humaine et comparée*. In press.

Rudin, W. and Hecker, H. (1976). Morphometric comparison of the midgut epithelial cells in male and female *Aedes aegypti* L. (Insecta: Diptera). *Tissue and Cell*, **8**, 459–470.

Rutledge, L. C., Hayes, D. E. and Ward, R. A. (1970). *Plasmodium cynomolgi*: sources of variation in susceptibility of *Anopheles quadrimaculatus*, *A. balabacensis*, and *A. stephensi*. *Experimental Parasitology*, **27**, 53–59.

Saf'janova, V. M. and Alekseev, A. N. (1967). Susceptibility of *Phlebotomus papatasi* Sc. and *Sergentomyia arpaklensis* Perf. to leptomonads of different serological groups experimentally. (In Russian). *Meditsinskaya Parazitologiya i Parazitarnye Bolezni*, **36**, 580–586.

Sergent, Ed., Sergent, Et., Lemaire, G. and Senevet, G. (1915). Hypothèse sur le phlébotome "transmetteur" et la tarente "réservoir du virus" du bouton d'Orient. *Annales de l'Institut Pasteur d'Algérie*, **29**, 309–322.

Shaw, J. J. and Lainson, R. (1972). Leishmaniasis in Brazil. VI. Observations on the seasonal variations of *Lutzomyia flaviscutellata* in different types of forest and its relationship to enzootic rodent leishmaniasis (*Leishmania mexicana amazonensis*). *Transactions of the Royal Society of Tropical Medicine and Hygiene*, **66**, 709–717.

Sherlock, I. A. and Sherlock, V. A. (1961). Sobre a infecção experimental de *Phlebotomus longipalpis* pela *Leishmania donovani*. *Revista brasileira de biologia*, **21**, 409–418.

Shortt, H. E. (1928). The life-history of *Leishmania donovani* in its insect and mammalian hosts. *Transactions of the 7th Congress of the Far Eastern Association of Tropical Medicine*, December 1927, Vol. III. Calcutta: Thacker's Press, 12–18.

Shortt, H. E. (1945). Recent research on kala-azar in India. *Transactions of the Royal Society of Tropical Medicine and Hygiene*, **39**, 13–41.

Shortt, H. E. and Swaminath, C. S. (1927). *Monocystis mackiei* n. sp., parasitic in *Phlebotomus argentipes* Ann. and Brun. *Indian Journal of Medical Research*, **15**, 539–552.

Shortt, H. E. and Swaminath, C. S. (1928). The method of feeding of *Phlebotomus argentipes* with relation to its bearing on the transmission of kala-azar. *Indian Journal of Medical Research*, **15**, 827–836.

Shortt, H. E., Barraud, P. J. and Craighead, A. C. (1926). The life-history and morphology of *Herpetosoma donovani* in the sandfly *Phlebotomus argentipes*. *Indian Journal of Medical Research*, **13**, 947–959.

Shortt, H. E., Craighead, A. C. and Swaminath, C. S. (1928). A brief résumé of recent kala-azar research with special reference to India. *India Journal of Medical Research*, **16**, 221–237.

Shortt, H. E., Smith, R. O. A., Swaminath, C. S. and Krishnan, K. V. (1931). Transmission of Indian kala-azar by the bite of *Phlebotomus argentipes*. *Indian Journal of Medical Research*, **18**, 1373–1375.

Sidhu, H. S. and Patton, R. L. (1970). Carbohydrates and nitrogenous compounds in the honeydew of the mustard aphid, *Lipaphis erysimi*. *Journal of Insect Physiology*, **16**, 1339–1348.

Smith, R. O. A., Lal, C., Mukerjee, S. and Halder, K. C. (1936). The transmission of *L. donovani* by the bite of the sandfly *P. argentipes*. *Indian Journal of Medical Research*, **24**, 313–316.

Smith, R. O. A., Halder, K. C. and Ahmed, I. (1940). Further investigations on the transmission of kala-azar. Part III. The transmission of kala-azar by the bite of the sandfly *P. argentipes*. *Indian Journal of Medical Research*, **28**, 585–591.

Smith, R. O. A., Halder, K. C. and Ahmed, I. (1941). Further investigations on the transmission of kala-azar. Part VI. A second series of transmissions of *L. donovani* by *P. argentipes*. *Indian Journal of Medical Research*, **29**, 799–802.

Snodgrass, R. E. (1935). "Principles of Insect Morphology". McGraw-Hill, New York.

Southgate, B. A. and Manson-Bahr, P. E. C. (1967). Studies on the epidemiology of East African leishmaniasis. 5. *Leishmania adleri* and natural immunity. *Journal of Tropical Medicine and Hygiene*, **70**, 33–36.

Southgate, B. A. and Oriedo, B. V. E. (1967). Studies on the epidemiology of

East African leishmaniasis. 3. Immunity as a determinant of geographical distribution. *Journal of Tropical Medicine and Hygiene*, **70**, 1–4.

Southwell, T. and Kirshner, A. (1938). On the transmission of leishmaniasis. *Annals of Tropical Medicine and Parasitology*, **32**, 95–102.

Strangways-Dixon, J. and Lainson, R. (1962). Dermal leishmaniasis in British Honduras: transmission of *L. brasiliensis* by *Phlebotomus species*. *British Medical Journal*, i, 297–299.

Strangways-Dixon, J. and Lainson, R. (1966). The epidemiology of dermal leishmaniasis in British Honduras. Part III. The transmission of *Leishmania mexicana* to man by *Phlebotomus pessoanus*, with observations on the development of the parasite in different species of *Phlebotomus*. *Transactions of the Royal Society of Tropical Medicine and Hygiene*, **60**, 192–207.

Strong, R. P. (1924). Investigations upon flagellate infections. *American Journal of Tropical Medicine*, **4**, 345–372.

Swaminath, C. S., Shortt, H. E. and Anderson, L. A. P. (1942). Transmission of Indian kala-azar to man by the bites of *Phlebotomus argentipes*, Ann. and Brun. *Indian Journal of Medical Research*, **30**, 473–477.

Symmers, W. St C. (1960). Leishmaniasis acquired by contagion; a case of marital infection in Britain. *Lancet*, i, 127–130.

Tanada, Y. (1967). Epizootiology and microbial control. *In:* "Comparative Pathobiology. I: Biology of the Microsporidia" (L. A. Bulla and T. C. Cheng, eds), pp. 247–379. Plenum Press, New York.

Tikasingh, E. S. (1975). Observations on *Lutzomyia flaviscutellata* (Mangabeira) (Diptera: Psychodidae), a vector of enzootic leishmaniasis in Trinidad, West Indies. *Journal of Medical Entomology*, **12**, 228–232.

Trager, W. (1974a). Nutrition and biosynthetic capabilities of flagellates: problems of *in vitro* cultivation and differentiation. *In:* "Trypanosomiasis and Leishmaniasis with Special Reference to Chagas' Disease", pp. 225–254. Ciba Foundation Symposium 20 (new series), Associated Scientific Publishers, Amsterdam.

Trager, W. (1974b). Discussion. *In:* "Trypanosomiasis and Leishmaniasis with Special Reference to Chagas' Disease", p. 248. Ciba Foundation Symposium 20 (new series), Associated Scientific Publishers, Amsterdam.

Van Handel, E. (1972). The detection of nectar in mosquitoes. *Mosquito News*, **32**, 458.

Vickerman, K. (1965). The identity of *Leishmania chamaeleonis* Wenyon, 1921. *Transactions of the Royal Society of Tropical Medicine and Hygiene*, **59**, 372.

Vickerman, K. (1976). The diversity of kinetoplastid flagellates. *In:* "Biology of Kinetoplastida", Vol. I (W. H. R. Lumsden and D. A. Evans, eds), pp. 1–34. Academic Press, London.

Wallace, F. G. (1966). The trypanosomatid parasites of insects and arachnids. *Experimental Parasitology*, **18**, 124–193.

Wallace, F. G. (1977). Developmental stages of trypanosomatid flagellates: a new terminology revisited. *Protozoology*, **3**, 51–56.

Ward, R. A. and Savage, K. E. (1972). Effects of microsporidian parasites on anopheline mosquitoes and malarial infection. *Proceedings of the Helminthological Society of Washington*, **39**, 434–438.

Ward, R. D. (1974). Granule formation in the accessory glands of a laboratory strain of *Lu. longipalpis* (Diptera: Phlebotomidae) from Ceará State, Brazil. *Transactions of the Royal Society of Tropical Medicine and Hygiene*, **68**, 171.

Ward, R. D. (1977a). New World leishmaniasis: a review of the epidemiological changes in the last three decades. *Proceedings of the XV International Congress of Entomology, August, 1976, Washington*, pp. 505–522.

Ward, R. D. (1977b). The colonization of *Lutzomyia flaviscutellata* (Diptera: Psychodidae); a vector of *Leishmania mexicana amazonensis* in Brazil. *Journal of Medical Entomology*, **14**, 469–476.

Ward, R. D. and Fraiha, H. (1977). *Lutzomyia umbratilis*, a new species of sand fly from Brazil (Diptera: Psychodidae). *Journal of Medical Entomology*, **14**, 313–317.

Ward, R. D. and Killick-Kendrick, R. (1974). Field and laboratory observations on *Psychodopygus lainsoni* Fraiha and Ward and other sandflies (Diptera: Phlebotomidae) from the Transamazônica highway, Pará State, Brazil. *Bulletin of Entomological Research*, **64**, 213–221.

Ward, R. D., Lainson, R. and Shaw, J. J. (1973). Further evidence of the rôle of *Lutzomyia flaviscutellata* (Mangabeira) as the vector of *Leishmania mexicana amazonensis* in Brazil. *Transactions of the Royal Society of Tropical Medicine and Hygiene*, **67**, 608–609.

Ward, R. D., Lainson, R. and Shaw, J. J. (1977). Experimental transmission of *Leishmania mexicana amazonensis* Lainson and Shaw between hamsters by the bite of *Lutzomyia flaviscutellata* (Mangabeira). *Transactions of the Royal Society of Tropical Medicine and Hygiene*, **71**, 265–266.

Wenyon, C. M. (1926). "Protozoology", Vol. I. Baillière, Tindall and Cox, London.

Wenyon, C. M. (1932). The transmission of *Leishmania* infections. A review. *Transactions of the Royal Society of Tropical Medicine and Hygiene*, **25**, 319–351.

Williams, P. (1966). Experimental transmission of *Leishmania mexicana* by *Lutzomyia cruciata*. *Annals of Tropical Medicine and Parasitology*, **60**, 365–372.

Williams, P. (1970). Phlebotomine sandflies and leishmaniasis in British Honduras (Belize). *Transactions of the Royal Society of Tropical Medicine and Hygiene*, **64**, 317–364.

Williams, P. and Coelho, M. V. (1978). Taxonomy and transmission of *Leishmania*. *Advances in Parasitology*, **16**, 1–42.

Young, C. J., Turner, D. P., Killick-Kendrick, R., Rioux, J. A. and Leaney, A. J. Fructose in *Phlebotomus ariasi* (Diptera: Psychodidae). In Press.

Young, D. G. and Lewis, D. J. (1977). Pathogens of Psychodidae (phlebotomine sand flies). *Bulletin of the World Health Organization*, **55**, Suppl. 1, 9–24.

Yuan, I. C., Chu, H. J. and Ho, E. A. (1943). Transmission of leishmaniasis to the Chinese hamster (*Cricetulus griseus*) by feeding of infected Chinese sandflies (*Phlebotomus chinensis*). *Chinese Medical Journal*, **62**, 204–206.

9

Immunity to *Trypanosoma* (*Herpetosoma*) Infections in Rodents

G. A. T. TARGETT

Department of Medical Protozoology,
London School of Hygiene and Tropical Medicine,
London, England

P. VIENS

Departement de Microbiologie et Immunologie,
Université de Montréal, Montréal, Canada

I.	Introduction	462
II.	Course of infection	462
III.	Non-immunological factors which determine the pattern of infection	463
IV.	Nature of the immune response	464
	A. Thymus dependency of the immune response . . .	464
	B. Immunodepressive treatment	465
	C. Passive transfer of immunity with serum and cells . .	466
	D. Trypanocidal antibodies and serological responses to infection	467
	E. Ablastin	468
V.	Antigens, antigenic variation and the cell surface . . .	472
VI.	Immunization	473
VII.	Persistence of infection	474
VIII.	Comment	475
IX.	References	476

I. Introduction

Trypanosomes of the subgenus *Herpetosoma* occur primarily as parasites of rodents (Molyneux, 1976), the important exception being *Trypanosoma* (*Herpetosoma*) *rangeli* which has a wide range of vertebrate hosts including man (D'Alessandro, 1976). Most of the other species show a marked host specificity and, generally, the mammalian hosts have infections which are patent for only a few weeks. There is no obvious pathogenicity, and an effective immune response brings about resolution of the parasitaemia and a lasting resistance to homologous reinfections.

This pattern of infection is intriguing whatever aspect of the host–parasite relationship is considered. Transmission of the trypanosome, for example, is essential for the survival of the parasite, yet the immune response of the host appears to restrict the time during which this can occur to only a short period. There may, of course, be subtle aspects of these host–parasite associations that we do not appreciate at present which ensure that transmission will occur at other times, and certainly the associations between parasite and host are generally well-established and finely balanced. In this respect they may be compared with many of the trypanosomes of medical and economic importance which, though pathogenic when parasites of man and/or domestic livestock, are often non-pathogenic in their natural hosts (e.g. *T. brucei* in game animals). A study of immunological interactions of this type is therefore an important aspect of attempts to devise immunological methods of control of trypanosome infections. There are, in addition, many conditions of stress on the host that can occur naturally and impair the balanced state to such an extent that *Herpetosoma* infections prove fatal.

In this review we shall consider in detail only the most recent studies on these parasites, as D'Alesandro (1970) has given a comprehensive account of much of the early work. This means that we shall be concerned with only two species of the *Herpetosoma*, *T. (H.) lewisi* and *T. (H.) musculi*, since other species have received little attention from an immunological point of view.

II. Course of infection

T. lewisi and *T. musculi* are effectively restricted in terms of vertebrate hosts to rats (*Rattus spp.*) and mice (*Mus musculus*) respectively. Though variations in parasitaemias are seen with different strains of both parasites and hosts, there are nevertheless features common to the infections. Reproduction by the parasites is restricted largely to the first few days of the infection. Multiplication takes place in the kidneys (Ormerod, 1963; Wilson, 1971) and in the peripheral circulation (D'Alesandro, 1970;

Targett and Viens, 1975a) and produces a rapid rise in blood para-sitaemia. An ablastic response by the host then curtails the reproduction. In *T. lewisi* infections there is good evidence for production of a try-panocidal antibody at about the same time; with *T. musculi* this has yet to be shown conclusively. The effect on *T. lewisi* infections is commonly to produce a dramatic fall in parasite numbers followed by a low-grade but stable level of infection lasting usually a few weeks, perhaps several months. During this period, only non-reproducing or "adult" trypano-somes are seen. In *T. musculi* infections the crisis does not bring about a sharp drop in parasitaemia, and the stable or plateau phase of infection during which, again, only "adult" trypanosomes are seen in the blood, is of shorter duration (Viens *et al.*, 1974a). With both species there is almost always a second immunological crisis which removes the trypanosomes from the blood (Targett and Viens, 1975b; D'Alesandro, 1970) and leaves the host aparasitaemic and immune to homologous challenge. Corradetti (1963) described the immunity of the rat to *T. lewisi* as com-plete and sterile but we have shown that small numbers of *T. musculi* parasites persist in the vasa recta of the kidneys of infected mice long after they have become aparasitaemic (Viens *et al.*, 1972; Targett and Viens, 1975a). However, we failed to show anything comparable in rats which had recovered from *T. lewisi* (Wilson *et al.*, 1973).

III. Non-immunological factors which determine the pattern of infection

It is difficult to separate the immunological and non-immunological determinants of infection because they are so closely related. As a simple illustration, the greater susceptibility of young rats to *T. lewisi*—to the point where many die while older animals always survive—is in part a measure of the immunological competence of the host. The same may be true with elevated parasitaemias brought about by dietary deficiencies (see D'Alesandro, 1970).

One interesting example of a greatly increased susceptibility to infec-tion is that occurring in pregnant mice infected with *T. musculi* (Kram-pitz, 1975). When exposed to infection 4–14 days post-conception, mice develop overwhelming parasitaemias with multiplication of the parasite occurring in the peripheral blood and the maternal circulation of the placenta. Infection may kill the host and will certainly produce abortion. The apparently uncontrolled development of the parasites is related to the presence of a developing placenta. It does not occur in mice infected before they become pregnant, during the last week of pregnancy or when lactating. Nor does the pregnancy induce relapses or apparently alter an established immunity. Krampitz (1975) suggests that the pregnant host may not produce or tolerate host responses which inhibit cell reproduction. Shaw and Dusanic (1973) showed that *T. lewisi* also develops preferentially in the placenta of a pregnant rat and there is some elevation of the blood parasitaemia, though it is not as marked or as sustained as with *T. musculi* in the mice.

Most of the trypanosomes of this subgenus show a marked host specificity and most studies, early and recent, indicate that development in a heterologous host is prevented because of the absence of some necessary factor and not because of immunological incompatibility. Thus, Lincicome and Francis (1961) found that *T. lewisi* would develop in mice providing these were given a daily supplement of rat serum. The parasite did not become adapted to the mouse, even after numerous passages, so there was clearly an essential element in the supplement. Greenblatt and others (see Greenblatt, 1975) have attempted to identify this factor, and Greenblatt (1975) speculates that it might be transferrin or haemopexin; he concludes also that the factor has a nutritional rather than an immunodepressive role. *T. musculi* will not normally develop in the rat, but, curiously, rat peritoneal cells were shown to promote and sustain growth of the mouse parasite *in vitro* (Viens *et al.*, 1977). Recent studies (Dwyer and D'Alesandro, 1976b) have shown that the surface coat of *T. musculi* is composed in large part of mouse serum proteins, especially IgG, and it is suggested that they serve to stabilize the parasite pellicular membrane. Trypanosomes in which the surface coat had been removed by trypsin treatment rapidly readsorbed mouse serum proteins on to the surface membrane, but they would also take up serum proteins from a variety of heterologous hosts. This implies a non-specific adsorbance without, in the case of *T. musculi*, specific receptors for mouse serum proteins. Dwyer and D'Alesandro (1976b) suggest, however, that, while heterologous proteins bind avidly to the pellicular membrane of the trypanosome, they do not have the membrane-stabilizing properties of the homologous proteins.

IV. Nature of the immune response

The non-pathogenic nature of infections in rats and mice is partly a consequence of the immune response, and the typical course of infection already described indicates that this is a complex process involving several stages.

A. THYMUS DEPENDENCY OF THE IMMUNE RESPONSE

T. musculi infections in T-lymphocyte-deprived CBA mice are initially the same as infections in intact animals, with a phase of rapidly increasing parasitaemia followed by an abrupt change to give rise to the plateau or stable phase of the parasitaemia. In intact mice this lasts about 10 days before the second crisis leaves the mouse aparasitaemic; in deprived mice the parasitaemia either remains relatively constant or increases slowly until the mouse dies, which is almost invariably the outcome of the infection. The time after inoculation when death occurs varies from about 40 days to more than one year (Viens *et al.*, 1974a; Targett and Viens, 1975a). Multiplicative forms of the parasite persist throughout the infection indicating that there is no ablastic response, yet there is clearly some regulatory mechanism operating on the trypanosomes in the T-cell-deprived mice, though it is not wholly effective.

Treatment of mice with antithymocyte serus (ATS) one day before and one, three and five days after inoculation with *T. musculi* produced an infection which was like that in T-cell-deprived mice although recovery occurred after a period of about 70 days (Viens *et al.*, 1974a). Spira and Greenblatt (1970) found that treatment of rats with ATS produced severe, often fatal, infections with *T. lewisi*, and Tawil and Dusanic (1971) showed that ALS treatment started 3 days before infection lead to death from the infection. They showed later (see Dusanic, 1975a) that if ALS treatment was begun after inoculation of parasites, even only 2 days later, the resulting parasitaemia was normal. In both series of experiments it was shown that the immunodepressive effects of ATS or ALS treatment were due in part to suppression of the ablastic response.

All the above results indicate that initiation of immune responses to *T. musculi* and *T. lewisi* is thymus dependent. In contrast, Hanson and Chapman (1974) could show no effect of neonatal thymectomy on *T. lewisi* infections.

B. IMMUNODEPRESSIVE TREATMENT

Very many immunodepressive procedures have been employed in animals infected with *T. lewisi* and it is worthwhile considering some of these briefly in relation to the mechanisms of immunity that are affected.

Splenectomy has a multiplicity of effects, and many early experiments were complicated by intercurrent infections (D'Alesandro, 1970). Thus, while there was some evidence that removal of the spleen produced increased parasitaemias in *T. musculi* infections and impairment of the ablastic response to both *T. musculi* and *T. lewisi*, the effect of splenectomy on uncomplicated *T. lewisi* in rats seemed on the whole to be slight (Dusanic, 1975a). Irradiation procedures similarly have many effects but give rise to elevated parasitaemias through suppression of trypanocidal and ablastic effects.

El-On and Greenblatt (1971) treated rats with cyclophosphamide shortly after inoculation with *T. lewisi* and at a time when its effect might be expected to be largely on B-lymphocytes. The treated group showed higher parasitaemias, increased mortality, a prolongation of the period of reproductive activity and a decrease in levels of IgG.

Taliaferro and D'Alesandro (1971) attempted to suppress antibody and in particular the reproduction-inhibiting responses by treatment with adenine which interferes with DNA synthesis. They produced some prolongation and some enhancement of reproductive activity.

The effect of corticosteroid treatment on infection was somewhat like that of ALS. Herbert and Becker (1961) found that it had no effect on parasitaemias in *T. lewisi*-infected rats but Sherman and Ruble (1967), by increasing individual doses and starting treatment 2 days before infection, produced much more severe infections. Patton and Clarke (1968) produced a similar effect with dexamethasone when treatment was begun 3 days before inoculation.

C. PASSIVE TRANSFER OF IMMUNITY WITH SERUM AND CELLS

Experiments involving passive transfer of serum carried out by Taliaferro and co-workers and by Coventry (see Taliaferro, 1924; Coventry, 1925; D'Alesandro, 1970) established humoral aspects of the immune response of rats to *T. lewisi* which are still widely accepted. We shall be discussing the nature of these humoral factors and the kinetics of their production later, but essentially it was shown that serum taken after the first crisis was trypanocidal for dividing parasites but not for adult forms whereas serum collected after the second crisis was trypanocidal for all stages of the parasite. Independently, a reproduction-inhibiting factor became demonstrable following infection, with a titre which was maximal immediately after the first crisis but declined thereafter. Taliaferro (1938) also showed that serum from mice which had recovered from *T. musculi* was trypanocidal and also inhibited reproduction. Patton (1972a) found that dexamethasone-treated rats could be protected against *T. lewisi* by immune cells and immune serum and also by non-immune cells and immune serum, indicating the essential aspect of the humoral factors. He also protected untreated rats with cells and serum from immune animals.

Serum and cells have been tested for their effects on *T. musculi* infections in mice by introduction before infection, during the reproductive stages of the parasitaemia and during the plateau phase. Serum from immune animals given prior to infection prolonged the pre-patent period and markedly reduced the parasitaemias (Viens et al., 1974a). Serum collected after the first crisis of infection was passively transferred to other mice in the early stages of patency; the effect was greatly to reduce the number of multiplicative forms in the blood and to inhibit DNA synthesis, with a consequent check on the parasitaemia, which never reached normal peak levels. Serum from animals which had recovered from infection had similar though slightly less marked effects. Interestingly, serum from T-cell-deprived infected mice had little effect on the numbers of circulating dividing forms but inhibited the development of the total parasitaemia for a while, i.e., the serum showed some trypanocidal but no ablastic activity (see below). The same experiments were performed with infected T-cell-deprived mice as recipients and there were clear inhibiting effects on multiplication of the parasite and hence on parasitaemia, but this lasted for only about 6 days (Viens *et al.*, 1974a).

In attempts to accelerate the rate of clearance of parasites from the infected host, serum and cells were passively inoculated during the plateau phase of infection. Perhaps not surprisingly because of the excess of antigen present, immune serum alone did not modify the pattern of infection (Viens *et al.*, 1974b). When immune or normal serum was inoculated at the same time as either adherent or non-adherent cells from mouse spleen or from the peritoneal cavity, the results were very clear. Infections were terminated most rapidly whenever non-adherent cells from immune hosts were inoculated (Targett and Viens, 1975b; Viens *et al.*, 1974b).

Further experiments involved adoptive transfer of immune spleen cells at the onset of *T. musculi* infections in T-cell-deprived mice. Unfractionated spleen cell populations had a strong protective effect and this was not reduced if the cells were treated with anti-θ antiserum *in vitro* prior to inoculation (Pouliot *et al.*, 1977). Thus, while the initiation of the immune response is clearly T-cell dependent (see above), its maintenance seems not to be so.

D. TRYPANOCIDAL ANTIBODIES AND SEROLOGICAL RESPONSES TO INFECTION

With the demonstration by passive-transfer experiments that the antibody responses at the first and second crises during *T. lewisi* infections are distinct from one another, the nature of the antibodies involved has been investigated. At both points in the infection, agglutinating activity *in vitro*, which correlates well with protective activity, has been demonstrated (Yasuda and Dusanic, 1969; D'Alesandro, 1970). D'Alesandro (1959) had produced supporting evidence for earlier observations that the first trypanocidal antibody was IgG, and the second IgM. In a later study he has confirmed this by showing that the agglutinin response to reproducing forms (the first trypanocidal antibody) is confined to the IgG fraction while the second agglutinating response is IgM (D'Alesandro, 1976). Before considering further any mechanisms other than agglutination which might be involved in the trypanocidal effects, it is worthwhile making some comparisons with the response of mice to *T. musculi*. Viens *et al.* (1974a) determined monospecific anti-*T. musculi* fluorescent antibody titres in infected T-cell-deprived and intact mice. In intact mice, IgG_1, IgG_2 and IgM antibodies appeared simultaneously following infection. The IgM quickly reached a plateau which was maintained for a long period. In infected deprived mice, total immunoglobulin and IgG_2 levels were lower than those of controls, and production of IgG_1 was suppressed for 35 days and reached only low levels thereafter. IgM antibody titres, on the other hand, were similar to those of the intact animals. This observation, combined with the parasitaemias seen in T-cell-deprived mice and the results of passive transfer experiments, lead Viens *et al.* (1975) to propose that the first trypanocidal antibody is IgM and is still produced in T-cell-deprived mice. This is a point of contrast with *T. lewisi* infections where the first crisis antibody is IgG. Viens *et al.* (1975) also failed to show any agglutinating activity in antisera from *T. musculi*-infected mice under conditions in which this was readily demonstrable with *T. lewisi* and rat sera. It seemed probable therefore that the trypanocidal effects here were mediated by some other mechanism.

D'Alesandro (1970) discusses evidence of several trypanocidal mechanisms operating in *T. lewisi* infections. Observations on actively and passively immunized hosts indicate an important role for phagocytic cells with assumed opsonic activity in the serum (Patton, 1972a). Taliaferro (1938) also demonstrated lysis of trypanosomes, especially with hyperimmune serum, and it seems likely that agglutination, opsonization and phagocytosis, and lysis may all occur as elements of the response *in vivo*. Precipitins to trypanosome extracts have also been demonstrated (D'Alesandro, 1972).

The sera from *T. musculi*-infected mice which failed to show any agglutinating activity nevertheless had a marked neutralizing effect on the parasites after *in vitro* incubation. Though the infectivity of the parasite stabilates was greatly reduced, the numbers of motile trypanosomes was the same at the end of the period of incubation in immune serum as at the beginning (Viens *et al.*, 1975). Dusanic (1975b) has shown, too, that *T. musculi* parasitaemias in complement-deficient mice are the same as those in mice with complete complement systems, implying that complement-dependent antibody-mediated lysis is not responsible for terminal elimination of the parasites.

E. ABLASTIN

1. Nature of the ablastic response

This has been referred to several times already, but since this aspect of the *Herpetosoma* infections has provoked more interest than any other it should be examined in some detail. What has been proposed, and supported for a long time, is that an antibody (ablastin) is produced during the course of infection which inhibits the reproduction activity of the trypanosomes without otherwise harming them (D'Alesandro, 1975).

2. Evidence for ablastic activity

Early studies on morphological changes (Taliaferro, 1932) and on protein and nucleic acid synthesis *in vivo* (Pizzi and Taliaferro, 1960; Taliaferro and Pizzi, 1960) have indicated that a factor is produced during infection which stops synthesis and division by the trypanosomes; more recent *in vitro* studies with *T. lewisi* (Patton, 1972b) and *T. musculi* (Trudel and Viens, unpublished observations) on the uptake of ³H-thymidine have supported this conclusion. Patton (1975) has also shown by *in vivo* labelling with ³H-thymidine that the shortest generation or doubling time for *T. lewisi* is 8 h. This occurred on day 3 of an infection, whereas, by day 5, the doubling time had become 24 h, in intact rats, and 12 h in rats treated with dexamethasone. Still further evidence came from autoradiographic experiments in which reproducing organisms which had been labelled with ³H-thymidine were placed in medium containing normal serum or ablastic serum. The latter greatly increased the time required to half the mean grain count, indicating that cell synthesis had been very much reduced.

There are some who have expressed doubts about the ablastin concept. Ormerod (1963) had suggested that production of trypanocidal antibodies directed against the juvenile and the adult forms could explain the phenomenon of inhibition of multiplication adequately, though he now concedes (Ormerod, 1975) that much recent evidence favours the existence of an inhibiting substance. Greenblatt and co-workers (see Greenblatt, 1975) were puzzled by the apparent inability to show ablastic activity with sera taken around the 5th day of patency, when it would be expected. This has been to a large extent answered by D'Alesandro (1975) who has shown that such activity is demonstrable *in vitro* from about the 4th day of infection. Greenblatt *et al.* (Greenblatt and Tyroler, 1971; Greenblatt, 1973; 1975) have also looked for other explanations of the fact that the trypanosome population in the blood became adult and non-dividing, and they have evidence of sequestration of parasites within the spleen with, perhaps, selection for dividing forms. This certainly deserves further study. Lajeunesse *et al.* (1975) also made an observation which bears on the evidence for ablastic activity. They found that, during experimentally induced infections, numerous trypanosomes remained and divided within the peritoneal cavity. The striking feature was that dividing forms persisted throughout the course of infection, i.e. long after they had disappeared from the blood. We shall come back to this point.

3. Ablastin and the immune response

Some direct and much indirect evidence indicates that ablastin has the characteristics of an antibody. D'Alesandro (1970) summarizes the early crude fractionation studies and discusses one of the properties which had caused so much doubt about the antibody nature of the substance, its apparent low avidity and consequent non-absorbability. Recent ultracentrifugation and gel filtration studies indicate however that it is an IgG antibody (Dusanic, 1975a). The antibody nature of ablastin is inferred, too, from immunosuppressive treatments in which the trypanocidal and reproduction-inhibiting effects can also be separated (Dusanic, 1975a). In addition, P. A. D'Alesandro and A. D. Clarkson, Jr. (personal communication) have now demonstrated that ablastin can be absorbed from serum or plasma. They found that *T. lewisi* trypanosomes used in previous absorption experiments already had ablastin bound to their surface coats at the time they were isolated from donor rats and could not therefore absorb more ablastin *in vitro*. On the other hand, trypanosomes isolated from hydrocortisone-treated rats did not have specific surface receptors blocked because ablastin production was suppressed as a result of the treatment. These trypanosomes would readily absorb-out ablastic activity *in vitro*.

In T-cell-deprived mice infected with *T. musculi* the ability to produce ablastin was shown to be impaired (Viens *et al.*, 1974a; Targett and Viens, 1975a), and, from further studies on the specific immunoglobulin changes occurring during infection, it was proposed that ablastin is an IgG$_1$ antibody (Viens *et al.*, 1974, 1975).

The presumptive evidence of its antibody nature is therefore strong and treatment with suitable antisera and enzymes—standard techniques for revealing antibody structure—should give conclusive proof (D'Alesandro, 1975).

4. The origin and localization of ablastinogen

One of the most intriguing aspects of the ablastin response is the nature of the stimulus which initiates its production, and the subsequent mode of action. Bawden (1975) has summarized what we know so far of the properties of the ablastinogen. He has some evidence that the antigen has protein components and suggests that it is a part of the plasma membrane of the trypanosome. D'Alesandro (1972) had shown that, though antigens (called exoantigens) were detectable in the plasma of rats during the course of an untreated *T. lewisi* infection, these did not include the ablastinogen, or indeed the antigens which stimulate the trypanocidal antibodies. Bawden (1974) was able to find ablastinogen in the plasma of infected rats that had been immunosuppressed by treatment with hydrocortisone and he suggests (Bawden, 1975) that this was because ablastinogen is located in filaments which are shed by the trypanosomes "as a normal course of events"; in immunocompetent rats these would be removed rapidly by phagocytic cells but in immunosuppressed animals they would not. *T. lewisi* is compared closely with *T. brucei* where release of filaments has been studied in more detail, but it is important to remember that even here there is still considerable doubt about the natural *in vivo* shedding of filaments which are so easily demonstrable *in vitro* (but see Ellis *et al.*, 1976).

Ablastinogen is present both in the juvenile (dividing) and the adult (non-reproducing) forms of the parasite, in the first case acting as the antigenic stumulus for ablastin production, but in the second presumably bound and neutralized by the ablastin.

5. Mode of action of ablastin

Nothing to compare with production of ablastin and the consequent inhibition of reproduction has so far been demonstrated with trypanosomes other than species of *Herpetosoma*. This implies a uniqueness about it, but both Ormerod (1975) and Patton (1975) suggest that there may not be anything unusual in the production of an inhibitor of reproduction but that the response to these inhibitors determines whether infections are pathogenic or non-pathogenic. We shall consider shortly how this relates to antigenic change by the parasite.

The presence of ablastin in the ambient seems to be essential to maintain the trypanosomes in a non-reproducing state; if the adult *T. lewisi* are transferred to a new host they begin reproducing at once. We have seen that the antigen which stimulates its production is thought to be located in the plasma membrane of the parasite (Bawden, 1975), and Patton (1975) has good evidence that it is inhibition of membrane function which is responsible for the check on reproduction. There are, of course, many metabolic changes associated with reproduction inhibition, notably the marked depression of protein and nucleic acid synthesis, but most of these are a sequel to the effect of ablastin. Patton (1975) showed that glucose uptake as a function of substrate concentration revealed comparable values for reproducing and ablastin-inhibited *T. lewisi*, i.e. their affinity for the substrate was similar, but there was evidence of a reduction in the number of transport sites in the inhibited trypanosomes. An effect on active transport was also indicated when addition of ablastic serum inhibited the outward flow of 2-deoxy-D-glucose from the trypanosome in the presence of glucose. Uptake of labelled thymidine was restricted too in ablastin-inhibited trypanosomes. In a series of elegant experiments Patton (1972b) found that a known transport inhibitor, ouabain, had an ablastic effect on *T. lewisi*. Ouabain acts, through Na^+ and K^+ stimulation, on ATPase, and Patton showed similar modes of action of the inhibitor and of ablastic serum from infected rats (Patton, 1975). He proposed that ablastin (IgG) causes direct inhibition of translocation of carbohydrates, of thymidine, and possibly of other substrates into *T. lewisi* and therefore arrests reproduction. Such a process is readily reversible.

A few observations are not easily explained in terms of inhibition by antibody alone. The persistence of a high rate of reproduction of *T. musculi* in the peritoneal cavity of mice at a time when multiplication in the blood has ceased and the ablastin titre is high has been mentioned already and is difficult to explain if the effect is due to an IgG antibody alone since this is likely to be present in the peritoneal fluid (Lajeunesse *et al.*, 1975). Similarly, the persistence for many months of dividing forms of *T. musculi* in the kidneys of mice (see below) occurs though the plasma contains ablastin (and trypanocidal antibody). D'Alesandro (1975) suggests that these populations should be tested for antibody resistance.

V. Antigens, antigenic variation and the cell surface

Surprisingly little is known of the antigens of the parasite which provoke the different phases of the immune response. Bawden (1975) recognized three antigenic compartments: (a) intracellular antigens, which consist primarily of antigens restricted to the cytoplasm and cell organelles and hence probably unimportant as stimulators of antibody; (b) plasma membrane antigens, found in the cell membrane and in the surface coat; and (c) extracellular antigens.

The ablastic effect produces at least two distinct populations of trypanosomes, one dividing and one non-dividing or adult, and antigenic analyses by Entner and Gonzales (1966) and Entner (1968) demonstrated changes in antigenicity of *T. lewisi* during the course of infection. They used freeze-thawed whole organisms as their source of antigen so it is not possible to say to which of the antigen compartments each antigen belongs. However, they showed three antigenically distinct stages of *T. lewisi*, the first two being part of the reproducing population while the third was associated with trypanosomes seen after reproduction has ceased. If one assumes that the antigens specific to each population are expressed by the living trypanosome, this fits well with the proposal that trypanocidal antibodies specific to dividing and adult forms are produced.

We see therefore evidence of antigenic variation, but of very limited duration (occurring only once or twice), the limiting factor being production of ablastin which inhibits any further multiplication. However, as Ormerod (1975) points out, the conversion factor for change from one antigenic type to another is an antibody, as it is with those trypanosomes (e.g., *Trypanozoon*, *Nannomonas*) which show continuous antigenic variation. D'Alesandro (1976) showed one probable difference between the

Herpetosoma and the salivarian trypanosomes. He demonstrated that agglutinins specific to reproducing and adult *T. lewisi*, respectively, were produced, but, most interestingly, he showed too that the reproducing variant had a surface agglutinogen which would react with and absorb agglutinins produced against the adult variant. However, this antigen on the reproducing variant does not appear to be immunogenic *in vivo*. The failure to demonstrate agglutinating activity in the serum of *T. musculi*-infected or immune mice by either direct or indirect means was also unexpected (Viens *et al.*, 1975), and, on available evidence, indicates a marked difference in surface antigen properties between *T. lewisi* and *T. musculi*.

The cell surface is presumably the location for most immunogens, though extracellular antigens may subserve an important role in stimulation of immune responses. Some detailed studies on the cell surface have recently been made with both *T. lewisi* and *T. musculi* though, as yet, there has been no attempt to try to relate chemical constitution to immunological function. Both species have a surface coat composed of a rather irregular fibrillar matrix, and studies on agglutination with polycationic dye compounds (Dwyer, 1975; Dwyer and D'Alesandro, 1976a) and with lectins (Dwyer, 1976; Dwyer and D'Alesandro, 1976b) showed the random distribution in the surface coat and in the pellicular and flagellar membranes of complex polyanionic carbohydrates similar or identical to α-D-mannose, N-acetylgalactosamine, N-acetylglucosamine and α-L-fucose. They were also present in the membranes of culture forms of *T. lewisi*. As mentioned earlier (p. 464) the surface coat is also composed in part of adsorbed host serum proteins (Dwyer and D'Alesandro, 1976b). There is clearly much of interest to be learned in trying to relate surface structure of these trypanosomes, adsorption of host serum proteins, production and expression of antigens, and the ablastic, serologic and protective immune responses of the host.

VI. Immunization

A strong immunity to homologous challenge has been produced by immunization with *T. lewisi* and *T. musculi* parasites which have been killed or attenuated (see D'Alesandro, 1970; Viens *et al.*, 1975). None of these studies has, however, involved attempts to characterize important antigens; the closest to this has been the very effective immunity to *T. lewisi* produced by immunization with "metabolic products" from the supernatant of cultures of bloodstream forms of the parasite in rat serum–saline mixtures (Thillet and Chandler, 1957). Irradiated vaccines, in which the parasites retain their motility (and their ability to divide *in vitro*) but are non-infective, were also very effective (Sanders and Wallace, 1966).

Cross-immunity tests have been few, but inoculation of live *T. lewisi* into mice produces partial resistance to subsequent challenge with *T. musculi* (Mühlpfordt, 1971; Dusanic, 1975a). However, attempts to modify infections with pathogenic trypanosomes by prior exposure of mice to *T. musculi* were unsuccessful (Viens *et al.*, 1975). Also, while the cross resistance between *T. lewisi* and *T. musculi* might indicate a degree of antigenic similarity, we should note the results of cross-immunity studies with unrelated parasites. On the one hand Cox (1975) showed that concurrent malaria infections can enhance *T. musculi* parasitaemias sometimes to fatal levels, presumably through immunodepression, but Meerovitch and Ackerman (1974) found that a pre-existing *Trichinella spiralis* infection greatly reduced a *T. lewisi* infection in rats even though, under other circumstances, *T. spiralis* has also been shown to be immunodepressive.

VII. Persistence of infection

Recovery from infection with *T. lewisi* or *T. musculi* leaves the host immune to homologous challenge, yet, in mice, a small population of *T. musculi* parasites remains in the immune host for many months, perhaps in some cases for life. So far they have been found only in the kidneys, more specifically in the vasa recta (Viens *et al.*, 1972) though there is nothing as yet to indicate whether this site is of special significance. However, an extensive search has failed to reveal parasites in other parts of the body. The kidney populations which have been found after infection of several strains of mice (outbred and inbred) pose interesting questions. What is their biological significance, assuming that they occur in natural infections? How do they survive in an immune host which can deal very effectively with a challenge infection (Viens *et al.*, 1975)? Are they in fact essential for the maintenance of the strong immunity?

The parasites are demonstrable by direct examination of kidney tissue, in histological sections and by inoculation of macerated kidney tissue into uninfected animals. We have made many attempts to release the parasites from the kidneys by immunosuppression of the host. The methods used have included secondary T-cell deprivation, X-irradiation and treatment with ATS and cyclophosphamide, all without success (Targett and Viens, unpublished results).

Viens *et al.* (1975) discuss some of the ways in which the trypanosomes might survive as an actively dividing population in what is apparently an immunologically hostile environment. The site in which they occur may first preclude an effective immune response, especially if it requires cell-to-cell contact. Even purely humoral responses may not function equally effectively in all parts of the circulatory system; the ionic composition of the plasma in the kidney might, as one example, be sufficiently different from that of the peripheral circulation to influence immunological reactions. Alternatively, changes in the parasite might ensure its survival. D'Alesandro (1975) suggested one possible change, a resistance by these parasites to ablastin and to trypanocidal antibodies. Antigenic variation, shown to be effective for survival of some species of malaria in an immune host (see Brown, 1976), might also occur, though our attempts to demonstrate antigenic differences between kidney and blood populations have not so far been successful.

As for their biological significance, it is possible that they serve to maintain the immunity at a high level through continuous release of small numbers of trypanosomes into the peripheral circulation. Other possibilities that we have suggested (Viens *et al.*, 1975) are that they release forms infective only to the flea vector or that they may effect oral transmission of infection through cannibalism by mice.

There are two points to be remembered in relation to these parasites. The first is that the kidney stages are probably an integral part of the life cycle and not an aberrant offshoot. Development in the kidneys occurs during the acute phase of infections with both *T. musculi* and *T. lewisi* (Ormerod, 1963), and, as D'Alesandro (1975) has noted, reproductive tissue stages are an integral part of the life cycle of many Stercoraria. This does not of course explain how these small numbers of parasites continue to survive and multiply within the immune host, but the second point to be remembered is that these are long-established host–parasite relationships in which the immune response is most likely to be as essential for survival of the parasite as for ridding the host of its invader.

VIII. Comment

Progress towards the development of vaccines which might be effective in preventing the diseases of man or livestock caused by salivarian trypanosomes is slow; in some cases the prospects for success seem remote. Yet, as we said at the beginning, these same organisms rarely if ever kill their natural hosts and there is little pathology associated with these infections. Infections with *Herpetosoma* species present in a broadly similar way and, although the basic elements of the humoral responses in these infections have been known for some time, we are only just beginning to understand those cellular events which necessarily precede and those which, almost certainly, are required to complement the antibody response. We are beginning to show something of the nature of an immune response which is an integral part of the host–parasite relationship, and this should serve to guide our attempts to modify the immune response in those infections (caused mainly by salivarian trypanosomes) where it not only fails to dictate the outcome of the infection, but often contributes to the imbalance which we recognize as pathogenesis and pathology, and which too often leads to death of the host. In this respect there are many fertile areas for comparative study. There is, for example, a need for detailed studies on histopathological changes during the course of the non-pathogenic infections for comparison with those occurring during trypanosome infections which are pathogenic. Allied to this is the effect of infection on the ability of the host to make other immunological responses. This has been examined in some detail with salivarian trypanosomes (Hudson et al., 1976), but the generalized immunodepressive effects of *Herpetosoma* infections are less well known (Albright et al., 1977).

The key to control of these infections is the ablastic response which regulates multiplication by the parasite. Alongside our attempts to develop vaccines for trypanosomes which prevent totally the development of the pathogen, we should perhaps try to induce artificially something like the controlled mutliplication that is the determining factor in infections with *T. lewisi, T. musculi* and related trypanosomes.

IX. References

Albright, J. F., Albright, J. W. and Dusanic, D. G. (1977). Trypanosome induced splenomegaly and suppression of mouse spleen cell responses to antigens and mitogens. *Journal of the Reticuloendothelial Society*, **21**, 21–31.

Bawden, M. P. (1974). *Trypanosoma lewisi*: characteristics of an antigen which induces ablastic antibody. *Experimental Parasitology*, **36**, 397–404.

Bawden, M. P. (1975). Whence comes *Trypanosoma lewisi* antigen which induces ablastic antibody: studies in the occult? *Experimental Parasitology*, **38**, 350–356.

Brown, K. N. (1976). Resistance to malaria. *In*: "Immunology of Parasitic Infections" (S. Cohen and E. H. Sadun, eds), pp. 268–295. Blackwell, Oxford.

Corradetti, A. (1963). Acquired sterile immunity in experimental protozoal infections. *In*: "Immunity to Protozoa" (P. C. C. Garnham, A. C. Pierce and I. Roitt, eds), pp. 69–77. Blackwell, Oxford.

Coventry, F. A. (1925). The reaction product which inhibits reproduction of the trypanosomes in infections with *Trypanosoma lewisi*, with special reference to its changes in titer through the course of the infection. *American Journal of Hygiene*, **5**, 127–144.

Cox, F. E. G. (1975). Enhanced *Trypanosoma musculi* infections in mice with concomitant malaria. *Nature, London*, **258**, 148–149.

D'Alesandro, P. A. (1959). Electrophoretic and ultracentrifugal studies of antibodies to *Trypanosoma lewisi*. *Journal of Infectious Diseases*, **105**, 76–95.

D'Alesandro, P. A. (1970). Nonpathogenic trypanosomes of rodents. *In*: "Immunity to Parasitic Animals", Vol. 2 (G. J. Jackson, R. Herman and I. Singer, eds), pp. 691–738. Appleton-Century-Crofts, New York.

D'Alesandro, P. A. (1972). *Trypanosoma lewisi*: production of exoantigens during infection in the rat. *Experimental Parasitology*, **32**, 149–164.

D'Alesandro, P. A. (1975). Ablastin: The phenomenon. *Experimental Parasitology*, **38**, 303–308.

D'Alesandro, P. A. (1976). The relation of agglutinins to antigenic variation of *Trypanosoma lewisi*. *Journal of Protozoology*, **23**, 256–261.

D'Alessandro, A. (1976). Biology of *Trypanosoma (Herpetosoma) rangeli* Tejera,

1920. *In:* "Biology of the Kinetoplastida", Vol. 1 (W. H. R. Lumsden and D. A. Evans, eds), pp. 327–403. Academic Press, London and New York.

Dusanic, D. G. (1975a). Immunosuppresion and ablastin. *Experimental Parasitology*, **38**, 322–337.

Dusanic, D. G. (1975b). *Trypanosoma musculi* infections in complement deficient mice. *Experimental Parasitology*, **37**, 205–210.

Dwyer, D. M. (1975). Cell surface saccharides of *Trypanosoma lewisi*. I. Polycation-induced cell agglutination and fine structure cytochemistry. *Journal of Cell Science*, **19**, 621–644.

Dwyer, D. M. (1976). Cell surface saccharides of *Trypanosoma lewisi*. II. Lectin-mediated agglutination and fine-structure cytochemical detection of lectin-binding sites. *Journal of Cell Science*, **22**, 1–19.

Dwyer, D. M. and D'Alesandro, P. A. (1976a). The cell surface of *Trypanosoma musculi* bloodstream forms. I. Fine structure and cytochemistry. *Journal of Protozoology*, **23**, 75–83.

Dwyer, D. M. and D'Alesandro, P. A. (1976b). The cell surface of *Trypanosoma musculi* bloodstream forms. II. Lectin and immunologic studies. *Journal of Protozoology*, **23**, 262–271.

Ellis, D. S., Ormerod, W. E. and Lumsden, W. H. R. (1976). Filaments of *Trypanosoma brucei*: some notes on differences in origin and structure in two strains of *Trypanosoma* (*Trypanozoon*) *brucei rhodesiense*. *Acta Tropica*, **33**, 151–168.

El-On, J. and Greenblatt, C. L. (1971). The effects of the immuno-suppressive agent cyclophosphamide on IgG levels and parasite number on experimental trypanosomiasis. *Israel Journal of Medical Science*, **7**, 1294–1298.

Entner, N. (1968). Further studies on antigenic changes in *Trypanosoma lewisi*. *Journal of Protozoology*, **15**, 638–640.

Entner, N. and Gonzales, C. (1966). Changes in antigenicity of *Trypanosoma lewisi* during the course of infection in rats. *Journal of Protozoology*, **13**, 642–645.

Greenblatt, C. L. (1973). *Trypanosoma lewisi*: electron microscopy of the infected spleen. *Experimental Parasitology*, **34**, 197–210.

Greenblatt, C. L. (1975). Nutritional and immunological factors in the control of infections with *Trypanosoma lewisi*. *Experimental Parasitology*, **38**, 342–349.

Greenblatt, C. L. and Tyroler, E. (1971). *Trypanosoma lewisi*: *in vitro* behaviour of rat spleen cells. *Experimental Parasitology*, **30**, 363–374.

Hanson, W. L. and Chapman, W. L. Jr. (1974). Comparison of the effects of neonatal thymectomy on *Plasmodium berghei*, *Trypanosoma lewisi* and *Trypanosoma cruzi* infections in the albino rat. *Zeitschrift für Parasitenkunde*, **44**, 227–238.

Herbert, I. V. and Becker, E. R. (1961). Effect of cortisone and x-irradiation on the course of *Trypanosoma lewisi* infection in the rat. *Journal of Parasitology*, **47**, 304–308.

Hudson, K. M., Byner, C., Freeman, J. and Terry, R. J. (1976). Immunodepression, high IgM levels and evasion of the immune response in murine trypanosomiasis. *Nature, London*, **264**, 256–258.

Krampitz, H. E. (1975). Ablastin: antigen tolerance and lack of ablastin control of *Trypanosoma musculi* during host's pregnancy. *Experimental Parasitology*, **38**, 317–321.

Lajeunesse, M. C., Richards, R., Viens, P. and Targett, G. A. T. (1975). Persistence of dividing forms of *Trypanosoma musculi* in the peritoneal cavity of infected CBA mice. *IRCS Medical Science*, **3**, 244.

Lincicome, D. R. and Francis, E. H. (1961). Quantitative studies on heterologous sera inducing development of *Trypanosoma lewisi* in mice. *Experimental Parasitology*, **11**, 68–76.

Meerovitch, E. and Ackerman, S. J. (1974). Trypanosomiasis in rats with trichinosis. *Transactions of the Royal Society of Tropical Medicine and Hygiene*, **68**, 417.

Molyneux, D. H. (1976). Biology of trypanosomes of the subgenus *Herpetosoma*. *In:* "Biology of the Kinetoplastida", Vol. 1 (W. H. R. Lumsden and D. A. Evans, eds), pp. 285–325. Academic Press, London and New York.

Mühlpfordt, H. (1971). Reaktion der maus auf serum behandlung und *Trypanosoma lewisi* infektion. *Zeitschrift für Tropenmedizin und Parasitologie*, **22**, 203–212.

Ormerod, W. E. (1963). The initial stages of infection with *Trypanosoma lewisi*: control of parasitaemia by the host. *In:* "Immunity to Protozoa" (P. C. C. Garnham, A. C. Pierce and I. Roitt, eds), pp. 213–227. Blackwell, Oxford.

Ormerod, W. E. (1975). Ablastin in *Trypanosoma lewisi* and related phenomena in other species of trypanosomes. *Experimental Parasitology*, **38**, 338–341.

Patton, C. L. (1972a). *Trypanosoma lewisi*: influence of sera and exudate cells. *Experimental Parasitology*, **31**, 370–377.

Patton, C. L. (1972b). Inhibition of reproduction in *Trypanosoma lewisi* by ouabain. *Nature New Biology*, **237**, 253–255.

Patton, C. L. (1975). The ablastin phenomenon: inhibition of membrane function. *Experimental Parasitology*, **38**, 357–369.

Patton, C. L. and Clarke, D. T. (1968). *Trypanosoma lewisi* infections in normal rats and rats treated with dexamethasone. *Journal of Protozoology*, **15**, 31–35.

Pizzi, T. and Taliaferro, W. H. (1960). A comparative study of protein and nucleic acid synthesis in different species of trypanosomes. *Journal of Infectious Diseases*, **107**, 100–107.

Pouliot, P., Viens, P. and Targett, G. A. T. (1977). T. lymphocytes and the transfer of immunity to *Trypanosoma musculi* in mice. *Clinical and Experimental Immunology*, **27**, 507–511.

Sanders, A. and Wallace, F. G. (1966). Immunization of rats with irradiated *Trypanosoma lewisi*. *Experimental Parasitology*, **18**, 301–304.

Shaw, G. L. and Dusanic, D. G. (1973). *Trypanosoma lewisi*: termination of pregnancy in the infected rat. *Experimental Parasitology*, **33**, 46–55.

Sherman, I. W. and Ruble, J. A. (1967). Virulent *Trypanosoma lewisi* infections in cortisone-treated rats. *Journal of Parasitology*, **53**, 258–262.

Spira, D. T. and Greenblatt, C. L. (1970). The effects of antithymocyte serum on *Trypanosoma lewisi* infections. *Journal of Protozoology*, **17**, (Supplement), 29.

Taliaferro, W. H. (1924). A reaction product in infections with *Trypanosoma lewisi* which inhibits the reproduction of the trypanosomes. *Journal of Experimental Medicine*, **39**, 171–190.

Taliaferro, W. H. (1932). Trypanocidal and reproduction-inhibiting antibodies to *Trypanosoma lewisi* in rats and rabbits. *American Journal of Hygiene*, **16**, 32–84.

Taliaferro, W. H. (1938). Ablastic and trypanocidal antibodies against *Trypanosoma duttoni*. *Journal of Immunology*, **35**, 303–328.

Taliaferro, W. H. and D'Alesandro, P. A. (1971). *Trypanosoma lewisi* infection in the rat. Effect of adenine. *Proceedings of the National Academy of Sciences, U.S.A.*, **68**, 1–5.

Taliaferro, W. H. and Pizzi, T. (1960). The inhibition of nucleic acid and protein synthesis in *Trypanosoma lewisi* by the antibody ablastin. *Proceedings of the National Academy of Sciences, U.S.A.*, **46**, 733–745.

Targett, G. A. T. and Viens, P. (1975a). Ablastin: control of *Trypanosoma musculi* infections in mice. *Experimental Parasitology*, **38**, 309–316.

Targett, G. A. T. and Viens, P. (1975b). The immunological response of CBA mice to *Trypanosoma musculi*: elimination of the parasite from the blood. *International Journal for Parasitology*, **5**, 231–234.

Tawil, A. and Dusanic, D. G. (1971). The effects of antilymphocytic serum (ALS) on *Trypanosoma lewisi* infection. *Journal of Protozoology*, **18**, 445–447.

Thillet, C. H. and Chandler, A. C. (1957). Immunization against *Trypanosoma lewisi* in rats by injections of metabolic products. *Science*, **125**, 346–347.

Viens, P., Targett, G. A. T., Wilson, V. C. L. C. and Edwards, C. I. (1972). The persistence of *Trypanosoma* (*Herpetosoma*) *musculi* in the kidneys of immune CBA mice. *Transactions of the Royal Society of Tropical Medicine and Hygiene*, **66**, 669–670.

Viens, P., Targett, G. A. T., Leuchars, E. and Davies, A. J. S. (1974a). The immunological response of CBA mice to *Trypanosoma musculi*. I. Initial control of the infection and the effect of T-cell deprivation. *Clinical and Experimental Immunology*, **16**, 279–294.

Viens, P., Pouliot, P. and Targett, G. A. T. (1974b). Cell-mediated immunity during infection of CBA mice with *Trypanosoma musculi*. *Canadian Journal of Microbiology*, **20**, 105–106.

Viens, P., Targett, G. A. T. and Lumsden, W. H. R. (1975). The immunological response of CBA mice to *Trypanosoma musculi*: mechanisms of protective immunity. *International Journal for Parasitology*, **5**, 235–239.

Viens, P., Lajeunesse, M. C., Richards, R. and Targett, G. A. T. (1977). *Trypanosoma musculi*: *in vitro* cultivation of blood forms in cell culture media. *International Journal for Parasitology*, **7**, 109–111.

Wilson, V. C. L. C. (1971). The morphology of the reproductive stages of *Trypanosoma* (*Herpetosoma*) *musculi* in C3H mice. *Journal of Protozoology*, **18** (Supplement), 43.

Wilson, V. C. L. C., Viens, P., Targett, G. A. T. and Edwards, C. I. (1973). Comparative studies on the persistence of *Trypanosoma* (*Herpetosoma*) *musculi* and *T.* (*H.*) *lewisi* in immune hosts. *Transactions of the Royal Society of Tropical Medicine and Hygiene*, **67**, 271.

Yasuda, S. and Dusanic, D. G. (1969). Comparative immunological studies on somatic and secretion-excretion products of bloodstream and culture forms of *Trypanosoma lewisi*. I. Protective immunity and the agglutinin response. *Journal of Infectious Diseases*, **119**, 562–568.

10

Virulence of Trypanosomes in the Vertebrate Host

W. J. HERBERT AND D. PARRATT*

*University Department of Bacteriology and Immunology,
Western Infirmary, Glasgow, Scotland*

I.	Introduction to virulence	482
	A. Definitions	482
	B. Evaluation	482
	C. Pathological basis	485
II.	Evolutionary aspects of virulence	486
	A. Evolutionary adaptation	486
	B. Identification of the natural host	487
III.	Virulence of a single species of trypanosome in different vertebrate hosts	491
	A. Range of virulence in different hosts	491
	B. Influence of body-size of the host	493
IV.	Virulence of different stocks of a single species	494
V.	Differences in virulence amongst the variable antigen types of a trypanosome serodeme	497
VI.	Changes in virulence following passage	500
	A. In laboratory animals or other "unnatural" hosts	500
	B. In "natural" hosts	502
VII.	Changes in virulence induced by drugs	504
VIII.	Variation in virulence following exposure to high ambient temperatures	504

* Present address: Department of Bacteriology, University of Dundee, Ninewells Hospital, Dundee, Scotland.

IX. General discussion 505
    A. How should the term "virulence" be defined? . . . 506
    B. Microorganismal multiplication and virulence . . . 506
    C. Mechanisms of trypanosome pathogenicity in relation to
    virulence 511
    D. Conclusion 514
X. Acknowledgements 514
XI. References 515

I. Introduction to virulence

A. DEFINITION

In this paper the term virulence will be taken to mean the capacity*
of a parasite to damage and to cause disease in its host. Two other
characters of a parasite, namely, infectivity and transmissibility, are
usually so closely associated with virulence that the latter is often confused with them. However, infectivity is not in any formal way related to
virulence, for virulence describes the pathogenic effects that are seen in
the host *after* infection has occurred. Thus many stercorarian trypanosomes appear to be highly infective but of negligible virulence. Similarly,
the transmissibility of the parasite depends on its availability to the vector,
whether or not it has damaged the host, together with such factors as its
stability outside of the host and its infectivity for a new host (Mims,
1976).

B. EVALUATION

A base-line for virulence from which excursions can be measured is
unfortunately, not yet available for any infection. It must, however, be
established in the future in order to clarify host–parasite relationships.
This will be difficult, especially in hosts in which the parasite is of negligible virulence, but it must be remembered that such hosts are the ones
most likely to provide information of practical value; where infection is
obvious and results in disease, the host–parasite relationship can be regarded as, of necessity, disturbed and thus less susceptible to useful
analysis.

The trypanosomes infecting vertebrates exhibit the full range of
virulence possible, that is, from the production of a rapidly lethal infection, to a commensal relationship that has no detectable deleterious

---

* It should be noted that though a highly virulent organism has a high *capacity* to
inflict damage on its host, it may not fully utilize this capacity in a particular instance.

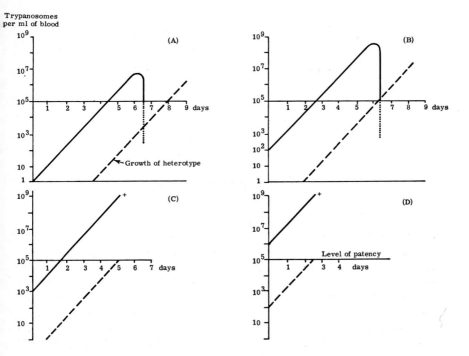

FIG. 1. Theoretical graphs showing the survival of mice infected by various doses of a trypanosome stock of high virulence: (A) 1 ID_{63} (B) 10^2 ID_{63} (C) 10^3 ID_{63} and (D) 10^6 ID_{63}. In each of the graphs it is assumed that by the sixth day of the infection the immune response will be sufficient to induce remission and that a parasitaemia exceeding 10^9 is lethal. The doubling time of the organism is taken as six hours. The graphs also show the growth of a heterotype that has appeared at a ratio of one organism to 10^4 homotype organisms (Van Meirvenne et al., 1975b). Thus in (A) remission is evident as a day on which no patent parasitaemia is detected, in (B) as a reduction in parasitaemia, whilst in (C) and (D) the mice die before remission occurs.

Note. In this chapter all original figures that show changes in parasitaemia are presented with the X axis at approximately the level of patency as detected on examination of twenty fields of a wet blood-film. By this convention, the important, but unseen growth of the organism and its heterotypes in subpatent parasitaemic numbers can be displayed for comment.

effects on the host. Except at these two extremes, virulence is difficult to quantify. Most evaluations reported are subjective and for these a five-point scale will be used employing the following adjectives: negligible, low, moderate, high and extreme.

In this nomenclature, extreme virulence means death within a week of infection; high, death within about a month; moderate, within several months; low, a chronic infection persisting, with symptoms, for some years, sometimes with recovery; negligible, a complete absence of clinical signs and symptoms. However, the meaning of these terms will, to some extent, be weighted in relation to the normal life-span of the infected animal, e.g. an infection persisting for months in the mouse and one lasting years in a cow, are equated as being of low virulence.

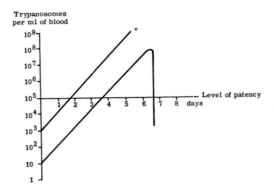

FIG. 2. Theoretical effect of a 2-log difference in the number of infective doses of a trypanosome stock used to infect mice. The organism appears to be extremely virulent in the mice given the larger doses ($+$ = death of the host) though with the lower dose it is evident that it is less virulent, the difference being magnified by the remission. In practice, low doses (of 10 or 100 ID_{63}) may rarely be given unless the infectivity of the original suspension is accurately known. Many experimenters are understandably reluctant to prepare a dose of 10 ID_{63}, which may involve making a hundred million-fold dilution of highly infected mouse blood. At such dilutions it is difficult to overcome the impression that one is injecting saline alone.

In some instances, numerical records are available, e.g. number of days from infection to death. However, such data may mislead when highly virulent materials are being considered because in these cases the length of survival will depend on the size of the infecting dose (Fig. 1).

When conventional "syringe-passage" methods of initiating an infection are used it is easy to give doses that vary enormously; for instance 1000 ID_{63} can be contained in one-twentieth of the volume of a drop of infected mouse blood. With two highly virulent stocks* a two log difference in dosage would produce the apparent difference illustrated in Fig. 2 though the stocks examined were similar. Even a careful standardization of the infecting dose in terms of the number of motile organisms in the inoculum may be misleading. Cunningham *et al.* (1963) have shown

* In this chapter terms such as stock, population, variable antigen type, primary isolation etc., conform to the definitions given in Chapter 15.

that trypanosomes can vary widely in their infectivity (up to a hundred fold) over the course of an infection though microscopically they appear to be equally motile at all stages (Fig. 3). Comparisons can, therefore, only validly be made amongst high and extremely virulent stocks if the infections have been initiated by known numbers of infective doses (Lumsden *et al.*, 1963) or, better, by single organisms.

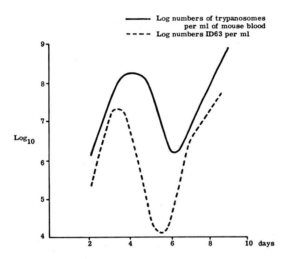

FIG. 3. Relationship of numbers of motile trypanosomes of *T. brucei* ssp., present in the blood of rats, to their infectivity, over the course of a relapsing infection. At the peak parasitaemia only one in one hundred of the organisms present is infective. Redrawn after Cunningham *et al.* (1963).

C. PATHOLOGICAL BASIS

The basis of the pathological effects of trypanosomiasis and thus the varied virulence of the causative trypanosomes is as yet poorly understood. In some circumstances the presence of enormous numbers of parasites ($>10^9$/ml) in the circulation can be shown to be directly and rapidly responsible for death, though in other instances large numbers (10^8–10^9/ml) can persist without any apparent immediate effect on the host. On the other hand, at the time of death in chronic infections very few organisms ($<10^5$/ml) may be found.

Many investigators have searched for a principal cause of pathogenesis for the disease such as a toxin with a clearly defined effect. A mechanism of this type can be shown to be a cause of death in special circumstances. Mice infected with the extremely virulent *T. brucei rhodesiense* variable antigen type ETat 2 (Lumsden and Herbert, 1975) die of hypoglycaemia when the parasitaemia exceeds 10^9/ml (Herbert *et al.*, 1975), although it should be noted that this is an artificial situation using extremely virulent organisms in an unnatural host. Also, other factors are evidently involved for the mice do eventually die even if their hypoglycaemia is corrected.

Natural infections most frequently present as a chronic and progressive dislocation of body functions of which weight-loss, anaemia, and blood protein aberrations are the most easily measurable disturbances. The picture is that of a contest in which both parasite and host wear each other out. The coup-de-grace may be effected by other parasites, the host's normal defence mechanisms against these having possibly been diverted to the trypanosomes. An immunosuppressive effect has been clearly demonstrated in trypanosomiasis (Greenwood et al., 1973).

Further, other parasitic organisms, present in what would normally be innocuous numbers, may be fatal in the debilitated animal, e.g. the blood taken by a few haematophagous nematodes, unnoticed in a healthy cow, may be an unacceptable proportion of the blood of an anaemic one and thus be the "straw that breaks the camel's back".

In the absence of evidence that the pathology seen in the disease is due to some direct toxic or destructive effect of the parasite, it may be postulated that many of the signs and symptoms seen in trypanosomiasis result from the host's immunological response to the parasite and to the antigens released by it. Any immunological reaction that causes overt self-inflected damage to the animal is known as a hypersensitivity reaction. A comprehensive review of hypersensitivity is presented by Gell et al. (1975) and it is evident that it is a factor of great importance in the pathology of many diseases.

The role of immunological hypersensitivity is most easily recognized when it follows stimulation by a non-reproducing agent, e.g. as in hayfever. If, as in trypanosomiasis, the organism can be readily found in large numbers in the body by simple examination, it may not be so evident that the pathogenic effects of the parasites reside in the hypersensitivity response that they evoke rather than in some direct damage caused by the organisms themselves. Instinct tends to insist that the mere presence of the parasites must be damaging. An extended discussion of immunological hypersensitivity in relation to trypanosome virulence is presented in Section IX of this chapter.

II. Evolutionary aspects of virulence

A. EVOLUTIONARY ADAPTATION

Trypanosomes can be divided into two groups if virulence to the host is used as the criterion. Firstly, those—mainly Stercoraria—that are host species-, or at least, host genus-specific and of negligible virulence.

Secondly, *T. cruzi* and most Salivaria, which can grow in a variety of different species, genera and even classes of host and exhibit the full spectrum of virulence in various members of these.

The groupings may be artificial, because the second comprises the trypanosomes of economic importance. These have been extensively investigated and their host range is therefore better known than is the case with the first. Every trypanosome species shows low or negligible virulence in at least a few of its possible hosts, or there exist some stocks of it that are of low virulence compared to the remainder.

It can be argued that the most "natural" host of a trypanosome is that in which it shows the lowest degree of virulence, for it is axiomatic that it is not to the advantage of any parasite to cause severe pathogenic effects in a host such as will rapidly cause death of the latter before onward transmission can take place. A long evolutionary relationship between parasite and host would be expected to result in the two living in harmony; also, due to mutual adaptation a restriction of the parasite to a small host range would be expected. High pathogenicity, on the other hand, suggests that, in evolutionary terms, the relationship is a more recent one (Hoare, 1972), e.g. *T. simiae* in the domestic pig.

When examining the distribution of any one trypanosome species amongst its various host species, it may be more valuable to identify those to which it is best adapted rather than those in which it is disease-producing. Where the former appear to be logically acceptable in an evolutionary sense, the information may be of epidemiological importance, i.e. they may be unexpected reservoir hosts. Where a host in which virulence is negligible appears to be aberrant on evolutionary grounds the situation is even more interesting and may yield clues of value for the control of disease-causing trypanosome infections.

B. IDENTIFICATION OF THE NATURAL HOST

Negligible virulence coupled with scanty parasitaemia and inefficient diagnostic (microscope search) techniques will result in an under-estimate of the host-range of many trypanosomes. Therefore, convenient new techniques for routinely recognizing very low host parasitaemias such as that of Lumsden *et al.* (1977) are important in enabling what may be more logically thought of as the "natural" hosts to be identified.

As an example, the host range of *T. brucei brucei* may be examined. This trypanosome shows moderate virulence in horses, dogs and camels, low virulence in sheep, goats and pigs, and low or possibly negligible virulence in humped cattle. Its natural hosts are, by most authors, assumed to be African "game" animals in which it is supposed, on inadequate evidence, to be of negligible virulence (Ashcroft *et al.*, 1959 and see Terry, Vol. 1, Chapter 11).

However, it has also been known for many years that this species can infect birds (Corson, 1931). Studies carried out in the present authors' laboratory, on a stock originating from primary isolation Lugala/55/

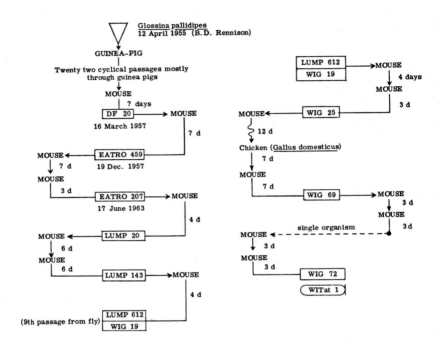

FIG. 4.   Pedigree of *T. brucei brucei* variable antigen type WITat 1. The stock from which this was derived appears to be that referred to by other authors as "Lugala 1". This identity is confirmed in the case of the work of Houba *et al.* (1969), as they state that they used organisms derived from stabilate EATRO 207. The primary isolation from which this stock was derived has provisionally been given the number LUGALA/55/EATRO/459. In the figure the pedigree up to stabilate LUMP 612 is set out as received from the World Health Organization cryobank at the Department of Medical Protozoology of the London School of Hygiene and Tropical Medicine. The conventional signs follow Lumsden *et al.* (1973), i.e., triangle = residence in vector; oblong box = cryopreserved stabilate; d = days; dotted line = isolation of a single organism; "wiggle" = observed antigenic variation; Royal cartouche = stabilate representing type-type of the variable antigen type. An additional convention has been added; this is a double box, e.g., that including LUMP 612 and WIG 19. This indicates that LUMP 612 was accessed to the Western Infirmary stabilate bank as WIG 19. LUMP = London University Medical Protozoology; WIG = Western Infirmary Glasgow. It may be noted that this stock appears to be inactivated by human serum and has proved non-infective when inoculated into human volunteers. The results of such tests should, however, be viewed with caution. (Since writing this, a human serum-resistant clone of this stock has been isolated following further passage in chickens).

EATRO/459*,† has shown that a clone population derived from it (variable antigen type WITat 1, Fig. 4) can regularly infect domestic chickens (*Gallus domesticus*). Infection can be initiated with a dose of 100 mouse ID_{63}, and the birds remain infected for at least 9 months. They show the same growth rate as controls and mature to lay eggs (Fig. 5). During this period the parasitaemia persists at about 3 organisms per ml of blood (R. Joshua, personal communication).

Duke (1933) showed that tsetse (*Glossina palpalis*) can be infected by feeding them on fowls carrying *T. b. rhodesiense* though onward transmission was not attempted. Nevertheless, a very low parasitaemia is no

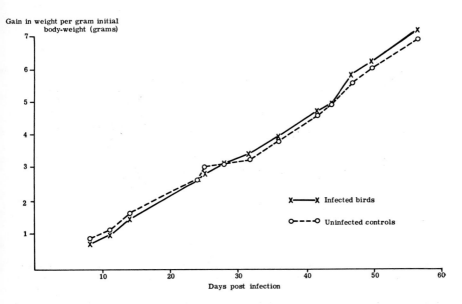

FIG. 5.   Mean growth rate of a group of six chickens (*Gallus domesticus*) that were infected with variable antigen type WITat 1 (derived from primary isolation LUGALA/55/EATRO/459) when the birds were 11 days old. The infection, as shown by xenodiagnosis in mice, persisted throughout the course of the experiment. The mean growth-rate of a similar control group of six uninfected chickens, kept in the same conditions, is also shown. (By courtesy of Dr. R. A. Joshua and Professor R. G. White.)

* Analysis of heterophil antibody responses indicates a possibility that this stock represents a subspecies of *T. brucei* that is distinct from *T. brucei brucei*, *T. b. rhodesiense* or *T. b. gambiense*. See also Chapter 11.

† The final digits in this (and other EATRO) primary isolation numbers are provisional but have been taken from the first designated stabilate made, see Fig. 4. This is the best that can be attempted at the time of writing owing to present difficulties in communicating with the East African Trypanosomiasis Research Organization. However, the number, as given, should enable a confident identification to be made of any laboratory-held stock for which a pedigree is available.

bar to successful transmission as can be deduced from the success of *T. theileri*, the ubiquitous stercorarian parasite of cattle throughout the world. Wells (1971) has shown that this organism is usually present at a level of less than one organism per ml of blood.

As, in general, *T. b. brucei* exhibits moderate to high virulence in mammals of many genera, it may be postulated that its persistence with negligible virulence in birds must indicate a very longstanding relationship with them. To extrapolate even further, could it be that the mutual adaptation is so good in this case because it goes back to the dinosaur ancestors of the birds (Ostrom, 1973)? The warm-blooded status of this whole ancestral line (Bakker, 1972) could have facilitated transfer to, and amongst, the comparably warm-blooded mammals. To follow such a thesis, the most natural hosts of *T. b. brucei* would have to be sought amongst the dinosaur relatives and descendants.

However, if on this argument the bird is adopted as a natural host of *T. brucei* the anomalous reaction of cattle (and African game) has to be explained. In this genus too, the organism appears to be able to persist without pathogenic effect. If trypanosomes and cattle have not had so long to become mutually adapted to each other as have trypanosome and bird then some physiological, biochemical or immunological peculiarity of host or parasite must be responsible. Some speculations on the rôle that immunological hypersensitivity may play in such a *modus-vivendi* are presented in Section IX of this chapter. On the other hand, of course, the argument may be reversed and the peculiarities sought in the bird. Furthermore, in the example taken there is, in fact, doubt as to the true subspecific identity of the *T. brucei* organism that so readily infects birds* (see Chapter 11). Evidently our knowledge of fundamental taxonomy is in many ways inadequate and, it is probably necessary to apply the latest techniques such as isoenzyme (Godfrey and Kilgour, 1976) and DNA (Newton, Vol. 1, Chapter 9) analysis to define accurately the identity of a trypanosome, before its natural hosts, or its comparative virulence in a range of hosts, can be discussed.

The example of *T. brucei* in the chicken illustrates the difficulties inherent in the identification of a "natural" host for any of the trypanosomes of economic importance. However, for convenience in this chapter, the natural hosts of the trypanosome species examined will be accepted as those normally quoted as such, i.e., largely the African game animals and domestic livestock from which the organisms can readily be recovered. Small laboratory animals whose wild relatives are uncommonly recorded as having been found infected will be treated as "unnatural" hosts.

---

* Following passage through chickens, a clone population that is resistant to the action of human serum has been isolated from this stock (Joshua *et al.*, 1978).

III. Virulence of a single species of trypanosome in different vertebrate hosts

A. RANGE OF VIRULENCE IN DIFFERENT HOSTS

Notwithstanding the discussion in the previous section on the effect of evolutionary relationships on the distribution of trypanosomes amongst their hosts, it would not be surprising to find that some species of host were entirely refractory to infection with certain trypanosomes merely because there were gross biochemical or physiological incompatibilities between the host and the parasite. Nevertheless, those Salivaria and Stercoraria that have been extensively studied because they cause disease in man and domestic animals are found to be able to infect many different host species. The virulence that they exhibit in domestic and laboratory hosts is summarized in Table 1.

The table gives the range of virulence that, in the opinion of the authors, is *most frequently* encountered. However, in all cases, reports of an exceptional virulence outwith that range exist. The exceptional being, of course, frequently the subject of notice just because it *is* unusual. In the table, virulence has been classified with an emphasis on survival time rather than external evidence of disease. This may be exemplified by comparing the effect of a stock of extreme virulence in the mouse, where no symptoms of infection may be seen until perhaps 5 minutes before death, when the animal suffers hypoglycaemic convulsion (Herbert *et al.*, 1975), compared with the miserably unhappy state of a rabbit, infected with the same stock, showing oedema, conjunctivitis, a staring coat etc. However, as the rabbit survives for a relatively long time, the stock can only be recorded as of moderate virulence in this species.

In most cases, reference has been made to original papers but where the information is in the general domain, or an exhaustive series of references would be needed for completeness, reference is made to Hoare's (1972) classical monograph.

The range of virulence of two species of trypanosome that infect man has not been recorded in Table I. *T. cruzi* and *T. rangeli* appear uniformly to show negligible or low virulence in all infected mammals, though *T. cruzi* can cause acute disease in young children (Hoare, 1972). The biology of the completely non-pathogenic trypanosome *T. rangeli* is exhaustively discussed by D'Alessandro in Volume 1, Chapter 8, and *T. cruzi* in animal hosts is discussed by Miles in Chapter 2 of the present volume.

It is tempting to associate the lack of virulence of these parasites with a tissue habitat (though evidence for this is not conclusive in the case of *T. rangeli*), and more especially with a possible lack of ability to undergo

Table 1. Relative virulence of seven trypanosome species of economic importance in domestic and laboratory animals and in man.

	T. brucei ssp.	*T. evansi*	*T. equiperdum*	*T. vivax*	*T. congolense*	*T. simiae*	*T. suis*
Horse	II–III (38)	I–III (26, 27)	II (14, 33)	II–IV (3, 5, 6, 7)	II–III (14)		
Donkey	II–III (37)		I–II (6, 14)	II–IV (3, 5, 6, 7)	II–III (14)		
Camel	II–III (14, 52)	II–III (26, 28, 52)		R–II (6, 52)	III (53)	III–V (15)	
European cattle		I (27, 30, 31)					
Zebu cattle	I–II (6, 36, 38)	I (27, 30, 31)	I (35)	III–IV (1, 2)	II–III (6, 7)	R–II (16, 17, 18)	R (14)
West African dwarf cattle				II–III (19, 20)	II–III (19, 20)		
Sheep	II (6, 38)		I (35)	II–IV (3, 4, 5, 6)	II–III (14)	II–III (15)	R (14)
Goat	II (6, 38)			II–IV (3, 4, 5, 6)	II–III (14)	III (51)	R (14)
Pig	II (8, 38)		I (35)	R–I (8)	I–II (8)	V (8)	III–IV (24, 25)
Dog	III (6, 38, 39)	III (26, 29)	III (14)	R (6)	R–III (14)	R (14)	R (14)
Cat	III (14)				R–III (14)		
Rabbit	II–III (41)		(III) (34)	(II) (9)		II–III (22, 23)	
Guinea pig		II (48)	(II) (34)				
Rat	III–(V) (14, 36)		R–(III) (34)	(III–IV) (11)	R–III (12,13)	R (14)	R (14)
Mouse	III–(V) (14, 40) II[2]	IV (32)	R–(III) (34)	(IV) (10)	R–III (12, 13)	R (14)	R (14)
Chicken	I (46, 47, 49)	I (Goose, 45)	I (50)				
Man	R[1] (14, 42, 43, 44) II[2]–III[3]			R	R		

Virulence is graded on a five point scale: I, negligible; II, low; III, moderate; IV, high; and V, extreme. (See section IB for a fuller description of this classification); R, resistant to infection. Bracketed Roman numerals indicate virulence of laboratory adapted stocks. Superscript numbers, *T. brucei* column only. [1] = *T. b. brucei*, [2] = *T. b. gambiense*, [3] = *T. b. rhodesiense*. Bracketed figures refer to the following references:
1. Lewis (1954). 2. Fairbairn (1953). 3. Rodhain et al. (1941). 4. Van Hoof et al. (1948). 5. Curasson and Mornet (1948). 6. Hornby (1953). 7. Hornby (1952). 8. Stephen (1966a). 9. Blacklock and Yorke (1913a). 10. Taylor (1968). 11. Desowitz and Watson (1952). 12. Binns (1938). 13. Bruce et al. (1913b). 14. Hoare (1972). 15. Pellegrini (1948). 16. Barnett (1947). 17. Peel and Chardôme (1954a). 18. Chardôme and Peel (1967). 19. Stephen (1966b). 20. Desowitz (1959). 21. Bruce et al. (1912). 22. Kinghorn and Yorke (1912). 23. Kinghorn et al. (1913). 24. Peel and Chardôme (1954b). 25. Ochmann (1905). 26. Barotte (1925). 27. Cross (1921). 28. Sergeant et al. (1918). 29. Gomez Rodriguez (1956). 30. Edwards (1926). 31. Hoare (1956). 32. Krijgsman (1933). 33. Hutyra et al. (1938). 34. Haig and Lund (1948). 35. Curasson (1943). 36. Godfrey and Killick-Kendrick (1961). 37. Godfrey (1966). 38. Stephen (1970). 39. Curson (1928). 40. McNeillage and Herbert (1968). 41. Gray (1965). 42. Rickman and Robson (1970).

antigenic variation. It is evident that gross pathological damage must not be rapidly induced by a parasite if it is to survive for many years in a single host. However, at the end of that time pathological processes resulting from the presence of the parasite may be detectable, e.g. amyloidosis in old cattle after lifetime infection with *T. theileri* (Wells, E. A., personal communication) and grossly abnormal splenic architecture in chickens chronically infected with *T. b. brucei* (Wallace *et al.*, 1976).

B. INFLUENCE OF BODY-SIZE OF THE HOST

Whatever may be the pathological basis of trypanosome virulence, consideration of differential virulence amongst a range of species must take into account their absolute body size. If the organism is able to divide at the same rate in a large and in a small animal then, assuming that the initial number of infecting organisms was the same, the number of parasites per ml of tissue will be much higher in the small than in the large animal at any moment in time thereafter. This difference will be especially important at the moment when the immune response is sufficiently developed to cause remission of the infection (Fig. 6), because the immune response would be expected to take the same length of time to develop in both. Any pathogenic effects, whether due to the

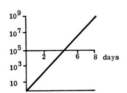

Growth of trypanosome population assuming one division every six hours
(a) Total numbers present in body

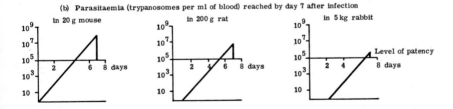

(b) Parasitaemia (trypanosomes per ml of blood) reached by day 7 after infection

FIG. 6.   Theoretical influence of body size of host on the development of a patent parasitaemia (and possibly on pathogenic potential) in a trypanosome infection initiated by a single organism. In the lower set of graphs it is assumed that an immune response at day 7 after infection has caused a remission of the parasitaemia.

organisms themselves or to immunological hypersensitivity, must be less severe at that time in the large animal due to the smaller weight of parasite per kg of host. Increased virulence seen on the transfer of a parasite of a domestic animal to a small laboratory animal must therefore be viewed in the context of size as well as of species difference.

Even amongst the small laboratory animals effects of size are evident. For instance, the extremely virulent *T. b. rhodesiense* variable antigen type ETat 2 inevitably kills mice (20–30 gm) in about 6 days, without remission. But in the rat (200 gm) it is overcome by the immune response before it reaches lethally pathogenic numbers and remission is seen. The reason may be that at the moment when the organism has multiplied to reach a total population of say 2×10^9 in either species, this will represent 10^9 per ml in mouse blood, but only 10^8 per ml in the rat's blood.

IV. Virulence of different stocks of a single species

The reports reviewed in this section suffer from a fundamental defect, a lack of information on the absolute identity of many stocks mentioned, especially those whose activity and virulence have been observed only in the field. Of stocks captured and held in laboratories, only a handful have published pedigrees so that the relationship of one laboratory's observations on any stock to those made in another laboratory is uncertain. Moreover, when cloning has not been carried out, there is no certainty that any population is not a mixture of several stocks of differing virulence, or even a mixture of different species (Oehler, 1913).

The recently introduced system of nomenclature for primary isolations and their derivatives (see Chapter 15) will greatly assist the laboratory situation. However, such identification is procedural rather than taxonomic and it is vital that the named primary isolates be then cloned and taxonomically identified and classified by isoenzyme (Godfrey and Kilgour, 1976), specific antigen, and heterophil antigen patterns. For instance, Dr. Joshua (personal communication) has observed that the heterophil antigen pattern of WITat 1 (Fig. 4) segregates it from other *T. brucei brucei* in the same way as the latter is segregated from *T. b. rhodesiense* and *T. b. gambiense* and as these latter are segregated amongst themselves (Parratt and Cobb, 1978; Chapter 11). Far from being merely a different stock, a derivative of LUGALA/55/EATRO/459 might therefore be considered to have the weight of a *T. brucei* subspecies.* On such considerations there may exist many more subspecies of *T. brucei*, our man-centred view of this group having so far led us to recognize differences between the *rhodesiense* and *gambiense* forms but to have lumped all the others together as *brucei brucei*. Or, on

* See footnote on p. 490.

the other hand, the differences between them all may overlap to the extent of reducing them merely to variant stocks.

It is a common observation that stocks of a single species, passaged in laboratory animals, vary considerably in the virulence that they exhibit. High virulence may, in such cases, be associated with the monomorphism that usually results from repeated syringe passage of *T. brucei* ssp. (see Section VI, A). But repeated syringe passage does not always result in increased virulence and similar differences are also seen in stocks of short passage history. For instance, *T. b. brucei* stocks originating from primary isolations* BUSOGA/60/EATRO/3 and LUGALA/69/EATRO/1244, the origins respectively of the ETat and GUTat serodemes, show high virulence; mice do not survive the first relapse parasitaemia. On the other hand, stocks of *T. b. brucei* originating from primary isolations LUGALA/55/EATRO/459 and SERENGETI/66/SVRP/10 show low or moderate virulence in mice. Similarly there are differences in the virulence of *T. congolense* stocks descended from primary isolations UHAYA/61/EATRO/13 and from stabilate GUP92—a stock of unknown history (GUP = Glasgow University Protozoology).

In some of these examples, high and extreme virulence can be explained by the presence in the serodeme of a character for high virulence that, in the ETat serodeme at least, appears to be expressed in association with certain antigenic types. The extreme virulence of variable antigen type ETat 2 (see Section V) is the obvious example (but see Fig. 10). However, clear differences in the virulence of different trypanosome stocks have been observed in the field.

Remarkable cases have been reported in which *T. b. gambiense* appears to be able to live in man without causing any symptoms, the organisms only being detected at routine examination (Sartory *et al.*, 1915; Cooke *et al.*, 1937; Harding and Hutchinson, 1948). As the reports concern infections in both Africans and Europeans, it seems unlikely that innate immunity or a residual immune response following previous infection, is responsible for the negligible virulence seen. On the other hand, as infections of negligible virulence in man do not appear to be widespread, it may be that the phenomenon is due to a superior ability of the patients to deal with the parasite than to infection with trypanosome stocks of special character. Better methods of diagnosis (Lumsden *et al.*, 1977, and Chapter 11 of this volume) could conceivably show that the reverse is true.

Similar reports, of negligible virulence or a carrier state, in man have been made in respect of *T. b. rhodesiense* (Conran, 1921; Lamborn and Howat, 1936; Davey, 1936; Blair, 1939) but in these cases also, the condition has been noticed in individuals and does not seem to be a general attribute of the trypanosome stock present in a particular geographical

---

* See second footnote on p. 489.

area. Apted (1970), however, concluded that there has been a general decline in the virulence of *T. b. rhodesiense* to man during the first half of this century. There is also some evidence for a continuous geographical distribution of stocks of *T. b. rhodesiense* of varying virulence. The virulence for man and for laboratory animals increasing from the southern part of East Africa, where mild infections are said to be common, northwards to Uganda where the disease is usually very acute (Apted, 1970; Ormerod, 1961).

Extraordinarily high virulence in trypanosome infections in man in the Lake Chad area in West Africa, where the organism responsible would be expected to be *T. b.* gambiense, have also been recorded. Duggan (1962) reported infections that were of *T. b. rhodesiense*-like virulence. Once again, however, one is faced with the problem of deciding what was in fact the true identity of the stock. Robertson and Baker (1957), faced with this problem during an epidemic of low virulence in the Acholi district of Northern Uganda, did not assume that the organism must have been a stock of *T. b. rhodesiense*. Instead, on the evidence of its negligible virulence to, or failure to infect, laboratory rodents and monkeys, they classified it as *T. b. gambiense*. The potential value of isoenzyme, or heterophile antibody analysis in such a situation is evident.

Turning to another species, Lewis (1954) demonstrated the existence of two stocks of *T. vivax*, of differing virulence, infecting cattle in Kenya. One of these, transmitted by *G. pallidipes*, was of high virulence, killing cattle in 30 days. The other produced a more chronic disease, the animals surviving for up to 160 days. This latter stock was transmitted by *G. fuscipes*. There seemed to be some association between the tsetse species responsible for transmission in that the virulence of the highly virulent stock was reduced when it was passed through *G. fuscipes*.

The virulence of *T. vivax* in cattle also seems to be related to its morphology, which may be an indication of the presence of different stocks, or even a marker of subspecificity. Hoare (1972) and Fairbairn (1953) noted that short forms are responsible for acute disease in both East and West Africa but that chronic cases in East Africa are found to be infected with long forms alone. Wenyon and Hanschell (1912) also considered that they could equate virulence with morphological differences between stocks of *T. b. rhodesiense* which were observed on passage in rats. In their view, the higher the proportion of posterior-nuclear forms seen, the greater the virulence. Hoare (1972) too, believes that there is some indication of a relationship between the length of *T. evansi* and its virulence. Thus mild disease is produced by the shorter forms in, e.g., North African horses; but an acute and fatal disease is produced in Soviet Middle Asia and India, where the longest forms are found.

V. Differences in virulence amongst the variable antigen types of a trypanosome serodeme

Rudolph Oehler, a pioneer in the use of defined populations in the study of trypanosomes (Oehler, 1913), reported that it was easier to prepare clones from some stocks than from others. He found (Oehler, 1914a) that with some stocks only one infection was obtained per twenty single organisms selected, whilst from others the proportion was one in five. These latter stocks were, he noted, the most virulent. Oehler's findings were not confirmed for over half a century, until McNeillage and Herbert (1968), preparing the ETat serodeme, noticed that it was much easier to obtain clones of some variable antigen types than of others. In the case of ETat 1, only one success was recorded in 23 attempts, whilst the ratio was between 4·5 : 1 and 2 : 1 in the case of ETat 2–6.

These reports refer, essentially to the *infectivity* of the organisms (see Section 1A). However, McNeillage and Herbert (1968) further observed that there was a striking difference between the virulence of the different clones that they had obtained. Mice inoculated with *single* organisms of the variable antigen types ETat 2, 3 or 5 always died in the first parasitaemic wave, remissions of these infections were never observed.* On the other hand, mice inoculated with single organisms of types ETat 1, 4 or 6 showed remissions, followed, usually, by relapse to one of the extremely virulent types so that they died in the first relapse. Thus it is possible to postulate that if mice were immunized against all of the extremely virulent variable antigen types, infection with this serodeme would result in a chronic relapsing infection. However, the link between virulence and variable antigen type is not inevitable. Dr. D. Barry has isolated two groups of clones all bearing the antigen AnTat 1, one group before and one after cyclical transmission. The former clones are extremely virulent, the latter produce at least one, sometimes more, relapses (Fig. 10).

It is tempting to ascribe these results to differences in growth rates. Thus the most virulent organisms are assumed to grow so fast that a lethal parasitaemia is reached, in the mouse, before the immune response has developed sufficiently to destroy them, or to inhibit their rate of multiplication (Ormerod, 1970). However, the behaviour of trypanosomes at the time of remission does not appear to confirm this hypothesis. In *T. brucei* sspp. infections in mice, remission occurs between day 5 and day 10, the day on which it is observed being related to the size of the infecting dose as shown in Table 2. If the hypothesis, that the growth rate is directly related to virulence, is true, it would be expected that an extremely virulent organism would bring about death before a remission could occur. However, this is not so; Table 3 shows that ani-

---

* These results refer to experiments carried out at room temperature. For a discussion of the modifications of virulence that are seen at high ambient temperatures, see Section VIII.

Table 2. Days in which remission of infection was observed in groups of mice infected with *T. brucei* spp. LUGALA/55/EATRO/459 stabilate WIG 25, the pedigree of which is shown in Fig. 4. The groups of mice were each given infective doses varying in tenfold steps, in an infectivity titration.

Number of infected mice observed	Mean dose ID_{63} per mouse	Mean day on which remission was observed	Range
6	501	5	5
6	50	6·7	6–8
5	5	7·2	6–8
3	0·5	7·3	7–10

Table 3. Day on which groups of mice infected with the extremely virulent stabilate WIG 3 of *T. b. rhodesiense* BUSOGA/66/EATRO/3 died. This stabilate is a defined population of variable antigen type ETat 2 whose pedigree is shown in Fig. 8. The groups of mice were given infective doses varying in tenfold steps in an infectivity titration.

Number of infected mice observed	Mean dose ID_{63} per mouse	Mean day on which found dead	Range
6	1000	6·3	6–7
6	100	7·6	7–8
6	10	7·8	7–8
4	1	8·5	8–9

mals infected with slightly larger doses of an extremely virulent trypanosome die after the time at which an immune response sufficient to destroy them *could* have occurred.

A study of the doubling times of trypanosomes of various degrees of virulence also leaves some doubt as to a full equivalence of virulence with growth rate. Table 4 presents the doubling times of several defined populations of trypanosomes each of which originated from a single organism. These were calculated on the assumption that logarithmic growth occurred from the time of administration of the originating organisms to the first parasitaemia measured; during this period the immune response could be expected to have had least effect. For the purposes of the present discussion, a more useful figure than the doubling time is the period required to reach a total parasitaemia of 10^9. In the mouse a parasitaemia of about this intensity appears to be lethal. The extremely virulent examples of variable antigen type AnTat 1 do reach this figure in the shortest time but the extremely virulent "Liverpool" strain clones require one and a half days longer. Moreover, clones which

Table 4. Growth parameters of *T. brucei* sspp. trypanosome populations in mice, each population having originated from the inoculation of a single organism.

Antigenic identity of clone	Number of clones observed	Measured mean doubling time (hours)	Remission observed in mouse infections initiated by a single trypanosome	Calculated time required to reach 10^9 organisms (days)
AnTat 1 pre-cyclic	6	5·29	No	6·59
AnTat 1 (post-cyclic)	5	5·70	Yes	7·10
ETat 2	3	5·74	No	7·15
WITat 3	1	5·74	Yes	7·15
WITat 4	1	5·78	No	7·20
WITat 2	5	5·94	Yes	7·40
Clone BA	1	6·37	Yes	7·94
Clone AP	1	6·42	Yes	8·00
Liverpool	2	6·49	No	8·09
WITat 1	1	6·73	Yes	8·38

[a]AnTat=Antwerp *Trypanozoon* antigenic type. ETat=Edinburgh *Trypanozoon* antigenic type. WITat=Western Infirmary *Trypanozoon* antigenic type.

The ETat 2 trypanosomes were obtained from a mouse that had been infected 2 days previously with stabilate WIG 41. This stabilate is one
mouse passage from LUMP 36 (Lumsden and Herbert, 1975) and two mouse passages from the type-type of variable antigen type ETat 2. The
pedigree of variable antigen type WITat 1 is shown in Fig. 4 and the data for growth rate in the table refers to the type-type itself. The clones
of WITat 2, 3, 4 and the two unidentified clones (AP and BA) were derived from the type-type of WITat 1 by passage and antigenic variation
in mice and chickens. These results are published with the kind permission of Dr. R. Joshua and Professor R. G. White.

The two groups of clones carrying the variable antigen AnTat 1 were derived from primary isolation MUVUBWE/66/EATRO/1125, and their
pedigrees are given by Van Meirvenne *et al.* (1975b) and Le Ray *et al.* (1977). One group (pre-cyclic) were derived from frequently syringe-
passaged material, and the other group (post-cyclic) immediately after tsetse fly transmission. It will be noted that there is a marked difference in
virulence between these. Data are also shown for two clones prepared from the classical, and extremely virulent, "Liverpool strain". The AnTat
and "Liverpool strain" results are published by the kind permission of Dr. David Barry.

In every case the doubling time was calculated from the time taken from cloning to the first patent parasitaemia that could be reliably estimated
by the matching method of Herbert and Lumsden (1976), i.e., greater than antilog 5·4 ml.

produce an infection of only moderate virulence in mice are distributed randomly amongst the extremely virulent ones. The simple explanation, that virulence is always porportional to the doubling-time does not, therefore, appear to be tenable. A more detailed examination of the shape of the growth curve of these variant antigen types in the mouse and, especially their relationship to and influence on, the rate of development of the immune response appears to be needed before a viable hypothesis for the observed differences can be proposed.

VI. Changes in virulence following passage

A. IN LABORATORY ANIMALS OR OTHER "UNNATURAL" HOSTS

The classical method for increasing the virulence of a pathogen for any host is by repeated, rapid, passage through that host. The effect observed may be explained by assuming that the most rapidly growing organisms, be they mutants or other variants, are preferentially transferred at each passage. However, as has been discussed in Section V, high virulence may not be due to rapid growth alone, which would be the ideal circumstance for this type of population change on sequential transfers.

Amongst the trypanosomes, rapid syringe passage, rather than cyclical passage through an insect vector, appears to be essential if an increase in virulence is to be obtained. Early investigators showed considerable interest in this aspect of the disease and have provided many reports. For instance, Mesnil (1912) passaged a stock of *T. b. gambiense* in rats. Initially they survived for 202 days, but after repeated passage for seven years, this was gradually reduced to 10 days. However, he noted that even at this extreme the stock was still less virulent than a stock of *T. b. rhodesiense* available to him. Sir David Bruce (Bruce et al., 1914a) passaged a *T. b. brucei* stock repeatedly through dogs and noted that it developed greatly increased virulence. Oehler (1914b) found that passaging *T. b. brucei* in mice increased its monomorphism and virulence so markedly that after 20 passages the animals died in 6-8 days without showing remission.

Other trypanosomes able to grow in laboratory animals also showed the same effect. Blacklocke and Yorke (1913b) found that the survival time of rats infected with *T. congolense* from a horse was initially about 89 days, but after 51 passages this was reduced to 9 days.

Syringe passage of a trypanosome stock in one species of host, and thus increasing the virulence of the stock to that species, might be expected to attenuate it in respect of a second species of host. Terry (1910), working with *T. evansi*, observed this effect. A stock of high virulence for mice became greatly attenuated in respect of them after being passaged for 6 months in guinea-pigs. In the latter, however, it greatly increased in virulence during this time.

Repeated passage does not, however, invariably bring about an increase in virulence. Laveran (1915a) passaged a stock of *T. b. gambiense* for 12 years in guinea-pigs during which time it became less virulent for them, eventually taking 9 months to kill the animals. A similar attenuation was observed by Darling (1912), working with *T. evansi.* In his experiments, guinea-pigs eventually survived for over a year, whilst still showing a low parasitaemia. It is well known that, following passage to laboratory animals, *T. vivax* is unable to survive once serum of the original host is withdrawn (Hoare, 1972). A reduction of ability to survive for more than a few passages in the laboratory host is also occasionally seen in *T. b. brucei* infections. For example, Gitatha (1968) isolated this subspecies from an infected African buffalo into mice. There was a reduction in the parasitaemia reached at each passage until the third, after which the stock was lost. Also, there are the somewhat bizarre experiments of Wendelstadt and Fellmer (1910) in which they passaged *T. b. brucei* through tortoises, lizards, beetles, and slugs before returning it to the rat. Their report was to the effect that, in addition to morphological changes, there was an increase in virulence.

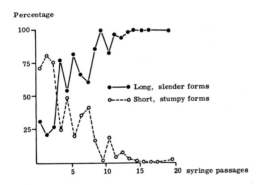

FIG. 7.   Development of monomorphism on rapid syringe passage of *T. brucei brucei* in rats. Redrawn after Bruce *et al.* (1914b).

The increase in virulence seen in *T. brucei* sspp. on passage is associated with the development of monomorphism, whether the passage is in mice (Allsopp *et al.*, 1969) or rats (Bruce *et al.*, 1914b) as is well shown in Fig. 7. In both hosts, almost complete monomorphism and the highest virulence was achieved after about 16–18 passages. In all large trypanosome populations, even those derived in the best conditions from a single organism, a minority are present that express characters different from those of the majority that have been selected for by the cloning process.

For instance, Van Meirvenne *et al.* (1975a, b) showed that heterotypes of many variant antigen types were present, in a proportion of about 1 : 10 000 in any putative defined variable antigen type population. Other characters, such as that for virulence, may be expressed in a similar proportion, and may in fact be genetically linked. It is easy, therefore, to conclude that a simple selective process, in which that part of the population that grows best in the host is transferred in ever more preferential numbers at each passage, can account for the observed increase in virulence. There will be natural selection for the forms that survive best when spread by the vector available, in this case a syringe. The observations provide no evidence that change in the genome has occurred or that mutants have been selected. Nevertheless the grossly reduced virulence of the "Tinde" stock (see below, Section VIb) on its return to sheep after extended passage in mice (Ashcroft, 1957b) would provide positive evidence for mutational change, whilst *T. b. rhodesiense*, passaged by Laveran (1915a) for 12 years in guinea-pigs without losing its resistance to human serum, is evidence against. Proof could only be obtained by a careful analysis of the change and this would require that each passage was effected with identified single organisms. However, the apparent regularity with which extreme virulence and monomorphism results from repeated syringe passage gives rise to a suspicion that the ability to effect this change is built into the genome of many trypanosome stocks. It may therefore be that different variable antigen types are operating those differing sections of their genome (operons) which give them their selective advantage *in vivo*.

B. IN "NATURAL" HOSTS

Field observations of trypanosomiasis have occasionally indicated that changes in virulence can be identified during the course of an epidemic. If an epidemic be assumed to result from the spread of a single stock, rather than from the activation of many different endemic ones, changes in virulence can be attributed to variation in that stock during cyclical passage. During the classical outbreak of sleeping sickness in Uganda at the turn of the century, an apparent increase in the virulence of *T. b. rhodesiense* was seen; the virulence being greater as the disease progressed northwards (Ormerod, 1961). This could have been due to the gradual predominance of an especially virulent line of a single stock. Or, on the other hand, it could have been a stock that was able to propagate more effectively, e.g. by being able to colonize tsetse better than the others.

Few experiments have been carried out to test the effect of repeated passage in a natural host. The most exhaustive is the "Tinde" experiment. This was carried out in Uganda where a stock of *T. b. rhodesiense*

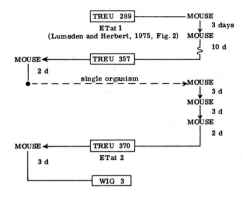

FIG. 8.   Pedigree of stabilate WIG 3. This was identified as being of variable antigen type ETat 2. Even though it is not descended from the type-type of ETat 2 it nevertheless possesses the same character of extreme virulence. TREU 289 is a 29th passage population derived from primary isolation BUSOGA/60/EATRO/3 and is in direct line from the type-type of ETat 1. The conventional signs follow the same scheme as those used in Fig. 4, q.v.

was maintained in sheep for 23 years as a line passaged by *G. morsitans* (Ashcroft, 1957a, 1959). When virulence was measured in terms of the length of life of rats infected with this stock by *Glossina* that had been fed on various hosts, it was found to be less virulent when obtained from the sheep than when obtained from antelopes or monkeys (in which it had been passaged). Moreover, on return of the stock from rat back to sheep no increased virulence was seen (Ashcroft, 1957b, 1959). However, syringe passage of the stock as a mouse line for 20 years caused it to become monomorphic and of extreme virulence for the mice killing them in 5–6 days. Sheep infected, by syringe, with this mouse line showed complete recovery from the infection in 30–35 days, whereas the sheep in which the fly line was continuing to be passaged invariably died (Ashcroft, 1957c, 1960).

A similar conservation of virulence, though over a much shorter period, has been shown for cyclically transmitted *T. vivax*. A highly virulent stock of this species examined by Lewis (1954) was found to retain its virulence to cattle, on transmission by *G. pallidipes*, over a period of 3 years. Even syringe passage of *T. vivax* through 39 goats over a period of 2½ years produced no variation in its virulence to this host, it uniformly killed them in 29–30 days. However, at the end of the passage sequence some change had occurred in that the stock was then said to be able to infect rabbits (Blacklocke and Yorke, 1913a).

Thus, despite the lack of definition, inevitable at present, of the field strains passaged in their natural hosts there seems no evidence of gross changes in virulence in these circumstances such as is seen when the organisms are syringe passaged in small laboratory rodents.

VII. Changes in virulence induced by drugs

Early work on the resistant forms of trypanosomes that appear after ineffective drug treatment reported them as being of varying virulence. Sometimes this was reduced (Browning, 1908; Moore et al., 1908) or, in other cases, their virulence was enhanced (Moore et al., 1908).

Apart from resistance, another effect of drugs can be the appearance of trypanosomes that, on light microscopy, appear to have lost their kinetoplast. Similar dyskinetoplastic forms may appear spontaneously particularly in stocks of T. evansi and in monomorphic lines (Vickerman and Preston, Vol. 1, Chapter 2). Some dyskinetoplastic stocks have been reported to be of lower virulence than the stock from which they originated. This effect has been reported for T. evansi and T. b. brucei (Laveran, 1911, 1915b) but Mühlpfordt (1964) found a shorter doubling time in dyskinetoplastic forms of T. evansi. He did not comment on their virulence but, as has been discussed above (Section V), this may not necessarily be associated with increased virulence.

Both the selection of resistant mutants and drug damage to the organism's DNA (and many trypanocidal drugs have an affinity for DNA) might be expected to result in the propagation of forms that, although efficient in that they could withstand the drug, might be inefficient in other respects. A decrease in virulence in such circumstances would then be the expected outcome.

VIII. Variation in virulence following exposure to high ambient temperatures

A moderating influence of high ambient temperature on the virulence of trypanosome infections appears first to have been reported by Oehler (1914b). He examined a stock of T. b. brucei that killed mice, kept at room temperature, in 6-8 days without remission. This same stock, in mice kept in an incubator at 35°C only produced an acute infection in about half of the animals, the others showed a chronic relapsing infection. These observations have been confirmed by the present authors (unpublished observations) and especially by Otieno (1972) who examined a defined population of the variable antigen type ETat 2. Examples of this variable antigen type, when derived from primary isolation BUSOGA/66/EATRO/3, seem always to show extreme virulence in mice. As noted in Section V above, a mouse infected with a single organism and kept at normal room temperature invariably dies without showing remission of the infection. However, mice similarly infected but kept in a hot room at between 35°C and 37°C exhibit a chronic relapsing infection. Moreover, the present authors, in association with Dr. R. F. MacAdam, have observed that the usual pathological changes seen in chronic trypanosomiasis in mice, e.g. an enlarged spleen and liver, are absent in these mice.

Thus, under the influence of high ambient temperature an extremely virulent trypanosome shows only moderate virulence. Whether the essential difference is in the response of the host or is a change in the behaviour of the parasite is unknown. The effect of high ambient temperature cannot be upon ETat 2 alone for there are many other equally virulent types in the ETat serodeme which would be expected to appear during the relapses in the chronic infection that are seen in mice kept at incubator temperature.

Otieno (1972) suggested that the effect observed resulted from low oxygen tension in the blood of the mice held at high ambient temperature, it having been reported (Fulton and Spooner, 1957) that freshly isolated strains differ from syringe passaged strains, in their oxygen requirements. The observed reduction in virulence was particularly apparent in the latter, which consume most oxygen.

An alternative hypothesis is that there is a change in the development of the trypanosome due to abolition of the temperature gradient that normally exists between the skin and the body core. In large animals, in the tropics, trypanosome parasitaemia as detected in the peripheral blood is known to vary at different times of the day and thus at different ambient temperatures. The body of a host within an incubator would be at core temperature throughout. It may be that in these circumstances an interruption to the normal development of the trypanosome population would take place, there being no cool skin (the site of vector transmission) available to stimulate proper development of the vector-infective stumpy forms. However, such an explanation, i.e. encouragement of the production of long thin trypanosomes, does not conform with what is otherwise known about such forms, for in monomorphic infections these seem extraordinarily virulent.

IX. General discussion

In this concluding section, three aspects of virulence are discussed. Firstly, the meaning of the term "virulence"; secondly, the mechanisms by which a trypanosome is able to multiply in the body of the host despite the host's defences; and thirdly, how, having multiplied, it inflicts damage on the tissues of that host.

A. HOW SHOULD THE TERM "VIRULENCE" BE DEFINED?

The current concept of virulence is solely that of a capacity to inflict damage to the host and this definition is adhered to throughout the present chapter. However, investigation of the natural history of any microbial infection ultimately centres on the interplay between the multiplying microorganism and the escalating defence against it. In this context, the attribute of the microorganism that is termed virulence could be defined as its ability to turn the balance in favour of itself, whether or not by so doing it inflicts damage on the host. But this may be a limited concept, for the most successful micro-organisms should be those which survive without seriously jeopardizing the life of the host; examples amongst the trypanosomes have been presented earlier.

Thus, during the preparation of this chapter it has become evident to us that there exist deficiences in the terminology at present employed to describe and classify pathogenic interactions between micro-organisms and their hosts. Further terms require to be introduced and the present ones more closely defined. For instance, in addition to our comment above we also have doubts, for example as to whether "high" virulence should imply early death of most hosts, or *eventual* death of all hosts from the infection even if this takes years to happen. Such queries can easily be multiplied and it is clear that improvement in the terminology would invigorate investigation into this vital area of host–parasite interaction.

B. MICRO-ORGANISMAL MULTIPLICATION AND VIRULENCE

As indicated in Section I, C above, there is no generally accepted evidence that trypanosomes (even the tissue dwelling forms) are themselves directly pathogenic even when present in large numbers. For example, parasitaemias of the order of 10^7–10^8 per ml can be tolerated, which implies that damage due to a toxin is an unlikely cause of the trypanosome's pathogenicity. It could, of course, be that only very small amounts of toxin are liberated and so a large number of organisms is required for its production. Against this is the fact that drug treatment at a late stage can effect a cure without apparent pathogenic sequelae. Also, a relatively small increase in the level of parasitaemia to 10^9 organisms per ml is frequently associated, in mice, with death. Indeed, in mice, death occurring at this point has been shown to be due to hypoglycaemia (Herbert *et al.*, 1975). Correction of the hypoglycaemic state, even in the terminal stages, can temporarily prevent a lethal consequence. It is tempting to postulate that the massive overgrowth of the trypanosomes uses more of the host's glucose than the latter can replace, a situation analogous to the ultilization of glucose by bacteria in the cerebrospinal fluid in pyogenic meningitis. The explanation for the hypoglycaemia could of course, be different, but this would not detract from the basic premise that trypanosomes in the mouse infection must multiply up to levels of 10^9 per ml before death occurs. The situation appears to be "all or nothing" in the sense that there is little *observable* evidence of host damage prior to the attainment of this order of host parasitaemia and it is therefore clearly of fundamental importance to consider the factors which allow this trypanosome overgrowth to occur.

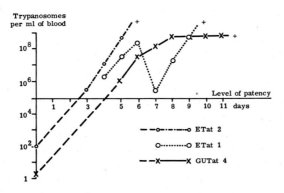

FIG. 9.   Three possible outcomes of the interaction between trypanosome and host. The data are taken from experiments in which individual mice had been infected with either: antilog 2·0 ID_{63} of stabilate WIG 41, variable antigen type ETat 2; or antilog 0·4 ID_{63} of stabilate WIG 84, variable antigen type GUTat 4; or an unknown number of infective doses of stabilate WIG 30, variable antigen type ETat 1. GUTat 4 has been isolated from a stock descended from primary isolate LUGALA/69/EATRO/1244. On day 10 of the GUTat 4 infection a trypanosome lysis test was carried out and the population of trypanosomes in the mouse was found to be over 99% GUTat 4. The dashed lines show theoretical growth from the infecting doses where this is known. The parasitaemias were estimated by the matching method of Herbert and Lumsden (1976). $+$ = death of host.

It would be expected that trypanosomes which were able to multiply most rapidly would reach levels of parasitaemia that were lethal faster than more slowly growing organisms. However, the evidence for this is poor (see Tables 2, 3 and 4). As indicated earlier, trypanosome rate of multiplication (mean doubling time) is not significantly different between highly virulent and poorly virulent clones. Moreover, the data in Table 2 imply that an immune response capable of effecting remission of *T. brucei brucei* infections in the mouse exists by the fifth or sixth day of infection. However, infection with an extremely virulent variable antigen type of *T. b. rhodesiense* only causes death of the host on the 7th or 8th day of infection (Table 2), that is, *after* an effective immune response should have been available.

In such circumstances it is very tempting to postulate the existence of a factor which "protects" the parasite from the developing immune response; the appearance of trypanosomes with new variable antigens, perhaps acting as a protective coat, has supported this idea. Nevertheless, there is ample evidence that the organisms comprising the bulk of the population do not change their surface antigen as their numbers increase. The small numbers of trypanosomes present as heterotypes, expressing other variable antigens on their surface, remain as a tiny proportion of the whole (Van Meirvenne *et al.*, 1975a), and these types also can be shown to be capable of being neutralized by antibody. Also only a few variable antigen types have a lethal or highly virulent potential in mice. The possession of a particular variable antigen type cannot therefore explain the differences in virulence of each type. Although there is evidence of an association between certain variable antigens (e.g., ETat 2) and high virulence, it seems probable that these factors (antigenic identity and virulence) will always be found to be independent characters. In the case of AnTat 1, this has now been clearly demonstrated (Fig. 10).

Returning to the question of multiplication rate, it must be remembered that the calculated values have been obtained from counts of trypanosomes in the blood taken at two (or more) different points in the infection. Such data allows the observable rate of multiplication to be determined but this is not necessarily the real rate. As the organism multiplies some of the organisms would be expected to be removed by the immune response or other mechanisms. The parasitaemia observed at any one time is, thus, an estimate of the residual organisms, not of the total mass produced, i.e. viable and multiplying organisms, plus non-viable organisms, plus organismal fragments in the process of elimination, plus already eliminated material. However, as death of the host occurs regularly at a fixed point (reflected, in mice, as a parasitaemia of about 10^9 per ml) it seems likely that the total mass is an important parameter. It may be seen, therefore, that a slowly-multiplying trypanosome cannot effect a change in mass from $\ell m/2$ to ℓm (where ℓm is the lethal mass) before the immune response has doubled its capacity. A rapidly multiplying organism, on the other hand, is easily able to achieve this. Indeed an organism can only increase its mass in a host if its rate of multiplication exceeds the rate of its destruction by the defences of the host. Furthermore, the rate of destruction must be directly related to the rate of increase in the immune responses (cellular, humoral and cell-mediated) of the host. But, as with most opposing factors in

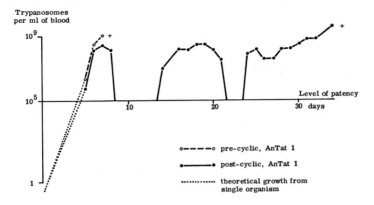

FIG. 10. Growth, in mice, of two clones recovered from a stock originating from primary isolation MUVUBWE/66/EATRO/1125, the origin of the AnTat serodeme. Both exhibit the variable antigen type, AnTat 1. The extremely virulent clone (doubling time 5·73 h, see Table 4) was obtained after repeated syringe passage of the stock. The moderately virulent clone (doubling time 6·34 h) was obtained after cyclical transmission of a similar, extremely virulent, clone through *Glossina* (Le Ray *et al.*, 1977). A separation of the characters responsible for antigenic identity and for virulence is thus demonstrated.

In each case, the infections shown were initiated by a single organism and the parasitaemias estimated by the matching method. The theoretical portions of the growth curves have their origins at half an organism per ml on the assumption that the blood volume of a mouse is about 2 ml. (Unpublished results, presented here by kind permission of Dr. David Barry.)

nature, the closer their convergence, the slower the convergence becomes. Thus the change from a mass of $\ell m/16$ to $\ell m/8$ will take place more quickly than the change from $\ell m/8$ to $\ell m/4$ and so on, because a greater proportion of organisms will be destroyed in the second period than in the first. It can thus be predicted that a lethal infection will take longer to end, because of the slow increase to lethal mass, than an infection that would remit at a smaller trypanosome mass. The data in Tables 2 and 3, although obtained from limited experiments, tend to support this view and we would suggest that the hypothesis given provides a reasonable explanation of an otherwise paradoxical situation.

There is, however, another important conclusion to be drawn from the data in Tables 2 and 3. Reference to Table 3 indicates that the higher the infecting dose, the sooner death occurs. This is to be expected as the increased dose enables the organism to reach the lethal mass more quickly thereby outstripping the immune response (Fig. 1). This is a basic tenet of microbiological thought which holds for all infections. However, on the same basis it would be expected that, for an organism that produces a remitting infection, remission would occur earlier with low doses than with high doses because the immune response in the low dose instance would be effective more quickly. Clearly the reverse is the case (Table 2), and this paradox can only be resolved if it is assumed that the immune response "paces" itself according to the rate which is set by the organisms.

We would suggest that the stimulus to develop the immune responses is the *rate* of expansion of microorganism mass and that the differences in virulence of different trypanosomes, as explained above, depends on their *rate* of multiplication in the host. Thus, it is possible to envisage many outcomes of experimental infection. A low infective dose of a relatively slowly multiplying trypanosome will stimulate a sluggish response with a prolonged infection leading eventually to remission. A higher dose of the same organism, because of the more rapidly expanding mass afforded by the high dose will stimulate a more vigorous response and result in earlier remission. Similarly, a high dose of virulent trypanosomes will stimulate a vigorous immune response but death will occur because the *rate* of increase of the response cannot exceed the rate of multiplication of the organism. A lower dose of the same trypanosome gives the host response a chance to catch up, but this amounts only to a prolongation of the interval to death because the rate of multiplication of the organism, as defined above, will always exceed the rate of increase of the immune response to it. Thus virulence may be seen as directly related to the rate of multiplication of the microorganism in the particular host. The variations described above influence only the *pattern* of disease produced, i.e. acute fatal, chronic fatal, acute remitting, chronic remitting, etc. Examples of these are shown in Figs. 9 and 10.

However, instead of continuing to expand a hypothesis founded on the theoretical ideas outlined above, it is wise to assess the practical aspects of the situation. It then appears that, at present, information vital to the argument is unavailable because details of multiplication rates *in vivo* are always based on observed trypanosomes only and therefore cannot be the *actual* rates (see above). Conversely, any *in vitro* determination of multiplication would remain suspect if only because the counter balance of the immune response was lacking. In order to overcome these defects, we would suggest that rather than attempt to assess the number of organisms by counting, methods be developed which can, by using a marker (biochemical, antigenic etc.), directly measure the total mass of organisms in the body of the host and thereafter the rate of increase of this mass. Techniques analogous to the recently-described immunoassay of *Candida albicans* antigen (Warren *et al.*, 1977) might be envisaged for this purpose. If similar techniques can be evolved to study the increasing response to the trypanosomes, the essential information necessary for a proper analysis of host–trypanosome interplay would then be available.

C. MECHANISMS OF TRYPANOSOME PATHOGENICITY IN RELATION TO VIRULENCE

In the course of the present review, various suggestions have been made to account for the differences in virulence reported, differences in growth-rates amongst variable antigen types and their influence on the rate of development of the immune response. However, as has been pointed out, there is, as yet, no generally accepted evidence that trypanosomes are themselves directly pathogenic even when present in large numbers after fast growth. Indeed their low, or moderate, virulence in many hosts is strong evidence to the contrary. None the less, they do often produce overt disease. We suggest that it is possible to explain the differences in pathogenicity observed, by the hypothesis that the most important factor in this is hypersensitivity.

The predominantly important types of hypersensitivity involved in our hypothesis are types II and III of Gell *et al.* (1975), i.e. cytotoxic and immune complex forms. Type I (anaphylactic hypersensitivity), which is responsible for diseases such as hay-fever and asthma, is unlikely to be involved to any great extent. This type is mediated by mast-cell sensitizing antibody largely of the IgE immunoglobulin class. This shows only a slight, probably insignificant, elevation in human infection (Herbert *et al.*, in preparation). Type IV, delayed hypersensitivity due to cell-mediated immunity, is, so far, ill-defined in salivarian trypanosome infections. There is, however, evidence for it in the form of lymphocyte accumulations and granulomatous lesions late in chronic *T. brucei* infections, when the parasite has spread to tissues other than blood (Losos and Ikede, 1972; Murray, 1974). Type II hypersensitivity, on the other hand, has been suggested as being responsible for the anaemia seen in the disease (Herbert and Inglis, 1973; Woo and Kobayashi, 1974). The mechanism proposed is similar to that operating in the disease fowl typhoid (Buxton, 1959). It is suggested that variable antigens released by the trypanosomes *in vivo* become coated on to the host's erythrocytes. At each remission of infection these antigen-coated erythrocytes are destroyed by antibody, simultaneously with the parasites. Repetition of the process as each variant arises could explain the chronic erythrocyte loss. In addition, reactive haemolysis at the time of remission may also cause additional loss of erythrocytes.

The major cause of tissue damage, however, is likely to be the complexes of antigen with antibody, which are repeatedly formed during the course of the disease (Boreham and Kimber, 1970). Such damage, due to "immune complexes" is classified by Gell and Coombs as Type III hypersensitivity. There is good general evidence from experimental models, and in human disease, that immune complexes are responsible for tissue damage, notably in the kidneys of the patient (McLean and Michael, 1974). It would be possible then for such complexes to be deposited in the arteries of tissues other than kidney, for instance the lungs and liver, with resultant damage. The damage is caused by activation of complement which induces chemotaxis of polymorphonuclear leucocytes to the site of immune complex deposition and their accumulation there. A focus of inflammation is thus produced (Goldstein and Weissmann, 1974).

The key factor in the precipitation of such damage is the relative proportion of antigen to antibody in the complex. Complexes that are formed in *slight* (4 to 10 times) antigen excess are particularly harmful, seemingly because they persist, and therefore are inflammatory, for long periods of time (Cochrane, 1965). Indeed, serum sickness, which can be thought analogous to trypanosomiasis in that antigen–antibody reactions occur in the circulation, has been shown to occur only when an excess of antigen is present (Dixon *et al.*, 1961). From the discussion in Section IX, A above, it follows that in trypanosomiasis the chances of the organism's multiplication exceeding the immune (antibody) response are always high. Thus with rapidly multiplying trypanosomes, the quantity of antigen lost from the organisms either naturally (exo- or released antigen) or following disintegration, is large, whereas with slowly multiplying organisms antigen becomes available much more gradually. In this latter case it is likely that antibody production will overwhelm the antigen output producing a remission of the disease and consequently obviating the possibility that an excess of antigen will persist for a prolonged period. Thus the former, rapidly multiplying, organisms will precipitate more immune-complex-mediated damage and therefore will be more pathogenic.

A second important aspect of immune-complex hypersensitivity is that the quantity of complex (of appropriate damaging type, i.e. antigen–antibody ratio) formed determines the *amount* of tissue damage which results. The greater the amount of complex that is formed the greater is the complement activation. This in turn leads to more polymorphonuclear leucocyte accumulation and more inflammatory damage. Clearly *some* immune complex damage follows *every* antigen–antibody interaction, although, as in the example given above, where the formation of complexes is limited to a short period the *absolute* quantity of complexes is small. If the infection is cured at this stage the resulting damage will be slight and quickly repaired. In trypanosomiasis, of course, the outcome is not so favourable because antigenic variation leads to a chronic remitting parasitaemia. The cumulative damage produced by many short episodes of immune complex formation is likely to be as great as the damage caused by one long episode, and ultimately the damage to the tissues will be enough to cause death.

Such premises enable the gross differences in virulence that are to be seen amongst the trypanosome infections, to be explained as follows:

1. An explosive outgrowth of the trypanosome population from immune restriction which precipitates fatal biochemical changes in the host. This is *not* an immunological hypersensitivity.

2. A rapid outgrowth which is insufficient to induce biochemical disaster but is sufficient to lead to massive immune complex formation and rapid death.

3. A slower outgrowth (of remitting infection by variant antigen types) which, over a long period, produces cumulative tissue damage and death.

4. Trypanosome growth that is contained and eradicated by a rapid immune response. In this instance there will be cure and little accumulation of immune complexes, perhaps resulting in an asymptomatic episode of infection.

Accepting these general mechanisms as a basis to explain the differences in outcome of various trypanosome infections it is possible to comment, from an immunological point of view, on the three unusual problems of virulence outlined earlier.

1. The rôle of common and heterophile antigens in the production of immunological damage (see also Chapter 11).

It is curious to note that the repeated release, in the early stages of a remitting infection, of large quantities of common antigens is unlikely to result in the production of damaging immune complexes. The common antigen will be released into the presence of existing antibody (at least after the first variant population has been destroyed so that antibodies to the internal antigens are stimulated) and will induce a rapid secondary response. The balance will therefore be one of continual antibody excess which is not of great danger.

However, late in the disease, due to antigenic competition and immunosuppression (Greenwood *et al.*, 1973) resulting from the need of the host to respond to the repeated appearance of new variable antigens, there will be a reduced ability to respond to the common antigens. In this situation, a disease-causing antigen–antibody ratio may appear. Complexes formed in this way will be particularly damaging as large quantities of the common antigens are released over a short period as each variable antigen type is destroyed. Such a situation can be envisaged to occur late in the course of the infection and will accelerate the pathogenic effect of the disease at this time.

2. Reduction in virulence of stocks in hosts kept at high ambient temperatures (Section VIII of this chapter)

In this case a key observation may be the lack of abnormal pathology seen in mice kept at elevated temperatures (R. F. MacAdam, personal communication). Thus it may be that no damaging immune complexes were formed because the rate of production of the trypanosome antigen kept exactly in step with the rate of antibody production.

3. Tolerance of birds to mammalian trypanosome infections

The low virulence of mammalian trypanosomes to birds may have nothing to do with our postulate of a long evolutionary relationship (Section II, B). The key factor could be the known rapid antibody response of birds. Not only may this lead to rapid removal of the organisms but also an equalization of the rates of production of antigen and antibody so that damaging complexes are not produced.

D. CONCLUSION

The authors conclude that trypanosome virulence is not merely a reflection of the aggressive nature and abilities of these highly sophisticated microorganisms. More important are their interactions with, and ability to stimulate, to control and, it might be said, to direct, the reactions of their host. These various aspects may be difficult to unravel but with the increasing availability of serodemes of organisms with defined characteristics and the development of techniques for quantitating antigens present *in vivo*, many of the suggestions made in this chapter could be tested. Confirmation, or otherwise, would be of great value in helping to explain the pathogenesis, not only of trypanosomiasis, but of other chronic infections and, also, of diseases resulting from repeated exposure to non-replicating antigens.

X. Acknowledgements

We are grateful to D. Barry, R. A. Joshua, W. H. R. Lumsden, D. Shipwright and K. Vickerman for provocative discussions on the subject of this paper. We are also very grateful to Dr. David Barry, Dr. R. A. Joshua and Professor R. G. White for permission to quote their unpublished results.

XI. References

Allsopp, B. A., Walker, P. J., Nguli, K. N. and Watts, J. M. A. (1969). Acquisition of monomorphism and change in drug sensitivity by strains of *T. rhodesiense* isolated from humans. *East African Trypanosomiasis Research Organization Report 1969*, p. 18.

Apted, F. I. C. (1970). The epidemiology of Rhodesian sleeping sickness. *In:* "The African Trypanosomiases" (H. W. Mulligan and W. H. Potts, ed.), p. 645. Allan and Unwin, London.

Ashcroft, M. T. (1957a). The continued infectivity to man of strains of *T. rhodesiense* maintained in animals. *East African Trypanosomiasis Research Organization Report 1956–57*, p. 33.

Ashcroft, M. T. (1957b). The influence of the host animal on the virulence of a strain of *T. rhodesiense*. *East African Trypanosomiasis Research Organization Report 1956–57*, p. 36.

Ashcroft, M. T. (1957c). A comparison between a syringe-passaged and a fly-transmitted line of the same strain of *T. rhodesiense*. *East African Trypanosomiasis Research Organizational Report 1956–57*, p. 34.

Ashcroft, M. T. (1959). The Tinde Experiment: A further study of the long-term cyclical transmission of *Trypanosoma rhodesiense*. *Annals of Tropical Medicine and Parasitology*, **53**, 137–146.

Ashcroft, M. T. (1960). A comparison between a syringe-passaged and a tsetse-fly-transmitted line of a strain of *Trypanosoma rhodesiense*. *Annals of Tropical Medicine and Parasitology*, **54**, 44–59.

Ashcroft, M. T., Burtt, E. and Fairbairn, H. (1959). The experimental infection of some African wild animals with *Trypanosoma rhodesiense*, *T. brucei* and *T. congolense*. *Annals of Tropical Medicine and Parasitology*, **53**, 147–161.

Baker, J. R., Sachs, R. and Laufer, I. (1967). Trypanosomes of wild mammals in an area northwest of the Serengeti National Park, Tanzania. *Zeitschrift für Tropenmedizin und Parasitologie*, **18**, 280–284.

Bakker, R. T. (1972). Anatomical and ecological evidence of endothermy in donosaurs. *Nature, London*, **238**, 81–85.

Barnett, S. F. (1947). *Trypanosomiasis in the pig*. Ph.D. Thesis, University of London. Quoted by Hoare (1972).

Barotte, J. (1925). Les trypanosomiases de l'Afrique du Nord. *Memoires de la Société des Sciences naturelles du Moroc*, **11**, 1. Quoted by Hoare (1972).

Binns, H. R. (1938). Observations on the behaviour in laboratory animals of *Trypanosoma congolense* Broden, 1904. *Annals of Tropical Medicine and Parasitology*, **32**, 425–430.

Blacklock, B. and Yorke, W. (1913a). *Trypanosoma vivax* in rabbits. *Annals of Tropical Medicine and Parasitology*, **7**, 563–568.

Blacklock, B. and Yorke, W. (1913b). The probable identity of *Trypanosoma congolense* (Broden) and *T. nanum* (Laveran). *Annals of Tropical Medicine and Parasitology*, **7**, 603–607.

Blair, D. M. (1939). Human trypanosomiasis in Southern Rhodesia. 1911–38. *Transactions of the Royal Society of Tropical Medicine and Hygiene*, **32**, 729–742.

Boreham, P. F. L. and Kimber, C. D. (1970). Immune complexes in trypanosomiasis of the rabbit. *Transactions of the Royal Society of Tropical Medicine and Hygiene*, **64**, 168–169.

Browning, C. (1908). Chemotherapy in trypanosome infections: an experimental study. *Journal of Pathology and Bacteriology*, **12**, 166–190.

Bruce, D., Harvey, D., Hamerton, A. E., Davey, J. B. and Lady Bruce (1912). The morphology of *Trypanosoma Simiae* sp. nov. *Proceedings of the Royal Society*, **85B**, 477–481.

Bruce, D., Harvey, D., Hamerton, A. E. and Lady Bruce (1913a). Trypanosomes of domestic animals in Nyasaland. I. *Trypanosoma Simiae* sp. nov. Part II. The susceptibility of various animals to *T. Simiae*. *Proceedings of the Royal Society*, **87B**, 48–57.

Bruce, D., Harvey, D., Hamerton, A. E. and Lady Bruce (1913b). Trypanosome diseases of domestic animals in Nyasaland. III. *Trypanosoma pecorum*. *Proceedings of the Royal Society*, **87B**, 1–25.

Bruce, D., Hamerton, A. E., Watson, D. P. and Lady Bruce (1914b). The trypanosome causing disease in man in Nyasaland. The naturally infected dog strain. Part II. Susceptibility of animals. *Proceedings of the Royal Society*, **88B**, 130–138.

Bruce, D., Hamerton, A. E., Watson, D. P. and Lady Bruce (1914b). The trypanosome causing disease in man in Nyasaland. The naturally infected dog strain, Part I. Morphology. *Proceedings of the Royal Society*, **88B**, 111–130.

Buxton, A. (1959). The *in vivo* sensitization of avian erythrocytes with *Salmonella gallinarum* polysaccharide. *Immunology*, **2**, 203–210.

Chardôme, M. and Peel, E. (1967). "Les trypanosomes transmis par *Glossina morsitans* au Bugesera" (Rwanda et Burundi). Brussels (Ad. Goemaere). Quoted by Hoare (1972).

Cochrane, C. G. (1965). The Arthus Reaction. *In:* "The Inflammatory Process" (B. W. Zweifach, L. Grant and R. I. McCluskey, ed.). Academic Press; New York and London.

Conran, P. (1921). Intermissions in trypanosomiasis. *British Medical Journal*, **1**, 916.

Cooke, W. E., Gregg, A. L. and Manson-Bahr, P. H. (1937). Recent experiences of mild or symptomless infections with *Trypanosoma gambiense* from the Gold Coast and Nigeria. *Transactions of the Royal Society of Tropical Medicine and Hygiene*, **30**, 461–466.

Corson, J. F. (1931). Direct infection of native fowls with *Trypanosoma rhodesiense*. *Journal of Tropical Medicine and Hygiene*, **34**, 109.

Cross, H. E. (1921). The course that surra runs in ponies, buffaloes and other animals. *Bulletin. Agricultural Research Institute, Pusa*, No. 99. Quoted by Hoare (1972).

Culwick, A. T. and Fairbairn, H. (1947). Polymorphism in *Trypanosoma simiae* and the morphology of the metacyclic forms. *Transactions of the Royal Society of Tropical Medicine and Hygiene*, **41**, 415–418.

Cunningham, M. P., van Hoeve, K. and Lumsden, W. H. R. (1963). Variable infectivity of organisms of the *T. brucei* subgroup during acute relapsing infections in rats related to parasitaemia, morphology and antibody response. *East African Trypanosomiasis Research Organization Report 1962–63*, p. 21.

Curasson, G. (1943). *Traité de protozoologie veterinaire et comparée*. **1**. *Trypanosomes*. Paris. Quoted by Hoare (1972).

Curasson, G. and Mornet, P. (1948). *Trypanosoma vivax-cazalboui*. *Revue d'Élevage et de Médecine Vétérinaire des Pays Tropicaux*, **2**, 225.

Curson, H. H. (1928). Nagana in Zululand. *13th and 14th Reports of the Director of Veterinary Education and Research of the Department of Agriculture of South Africa*. Pt. 1, p. 309. Quoted by Hoare (1972).

Darling, S. T. (1912). Reduction of virulence in a strain of *Trypanosoma hippicum* selected from a guinea-pig. *Bulletin de la Société de Pathologie Exotique*, **5**, 184–187.

Davey, J. B. (1936). Trypanosomiasis. *British Medical Journal*, **1**, 1321–1322.

Desowitz, R. S. (1959). Studies of immunity and host-parasite relationships. 1. The immunological response of resistant and susceptible breeds of cattle to trypanosomal challenge. *Annals of Tropical Medicine and Parasitology*, **53**, 293–313.

Desowitz, R. S. and Watson, H. J. C. (1952). Studies on *Trypanosoma vivax*. III. Observations on the maintenance of a strain in white rats. *Annals of Tropical Medicine and Parasitology*, **46**, 92–100.

Dixon, F. J., Feldman, J. D. and Vazquez, J. J. (1961). Experimental glomerulo-nephritis: the pathogenesis of a laboratory model resembling the spectrum of human glomerulonephritis. *Journal of Experimental Medicine*, **113**, 899–919.

Duggan, A. J. (1962). A survey of sleeping sickness in Northern Nigeria from the earliest times to the present day. *Transactions of the Royal Society of Tropical Medicine*, **56**, 439–480.

Duke, H. L. (1933). The domestic fowl of Uganda as a host for trypanosomes of the *brucei* group. *Parasitology*, **25**, 171–191.

Edwards, J. T. (1926). The chemotherapy of surra (*Trypanosoma evansi*) infections of horses and cattle in India. *Transactions of the Royal Society of Tropical Medicine and Hygiene*, **20**, 10–71.

Fairbairn, H. (1953). Studies on *Trypanosoma vivax*. IX. Morphological differences in strains and their relationship to pathogenicity. *Annals of Tropical Medicine and Parasitology*, **47**, 394–405.

Fairbairn, H. and Culwick, A. T. (1949). The differentiation of the polymorphic trypanosomes. *Annals of Tropical Medicine and Parasitology*, **43**, 90–95.

Fulton, J. D. and Spooner, D. F. (1957). Comparison of the respiratory activity of an old and of a freshly isolated strain of *Trypanosoma rhodesiense*. *Annals of Tropical Medicine and Parasitology*, **51**, 417–421.

Gell, P. G. H., Coombs, R. R. A. and Lachmann, P. J. (1975). "Clinical Aspects of Immunology", 3rd ed., p. 761. Blackwell Scientific Publications.

Gitatha, S. K. (1968). Trypanosome isolation from various hosts. *East African Trypanosomiasis Research Organization Report, 1968*, p. 13.

Godfrey, D. G. (1966). The course of infection with a strain of *T. brucei* in donkeys. *Annual Report of the Nigerian Institute for Trypanosomiasis Research, 1966*, p. 40.

Godfrey, D. G. and Kilgour, V. (1976). Enzyme electrophoresis in characterizing the causative organism of Gambian trypanosomiasis. *Transactions of the Royal Society of Tropical Medicine and Hygiene*, **70**, 219–224.

Godfrey, D. G. and Killick-Kendrick, R. (1961). Bovine trypanosomiasis in Nigeria. I. The inoculation of blood into rats as a method of survey in the Donga Valley, Benue Province. *Annals of Tropical Medicine and Parasitology*, **55**, 287–297.

Goldstein, I. M. and Weissmann, G. (1974). Cellular and humoral mechanisms in immune complex injury. *Progress in immunology II*, **5**, 81–90.

Gomez Rodrigues, R. J. (1956). Estudio de la tripanosomiasis natural del canino (*Canis fam.*) en Venezuela. *Revista de Medicina Veterinaria y Parasitologia (Caracas)*, **15**, 63. Quoted by Hoare (1972).

Gray, A. R. (1965). Antigenic variation in clones of *Trypanosoma brucei*. 1. Immunological relationship of the clones. *Annals of Tropical Medicine and Parasitology*, **59**, 27–36.

Greenwood, B. M., Whittle, H. C. and Molyneux, D. H. (1973). Immunosuppres-

518   W. J. HERBERT AND D. PARRATT

sion in Gambian trypanosomiasis. *Transactions of the Royal Society of Tropical Medicine and Hygiene*, **67**, 846–850.

Haig, D. A. and Lund, A. S. (1948). Transmission of the South African strain of dourine to laboratory animals. *Onderstepoort Journal of Veterinary Science*, **23**, 59–61.

Harding, R. D. and Hutchinson, M. P. (1948). Sleeping sickness of an unusual type in Sierra Leone and its attempted control. *Transactions of the Royal Society of Tropical Medicine and Hygiene*, **41**, 481–512.

Herbert, W. J. and Inglis, M. D. (1973). Immunization of mice against *T. brucei* infection by the administration of released antigen adsorbed to erythrocytes. *Transactions of the Royal Society of Tropical Medicine and Hygiene*, **67**, 268.

Herbert, W. J. and Lumsden, W. H. R. (1976). *Trypanosoma brucei*: A rapid "matching" method for estimating the host's parasitaemia. *Experimental Parasitology*, **40**, 427–431.

Herbert, W. J., Mucklow, M. G. and Lennox, B. (1975). The cause of death in acute murine trypanosomiasis. *Transactions of the Royal Society of Tropical Medicine and Hygiene*, **69**, 4.

Hoare, C. A. (1956). Morphological and taxonomic studies on mammalian trypanosomes. VIII. Revision of *Trypanosoma evansi*. *Parasitology*, **46**, 130–172.

Hoare, C. A. (1972). "The Trypanosomes of Mammals". Blackwell Scientific Publications, Oxford.

Hood, Mary N. (1949). *Trypanosoma equiperdum*, *Trypanosoma brucei* and *Trypanosoma hippicum* infections in avian hosts. *American Journal of Tropical Medicine*, **29**, 379–387.

Hornby, H. E. (1952). "Animal Trypanosomiasis in Eastern Africa. 1949". London: H.M.S.O.

Hornby, H. E. (1953). Unpublished manuscript, quoted by Hoare (1972).

Houba, V., Brown, K. N. and Allison, A. C. (1969). Heterophile antibodies, M. antiglobulins and immunoglobulins in experimental trypanosomiasis. *Clinical and Experimental Immunology*, **4**, 113–123.

Hutyra, F., Marek, J. and Manninger, R. (1938). "Special Pathology and Therapeutics of the Diseases of Domestic Animals", 4th edn. London: Ballière.

Kinghorn, A. and Yorke, W. (1912). Trypanosomes obtained by feeding wild *Glossina morsitans* on monkeys in Luangwa Valley, Northern Rhodesia. *Annals of Tropical Medicine and Parasitology*, **6**, 317–323.

Kinghorn, A., Yorke, W. and Lloyd, L. (1913). Final report of the Luangwa sleeping sickness commission of the British South Africa Company 1911–1912. *Annals of Tropical Medicine and Parasitology*, **7**, 183–329.

Krijgsman, B. J. (1933). Biologische Untersuchungen ueber das system: Witstier-Parasit. I u II Teil: Die Entwicklung von *Trypanosoma evansi* in Mous und Ratte. *Zeitschrift für Parasitenkunde*, **5**, 592–602.

Lamborn, W. A. and Howat, C. H. (1936). A possible reservoir host of *Trypanosoma rhodesiense*. *British Medical Journal*, **1**, 1153–1155.

Laveran, A. (1911). Contribution a l'étude du *Trypanosoma brucei* sans blépharoplaste de Werbitzki. *Bulletin de la Société de Pathologie Exotique*, **4**, 233–239.

Laveran, A. (1915a). Au sujet d'un *Trypanosoma gambiense* qui, conservé depuis 12 ans chez des animaux, est resté-resistant au serum humain. *Bulletin de la Société de Pathologie Exotique*, **8**, 442–446.

Laveran, A. (1915b). Sur les varietés acentrosomiques artificielles des trypanosomes. *Comptes Rendus des Séances de l'Academie des Sciences, Paris*, **17**, 543–546.

Leese, A. S. (1927). "A Treatise on the One-humped Camel in Health and Disease". Haynes, Stamford, Lincs.

Leese, A. S. (1933). First supplement to: "A Treatise on the One-humped Camel". Leese, Guildford.

Le Ray, D., Barry, J. D., Easton, C. and Vickerman, K. (1977). First tsetse fly transmission of the "AnTat" serodeme of *Trypanosoma brucei*. *Annales de la Société Belge de Medecine Tropicale*, **57**, 369–381.

Lewis, E. A. (1954). Notes on *Trypanosoma vivax*: its transmission by tsetses and by syringe passage. V. *Meeting of the International Scientific Committee on Trypanosomiasis Research. Pretoria*, p. 85.

Losos, G. J. and Ikede, B. O. (1972). Review of pathology of diseases in domestic and laboratory animals caused by *Trypanosoma congolense*, *T. vivax*, *T. brucei*, *T. rhodesiense* and *T. gambiense*. *Veterinary Pathology*, **9**, supplement.

Lumsden, W. H. R. and Herbert, W. J. (1975). Pedigrees of the Edinburgh *Trypanosoma* (*Trypanozoon*) antigenic types (ETat). *Transactions of the Royal Society of Tropical Medicine and Hygiene*, **69**, 205–208.

Lumsden, W. H. R., Cunningham, M. P., Webber, W. A. F., van Hoeve, K. and Walker, P. J. (1963). A method for the measurement of the infectivity of trypanosome suspensions. *Experimental Parasitology*, **14**, 269–279.

Lumsden, W. H. R., Herbert, W. J. and McNeillage, G. J. C. (1973). "Techniques with Trypanosomes". Churchill Livingstone, Edinburgh & London.

Lumsden, W. H. R., Kimber, C. D. and Strange, M. (1977). *Trypanosoma brucei*: detection of low parasitaemias in mice by a miniature anion-exchanger/centrifuge technique. *Transactions of the Royal Society of Tropical Medicine and Hygiene*, **71**, 421–424.

McLean, R. H. and Michael, A. F. (1974). Activation of the complement system in renal conditions in animals and man. *Progress in Immunology II*, **5**, 69–79.

McNeillage, G. J. C. and Herbert, W. J. (1968). Infectivity and virulence of *Trypanosoma* (*Trypanozoon*) *brucei* to mice. 2. Comparison of closely related trypanosome antigenic types. *Journal of Comparative Pathology*, **78**, 345–349.

Mesnil, F. (1912). Variations de virulence du *Trypanosoma gambiense* de deux origines humaines. *Bulletin de la Société de Pathologie Exotique*, **5**, 375–380.

Mesnil, F. and Blanchard, M. (1912). Infections des poules dues aux *Trypanosoma gambiense* et *Tryp. rhodesiense*. *Comptes Rendus des Séances de la Société de Biologie (Paris)*, **72**, 938–940.

Mesnil, F. and Martin G. (1906). Sur la receptivité des oiseaux aux *trypanosomes* pathogènes pour les mammifères. *Comptes Rendus des Séances de la Société de Biologie (Paris)*, **60**, 739–741.

Mims, C. A. (1976). "The Pathogenesis of Infectious Disease". Academic Press, London.

Moore, B., Nierenstein, M. and Todd, J. L. (1908). Notes on the effects of therapeutic agents on trypanosomes in respect to (a) acquired resistance of the parasite to the drug; and (b) changes in virulence of the strains after escape from the drug. *Annals of Tropical Medicine and Parasitology*, **2**, 221–226.

Mühlpfordt, H. (1964). Die Generationsdauer verschiedener Trypanosomenarten. *Zeitschrift für Tropenmedizin und Parasitologie*, **15**, 145–153.

Murray, M. (1974). The pathology of African trypanosomiases. *Progress in Immunology II*, **4**, 181–192.

Ochmann, R. (1905). Trypanosomiasis bein Schweine. *Berliner Tierartzliche Wochenschrift*, **21**, 337–338.

Oehler, R. (1913). Ueber die Gewinnung reiner Trypanosomenstämme durch Einzellenübertragung. *Centralblatt für Bakteriologie Parasitenkunde und Infections-krankheiten, I, Ab. Orig.*, **67**, 569–571.

Oehler, R. (1914a). Untersuchungen über den Dimorphismus von *Trypanosoma brucei*. *Zeitschrift für Hygiene und Infektionskrankheiten*, **77**, 356–370.

Oehler, R. (1914b). Der Dimorphismus des *Trypanosome brucei* bei experimenteller Behandlung. *Zeitschrift für Hygiene und infectionskrankheiten*, 78, 188–192.

Ormerod, W. E. (1961). The study of volutin granules in trypanosomes. *Transactions of the Royal Society of Tropical Medicine and Hygiene*, 55, 313–327.

Ormerod, W. E. (1970). Pathogenesis and pathology of trypanosomiasis in man. *In:* "The African Trypanosomiases" (H. W. Mulligan, ed.), p. 587. Allen and Unwin, London.

Ostrom, J. H. (1973). The ancestry of birds. *Nature, London*, 242, 136.

Otieno, L. H. (1972). Influence of ambient temperature on the course of experimental trypanosomiasis in mice. *Annals of Tropical Medicine and Parasitology*, 66, 15–24.

Peel, E. and Chardôme, M. (1954a). Étude experimentale de souches de *T. simiae* Bruce 1912, transmises par *Glossina brevipalpis* du Mosso (Urundi). *Annales de la Société Belge de Médecine Tropicale*, 34, 345–360.

Peel, E. and Chardôme, M. (1954b). *Trypanosoma suis* Ochmann, 1905—trypanosome monomorphe pathogène de mammifères, evoluant dans les glandes salivaires de *Glossina brevipalpis* Newst. Mosso (Urundi). *Annales de la Société Belge de Médecine Tropicale*, 34, 277–295.

Pellegrini, D. (1948). *Trypanosoma simiae* (Bruce) infection of the camel. *East African Agricultural Journal*, 13, 207–210.

Rickman, L. R. and Robson, J. (1970). The testing of proven *Trypanosoma brucei* and *T. rhodesiense* strains by the blood incubation infectivity test. *Bulletin of the World Health Organization*, 42, 911–916.

Robertson, D. H. H. and Baker, J. R. (1957). A strain of *Trypanosoma gambiense* isolated from a case in Northern Uganda. *East African Trypanosomiasis Research Organization Report 1956–57*, p. 15.

Rodhain, J., van Goidsenhoven, C. and van Hoof, L. (1941). Étude d'une souche de *Trypanosome cazalboui* (*vivax*) du Ruanda. *Memoires de l'Institut r. Colonial Belge* (*Section des Sciences Naturelles et Médicales*), 11, 1. Quoted by Hoare, 1972.

Sartory, A., Lasseur, P. and Brissaud, H. (1915). Un cas de trypanosomiase chez un homme ayant quitté l'Afrique depuis huit ans. *Bulletin de l'Académie de Médecine* (*Paris*) 3rd ser., 73, 631–633.

Sergent, E., Sergent, E., Foley, H. and Lheritier, A. (1918). De la mortalité dans le Debab, trypanosomiase des dromadaires. *Bulletin de la Société de Pathologie Exotique*, 1, 568–570.

Stephen, L. E. (1966). "Pig Trypanosomiasis in Tropical Africa". Commonwealth Bureau of Animal Health. Review Series, No. 8.

Stephen, L. E. (1966). Observations on the resistance of West African N'dama and Zebu cattle to trypanosomiasis following challenge by wild *Glossina morsitans* from an early age. *Annals of Tropical Medicine and Parasitology*, 60, 230–246.

Stephen, L. E. (1970). Clinical manifestations of the trypanosomiases in livestock and other domestic animals. *In:* "The African Trypanosomiases" (H. W. Mulligan, ed.). Allen and Unwin, London.

Taylor, A. E. R. (1968). Studies on the rodent strain of *Trypanosoma vivax*. *Annals of Tropical Medicine and Parasitology*, 62, 375–381.

Terry, B. T. (1910). An attenuated surra of Mauritius with immunity tests after recovery. *Journal of Experimental Medicine*, 12, 176–181.

Terry, B. T. (1911). Trypanosomiasis in monkeys (*Macacus rhesus*) in captivity. *Proceedings of the Society for Experimental Biology and Medicine*, 9, 17–18.

Van Hoof, L., Henrard, C. and Peel, E. (1948). Quelques observations sur les trypanosomiase des grandes mammifères au Congo Belge. *Acta Tropica*, 5, 327–344.

Van Meirvenne, N., Janssens, P. G. and Magnus, E. (1975a). Antigenic variation in syringe passaged populations of *Trypanosoma* (*Trypanozoon*) *brucei*. I. Rationalization of the experimental approach. *Annales de la Société Belge de Médecine Tropicale*, **55**, 1–23.

Van Meirvenne, N., Janssens, P. G., Magnus, E., Lumsden, W. H. R. and Herbert, W. J. (1975b). Antigenic variation in syringe passaged populations of *Trypanosoma* (*Trypanozoon*) *brucei*. II. Comparative studies on two antigenic type collections. *Annales de la Société Belge de Médecine Tropicale*, **55**, 25–30.

Wallace, L. E., White, R. G. and Herbert, W. J. (1976). Massive segregation of B-cells in the germinal centres of the spleen of trypanosome-infected birds. *Transactions of the Royal Society of Tropical Medicine and Hygiene*, **70**, 279.

Warren, R. C., Bartlett, A., Bidwell, D. E., Richardson, M. D., Voller, A. and White, L. O. (1977). Diagnosis of invasive candidosis by enzyme immunoassay of serum antigen. *British Medical Journal*, **1**, 1183–1185.

Wells, E. A. (1971). Studies on *Trypanosoma theileri*-like trypanosomes of cattle. II. The characteristics of infection in a single Ayrshire cow. *British Veterinary Journal*, **127**, 470–475.

Wendelstadt, P. and Fellmer, T. (1910). Einwirkung von Kaltblüterpassagen auf Nagana -und Lewisi-Trypanosomen. II. Mitteilung. *Zeitschrift für Immunitatsforschung und Experimentelle Therapie*, **5**, 337–348.

Wenyon, C. M. and Hanschell, H. M. (1912). Notes on *Trypanosoma rhodesiense* from three cases of human trypanosomiasis. *Journal of the London School of Tropical Medicine*, **2**, 34–35.

Willett, K. C. (1970). Epizootiology of trypanosomiasis in livestock in East and Central Africa. *In:* "The African Trypanosomiases" (H. W. Mulligan, ed.), Allen and Unwin, London.

Woo, P. T. K. and Kobayashi, A. (1975). Studies on the anaemia in experimental African trypanosomiasis. 1. A preliminary communication on the mechanism of the anaemia. *Annales de la Société Belge de Médecine Tropicale*, **55**, 37–45.

Addendum

Joshua, R. A., Herbert, W. J. and White, R. G. (1978). Acquisition by *Trypanosoma brucei brucei* of potential infectivity for man by passage through birds. *Lancet*, **1**, 724–725.

Parratt, D. and Cobb, S. J. (1978). Heterophile antibody to red cells in human trypanosomiasis. *African Journal of Medical Science*, **7**, 57–64.

11

Heterophile Antibodies in Trypanosome Infections

D. PARRATT* and W. J. HERBERT

*Department of Bacteriology and Immunology,
(University of Glasgow),
Western Infirmary, Glasgow G11 6NT, Scotland*

I.	Introduction	524
II.	The nature of heterophile antigens	524
III.	The nature of heterophile antibodies	528
IV.	Heterophile erythrocyte antibodies in human trypanosomiasis .	530
	A. Introduction	530
	B. Differentiation of the heterophile response in *Trypanosoma brucei gambiense* and *T. b. rhodesiense* infections . . .	532
V.	Antibody specificity of the elevated immunoglobulin levels seen in trypanosomiasis	533
VI.	Application of heterophile antibodies for the diagnosis of trypanosomiasis	535
VII.	Heterophile antibodies in trypanosomiasis caused by *Trypanosoma* species other than *T. brucei* sub-species *gambiense* and *rhodesiense*	537
VIII.	Conclusions	539
	A. Diagnostic significance	539
	B. Biological significance	541
IX.	Acknowledgements	542
X.	References	542
XI.	Appendix I	544
XII.	Appendix II	544

* Present address: Department of Bacteriology, Ninewells Hospital, Dundee.

I. Introduction

In the course of many infectious diseases, antibodies appear in the host which are found to react strongly with antigens from species of plants, animals or microorganisms that are entirely unrelated to the parasite responsible for the infection. These antibodies have, therefore, the appearance of "rogue" antibody, are considered to be non-specifically derived and are thus termed "heterophile" antibody. It is often assumed that they represent a response to antigens of tissues damaged in the process of infection, as for example in malaria, where heterophile antibodies to erythrocyte antigens are thought to result from the destruction of the host's erythrocytes by the parasite (Faulk and Houba, 1973). In contrast, the heterophile antibody to sheep erythrocytes produced during the course of infectious mononucleosis in man (infection with Epstein–Barr virus, EBV) is so specific that its detection has been used for diagnosis of this disease for many years. The mechanism of production of this latter heterophile antibody is poorly established, although it is not produced by the human in any circumstance other than in infectious mononucleosis. This apart, the antibody does not appear to be produced in response to the EBV antigens. Such an antibody has a high degree of disease specificity (and is therefore useful for the diagnosis of the disease) but a poorly defined antigen specificity in the sense that the antigen stimulating its production cannot be easily identified; the antibody is fortuitously detected by the use of sheep erythrocytes.

The main intention of the present chapter is to consider the heterophile antibodies produced by trypanosome infections with respect to:

(a) Disease specificity: i.e. their usefulness as diagnostic markers of particular infections.

(b) Antigen specificity: i.e. the source and nature of the antigens which stimulate their production.

There are, however, features common to most heterophile antigens and heterophile antibodies, regardless of their derivation, and these aspects will be discussed in the two preliminary sections.

II. The nature of heterophile antigens

Heterophile antigens can be defined as antigens occurring in the tissues of many different species of animals, plants, or microorganisms, that show extensive cross-relationship due to structural similarities. A simple example concerns human blood group A substance, antibody to which cross-reacts well with polysaccharide material extracted from Type 14 pneumococcus (*Streptococcus pneumoniae*). There is no ready explanation for the cross reactivity in such a case where man and the pneumococcus are so unrelated, although it can be surmised that the cross reaction is due either to coincidence or to the persistence of a cellular component as an antigen from a common ancestor at some distant point in evolution.

The latter aspect receives some support from the finding that well-recognized heterophile antigens (e.g., Forssman antigen) have been shown to be basic constituents of cell walls or cell membranes (Boyd, 1956; Humphrey and White, 1970) and are components of those structures which perform important functions and therefore probably impart survival advantages. Substances such as these would tend to persist during evolution, although it is possible that some ancestral forms would lose the antigen or replace it by a similar substance. In this way any single antigen might eventually become widely and randomly distributed in present-day life forms, with analogous antigens in other species. Inevitably, the process of defining the species distribution of heterophile antigens is arduous, and those antigens whose distribution is well-defined have only been the subject of research because their chance discovery was coincident with a useful diagnostic or scientific application. In contrast, the chemical definition of some heterophile antigens is advanced. This is particularly so for the Forssman antigen(s), and it has become clear in this case that the receptor is in fact a hapten, composed of glycolipid (Fraser and Mallette, 1974).*

This means that a basic molecule containing the hapten may show little chemical variation between species whilst the specificity of its antigenic reaction, determined by the hapten(s), may be different. In this way, it is possible to envisage Forssman positivity and Forssman negativity in molecules which are chemically very similar in, for example, the erythrocytes of horse and rabbit respectively. Further, with the reverse case, minor changes of specificity would be expected to follow small structural changes of the hapten and this has been shown to be the case with the Forssman system (Fraser and Mallette, 1974). Nevertheless, of importance here is the recently advanced concept that antibodies may have more than one specificity and therefore may be reactive with as many as a hundred different antigens by virtue of the structural similarity (but not identity) of the latter (Richards et al., 1975). Heterophile antigen–antibody systems could, according to this idea, represent the several different (antigen) specificities encompassed by the same antibody, rather than a reaction of antibody with two identical antigens from

---

* Though it follows that the Forssman reactant should now be termed Forssman hapten, the more familiar term Forssman antigen will be retained in the remainder of this chapter. Antigen is the preferred term when considering heterophile responses though the specificity of such responses, as in the case outlined above, probably depends on hapten groups. It should also be noted that even though the heterophile antigenic determinants behave as haptens they are not similar to the classical chemical haptens such as nickel.

different species. The resolution of this problem justifies a thorough study of heterophile systems with the possibility that further valuable diagnostic procedures might be found.

In the investigation of heterophile systems it is necessary to ensure that each system is adequately defined in terms of the species of plant, animal or microorganism which provides the antigen, and the species from which the detecting antibody is obtained. Also important is information as to possible chemical or physical modification of an antigen during its extraction or demonstration. A theoretical example will demonstrate the importance of these aspects (Fig. 1). A heterophile antibody, a′ is produced during some disease process in animal species X and is detected by agglutination of cells taken from an animal species B (different from species X). Antigen A, which stimulates the antibody a, must therefore be a natural antigen in animal species B. A second antibody, of specificity a′ might be obtained from species X in response to Antigen A′ which reacts with cells from another species C. If species C has antigen A in addition to A′ it can provide cells agglutinable by both antibodies a and a′.

Cursory investigation of this kind of system can fail to recognize that cells from a certain species (C in this example) carry more than one heterophile antigen, or can fail to differentiate the two antibodies (a and a′) correctly. The latter distinction only becomes clear when cells from species B and C are used concurrently, or by absorption of antiserum from infected animal X (which contains both a and a′ antibodies) with cells from species B and C independently, to establish which activity is removed by each cell. In this way, the antibodies produced (by species X) can be defined in terms of their patterns of reaction. Furthermore, suppose that the reason for the production of antibodies a and a′ by animal species X was infection by a microorganism which introduced the antigens A and A′. The same organism infecting hosts B and C would be expected to induce antibody a in the former species, but neither a nor a′ in the latter as this species possesses both the heterophile antigens A and A′ and is therefore tolerant to them. Similarly, species B will not respond to antigen A. The puzzle may, however, be compounded, in that the cells from species B and C contain many other antigens and it is possible for a completely different antigen (D) to be introduced by the microorganism, which whilst not stimulating antibody in species X or B can initiate an antibody response in species C and such an antibody can be directed against the red cells of either species X or B. This antibody, d, could be confused with antibodies a and a′.

Advantage can be gained by extending the tests to include cells from many other species. In the example above, antigen A was only demonstrated in the cells of two species, B and C, and was absent in one, X. If the presence of the antigen is demonstrated in a further four species and

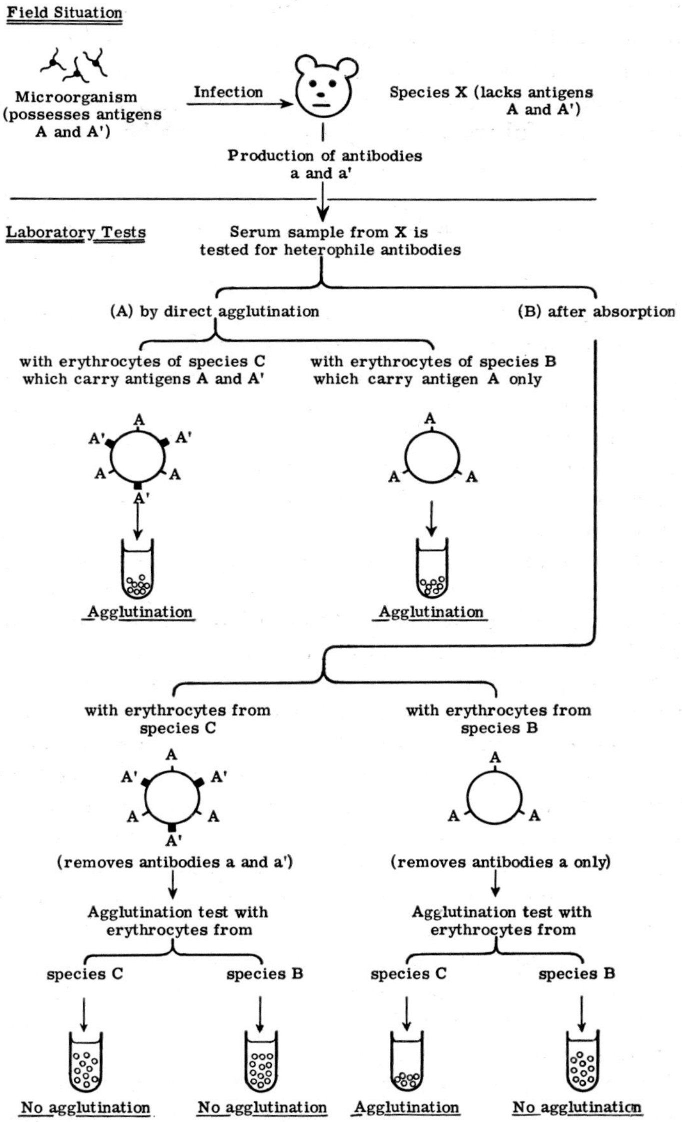

FIG. 1. Agglutination and absorption patterns of the serum of an animal species X when suffering from infection with a given microorganism. The serum of animal species X is tested with erythrocytes taken from animal species B and C. Species X, B and C are all different from one another.

its absence in three others, the antigen has been more thoroughly characterized and its typing is more accurate.

Thus, clearly, each heterophile antibody must be defined in terms of the species against which it reacts and the species which produces it. Only by such careful work can misinterpretations be avoided, and new heterophile systems discovered.

III. The nature of heterophile antibodies

Heterophile antibodies have important characteristics other than that of their ability to cross react with heterophile antigens. They are usually agglutinating and complement-fixing antibodies, are of high molecular weight, and are susceptible to dissociation with 0·05 M 2-mercapto-ethanol; these are features typical of IgM antibody. Where careful studies have been carried out to establish the immunoglobulin type, it has been shown that the heterophile antibodies are exclusively IgM (Wilkinson and Carmichael, 1964; Houba et al., 1969). IgG and IgA antibodies of the same specificities do not seem to be formed. This in itself is intriguing, in that antibody synthesis in most immune responses switches from IgM to IgG in its earliest stages (Uhr and Finkelstein, 1967). This switch is dependent on the availability of complement, and is under thymus influence. Thus it has been shown that sheep erythrocytes can elicit both IgM and IgG antibody when injected into normal chickens, but only IgM antibody in complement-depleted birds (Nielsen and White 1974). It may be that the characteristics of heterophile antibodies as defined above are determined by the handling of the antigen (in the presence or absence of complement) rather than some peculiarity of the antigen itself. It is, however, fortunate that heterophile antibodies are IgM in type, for their property of efficient agglutination has allowed their detection by simple direct saline agglutination procedures. In this type of test, heated serum (56°C for 30 min.) is reacted at various dilutions with a saline suspension of the appropriate cells (usually 1–2% v/v) and incubated for 1–2 h. The amount of antibody present is thus quantitated by determining the highest dilution of serum which produces agglutination (easily observed by the naked eye) of the cells. The simplicity and economy of such tests, combined with high specificity in some situations, has led to their widespread use as standard tests for the diagnosis of human disease (see Table 1).

The straightforward nature of these tests, however, does not appear to have provided an inducement to investigation of the nature of the stimulus to heterophile antibody production, which remains poorly understood (see Section I above). A further difficulty arises from the manifold modifications of these simple tests; incubation times, quantities and concentrations of reactants, diluents, and methods of absorption

Table 1. Heterophile antibody tests used in the diagnosis of human disease

Disease	Responsible agent	Source of the heterophile antigen	Diagnostic procedure
1. Infectious mono-nucleosis	Epstein–Barr virus	Horse and sheep erythrocytes	Paul–Bunnell agglutination test
2. Atypical pneumonia	*Mycoplasma pneumoniae*	Human erythrocytes	Agglutination at 4°C
		Streptococcus M.G.	Agglutination
3. Epidemic typhus	*Rickettsia prowazekii*	Proteus OX19	⎫
Scrub typhus	*Rickettsia tsutsugamushi*	Proteus OXK	⎬ Weil-Felix reaction
Tick-borne fevers	*Rickettsia rickettsii*	Proteus OX19 and OX2	⎭

vary widely between different investigators. In short, there is little uniformity or standardization of method. Particularly, this is a feature of investigations of trypanosome-associated heterophile antibodies, where, with few exceptions, it has been unusual to report a detailed methodology. A summary of the authors' techniques are given in Appendix II to this chapter.

Finally, it should be noted that heterophile antibody does not always agglutinate the "target" cells satisfactorily. This is the case with some erythrocyte/anti-erythrocyte systems where the failure to agglutinate is due to a "hidden" antigen which is presumed to be "recessed" in the deeper layers of the cell wall. This concept has been elaborated for the Forssman antigen of bovine cells by Coombs et al. (1961). In this and similar situations the antigen–antibody interaction can be shown by complement fixation, or, if the antibody satisfactorily agglutinates a second type of cell, by showing loss of that agglutinability following absorption of the serum by the non-agglutinated cells.

IV. Heterophile erythrocyte antibodies in human trypanosomiasis

A. INTRODUCTION

Investigations of heterophile antibodies in human trypanosomiasis over the past 30 years have yielded a confused picture. Henderson-Begg (1946) demonstrated agglutinins to sheep erythrocytes in the serum of patients with *T. b. gambiense* infection. Houba and Allison (1966) found heterophile sheep erythrocyte antibodies in human *T. b. rhodesiense* infections but not in *T. b. gambiense* infection. More recently, Houba *et al.* (1969) showed that monkeys (*Macaca mulatta*) infected with *T. b. rhodesiense*, *T. b. gambiense* or *T. b. brucei* (the latter originating from primary isolate LUGALA/55/EATRO/459) developed antibody to sheep erythrocytes. Parratt and Cobb (1978) in a retrospective examination of sera from *T. b. gambiense* and *T. b. rhodesiense* infections, found that heterophile antibodies to sheep erythrocytes were restricted to the latter infections. In the theoretical examples given earlier in the present chapter it became clear that definition of each heterophile antibody on the basis of its reactivity with erythrocytes of different species was essential, as indeed was consideration of the species producing the antibody. The confused picture in human trypanosomiasis may be partly due to restriction to one erythrocyte type (sheep), and partly to the investigation of antibody from two different species of infected host (man and monkey). In Table 2, some of the important agglutination reactions of human sera are listed and it will be seen that there is a difference in the pattern of reaction of sera from *T*.

Table 2. The principal agglutination and absorption patterns of some heterophile anti-erythrocyte antibodies

Erythrocytes employed in agglutination test	Human antibody of types			
	Classical Forssman	Infectious mononucleosis induced	T. b. rhodesiense induced	T. b. gambiense induced
Horse	+++	+++	− or ±	− or ±
Sheep	+++	++	+	− or ±
Rabbit	−	+	+++	++
Rat	−	?	+++	++
Guinea pig	−	?	+	+
Cells used for absorption	Agglutinins for sheep (or rabbit) erythrocytes after absorption			
Guinea pig kidney (T)	Absorbed	Not absorbed	Absorbed	Absorbed
Bovine erythrocytes (T)	Absorbed	Absorbed	Absorbed	Absorbed

+++—Very strong agglutination; ++—strong agglutination; +—slight agglutination; ±—weak agglutination at high serum concentrations; −—no agglutinations; ?—results equivocal. Absorptions—refer usually to absorption of sheep erythrocyte agglutinins, or of rabbit erythrocyte agglutinins in the case of $T.b.$ gambiense induced antibody.

b. rhodesiense and *T. b. gambiense* infections; and that both reactions differ from the patterns for Forssman antibody and for the antibody associated with infectious mononucleosis. Using the range of erythrocyte species listed, the patterns are clear, whereas the use of sheep erythrocytes (SRBC) alone, even with the accepted absorptions against guinea-pig kidney cells and bovine erythrocytes, does not allow adequate differentiation.

The *T. b. rhodesiense*-induced antibody is produced early after infection in humans and peak levels are observed after 10–14 days, following which the antibody declines and disappears within 6–8 weeks (Herbert *et al.*, 1979). It should be noted that in the patient described by Herbert *et al.* (1979) therapy was instituted at an early stage and this may have shortened the heterophile antibody response. In similar infections in monkeys, Houba *et al.* (1969) showed that the heterophile antibodies persisted for as long as the trypanosomes remained and disappeared only after appropriate treatment of the infection. More recent work in our laboratory using chickens infected with a stock of *T. b. brucei* originating from primary isolation LUGALA/55/EATRO/459 has confirmed that the production of heterophile antibodies does continue throughout the course of trypanosome infection.

B. DIFFERENTIATION OF THE HETEROPHILE RESPONSES IN *TRYPANOSOMA BRUCEI RHODESIENSE* and *T. B. GAMBIENSE* INFECTIONS

Heterophile antibody against sheep erythrocytes induced by *T. b. rhodesiense* infection in man, has been shown to be completely absorbed by guinea-pig kidney (GPK) cells and by heated bovine erythrocyte (HBE) suspensions (Parratt and Cobb, 1978) and therefore has the outward appearances of Forssman antibody (Table 2). However, the antibody agglutinates rabbit and rat erythrocytes (both Forssman antigen negative) and does not agglutinate horse erythrocytes (Forssman antigen positive). In fact the *T. b. rhodesiense* heterophile antibody with the characteristics shown in Table 2 has been shown to be a mixture of two specificities, one reactive with an antigen designated F′,* present on sheep, rabbit, rat and guinea-pig erythrocytes, and a second, reactive with an antigen R, found on rabbit and rat erythrocytes only.† The full reactions of these two antibodies (F′ and R) are shown in Table 3. Thus

---

* The designations of the heterophile antigens discussed in this chapter (i.e. R, R_2, F′ and F″) are those used in the authors' laboratory. No agreed or suggested nomenclature exists and it is probable that these antigens have not been reported before in any context. R, is named after rat and rabbit; R_2, rat reactive; F′ (F prime), Forssman-like, number one; F″ (F prime prime) Forssman-like number two.

† Note that R is probably partially expressed on guinea pig erythrocytes as shown by their weak agglutination.

Table 3. Characteristic agglutination patterns of human antibodies to F' and R, induced by *T. b. rhodesiense* infection.

Antibody	Horse	Reaction with erythrocytes of: Sheep	Rabbit	Rat	Guinea pig
anti F'	—	+ +	+ +	+ +	+ +
anti R	—	—	+ + +	+ +	+
Complete serum, i.e., anti F' and anti R	—	+ +	+ + + +	+ + +	+ + +
Serum absorbed with sheep erythrocytes[a]	—	—	+ +	+	+
Serum absorbed with rabbit erythrocytes[a]	—	—	—	—	—

+ + + + and + + + : Very strong agglutination; + + : strong agglutination; + : slight agglutination; — : no agglutination.   [a]Absorption carried out at 37°C for 1 h and thereafter 12 h at 4°C (room temperature) with equal volumes of serum and washed, packed erythrocytes.

serum containing *T. b. rhodesiense*-induced heterophile antibodies will agglutinate erythrocytes from all the above mentioned species and the agglutinating activity can only be fully removed by absorption with rabbit erythrocytes. In theory, rat or guinea-pig erythrocytes should be capable of absorbing the antibody but in practice they are much weaker than the rabbit cells in this respect.

T. b. gambiense infection in man stimulates heterophile erythrocyte antibodies with the specificity of the anti-R antibody described above. Thus the serum from these patients agglutinates rabbit and rat erythrocytes to high titre and may be weakly reactive with guinea-pig erythrocytes but fails to agglutinate either sheep or horse erythrocytes. Furthermore, the titre of antibody to rabbit cells is, in general, lower than that found for serum from *T. b. rhodesiense* cases, probably because the second antibody (anti-F') in the latter patients fortifies the agglutination response to these erythrocytes (Parratt and Cobb, 1978).

V. Antibody specificity of the elevated immunoglobulin levels seen in trypanosomiasis

On the basis of identification of two distinct heterophile antibodies in African trypanosomiasis (anti-F' and anti-R) it seemed reasonable to suggest that the aetiologically important organisms *T. b. rhodesiense* and *T. b. gambiense* were introducing the analogous antigens F' and R. Thus *T. b. rhodesiense* is considered to possess F' and R, whereas *T. b. gambiense* possesses only R (Parratt and Cobb, 1978). This simple explanation however introduces an important conceptual problem in that some investigators have considered the heterophile antibody in trypanosomiasis to be a manifestation of an anamnestic response (Houba *et al.*, 1969;

MacKenzie *et al.*, 1972; MacKenzie, 1973). Thus the trypanosome would stimulate antibody of widely varying specificity in a non-specific manner including antibodies to erythrocytes. In this sense the organism would act in a similar way to B-lymphocyte mitogens. Indeed, in acute trypanosomiasis, many other types of antibody are reported to be produced including rheumatoid factor, antinuclear factor, syphilis-associated antibodies and antibodies to *Brucella* organisms, and these probably contribute to the enormous increase of total serum IgM frequently observed (Mattern *et al.*, 1961; Houba *et al.*, 1969).

Herbert *et al.* (1979), however, investigated an accidental infection of a European laboratory worker, who subsequently developed high IgM levels, and heterophile antibodies to sheep erythrocytes (SRBC), but had no autoantibody or antibody to *Brucella* or *Salmonella* organisms and was repeatedly negative in serological tests for syphilis. The authors therefore argued that the increased IgM comprised the heterophile antibody and antibody which had been formed against specific antigens of the trypanosomes.

Significant amounts of the total IgM, however, could not be absorbed from the serum by means of concentrates of the trypanosome stock which produced the patient's infection, a similar finding to that described by Houba *et al.* (1969) who studied experimental trypanosome infections in monkeys. Thus, whilst some IgM could be accounted for by heterophile SRBC antibody, the greater part was "lost" and the authors (Herbert *et al.*, 1979) postulated that the "lost" antibody might be directed against many different variant antigens which were not represented in the concentrates used for absorption. This idea does not allow for a B-lymphocyte mitogen-like effect of a non-specific type as previously postulated (Houba *et al.*, 1969; Terry *et al.* 1973; Hudson *et al.* 1976) and hence a different explanation is required for the formation of the autoantibodies and antibody to microbial agents described by other investigators.

In the case of the autoantibodies, it seems to us not unreasonable to consider their formation to be a response to self-antigens uncovered as a direct result of tissue damage by the trypanosomes. If this is the case, more severe, or longer lasting, trypanosome infections would lead to a greater tendency to autoantibody formation. Thus, in the patient described by Herbert *et al.* (1979), the absence of autoantibodies may simply reflect the fact that diagnosis and treatment were rapid. In fact, this isolated, but well studied, case supports the idea of damage-induced autoantibody but does not substantiate the non-specific B-lymphocyte mitogen theory (see above) according to which any trypanosome infection, by providing the non-specific stimulation, would be expected to result in autoantibody formation.

The anti-microbial antibodies are more difficult to explain but may follow reactivation of intercurrent chronic infections, the reactivation being due to the debility induced by the trypanosome infection. Clearly, where intercurrent disease does not exist, as in the case described by Herbert *et al.* (1979), there will be no response towards other microbial antigens.

With the present interest in immune responses to infection, particularly in trypanosomiasis, satisfactory explanations of serological abnormalities as described above must be sought, and thorough study of the heterophile erythrocyte antibodies in African trypanosomiasis may provide a novel avenue by which to approach the problem. At present we would favour the idea that the heterophile antibodies represent, as indicated earlier, a response to antigens possessed by and therefore introduced by the trypanosomes. The antibody responses are thus classically-speaking "specific responses". The evidence in favour of this is as follows: Firstly, antibody to erythrocytes increases and decreases in parallel with specific trypanosome antibody, implying a close relationship with the infection (Henderson-Begg, 1946; Muniz and Dos Santos, 1954; Houba *et al.*, 1969) and persists for as long as the trypanosome infection persists. Secondly, heterophile antibodies can be absorbed by trypanosomes of the appropriate type (Houba *et al.*, 1969; Herbert *et al.*, 1978).* In addition heterophile antibodies of different erythrocyte specificities are produced by different trypanosome species, implying that the antigens introduced by the organisms are constant features of each species or subspecies of parasite (Parratt and Cobb, 1978).

VI. Application of heterophile antibodies for the diagnosis of trypanosomiasis

If the heterophile antibody responses are to be regarded as specific rather than non-specific their study is likely to be valuable in the diagnosis of trypanosomiasis. The difficulties in the diagnosis of trypanosomiasis, both in the sense of identifying infection, and of identifying the causative species of organism, centre on the epidemiology of the disease. The diagnosis of infection in an individual host is not usually difficult if overt disease is present, but if the organism shows negligible virulence in some individuals it may be difficult to prove them carriers. The problems of identifying a source for either type of infection are formidable. This is because the separation and identification of individual species of trypanosome is time-consuming and requires considerable expertise (Vickerman, Volume 1, Chapter 1) and also because identification by antigenic typing is confused by antigen variation (Gray and Luckins, Volume 1, Chapter 12) and the new isoenzyme (Godfrey and Kilgour,

---

* As noted above, p. 534, significant weights of the total elevated IgM were not removed on absorption but, after absorption, the remaining IgM did not contain any antibody reactive with the range of erythrocytes tested.

1976) and DNA (Newton, B.A. Volume 1, Chapter 9) techniques are still under development. For these reasons the epidemiological picture of trypanosomiasis is incomplete.

It follows that if a particular species of trypanosome, by causing an infection of a certain host species, induces in the latter an heterophile erythrocyte response which has a recognizable pattern, the response can be used to "map" the progress of the infection through a community. The difference in pattern of the heterophile responses of the human to *T. b. gambiense* and *T. b. rhodesiense* would appear sufficient to demarcate trypanosomiasis due to these two organisms and the techniques required are simple enough for large surveys. This does, however, require careful elucidation of the various patterns of heterophile response particularly if the same approach was used to delineate a reservoir of infection in a different animal species. If, for argument's sake it was essential to determine whether rabbits harboured *T. b. rhodesiense* under natural conditions, the tests outlined above for infection of man by this organism would not be useful, as the rabbit, by virtue of its possession of antigens F' and R, would be tolerant to them and thus would not be able to respond to these antigens even if they were introduced by trypanosomes. Rabbits might on the other hand, respond to other heterophile antigens introduced by the organism.* Heterophile erythrocyte antibodies have been described in the serum of several hosts other than man during infection with various trypanosome species (see Appendix I for list and references).

An example of the necessity for accurate specification can be found in the comparison of *T. b. gambiense* and *T. b. rhodesiense* infection in man and monkeys. As indicated above, humans infected with *T. b. rhodesiense* produce antibody to two antigens, F' and R, whereas those with *T. b. gambiense* infection produce antibody to R only (Parratt and Cobb, 1978). Consequently *T. b. rhodesiense* induces antibody to sheep erythrocytes (F'-bearing) whereas *T. b. gambiense* does not induce this antibody in humans (Table 2). It follows that humans do not possess either F' or R as naturally occurring antigens and this has been recently confirmed by direct experiment (Parratt and Herbert unpublished observations). In contrast, *T. b. gambiense* and *T. b. rhodesiense* both induce antibody to sheep cells in experimental infection of monkeys (Houba *et al.*, 1969). It seems, therefore, that monkeys must be responding to a further, as yet unidentified antigen, present on *T. b. gambiense* and on the sheep erythrocyte. This follows because the anti-SRBC antibody cannot be anti-F' (the human response to *T. gambiense* shows that F' is not available on these organisms) and yet the activity (anti-SRBC) cannot be attributed to antibody to R as sheep erythrocytes do not possess this antigen. With

---

* Rabbits have, of necessity been used in this argument, as nothing is known about the antigens carried by animals of epidemiological importance, such as bushbuck.

regard to the R antigen, the work of Houba and colleagues (Houba *et al.*, 1969) shows the same results as our own findings (Parratt and Cobb, 1978), namely that anti-R antibody (which can be stimulated by both *T. b. gambiense* and *T. b. rhodesiense*) reactive with rabbit cells, can be effectively removed from the serum by absorption with rabbit and rat erythrocytes, but not by sheep erythrocytes. It would be reasonable therefore to postulate that the monkey responded to a second sheep antigen F″ carried by *T. b. gambiense* which does not induce a human response because the human carries the same antigen.

Thus, the similarity at a superficial level between the response in man and monkeys probably has genuine differences, and requires a full and careful analysis. Houba and Allison (1966) originally stated that *T. b. gambiense* infection in man did not induce sheep erythrocyte antibodies, but modified this opinion, in the light of their later work (Houba *et al.*, 1969) with experimental monkey infections, by suggesting that human anti-sheep erythrocyte antibodies were not found in the early survey because of sampling difficulties. In our opinion it seems likely that the human and the monkey respond in a similar but different way to the antigens of *T. b. gambiense* (and possibly other trypanosomes also).

VII. Heterophile antibodies in trypanosomiasis caused by *Trypanosoma species* other than *T. brucei* sub-species *gambiense* and *rhodesiense*

Heterophile antibodies to erythrocytes are produced also in infections due to trypanosomes other than *T. b. gambiense* and *T. b. rhodesiense*. Notably, *Trypanosoma cruzi* infection in man produces anti-SRBC antibody (Muniz and Dos Santos, 1950) and although little is known of the range of specificity of this antibody (i.e., its reactions with erythrocytes of other species), there are many features which are similar to the pattern in salivarian trypanosome infections. Thus, the heterophile antibody is produced rapidly to a high titre during early, acute illness and declines to lower levels when the disease becomes chronic. In general, higher antibody titres to *T. cruzi* (culture forms) are associated with higher anti-erythrocyte titres. The heterophile antibody can be fully absorbed by suspensions of guinea-pig kidney cells, but only partially absorbed by heated bovine erythrocytes, characteristics which are similar to the *T. b. gambiense*- and *T. b. rhodesiense*-induced heterophile antibodies. However, *T. cruzi* antigen does not absorb the erythrocyte antibody (Muniz and Dos Santos, 1950) whereas *T. b. gambiense* and *T. b. rhodesiense* absorb the heterophile antibodies which they induce (Houba *et al.*, 1969; Herbert *et al.*, 1979). The difference may be due to the fact that the latter studies used animal-passaged trypanosomes for absorption, whereas Muniz and Dos Santos (1954) used culture forms in their experiments with *T. cruzi*. As the antigen pattern of culture forms is different from the pattern of bloodstream forms (see Gray and Luckins, Volume 1, Chapter 12) it seems possible that the heterophile antigens may have been lost or were poorly expressed in the culture forms used for absorption. However, with the limited information at present available it is not possible to present a balanced comment and it remains conceivable that the antibodies formed in response to *T. cruzi* are quite different from those induced by the other organisms.

Recently, collaborating with Dr. R. Joshua, we have observed another heterophile antibody response, in chickens infected with a defined population of trypanosomes designated variant antigen type WITat 1. This variant antigen type was derived from a stock* originating from primary isolation LUGALA/55/EATRO/459, the pedigree of which is presented in Fig. 4 of Chapter 10. This organism, thought originally to be *T. b. brucei*, shows characters that may possibly differentiate it as a subspecies of *T. brucei* other than the three generally recognized. Infection of chickens (*Gallus domesticus*) with WITat 1 induces antibody which will agglutinate the erythrocytes of sheep, guinea-pig and rabbits but not those of the horse. Thus it has the characteristics of antibody to the F′ antigen (see above) and this has been confirmed by absorption studies (Parratt and Herbert, unpublished data). The finding of this antibody is important for several reasons. Firstly, it is unusual to observe agglutinating antibody, against any antigen, in the chicken for longer than 7–10 days unless some feature is present, e.g. complement depletion, which interferes with the "switch" from IgM to IgG synthesis (Nielsen and White, 1974). In some of the chronically infected chickens the anti-erythrocyte agglutinins were maintained at high titre for up to 120 days. Thus further examination of this model may reveal the nature of the interference with the immune response, and this may lead to a better understanding of the reasons for the increased levels of IgM seen in many species during trypanosome infection. Secondly, examination of the chicken antibodies formed in the response to WITat 1 provided direct confirmation of the early findings obtained with human sera from *T. b. rhodesiense* infections. These human sera had F′ (and R) antibody and it could be predicted that the human was not a carrier of antigen F′ or antigen R. Indeed, the chicken sera with strong agglutinins for F′-carrying erythrocytes, failed to agglutinate human erythrocytes. Similarly, it could be predicted that WITat 1 would not induce anti-F′ antibody in the guinea-pig (F′-positive species) and this also has been confirmed by direct experiment. Interestingly WITat 1 infection in guinea-pigs induced a further heterophile antibody reactive only with rat erythrocytes. This has been designated anti-R_2 antibody and the

---

* Terms such as "stock", "variant antigen type", "Primary isolation" are used in this chapter with the meanings ascribed to them in Chapter 15 of this volume.

organism WITat 1 can be tentatively given the antigen pattern F′, R_2 +ve/R -ve, thus differentiating it from *T. b. gambiense* (R +ve/F′, R_2 -ve) and *T. b. rhodesiense* (F′, R +ve/R_2 -ve).

Thirdly, the findings outlined above provide a useful means of monitoring experimental infection, even at subpatent levels (about 3 organisms/ml in the chicken), by means of simple haemagglutination tests, and might find application in the detection of the carrier state in human trypanosomiasis (see Section VI above).

Heterophile erythrocyte antibodies associated with several other trypanosome infections have also been described. Thus Schindler (1973) reported high titres of antibody to erythrocytes in cattle infected with *T. congolense* and Clarkson *et al.* (1975) observed increases of antibody to chicken, rabbit and human erythrocytes during *T. vivax* infection in cattle. We have observed high titre heterophile antibodies to horse erythrocytes in the serum of a camel infected with *T. evansi* (Parratt and Herbert, unpublished data). These examples show that the phenomenon of heterophile antibody production is common in many trypanosome infections which further supports the postulate that their production is due to specific immunity rather than non-specific stimulation of already existing antibody responses. There is one notable absence from the list of trypanosome infections in which heterophile responses have been observed, namely *T. b. brucei* infection in cattle. Recourse to the literature does not make clear whether heterophile antibodies do not occur in this situation or whether they have simply been ignored or missed due to the concentration of effort on other aspects of the disease. We have examined sera from a small number of cattle with proven *T. b. brucei* infection and have failed to demonstrate any heterophile erythrocyte antibody (Parratt and Herbert, unpublished data). These results are in marked contrast, if supported by further investigation, to the *T. congolense* and *T. vivax* infections noted above, and demonstrate further the specific nature of the heterophile response. The lack of a heterophile response to *T. b. brucei* in cattle, may also be relevant to its negligible virulence in this host, an aspect discussed further in Chapter 10.

VIII. Conclusions

The significance and importance of heterophile erythrocyte antibodies in the study of trypanosome infections can be considered under two broad headings, namely diagnostic significance and biological significance.

A. DIAGNOSTIC SIGNIFICANCE

Although tests for the demonstration of erythrocyte antibodies have not been widely used in diagnosis in the past, there is now sufficient evidence, as reviewed here, to justify a trial of haemagglutination procedures in trypanosomiasis. In this we agree with the conclusions of Houba *et al.* (1969). Different trypanosome species appear to induce different patterns of heterophile response, and therefore recognition of the pattern of response rather than simply the demonstration of heterophile antibody, could provide valuable diagnostic information. The Paul–Bunnell test provides a useful corollary. The latter test had been the diagnostic procedure of choice in infectious mononucleosis for many years on an empirical basis, prior to the identification of the Epstein–Barr virus as the aetiologically important agent in this disease. The Paul–Bunnell test remains the most commonly used diagnostic procedure in the disease but the study of specific antibody responses (to EB virus) has led to a clearer understanding of the nature of infectious mononucleosis. The same may be envisaged in trypanosomiasis where the heterophile antibody tests could be used as screening procedures to establish or support the diagnosis, and give preliminary clues as to the possible causal organism, after which more detailed information could be obtained with tests using the relevant trypanosomes. The attractions of tests for heterophile antibodies are simplicity of operation, low cost and ease of acquisition of reagents. It is even possible that the tests could be performed as slide tests or adopted to reagent impregnated cards as has been done commercially with the Paul–Bunnell test.

Further investigation is clearly required to determine the usefulness of these tests in clinical practice and it is important that this work be carried out in a controlled manner. There is in our view a need to establish standard test procedures, using well defined reagents, and to develop a system of receptor designation (not necessarily the one which we have followed) which is clear and informative. Without care of this kind, valuable data may be overlooked. In this respect we would suggest that the inadequate definition of heterophile responses in the past has, in large part, been due to the conflicting results obtained by different investigators, each of whom has used a technique and nomenclature peculiar to themselves alone.

A further interesting aspect is whether serial measurement of heterophile antibody can be prognostically useful, once a diagnosis of trypanosomiasis has been established. As indicated earlier in this chapter, there is evidence that the heterophile antibody persists for as long as the trypanosomes persist and it may be possible by measuring the level of these antibodies to monitor the progress of infection during subpatent stages during therapy. Here again the ease of the heterophile antibody test would be an advantage, and this aspect is currently being assessed in our laboratory.

B. BIOLOGICAL SIGNIFICANCE

The biological significance of heterophile antibodies in trypanosomiasis depends on their origin. Two possible origins are (a) that the antibodies arise as a result of non-specific stimulation of antibody producing cells (B-lymphocytes and plasma cells) or (b) that they represent antibody formed against new antigens introduced during the infection. The reasons for and against each of these hypotheses have been given earlier but briefly it can be stated at this point that there is considerable evidence of trypanosome-induced specificity in these responses (Houba *et al.*, 1969; Parratt and Cobb 1978), and little direct proof of the validity of the first hypothesis. One crucial test of any substance thought to be a non-specific stimulator of lymphocytes (mitogen) is to allow the substance to react with the cells in an *in vitro* system. Direct stimulation of a non-specific type can then be determined according to the degree of cellular transformation and such tests are commonly employed using phyto-haemagglutinin, pokeweed mitogen and the B-lymphocyte mitogen, endotoxin. As far as we are aware analogous experiments using trypanosomes or trypanosome products have not clearly demonstrated this effect and in the absence of this type of information it is probably not prudent to interpret the heterophile antibody responses as "non-specific".

On the other hand the biological role of the heterophile antibodies as part of a "specific" response to trypanosome infection is not clear. The fact that the antibodies to erythrocytes are of IgM type, strongly complement fixing, and are absorbed by intact trypanosomes (Houba *et al.*, 1969) makes it reasonable to assume that they are capable of destroying the parasite, and thus may be important in protecting the host from infection. However, the antibodies are produced quickly after infection and maintained at high titre throughout the period of infection (Dos Santos, 1964; Houba *et al.*, 1969) without any apparent protective benefit. It seems likely then that the heterophile antigens of the trypanosome are "protected" from exposure to the antibodies and it is possible that the surface glycoprotein material of the parasite which is thought to contain the variable antigens (see Vickerman; Volume 1, Chapter 1), provides this protection. It could be anticipated that once antibody to the variable antigens had been formed this protective coat might be breached* thus allowing the heterophile antibodies access to the cell membrane to effect destruction of the organism. As the heterophile antibody persists for some time, only organisms which had a new and different variable antigen coat could survive and multiply and these in turn would be neutral-

---

* Perhaps by aggregation of the variable antigen to form "patches" and "caps" analogous to those seen when other cells, e.g. lymphocytes, are exposed to antibody. Capping has been observed, *in vitro*, on trypanosomes (Barry, 1975).

ized and then eliminated. Indeed, the ordered sequence and control of variable antigen production by trypanosomes (see Gray and Luckins, Volume 1, Chapter 12) indicates a highly evolved adaptive process on the part of the parasite. As heterophile antigens are both commonly represented in the animal kingdom and are powerful immunogens, we would suggest that they may have provided a strong stimulus to trypanosomes to evolve the "protective" variable antigens. Any parasite without this protection would, by virtue of its inherent heterophile antigens (probably in the form of important cell wall components), be susceptible to any naturally occurring antibody in animals devoid of the same antigen. This would limit the range of hosts available for the parasite. Low titres of naturally occurring antibodies to erythrocyte antigens (both extra- and intra-species) are common in most animals and are thought to follow minor exposure to the antigens early in life (Humphrey and White, 1970).

The specificities of such antibodies, however, vary from species to species, according to the antigenic make-up of the responding animal itself, and this may determine which species of host are successfully parasitized by the trypanosome. Accordingly, it could be that the "signal" for the trypanosome to produce its variable coat material might be the existence of natural heterophile antibody in small amounts. In the absence of the "signal", as for example in the insect vector, production of variable coat material would cease.

Whether heterophile erythrocyte antibodies can and do perform the functions elaborated above is conjecture, but there is sufficient evidence as reviewed in this chapter, to consider them specific and important features of trypanosome infections, worthy of more detailed investigations.

IX. Acknowledgements

The authors wish to acknowledge the help and useful discussion afforded to them by colleagues in the University Department of Bacteriology and Immunology, Glasgow. Particularly, we are indebted to Dr. Susan Cobb and Dr. Richard Joshua for the part they have played in investigating heterophile antibodies and to Dr. Hamish Mackenzie for his assistance in procuring reagents for these studies.

X. References

Barry, D. (1975). "Capping" of surface antigens on *Trypanosoma rhodesiense*. *Journal of Protozoology*, **22**, 49A.
Boyd, W. C. (1956). "Fundamentals of Immunology". Interscience Publishers Ltd., New York, London.

Clarkson, M. J., Penhale, W. J. and McKenna, R. B. (1975). Progressive serum protein changes in experimental infections of calves with *Trypanosoma vivax*. *Journal of Comparative Pathology*, **85**, 397–410.

Coombs, R. R. A., Coombs, A. M. and Ingram, D. G. (1961). "The Serology of Conglutination and its Relation to Disease". Blackwell Scientific Publications, Oxford.

Cruickshank, R. (1965). "Medical Microbiology", 11th Ed. E & S Livingstone Ltd., Edinburgh and London, pp. 912–914.

Faulk, W. Page and Houba, V. (1973). Immunological reactions with chromic chloride-treated erythrocytes. *Journal of Immunological Methods*, **3**, 87–98.

Fraser, B. A. and Mallette, M. F. (1974). Structure of Forssman hapten glycosphingolipid from sheep erythrocytes. *Immunochemistry*, **11**, 581–593.

Godfrey, D. G. and Kilgour, V. (1976). Enzyme electrophoresis in characterizing the causative organism of gambian trypanosomiasis. *Transactions of the Royal Society of Tropical Medicine and Hygiene*, **70**, 219–224.

Henderson-Begg, A. (1946). Heterophile antibodies in trypanosomiasis. *Transactions of the Royal Society of Tropical Medicine and Hygiene*, **40**, 331.

Herbert, W. J., Parratt, D., Van Meirvenne, N. and Lennox, B. (1979). An accidental laboratory infection with African trypanosomes of a defined stock. II: Studies on the serological response of the patient and the identity of the infecting organism. (Submitted for publication.)

Houba, V. and Allison, A. C. (1966). M-antiglobulins (rheumatoid factor-like globulins) and other gammaglobulins in relation to tropical parasitic infections. *Lancet*, **1**, 848–852.

Houba, V., Brown, K. N. and Allison, A. C. (1969). Heterophile antibodies, M-antiglobulins and immunoglobulins in experimental trypanosomiasis. *Clinical and Experimental Immunology*, **4**, 113–123.

Hudson K. M., Byner, C., Freeman, J. and Terry, R. J. (1976). Immunodepression, high IgM levels and evasion of the immune response in murine trypanosomiasis. *Nature, London*, **264**, 256.

Humphrey, J. H. and White, R. G. (1970). "Immunology for Students of Medicine", 3rd ed. Blackwell Scientific Publications, Oxford and Edinburgh.

Klein, F. and Mattern, P. (1965). Rheumatoid factors in primary and reactive macroglobulinaemias. *Annals of Rheumatic Disease*, **24**, 458.

MacKenzie, A. R. (1973). The "non-specific" immune response in young rabbits infected with *Trypanosoma brucei*. *Transactions of the Royal Society of Tropical Medicine and Hygiene*, **67**, 269.

MacKenzie, A. R., Boreham, P. F. L. and Facer, C. A. (1972). Non-trypanosome specific components of the elevated IgM levels in rabbit trypanosomiasis. *Transactions of the Royal Society of Tropical Medicine and Hygiene*, **66**, 344–345.

Mattern, P., Masseyeff, R., Michel, R. and Peretti, P. (1961). Etude immunochimique de la β_2 macroglobuline des serums de malades atteints de trypanosomiase Africaine a *T. gambiense*. *Annales de l'Institut Pasteur (Paris)*, **101**, 382–388.

Muniz, J. and Dos Santos, M. C. F. (1950). Heterophile antibodies in American trypanosomiasis: the presence of heterogenetic component(s) in the antigenic structure of the *Schizotrypanum cruzi* shown by "conditioned haemolysis" reaction. *O Hopital*, **38**, 163.

Nielsen, K. H. and White, R. G. (1974). Effect of host decomplementation on homeostasis of antibody production in fowl. *Nature, London*, **250**, 927.

Parratt, D. and Cobb, Susan J. (1978). Heterophile antibody to red cells in human trypanosomiasis. *African Journal of Medicine and Medical Sciences*, **7**, 57–64.

Richards, F. F., Konigsberg, W. H., Rosenstein, R. W. and Varga, J. M. (1975). On the specificity of antibodies. *Science*, **187**, 130–137.

Schindler, R. (1973). Experiments with serological methods on the differential diagnosis of trypanosomiasis in cattle in Africa south of the Sahara. *Transactions of the Royal Society of Tropical Medicine and Hygiene*, **67**, 290.

Terry, R. J., Freeman, Joan, Hudson, K. M. and Langstaffe, J. A. (1973). Immunoglobulin M production and immunosuppression in trypanosomiasis: a linking hypothesis. *Transactions of the Royal Society of Tropical Medicine and Hygiene*, **67**, 263.

Uhr, J. W. and Finkelstein, M. F. (1967). The kinetics of antibody formation. *Progress in Allergy*, **10**, 37–83.

Wilkinson, P. C. and Carmichael, D. S. (1964). Immunochemical characterization and serologic behaviour of antibodies against red cells in infectious mononucleosis. *Journal of Laboratory and Clinical Medicine*, **4**, 529.

XI. Appendix I

List of heterophile antibodies associated with trypanosomiasis

	Heterophile antibodies specific for	Produced by	After infection by	Reference
(1)	Rabbit and sheep erythrocytes	Human	*T. b. rhodesiense*	Parratt and Cobb (1978) Houba and Allison (1966)
(2)	Rabbit erythrocytes	Human	*T. b. gambiense*	Parratt and Cobb (1978)
(3)	Rabbit and sheep erythrocytes	Monkey (*Macacca mulatta*)	*T. b. rhodesiense*, *T. b. gambiense* and *T. b. brucei*	Houba *et al.* (1969)
(4)	Sheep erythrocytes	Rabbit	*T. b. brucei*	MacKenzie (1973)
(5)	Sheep erythrocytes	Human	*T. cruzi*	Muniz and Dos Santos (1950)
(6)	?	Cattle	*T. congolense*	Schindler (1973)
(7)	Chicken, rabbit and human erythrocytes	Cattle	*T. vivax*	Clarkson *et al.* (1975)
(8)	Sheep, guinea pig and rabbit erythrocytes	Chicken	*T. b. ? brucei* (WITat 1)	See Chapter text

XII. Appendix II
Authors' technical methods

Haemagglutination tests are usually carried out in plastic microtitre plates, and only occasionally as tube tests. When the latter are used the format of the test parallels that described for the Paul–Bunnell test in *Medical Microbiology* (Cruikshank, 1965). In the plate tests, sera are tested neat and at dilutions to approximately 1 in 5000, in 0·1 ml volumes. 0·15 m NaCl is used for dilution. 0·1 ml of 2% erythrocyte suspension is added to each well, the plates are shaken and incubated at 37°C for 2 h followed by 18 h at room temperature (18–20°C). Saline suspensions of the erythrocytes, in the absence of serum, are included in each test to control any autoagglutinability of the erythrocytes. The end point of agglutination is read by naked eye examination of the pattern of cells in each well. For confirmation, the plate is tilted gently to an angle of 45° and is re-examined after 1 minute. Agglutinated cells remain firmly fixed in position whereas non-agglutinated cells disperse from a neat circular "button" into a comma-shaped streak.

Absorptions of sera are carried out by mixing equal volumes of a 1 in 8 or 1 in 16 dilution of serum and of packed erythrocytes of the appropriate type. The mixtures are incubated at 37°C for 1 h and 4°C for a further 12 h. After centrifugation to retrieve the serum the appropriate haemagglutination test is repeated and if agglutination of the cells used in the absorption remains (or is not significantly reduced), the serum is further absorbed and retested.

12

Pathogenesis of *Trypanosoma cruzi* Infections*

W. L. TAFURI

Department of Pathology and Electron Microscopy Centre,
School of Medicine, Federal University of Minas Gerais,
Belo Horizonte, Brazil

I.	Pathogenetic concept. Parasite- and host-dependent factors playing a role in the pathogenesis of *Trypanosoma cruzi* infections .	547
	A. Parasite-dependent factors	548
	B. Host-dependent factors	550
II.	Natural history of *T. cruzi* infections	552
	A. The acute phase of *T. cruzi* infections	553
	B. The chronic phase of *T. cruzi* infections	591
III.	Lesions of the central nervous system in *T. cruzi* infections .	607
IV.	Concluding remarks	609
V.	Acknowledgements	609
VI.	References	610

I. Pathogenetic concept. Parasite- and host-dependent factors playing a role in the pathogenesis of Trypanosoma cruzi infections

This chapter concentrates on the formation of the lesions induced by *Trypanosoma cruzi* and analyses the mechanisms likely to be involved in the process. The data so far accumulated indicate that these mechanisms are multiple and dependent on various factors that may qualitatively or quantitatively interfere with the development of *T. cruzi* infection.

* Work supported by the National Research Council and the Research Council of the Federal University of Minas Gerais, Brazil.

A. PARASITE-DEPENDENT FACTORS

1. Polymorphism

Chagas (1909) and other investigators (Brener and Chiari, 1963, 1965; Brener, 1973) have reported the presence of different bloodstream forms of *T. cruzi* trypomastigotes in humans and in experimental animals; slender, broad and stout form trypomastigotes have been described (Brener, 1973), but their biological significance is still unknown. Indirect evidence showing that the predominance of one of the three forms may have a special biological significance was provided by Brener and Chiari (1971) in their studies on the effects of immunosuppressive agents in experimental chronic Chagas' disease. According to Brener (1973) the slender forms are more infective, inducing higher parasitaemia and lethality. The presence of these different bloodstream trypomastigote forms could represent a pool of different strains, and variation in these pool populations may explain certain epidemiological differences observed in *T. cruzi* infections (Lambrecht, 1965; Brant, 1966).

2. Tropism

Although *T. cruzi* may parasitize all cell types, observations in experimental and human infections have shown that some strains are predominantly myotropic (Andrade and Andrade, 1966), while others are reticulotropic (Taliaferro and Pizzi, 1955). Marked differences in the intensity of cellular parasitism were observed in the autonomic and central nervous system of albino mice inoculated with different *T. cruzi* strains (Tafuri and Brener, 1966a; Amaral *et al.*, 1975).

3. Cell penetration and virulence

In vitro experiments (Nogueira and Cohn, 1976) have shown that the penetration of epimastigotes and amastigotes into cells is by endocytosis. The parasites are initially surrounded by a membrane that separates them from the cytoplasmic organelles; this is usually present for up to 2 hours after penetration and shows as a clear halo. Later on the membrane is fragmented and the parasites set free in the cytoplasm. *In vivo*, the mechanism of cell penetration by *T. cruzi* remains obscure. The intracellular epimastigote forms multiply by binary division each 12 hours (Meyer and Oliveira-Musachio, 1948), to reach a maximum of about 500 parasites, i.e. about 9 generations (Dvorack, 1976), before causing the rupture of the cell. Not all amastigotes are transformed into trypomastigotes; electron microscopic studies of mice myocardium inoculated with different *T. cruzi* strains (Brener *et al.*, 1969) showed that about 15% of the amastigotes degenerated while the remainder induced cytoplasmic lysis of the host cell. As the development and severity of *T. cruzi*-induced lesions may be partially dependent on this phenomenon, it is necessary to determine the death rate of amastigotes of different strains in different host cells. The most virulent strains would be expected to be those displaying highest penetration capacity (slender forms) and highest lethality rate; in fact a high number of dead parasites and cells, as well as high amounts of antigens or inflammatory mediators induce more severe local and systemic responses (Tafuri, 1975). This concept of virulence differs from that based on parasitaemic curve and death of experimental animals.

4. Antigenic constituents

T. cruzi antigens have not yet been thoroughly investigated, but three types of antigen indentified by Nussenzweig *et al.* (1963) and by González-Cappa and Kagan (1969) could possibly be related to different clinical forms of Chagas' disease. According to Teixeira *et al.* (1975) various fractions of *T. cruzi* particulate subcellular antigens inoculated into rabbits induced microscopic lesions similar to those resulting from the inoculation of live parasites. These authors proposed that the lesions in the chronic Chagas' disease might be induced by a mechanism of delayed hypersensitivity to *T. cruzi* antigens.

5. Number of *T. cruzi* inoculated

Silva and Nussenzweig (1953) and Brener and Chiari (1963) showed that the severity of the infection and the survival rate of animals are dependent on the number of *T. cruzi* inoculated. According to Lima-Pereira (1976a), the inoculation of large numbers of *T. cruzi* produced high levels of parasitaemia with discrete cellular infiltration. This could be explained by the liberation of a large amount of antigenic material not of parasite origin which, by overloading the immune system would lead to a depression of the immunological response. Nevertheless, strains considered as highly virulent may give rise to severe infections with high mortality rates, even when a very small inoculum (Pizzi, 1961), or even a single trypanosome (Brener, personal communication) are used. In man, the relatively small number of observed cases of acute Chagas' disease is in sharp contrast with the high incidence of the chronic disease in endemic areas. This could be due either to the number of trypanosomes inoculated (Romãna and Terracini, 1945), or to the low virulence of the strains (Andrade, 1973).

6. Virulence attenuation

Brener *et al.* (1974) detected no decrease in the virulence of different *T. cruzi* strains sub-passaged in mice for 8 years, nor were changes observed in the parasitaemia, infectivity or polymorphism of these parasites.

B. HOST-DEPENDENT FACTORS

Regarding the host, some factors were observed to interfere with the parasite susceptibility and with the development and severity of *T. cruzi* infections, the most relevant among them being the following:

1. Sex and age

Whether the sex of an experimental animal has any influence on the outcome of an infection with *T. cruzi* is unclear. Hauschka (1947) showed that the male is more susceptible to infection than the female, whereas Streber (1950) suggested that the female is more susceptible. Silva and Nussenzweig (1953) and Brener (1961) observed that the sex of the animal had no effect on the level of parasitaemia and survival. The longer survival of infected female mice, as compared with that of the males observed by Hauschka (1947), is probably due to the more intense immunological response of the female, possibly related to their larger and heavier thymus and spleen (Lima-Pereira, 1976b). On the other hand, human findings indicate that children and adolescents are more susceptible than adults and the aged. The same is also true of experimental animals (Pizzi, 1957).

2. Genetic constitution

The important role played by the host genetic constitution, in the response to *T. cruzi* infection is shown by the data reported by various researchers. Pizzi *et al.* (1948/1949) suggested that the intensity of the inflammatory reaction, the parasitaemia level, and the mortality rate of infected mice are largely dependent on the genetic makeup of the mice. Some strains of mice are very susceptible to *T. cruzi* infection while others are resistant (Pizzi *et al.*, 1948/1949). Paulino da Costa (1976) showed that resistance to infection is probably related to many factors such as phagocytosis and lysis of the *T. cruzi* infective forms (Dias, 1933; Rubio, 1956) and the lytic activity of serum on the epimastigotes and trypomastigotes (Rubio, 1956; Warren and Borsos, 1959). Metacyclic forms obtained from triatomines survive only for about 17 minutes when mixed with human serum (Wood, 1953). This finding seems to indicate that, after penetration into the skin and eye conjunctiva, infective forms of *T. cruzi* can be destroyed by antiparasitic substances already present in the blood serum. The higher incidence of inoculation "Chagoma" in children, as compared with other age groups, may then be explained by the low level of antiparasitic substances in their blood.

3. Species

It is well known that some animals (e.g. poikilothermic vertebrates and birds) are markedly resistant to *T. cruzi* infections.

4. Effects of immuno-suppressors. Interferon

Steroid hormones, especially cortisone, elevate both blood stream parasitaemia and cellular parasitism during the acute phase of *T. cruzi* infection (Rubio, 1954). This effect of cortisone, however, has not been observed in the chronic phase of the infection (Brener and Chiari, 1963). There is evidence to show that interferon induces an increase of *T. cruzi* infection in mice (Martinez-Silva *et al.*, 1970), and that use of the various chemical and physical immuno-suppressive agents results in increases in the parasitaemia, the mortality rate and in the intensity of myocarditis of infected animals (Kumar *et al.*, 1970). *In vitro*, high levels of human interferon did not affect the growth of several *T. cruzi* strains (Golgher *et al.*, 1976). Increase in the parasitaemia, exacerbation of the inflammatory reaction and intensification of tissue injuries were observed in human cases of chronic Chagas' disease associated with immuno-suppressive diseases (Almeida *et al.*, 1974b). Similar findings were observed by Brener and Chiari (1971) after irradiation and cyclophosphamide treatment of *T. cruzi*-infected mice. It has been shown that mice infected with *T. cruzi* have depressed cellular and humoral immunological response to antigens not related to the parasite (Clinton *et al.*, 1975; Lima-Pereira, 1976a, b), the mechanism responsible for such decrease being still obscure. As suggested by Lima-Pereira (1976b), the decrease in the immunological response is not related to the lymphocytolysis which occurs in the thymus and spleen during the infection. A study of the mechanism involved in immuno-depression during *T. cruzi* infection, as well as a critical analysis of the relationship between the level of immunosuppression and the intensity of the lesions induced, would lead to a better understanding of the pathogenesis of the lesions occurring during the various developmental stages of infection.

5. Re-infection

The influence of repeated infection on the progress of Chagas' disease is not clear. Macedo (1973) showed that individuals living in triatomine-infested houses had more severe forms of the disease and that their mortality rate was higher than that of patients living in non-infested houses. Similarly, Chagas (1935), Prata (1955) and Rodrigues da Silva (1966) have suggested that repeated infection may possibly be one of the factors responsible for the more rapid onset both of the parasitaemia and the severity of cardiopathy observed in some cases.

6. Nutritional factors

The parasitaemia is higher and the lesions more severe in experimental animals with deficiency of vitamins B and A (Yaeger and Miller, 1960; Yaeger et al., 1963). Some authors have suggested that nutritional deficiency may be one of the factors responsible for the differences in the clinical manifestations of Chagas' disease in various Brazilian areas (Costa and Costa, 1960; Chapadeiro et al., 1964; Barbosa et al., 1970).

7. Temperature

Lowering of the body temperature has an intensifying effect on the severity of infection in experimental animals (Kolodny, 1939, 1940). Dvorack (1976) observed a direct relationship between the host temperature and the penetration of its cells by the parasites in the range from 29° to 35°C and suggested that natural infection occurs efficiently only over a narrow temperature range on the vertebrate surface. Temperatures above 35°C have a rate limiting effect on cell penetration.

II. Natural history of T. cruzi infections

American trypanosomiasis can be congenital or acquired. The latter is better known and presents at least two main forms: the cardiac forms and the digestive forms, the latter represented in Brazil by megaoesophagus and megacolon. Despite the extensive studies already conducted, much more investigation is still required in order to establish the natural history of the disease on a solid basis. The long asymptomatic period between the initial infection (inoculation "*Chagoma*") and the clinical manifestation of the disease chronic phase constitutes "a missing link in the natural history of the disease" (Almeida-Prado, 1959). The lack of scientific data on this cryptic period in the development of Chagas' disease is reflected in its classification into two forms: the acute phase, which comprises the changes appearing a few days after inoculation with *T. cruzi*, and the chronic phase, which occurs years later and can be symptomatic or asymptomatic.

What sort of changes does the host undergo after the end of the acute phase and the beginning of the chronic one? What are the factors responsible for the presence of distinct anatomical features, observed in the chronic phase of the disease, leading to the appearance of either the cardiac or the digestive form? To answer these questions and fill the gaps in our knowledge of the changes observed between the acute and chronic phases, various pathogenetic theories have been proposed.

Köberle's theory constituted a turning point in the study of the pathogenesis of Chagas' disease and opened new avenues for its exploration. From his investigations in humans and experimental animals

(Köberle and Nador, 1955; Köberle, 1956a, b, 1957, 1959, 1960, 1961, 1967, 1968), he concluded that the changes observed in the acute and the chronic phases of the disease could not be explained by a single pathogenetic mechanism. According to his findings, two different pathological processes are involved: (*a*) Chagas' disease proper, characterized by an acute septicaemic phase followed by a chronic phase with low parasiaemia; (*b*) Chagas "pathies" (the conditions resulting from lesions in the autonomic nervous system) occurring in the acute phase and leading to the death of ganglia nerve cells and the consequent denervation of the hollow organs. Thus, the destruction of the parasympathetic nervous system generally undergone in the disease acute phase can account for the functional alterations observed later on, constituting the *primum movens* of the "pathies" that appear in the chronic phase. Although Köberle's work defines, on firm anatomical basis, some of the changes which occur in the development of Chagas' disease and serves to fill the gap between the acute and the chronic phases, neither the whole sequence of events nor the mechanisms responsible for them are known and clearly understood. The findings that follow, observed in human and experimental trypanosomiasis, will help clarify some of the pathogenetic mechanisms of the lesions and suggest that other factors may be playing an equal or even more important role in the pathogenesis of this disease.

A. THE ACUTE PHASE OF *T. CRUZI* INFECTIONS

T. cruzi may parasitize any cell type in humans and experimental animals, but cellular parasitism is more frequent in the histiocytes, fibroblasts, central and peripheral neuroglia, smooth-muscle cells, cardiac-muscle cells and skeletal-muscle cells (Figs 1, 2). The causes of this cell tropism are not clear. Nogueira and Cohn (1976) reported that the presence of a protease-sensitive component in the macrophage plasma membrane is necessary for the uptake of *T. cruzi* and that such membrane component could also exist in other cell types, determining the tropism of *T. cruzi* for different tissue cells. The normal-looking intracellular *T. cruzi* forms induce partial lysis of the cytoplasmic organelles around the parasite, forming an electron-clear vacuole (Fig. 2). At this stage, no further changes in the cytoplasm or the nuclei of the parasitized cells are detectable by electron microscopy, nor is any inflammatory reaction observed (Figs 1, 2). However, when the parasites inside the cells and those free in the interstitium degenerate and die (Fig. 3), an acute focal inflammatory reaction develops in their vicinity (Fig. 4). The non-parasitized cells in the neighbourhood of these inflammatory foci show different levels of damage, and some of them die presenting the peculiar characters of cellular necrosis. Thus, the inflammatory reaction may possibly be induced by mediators of chemical inflammation released either from the damaged host-cells or from the degenerated lysed para-

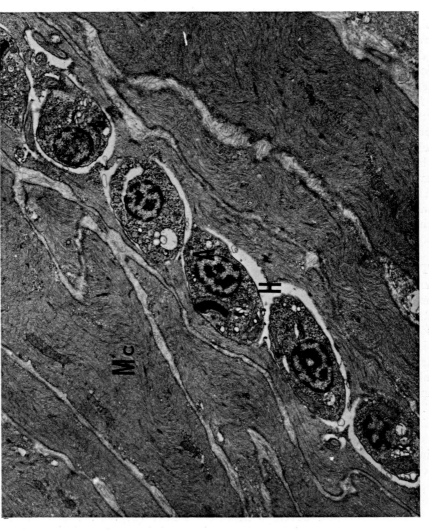

FIG. 1. Acute phase of *T. cruzi* infection. Mouse colon. Healthy amastigotes
(A) inside of smooth-muscle cells. Halo around parasite (H). Non-parasitized

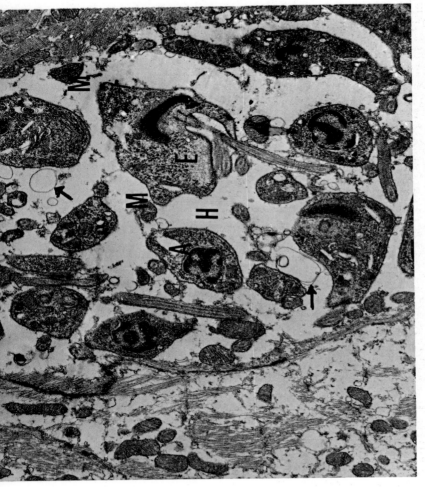

FIG. 2. Acute phase of *T. cruzi* infection. Mouse heart. Normal amastigotes (A) and epimastigotes (E) inside cardiac muscle cell. Clear space (H) around parasite. Mitochondria (M) partially preserved and cell debris inside clear digestive vacuole (arrows). × 18 000.

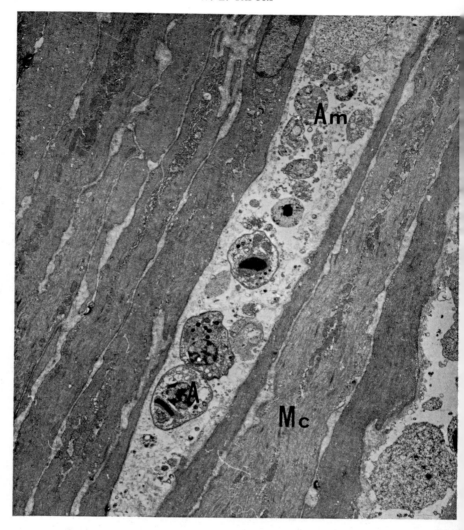

FIG. 3. Acute phase of *T. cruzi* infection. Mouse colon. Amastigotes (A) in different stages of degeneration are seen in widened intercellular space. Lysis of the interstitium structural components and formation of amorphous masses (Am). Smooth muscle cells (Mc) displaying normal aspect. × 7200.

sites, which then cause degenerative changes and the consequent death of normal non-parasitized host-cells in the vicinity of the inflammation foci. As cellular parasitism happens by chance, it is not difficult to understand the cause of the irregular distribution of the lesions in parasitized tissue or organs. Therefore, the appearance of different anatomo-

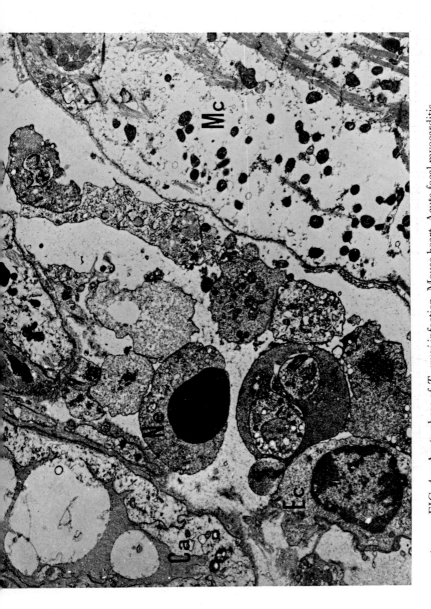

FIG. 4. Acute phase of *T. cruzi* infection. Mouse heart. Acute focal myocarditis. Swelling of capillary endothelial cells (Ca). Interstitial oedema. Infiltrative inflammatory cells (Ec), some of them presenting necrosis (Ne). Swelling of cardiac muscle cells (Mc). × 28 000.

clinical forms of the disease in the chronic phase could possibly be related to the intensity of the lesions induced in the acute phase.

1. Lesions of the Autonomic Nervous System (ANS)

The lesions of the sympathetic and parasympathetic nervous system, as observed by optical microscopy in the acute and chronic phases, are similar in man and in experimental animals. In the acute phase, the lesions in the superficial cardiac plexus, in the cervical, coeliac and lumbar ganglia, in the intramural ganglia of hollow organs (oesophagus, intestine, urinary bladder, ureter, etc) as well as those in the lungs and other organs are as follows:

(a) Presence of apparently normal parasites in the Schwann cells, in the capsular fibroblasts of both ganglia and sheath of extraganglionic nerve fibres, as well as in the peripheral nerves, with no surrounding inflammatory reaction.

(b) Periganglionitis and ganglionitis, neuritis and perineuritis, usually in disseminated (and sometimes systematized) foci with monocytic infiltration and rare granulocytes (Figs 5 and 6).

(c) Degenerative changes of neurons (chromatolysis, acute swelling) and nerve fibres; these can differ in severity from slight damage up to death and necrosis of the nerve cells (pyknosis and karyolysis) (Fig. 6). The lesions above were unpredictable and randomly distributed (in mice or other animals with infections of different durations) and, therefore, altered and apparently normal ganglia were frequently observed side by side. Furthermore, normal and degenerated or necrotic neurons were also seen next to one another in the same ganglion. However, an inflammatory process was always observed in the ganglia (ganglionitis) or in the surrounding tissues (cellulitis and myositis).

Although the changes undergone by the ANS are well defined at the optical microscope level, there is still great controversy on the pathogenetic mechanism leading to these changes. Köberle (1956a) postulated that a toxin or an enzyme released from dead parasites in the intercellular space caused the destruction of the neurons. Lisboa-Bittencourt (1960) proposed that neuronal destruction was induced by a direct mechanism (ganglionitis) and not indirectly as suggested by Köberle. Lopes (1965) observed an inflammatory reaction in the epicardiac adipose tissue (cellulitis) that extended to the ganglia (periganglionitis and ganglionitis), and induced partial or total destruction of ganglion structure with consequent reduction in the number of neurons. These findings are in agreement with those of Tafuri and Raso (1962) and Tafuri and Brener (1966a, b, 1967) in experimental *T. cruzi* infections of mice. Andrade and Andrade (1966), trying to determine which of the two hypothetical mechanisms of neuronal destruction was the more accurate, used two groups of mice experimentally infected with *T. cruzi*, the inflammatory reaction of one group being blocked by prior treatment with cortisone. The neuronal lesions were found to be in direct correlation with the inflammatory process in the vicinity of the ganglia. In those mice in which inflammatory reaction had been suppressed by cortisone, no neuronal lesions were observed, indicating that the inflammatory reaction in and around the ganglia play a dominant role in the destruction of neurons. Teixeira *et al.* (1975), working with rabbits infected with live forms of *T. cruzi* or inoculated with antigenic fractions of the parasite, observed that lysis of the neurons was related to the periganglionar lymphocytic infiltration, and suggested that the destruction of parasympathetic neurons could be caused by lymphocytes sensitized by *T. cruzi* antigens exerting a cytotoxic effect on the neurons.

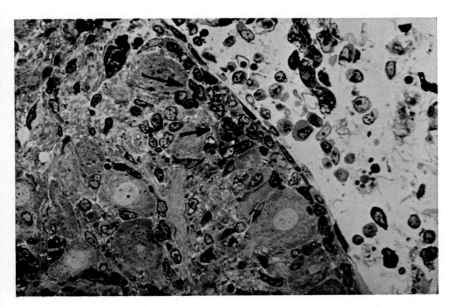

FIG. 5. Acute phase of *T. cruzi* infection. Sympathetic ganglion. Acute periganglionitis and ganglionitis. Diffuse infiltration of mononuclear cells in the ganglion periphery and discrete focal infiltration (arrows) inside of ganglion. Neuron and neuroglial cells showing normal morphological characters. × 320.

Electron microscopy showed that, both in the acute and the chronic phases of *T. cruzi* infection, lesions can be found in ANS neurons, in satellite and Schwann cells, in myelinic and amyelinic fibres and in periganglionar and interstitial connective tissue.

The lesions are systematized and always associated with degenerated *T. cruzi* amastigotes inside or outside the cells, with or without local inflammatory reactions (Figs 7 and 8). The changes in the nuclei of the

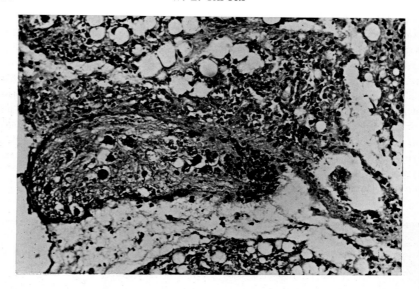

FIG. 6. Acute phase of *T. cruzi* infection. Mouse sympathetic ganglion. Acute necrotizing ganglionitis, periganglionitis and cellulitis. × 150.

neurons are less conspicous than those in the perikaryon. In areas of intense focal ganglionitis, there may be marked changes in nuclear structure, with disappearance or shrinkage of the nuclear membrane. The cytoplasmic changes vary in intensity, the lesions being severe in some neurons and discrete in others.

The following changes are generally observed:

(*a*) Swelling, cristolysis and vacuolization of mitochondria;

(*b*) Dilatation of the Golgi complex;

(*c*) Increase in the number of secondary lysosomes in the neurons of the most severely damaged ganglia;

(*d*) Peripheral chromatolysis;

(*e*) Rare presence of parasites in the parasympathetic and sympathetic neurons, their occurrence, however, being more frequent in the former than in the latter neurons (Figs 9 and 10).

The lesions in the intra- or extraganglionar nerve fibres are irregular in distribution and variable in intensity. They are directly related to the presence of degenerated parasites and focal inflammatory reaction (periganglionitis, ganglionitis, cellulitis or myositis), but may also be found in areas where the above changes have not occurred. The ultrastructural alterations most frequently observed are:

(*a*) Lysis of microtubules and neurofilaments;

(*b*) Swelling, vacuolization and lysis of the mitochondrial cristae;

(*c*) Swelling of the axoplasm, fragmentation of the axolemma, and the presence of osmiophilic electron-dense inclusions between the neuro-filaments;

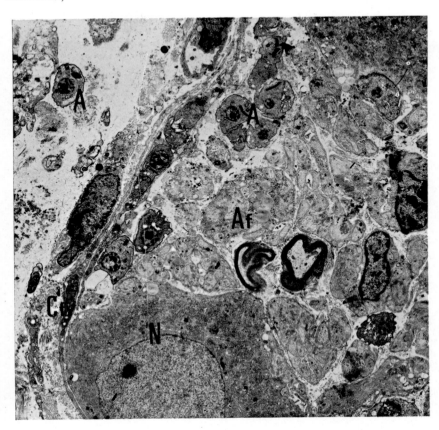

FIG. 7. Acute phase of *T. cruzi* infection. Mouse sympathetic ganglion. Normal and degenerated amastigotes (A) inside and outside the ganglion. Severe changes in amyelinic nerve fibres (Af). Dissociation of interstitial structures. Normal neurons (N). Capsular fibroblast (Cf). × 4500.

(*d*) Lysis of the myelin sheath shrinkage of the axon (Figs. 11, 12, 13).

The satellite and the Schwann cells are frequently parasitized by amastigotes. Around well-preserved and normal-looking *T. cruzi* forms, only minor cytoplasmic changes are found, no alterations in the other cellular organelles being detected. In these cells vacuole formation occurs, but no electron-dense material or limiting membrane are found around the parasites. The remaining cytoplasm and the nucleus of the parasitized cells, as well as the cells in the vicinity, show no alterations. However, in the sites where parasites have degenerated, marked alterations

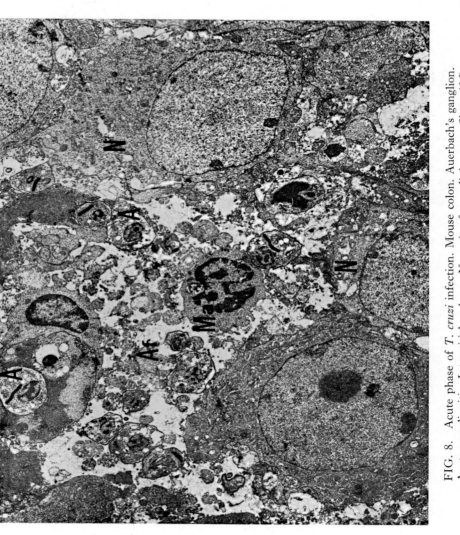

FIG. 8. Acute phase of *T. cruzi* infection. Mouse colon. Auerbach's ganglion. Acute ganglionitis. Interstitial oedema. Necrosis of amyelinic nerve fibres (Af). Macrophages (Ma) and degenerated amastigotes (A) in the interstitium. Partially

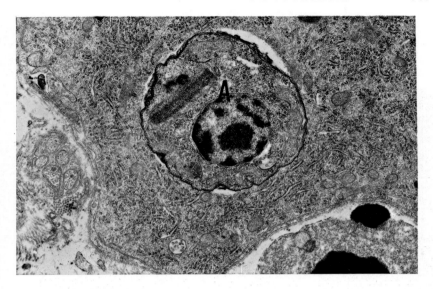

FIG. 9. Acute phase of *T. cruzi* infection. Mouse sympathetic ganglion. Well-preserved neuron with amastigote (A) inside. × 10 000.

can be seen not only in the parasitized satellite cells, but also in the neuron, in the fibres and in the adjacent interstitium, where focal acute inflammatory reaction then develops. It would appear, therefore, that the injuries to the satellite and Schwann cells are directly related to the cellular parasitism (Fig. 14) and to the focal inflammatory reaction which develops around them. The alterations observed in the neurons may also be directly related to the degenerative changes occurring in the satellite cells. On the whole, the lesions observed in the neuroglial cells were as follows:

(*a*) mitochondrial swelling and vacuolization;

(*b*) dilatation of the endoplasmic reticulum;

(*c*) lysis of the gliofilaments;

(*d*) presence of secondary lysosomes, vacuoles and amorphous, electron-dense inclusions in the cytoplasm of the altered cells (Fig. 14).

Intra- and extraganglionic capillaries and venules close to the inflammatory foci and in areas not topographically related, show intense swelling in their endothelial cells and lumen reduction (Fig. 23). Furthermore, they also showed the following alterations:

(*a*) widening of intercellular spaces;

(*b*) rupture of the plasma membrane;

(*c*) thickening of the basal membrane, alterations of the ground substance and presence of inflammatory cell infiltration. Parasitism of

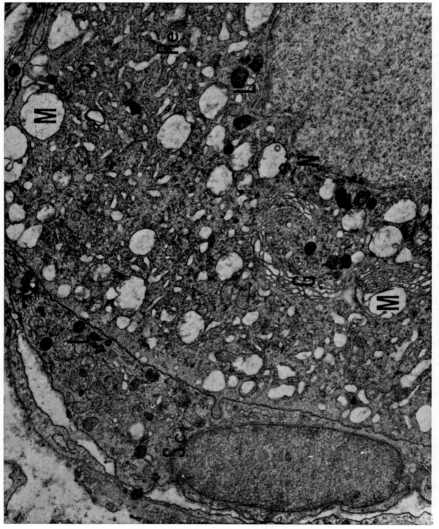

FIG. 10. Acute phase of *T. cruzi* infection. Mouse subepicardial ganglion. Neuron (N). Swelling and vacuolization of mitochondria (M). Dilation of the endoplasmic reticulum (Re). Partial chromatolysis. Golgi complex (G). Lysosomes

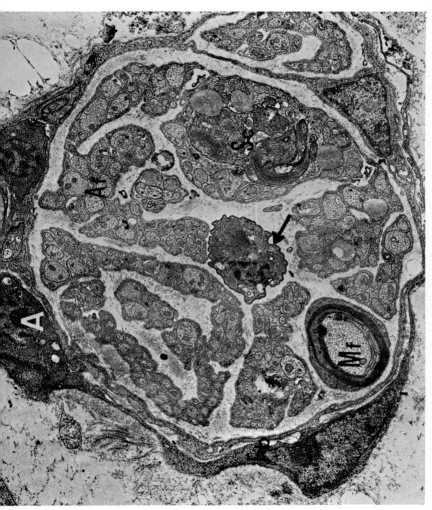

FIG. 11.   Acute phase of *T. cruzi* infection. Mouse sympathetic nerve. Amastigotes (A) inside capsular fibroblasts (Fb) in the Schwann cell (Sc) and in the interstitium (arrow). Myelinic (Mf) and amyelinic (Af) nerve fibres displaying normal aspect. × 3600.

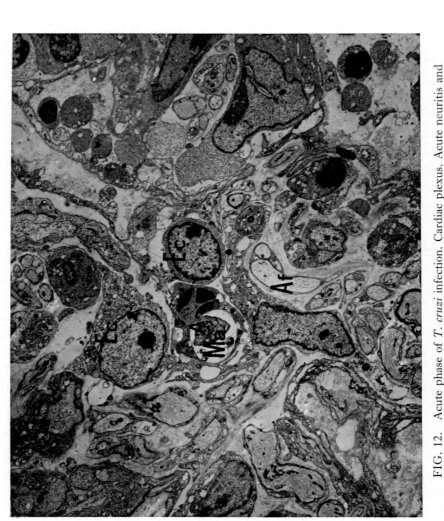

FIG. 12. Acute phase of *T. cruzi* infection. Cardiac plexus. Acute neuritis and perineuritis. Inflammatory infiltrative cell (Ec) in the interstitium. Amyelinic nerve fibres (Af) dissociated by oedema. Degenerated macrophage (Ma) with

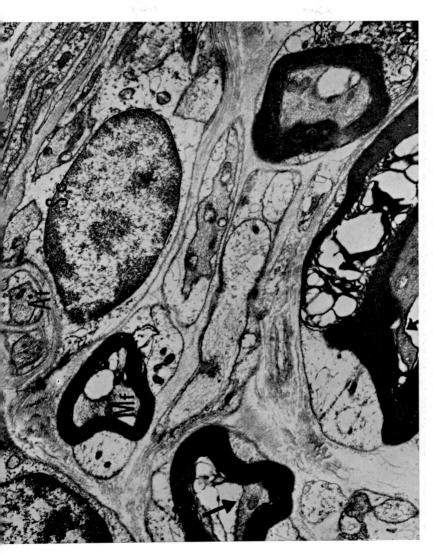

FIG. 13. Acute phase of *T. cruzi* infection. Cardiac plexus. Bundle of amyelinic (Af) and myelinic (Mf) nerve fibres with lysis of mitocrotubules and neurofilaments. Axonal shrinkage (arrows). Schwann cells (Sc). × 28 000.

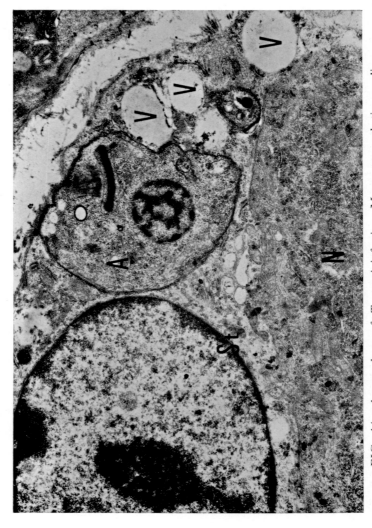

FIG. 14. Acute phase of *T. cruzi* infection. Mouse sympathetic ganglion. Satellite cells (St) with amastigote (A) inside; lysis of glioflaments and vacuoles (V). Well-preserved perikarion of neuron (N). × 10 000.

venules, smooth-muscle cells and arteriole walls was only occasionally observed.

Macrophages are the most intensely parasitized cells, and this fact has led many investigators to propose that macrophages play an important role in the host response to *T. cruzi* infection (Souza-Campos, 1929; Dias, 1932; Torres and Duarte, 1948; Taliaferro and Pizzi, 1955; Pizzi and Rubio, 1955 and others). Recently, many studies on parasite–macrophage interaction have been conducted both *in vitro* (Behbehani, 1971; Dvorack and Schmunis, 1972; Milder *et al.*, 1973; Nogueira, 1974; Nogueira and Cohn, 1976) and *in vivo* (Scorza and Scorza, 1972a, b). The results of these studies have been somewhat contradictory as concerns the mechanism of *T. cruzi* penetration and intracellular multiplication in the macrophages.

Two forms of phagocytosis occur: the immediate, taking place before the development of an immunological response, and the mediate, occurring after an immunological response is established. The first one, the immediate, is performed with little or no opsonization of the material to be phagocytosed. The second, the mediate, always takes place after the opsonization of the phagocytosed material. The mechanism of phagocytosis seems to be similar in both cases and can be arbitrarily divided into four steps: (1) migration of the phagocytes to the vicinity of the material; (2) identification and contact; (3) incorporation of the material into the phagocyte; (4) digestion.

After *T. cruzi* has entered the macrophage, the following may happen: (*a*) The amastigotes remaining in the macrophage cytoplasm are enveloped by the digestive vacuole membrane (Fig. 15 A, B, C).
(*b*) Binary multiplication of amastigotes not surrounded by involutory membrane (Fig. 16 A).
(*c*) Death and lysis of the parasites and/or the host cell (Fig. 16 B).

These observations seem to indicate that two types of macrophage are involved in the response to *T. cruzi* infection: macrophages previously sensitized by lymphocytes and non-sensitized macrophages. The former would have the function of ingesting and digesting *T. cruzi*, whereas the latter would act as host cells where the intracellular development of *T. cruzi* takes place. *In vitro* experiments have shown that epimastigotes are killed and digested inside the phagolysosome of macrophages (Nogueira and Cohn, 1976). Lima-Pereira and Sassine (1976) showed that peritoneal macrophages from mice infected with *T. cruzi* have increased phagocytic activity.

Nevertheless, the presence of dead parasites in the interstitium suggests the existence of another mechanism for parasite destruction, possibly of humoral nature.

There being no recognition of the antigen by the sensitized macrophages, non-specific-growth inhibition will probably not occur. In this

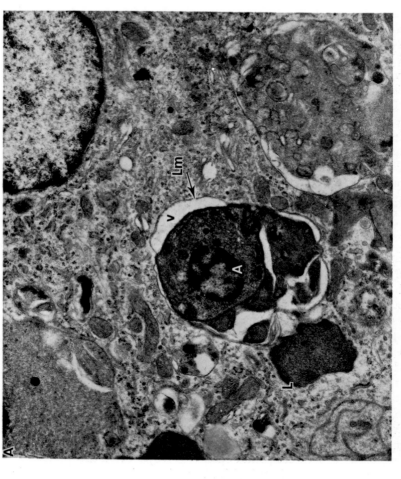

FIG. 15A. Acute phase of *T. cruzi* infection. Mouse heart. Sequential alterations in macrophages of the infiltrate. Phagolysosome formation. Lysosome (L),
limiting membrane (Lm). Amastigote (A). Cell debris inside the vacuole (V).
× 12 000.

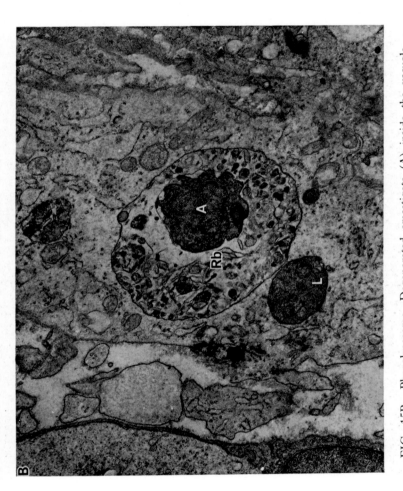

FIG. 15B. Phagolysosome. Degenerated amastigote (A) inside the vacuole. Residual bodies (Rb). Lysosome (L). × 12 000.

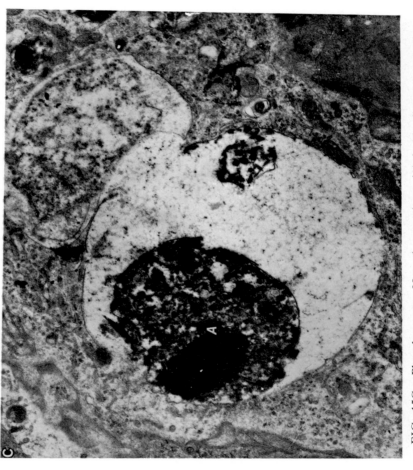

FIG. 15C. Phagolysosome. Necrotic amastigote (A) inside digestive vacuole. × 12 000.

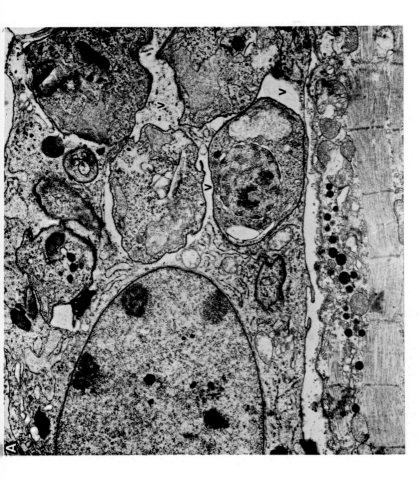

FIG. 16A. Acute phase of *T. cruzi* infection. Mouse heart. (A) Macrophage with many parasites inside. Absence of limiting membrane around the vacuole (V). × 18 000.

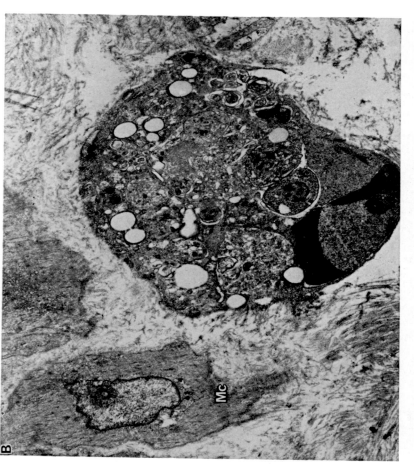

FIG. 16B. Necrotic macrophage with degenerated parasites in the cytoplasm. Smooth muscle cells (Mc) and interstitium displaying normal morphological feature. × 7200.

case, the trypomastigotes and the transition forms of *T. cruzi* escape from the phagocytic vacuoles and multiply in the cytoplasm. When released from parasitized cells, the amastigotes, like the trypomastigotes, display their ability to penetrate and multiply in other cells (Nogueira and Cohn, 1976). In our experiments, only amastigote and epimastigote-forms were found inside macrophages. In the interstitium, however, the three *T. cruzi* forms were present.

Intra- and extraganglionic fibroblasts are frequently parasitized, the alterations observed being similar to those seen in the Schwann cells.

In the peri- and intraganglionic inflammatory foci, the neurons and the nerve fibres are markedly dissociated by oedema and by the infiltration of inflammatory cells (monocytes, histiocytes, lymphocytes) and by neutrophile granulocytes. Many of the infiltrative cells, as well as the parasites in the interstitium degenerate and die. The mechanism causing these infiltrative cells to die abruptly in the inflammatory foci are so far not known (Fig. 17 A, B).

The alterations observed after *T. cruzi* infection in the vesicular component of the intramural nervous plexus of the hollow organs are now described, and their probable role in the pathogenesis of *T. cruzi* infection analysed.

In the perikaryon of the neurons and along the axons and their terminations agranular and granular vesicles of variable diameter are frequently found (Fig. 18 A, B). According to their size and content they may be classified as:

(*a*) synaptic vesicles (De Robertis and Bennet, 1954; Palade and Palay, 1954);

(*b*) clear vesicles (Hager and Tafuri, 1959a, b), also known as agranular vesicles;

(*c*) granular vesicles (Hager and Tafuri, 1959a, b; Grillo and Pallay 1962; Tafuri, 1964);

(*d*) large opaque vesicles, larger than the granular vesicles and called purinergic (Burnstock, 1972).

Although the function of those vesicles is not known, the marked morphological alterations of their components observed in congenital megacolon (Tafuri *et al.*, 1974b), in megaoesophagus and megacolon from Chagas' disease (Hial *et al.*, 1973), as well as changes in their numbers induced by scorpion toxin (Tafuri *et al.*, 1974a), have opened new perspectives for the study of their function and role in the pathogenesis of Chagas' disease lesions.

A quantitative study of granular and agranular vesicles in the axons of the Auerbach's plexus of the colon of both normal mice and mice infected with *T. cruzi* (acute infection) has demonstrated a marked reduction in the number of vesicles (especially of the granular ones) in the latter mice, as compared with that of the former (Almeida *et al.*, 1976).

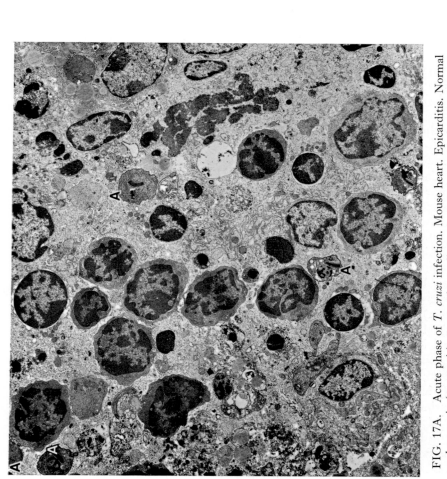

FIG. 17A.   Acute phase of *T. cruzi* infection. Mouse heart. Epicarditis. Normal and necrotic (apoptosis) mononuclear cells in the infiltrate. Degenerated amastigotes (A) in the interstitium. Capillary (Ca). Amorphous masses (Am)   × 3600

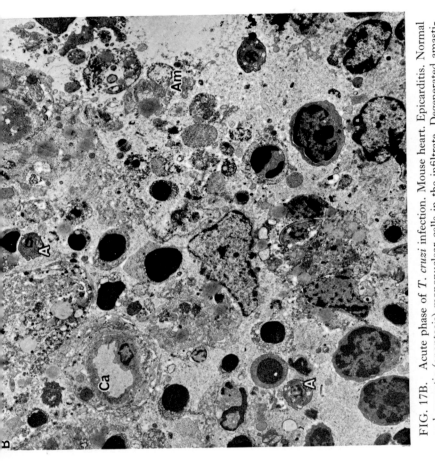

FIG. 17B. Acute phase of *T. cruzi* infection. Mouse heart. Epicarditis. Normal and necrotic (apoptosis) mononuclear cells in the infiltrate. Degenerated amastigotes (A) in the interstitium. Capillary (Ca). Amorphous masses (Am). × 3600.

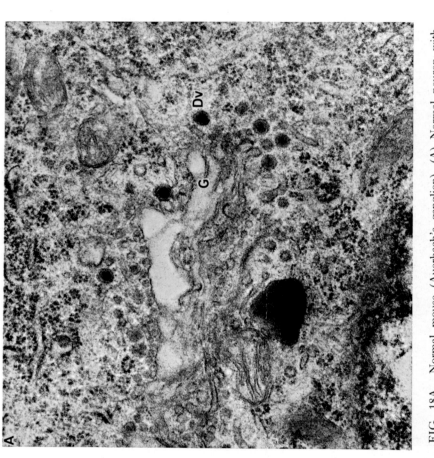

FIG. 18A. Normal mouse (Auerbach's ganglion). (A) Normal neuron with granular dense vesicles (Dv) close to the Golgi complex (G). × 28 000.

This decrease in the number of vesicles according to our observations could be due to:

(*a*) swelling of the axons;

(*b*) decrease in the synthetic activity of the perikaryon region of the neurone as a consequence of the lesion produced by the parasite and the inflammation that it causes;

(*c*) rupture of the vesicles;

(*d*) release of the granular vesicles contents (Fig. 19).

It has been shown that scorpion toxin induces a marked reduction in the number of granular vesicles in the Auerbach's plexus of the rat ileum as is found in acute experimental *T. cruzi* infections (Tafuri *et al.*,

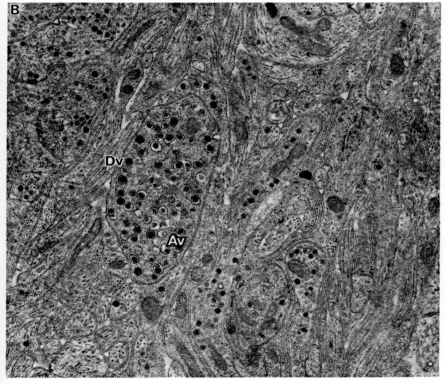

FIG. 18B. Dense granular (Dv) and agranular (Av) vesicles of amyelinic nerve fibre. × 18 000.

1974a). On the other hand, isolated rat and guinea-pig ileum treated with toxin also release acetylcholine and catecholamines (Diniz and Torres, 1968; Cunha-Melo *et al.*, 1970, 1973). These findings partially explain

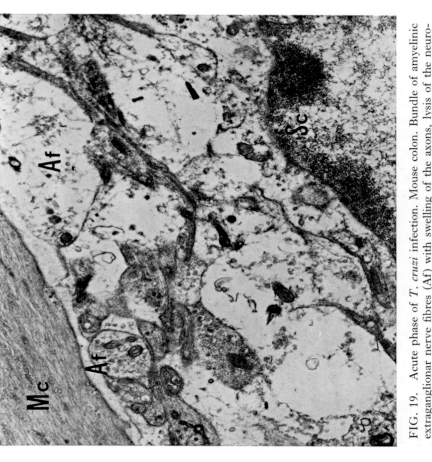

FIG. 19. Acute phase of *T. cruzi* infection. Mouse colon. Bundle of amyelinic extraganglionar nerve fibres (Af) with swelling of the axons, lysis of the neurofilaments and neurotubules and decrease of the vesicular component. Schwann cell (Sc). Smooth muscle cell (Mc). × 28 000.

the contraction and the relaxation induced in the ileum, but do not explain the contraction of atropine-treated preparations, which is assumed to be due to the release of substance P (Cunha-Melo *et al.*, 1973; Freire-Maia *et al.*, 1976a, b). This hypothesis was reinforced by experiments showing reduction of substance P content in the rat gut, after toxin injection (Hial and Diniz, 1971).

In the dilated segment of congenital megacolon (Tafuri *et al.*, 1974b) and in Chagas megaoesophagus and megacolon (Hial *et al.*, 1973), increases in the level of substance P in the muscular layers and in the number of granular vesicles of Auerbach's plexus were observed. In the narrow segment of congenital megacolon substance P is markedly decreased. Both findings indicate that the dense granular vesicles may contain, among other things, substance P. Nilsson *et al.* (1975) showed, by immunochemical methods, the presence of substance P in the Auerbach's plexus of the rabbit colon.

As we have shown (Almeida *et al.*, 1976), extracts made from muscle layers of mice with acute *T. cruzi* infections induced contraction of isolated guinea-pig ileum, similar to that evoked by bradykinin and substance P. However, the degree of contraction induced by extracts made from the intestines of *T. cruzi*-infected mice was far less intense than that induced by extracts from the colon of normal mice. It was demonstrated that substance P and extracts from the mouse colon induced contraction of isolated rat duodenum immersed in a bath containing Tyrode's solution with atropine, while bradykinin induced relaxation, indicating that in the mouse colon there is a substance capable of inducing contraction of the intestinal smooth muscle similar to that produced by substance P.

Machado *et al.* (1975; Machado and Machado, 1976) showed, however, that in the acute phase of experimental rat *T. cruzi* infection, a marked decrease in the heart noradrenaline content occurs, and that in the chronic phase of the infection, the level of heart noradrenaline is similar to that of control normal rats, thus indicating that the lesions induced in the sympathetic nerves of the heart in the acute phase of the infection, have completely recovered in the chronic phase.

It seems probable that the granular vesicles contain catecholamines and substance P, and that in the acute phase of Chagas' disease a decrease in the number of these vesicles and in the concentrations of heart and intestine mediators occurs.

2. Lesions of the heart and the digestive tract

The myocardium inflammatory changes induced by *T. cruzi* are perhaps the most severe known forms of myocarditis, both in man and in experimental animals. By optical microscopy, the lesions observed in the acute phase are as follows:

(*a*) Intense parasitism of the cardiac-muscle cells, subepicardiac-adipose-tissue histiocytes and interstitial-connective-tissue cells.

(*b*) Multiplication of the parasites inside the host cells leading to their rupture and release of the parasites into the interstitium. No inflammatory reaction is observed while the parasites from the host cells are healthy (Vianna, 1911).

(*c*) Focal acute inflammatory reaction in the areas of the interstitium where degenerated parasites are found.

(*d*) Inflammatory cellular infiltration most frequently composed of monocytes, histiocytes and granulocytes. The inflammatory cells accumulating in the endomysium and between the muscle cells, thus widening the space between the muscle cells as well as between the cells and the capillaries. This pattern is not found in other types of myocarditis and resembles phlegmonous inflammation, especially when numerous neutrophil granulocytes are found in the infiltrate.

(*e*) Degenerative changes of the non-parasitized myocardial cells in the neighbourhood of the inflammatory foci.

(*f*) Intense interstitial oedema.

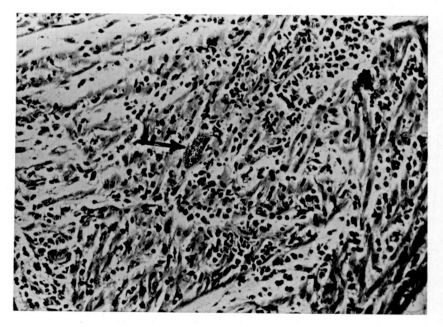

FIG. 20.   Acute phase of *T. cruzi* infection. Human acute myocarditis. Nests of parasites (arrow) inside the cardiac muscle cell. Intense inflammatory infiltrate with dissociation of the cardiac muscle cells that appear hypotrophic and degenerated. × 200.

(g) Inflammatory reaction and degenerative changes of the cardiac conducting system (Torres, 1941; Andrade, 1973). This is generally detected as extensive inflammatory infiltration of the bundle of Hiss, usually more intense in the right branch.

(h) Periganglionitis and ganglionitis (Figs 20 and 21).

The lesions induced by *T. cruzi* in the oesophagus and gastrointestinal tract are predominantly located in the muscle layers and in the intramural nervous plexus. In the oesophagus and intestine, as in the heart, focal myositis is observed around degenerated amastigotes in the interstitium. In the chronic phase of *T. cruzi* infection, megaoesophagus and megacolon may be observed.

By electron microscopy two types of lesions are found: one is induced by cellular parasitism and the other is not. In the latter case, the damaged cells are directly or indirectly related to inflammatory foci. When there is cellular parasitism, the lesions are more severe and extend to a larger number of cells. Intracellular parasites are observed from the 5th day after infection in experimental animals. In most cells the parasites display normal morphological features, although in about 15% of them clear morphological evidence of degenerative changes and cell death can be detected.

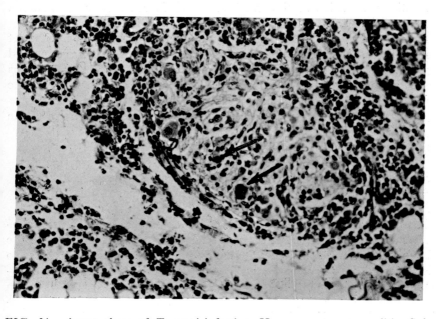

FIG. 21.   Acute phase of *T. cruzi* infection. Human acute myocarditis. Subepicardial ganglion. Cellulitis, periganglionitis and ganglionitis. Degenerative changes of the neurons (arrows). × 200.

In the myocardial cells where *T. cruzi* forms display normal morphological features, the following can be observed:

(*a*) Lysis of the myofibrils and the sarcoplasma around the parasites. The degree of myofibril destruction is directly related to the number of parasites present.

(*b*) The parasites are surrounded by a clear vacuole with no limiting membrane.

(*c*) In the vacuoles membrane debris and free mitochondria are found in addition to the amastigote and epimastigote forms of *T. cruzi*.

(*d*) The nuclei and other non-digested cytoplasmic areas appear normal.

(*e*) No changes are observed in the neighbourhood of parasitized cells (Fig. 2).

In the smooth-muscle cells and in myocardial cells containing degenerated parasites, the following changes are observed:

(*a*) Oedema of the sarcoplasm with dilatation of the endoplasmic reticulum.

(*b*) Presence of amorphous osmiophilic masses with lamellar structure.

(*c*) Myofibrils with granular appearance and partial blurring of their fine structure.

(*d*) Swelling, vacuolization and cristolysis of the mitochondria. In the neighbourhood of damaged cells containing degenerated parasites marked alterations of the interstitium with cellular inflammatory infiltration can be seen (Fig. 4).

In the vicinity of inflammatory foci or near degenerated parasites set free in the interstitium, the non-parasitized muscle cells undergo marked degenerative changes (Fig. 4). These damaged cells are more numerous than the parasitized cells and their lesions usually more severe. The following changes are then observed:

(*a*) Intracellular oedema and dilatation of the cisternal profiles of the endoplasmic reticulum.

(*b*) Disorganization and lysis of the myofibrils.

(*c*) Dissociation of the myofibrils with rupture of the sarcomere.

(*d*) Presence of amorphous osmiophilic masses and myelinic figures.

(*e*) Stretching and rupture of the plasma membrane.

(*f*) Necrosis of the muscle cells.

In the myocardium the most severe lesions are observed in the subepicardiac muscle cells close to infiltrative cells (Fig. 22). The connective tissue, the ground substance, the collagen and the elastic fibres close to degenerated cells are markedly altered. The capillaries in the inflammatory foci or in their vicinity show changes similar to those observed in the capillaries of the subepicardiac ganglia. The myocardial cells adjacent to these capillaries show discrete alterations, especially swelling and focal myocytolisis (Fig. 23).

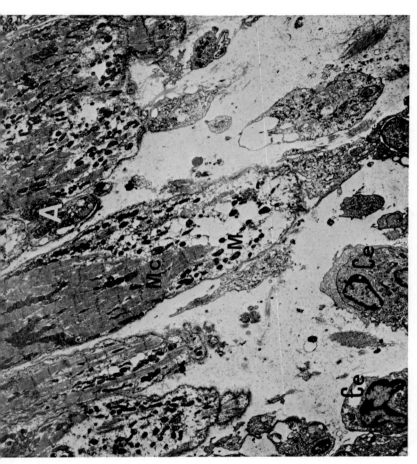

FIG. 22. Acute phase of *T. cruzi* infection. Mouse heart. Acute myocarditis. Interstitial oedema, cellular inflammatory infiltration (Ce). Degenerated amastigotes (A) in the interstitium. Subepicardiac muscle cells (Mc) with cytoplasmic swelling and dissociation of myofibrils. Mitochondria (M), × 4 500.

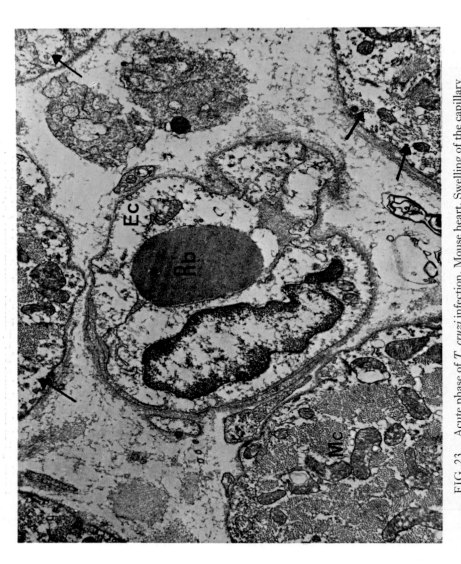

FIG. 23. Acute phase of *T. cruzi* infection. Mouse heart. Swelling of the capillary endothelial cells (Ec). Cardiac muscle cells (Mc): swelling of the sarcoplasm and

3. Pathogenesis

Our findings (Tafuri and Raso, 1962; Tafuri and Brener, 1966a, b; Tafuri and Maria, 1970; Tafuri *et al.*, 1973a, b; Tafuri, 1970, 1971, 1975; Lopes *et al.*, 1976) indicate that in experimental animals as well as in man, *T. cruzi* induced lesions vary in their distribution and severity. This variability in the distribution of the lesions is clearly observed among the different animals of the same experimental groups. Furthermore, even in the same experimental animal the lesions vary in intensity in the different foci. Thus some highly injured neurons are seen close to completely normal ones. The cellular lesions are either directly related to the parasitism or indirectly connected with it by the inflammatory process or the capillary lesions. The cellular lesions related to the inflammatory process are usually more severe than those directly induced by cellular parasitism.

Electron microscopic studies have demonstrated that the lesions in the sympathetic and parasympathetic ganglia of the hollow organs (heart, oesophagus, colon) have a random, irregular distribution. Parasites are frequently seen in the Schwann cells, in the fibroblasts and in the ganglia histiocytes. Parasitism of the neurons is not frequently observed. Parasites are more frequently found in the sympathetic than in the parasympathetic ganglia. This is possibly due to the fact of the former ganglia having in their structure blood vessels and connective tissue which are missing in the latter. Necrotizing ganglionitis is sometimes observed (Fig. 8), indicating local hypersensitive reaction possibly related to the release, in these foci, of larger amounts of antigenic material. The neurons, the nerve fibres and the Schwann cells more severely damaged are related either indirectly to ganglionitis and periganglionitis, or directly to degenerated parasites inside or outside the cells. Nevertheless, damaged nerves and nerve fibres are observed not to be directly related to the inflammatory process (Figs 11, 12, 13). As shown in Fig. 24, the nerves and ganglia of Auerbach's plexus can be damaged as a whole even when not all of its ganglia are injured.

Many questions require answering before a clear understanding of the presence of lesions in the acute stage of *T. cruzi* infections may be reached:

(*a*) The relationship between ANS lesions and those of the muscle cells.
(*b*) The relationship between the alterations of the connective tissue and those of the muscle cells.
(*c*) The nature and mechanism of ultrastructural changes in parasitized and non-parasitized cells.
(*d*) The mechanisms of ultrastructural lesions in capillaries and veins, in the ground substance and in other components of the connective tissue not related with the inflammatory foci. So far, it has not been possible to define clearly the relationship between the lesions, blood capillaries, and

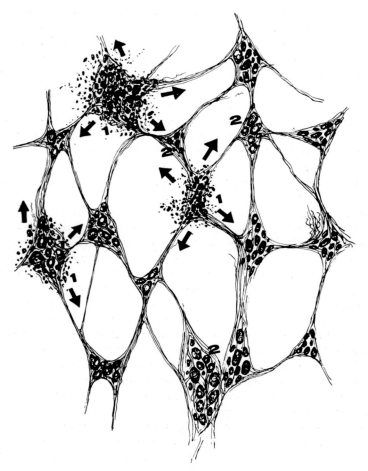

FIG. 24. Acute phase of *T. cruzi* infection. Schematic drawing of the Auerbach plexus of mouse colon. 1. Acute periganglionitis and ganglionitis. 2. Non-parasitized ganglia liable to be injured because of their synaptic interrelation with damaged ganglia.

the alterations of muscle cells and ganglia neurons. However, the analysis of ultrastructural data from *T. cruzi* acute infection has helped clarify some of the above questions (Tafuri, 1975). Electron microscopy has demonstrated:

(*a*) The severely damaged muscle cells are more frequently directly related to the focal inflammatory process or to degenerated parasites. The cells containing normal parasites are less damaged.

(*b*) The clear vacuole, lacking a limiting membrane, formed around the parasites in the cytoplasm is probably due to the action of lytic enzymes of parasite origin (Fig. 2). Electron microscopy findings indicate that the host cell degradation products are used by the parasites in their nutrition. There is also some indication that protoplasmic components of host cells may be incorporated by the parasites through the cystostome (Maria, personal communication). These findings seem to explain why when the parasites degenerate and die the clear vacuoles are no longer visible, severe degenerative changes having taken place. The so-called "parasitic cysts" or "pseudocysts" observed by optical microscopy, are shown by electron microscopy to correspond to focal digestion of the host cell cytoplasmic organelles.

Sanabria (1969) showed that *T. cruzi* has lysosomes and that acid phosphatase activity is also present in the clear multivesicular vacuoles of the parasite Golgi complex. Scorza (1972) showed that, eleven days after *T. cruzi* inoculation into rats, the parasitized heart-muscle cells display decreased oxidase and ATPase acitivities, while the diaphorases and phosphatases were increased. He also reported that the epimastigotes secrete acid phosphatases which diffuse into the cytoplasm and induce mitochondrial changes. The activated macrophages digest the parasites and release acid phosphatases and aminopeptidases into the intercellular space. The hydrolytic enzymes released induce interstitial oedema and lesions of the subepicardiac parasympathetic neurons, with consequent necrosis and destruction of some of them. Delgado (1968) in Scorza *et al.* (1972) correlated the activities of the acid phosphatases and amino-peptidases in amastigotes with the decrease of ATPase of the heart-muscle cells. He also correlated the alterations of alkaline phosphatase activity with vascular permeability.

(*c*) In the vicinity of degenerated parasites, there always occurs a focal inflammatory reaction, with lesions of the connective tissue and muscle cells. The focal inflammatory reaction is characterized by infiltration of mononuclear cells and a few neutrophils; there is also severe oedema, with dissociation of the collagen fibres and widening of the spaces between the muscle cells (Figs 4 and 22).

(*d*) The random distribution of the parasites in the heart and other organs determines the random nature of the focal inflammatory reaction and the randomness of the lesions in the sympathetic and parasympathetic ganglia, secondary to myositis and cellulitis. *Thus, most ganglia lesions are not due to special* T. cruzi *tropism to the nervous tissue, but are directly dependent on the inflammatory changes elicited in the muscle (myositis) and adipose tissue (periganglionary cellulitis reaching the ganglia).* Lopes (1965) proposed this as the main mechanism by which ganglia neurons in atrial walls of human heart are destroyed.

(*e*) Some of the changes observed in muscle cells may be secondary to lesions of the autonomic or intramural nervous system. Furthermore, one cannot exclude the possibility of some muscle-cell lesions being due to alterations in the capillaries, leading to decreased cellular metabolism and hypoxia. MacClure and Poche (1960) observed oedema of the endothelial cells of capillaries, with lumen decrease and presence of fibrin thrombus. These authors suggested that the lesions of the heart muscle cells could be due to the toxic effects of substances secreted by the parasites, and hypoxia induced by alteration in the capillary permeability. These changes, together with those observed in the endothelial cells, the basal membrane and in connective tissue ground substance, may be responsible for the lesions found in the muscle cells.

The impulse conducting system of the heart is severely damaged in acute experimental and human trypanosomiasis. According to Andrade (1974), the lesions found in young dogs infected with *T. cruzi* are as follows:

(*i*) acute inflammation and severe damage of the sino-atrial nodule;

(*ii*) intense parasitism and inflammatory changes in the atrio-ventricular nodule;

(*iii*) focal inflammatory changes of the bundle of Hiss.

Parasites are frequently found in its muscle cells. The right branch is usually more severely injured than the left one. Purkinje cells are frequently parasitized, displaying focal inflammatory reaction around them. According to Andrade (1974), the most severe lesions are found in the atrium, which is in agreement with our own findings with mouse, rat and man. This fact could explain why the sino-atrial nodule is usually more severely damaged. Andrade and Andrade (1966) and Anselmi *et al.* (1967) demonstrated that, in experimental Chagas' myocarditis, the lesions are more severe in the atrium, progressively decreasing in intensity towards the ventricle wall.

In short, ANS injuries in the acute stage of *T. cruzi* infection are dependent on the following factors:

(*a*) Parasitism of the Schwann cells, satellite cells and ganglia capsular fibroblasts. Parasitism of the parasympathetic neurons is rare, the sympathetic neurons being more frequently parasitized.

(*b*) Ganglionitis and periganglionitis.

(*c*) Injury of the neurons. These cells may undergo changes induced either directly by the parasitism and the inflammation, or indirectly through the lesions of the Schwann and satellite cells and axonal degeneration.

(*d*) Injury of the nerve fibres whose alterations are due to the following factors:

(*i*) ganglionitis, periganglionitis and perineuritis;

(*ii*) inflammation of the muscle (myositis, myocarditis) and the subepicardiac adipous tissue (cellulitis), reaching the neural network.

(*e*) Parasitism of the ganglionic cells.

(*f*) Changes in the ganglionic cells elicited through lesions of the Schwann and satellite cells and the axons.

(*g*) Lesions of the Schwann and satellite cells influencing the intraganglionic nerve fibres as well as the extraganglionic neural network (Fig. 24).

(*h*) Lesions of the heart impulse conducting system.

(*i*) Lesions of the interstitial components.

B. THE CHRONIC PHASE OF *T. CRUZI* INFECTIONS

Most work on experimental *T. cruzi* infections is concerned with the acute stage of the disease, when the parasitaemia is high and the course of the infection usually fatal (Tafuri and Raso, 1962). In regions where Chagas' disease is endemic the occurrence of naturally infected animals is frequent. This fact was reported by Chagas in his pioneer work (1909). Köberle (1957) detected megaoesophagus, megacolon and megabladder in several naturally infected dogs, and attributed enteromegaly to the infection. Okumura and Correa-Neto (1961) succeeded in inducing megaoesophagus and megacolon in dogs and mice chronically infected with *T. cruzi*. Guimarães and Miranda (1959) described a case of megaoesophagus in a rhesus monkey ten years after inoculation, and observed amastigote nests in its *muscularis mucosae*. Dias (1934) showed that the albino *Rattus norvegicus* is quite susceptible to *T. cruzi* infection, thus constituting a good experimental model for the study of both acute and chronic stages. The age of the animal is important, as young animals (18 days old) (Kolodny, 1940) are less resistant to infection than older ones (above 100 days) (Pizzi *et al.*, 1953). According to Vichi (1964a, b), 30-day-old animals die in the acute stage between the 16th and the 22nd day of infection. However, Gomez de Alcantara (1959) working with 19- and 25-day-old rats found that the mortality rate reached 60% between the 16th and 25th day of infection. The remaining 40% survived for over 8 months. Scorza and Scorza (1972a, b), in accordance with Pizzi *et al.* (1953), showed that 40-day-old rats did not die in the acute stage and that after the 18th day of infection no parasites could be found in their tissues. Yet we find diffuse pericarditis, myocarditis and endocarditis, with a predominating plasmo-histiocytic infiltration. According to the same authors, on the 29th day of infection the vascular and infiltrative phenomena almost disappeared and then only lymphocyte foci could be observed in the atria. No parasitism was detected, the infection sequelae being of discrete intensity. These results agree with our data from experiments on this animal. Nevertheless, in the few albino mice (*Mus musculus*) that survived the acute stage (Tafuri and Brener, 1966a), *T. cruzi* was seen to continue multiplying in their tissues, albeit at a slower rate, over 90 to 510 days after infection, thus giving rise to degenerative and inflammatory lesions similar to those found in the acute stage; however the intensity and the type of the cellular infiltration differed. Although few parasites were observed, the inflammation, whether focal or diffuse, was intense and the infiltration predominantly lymphoplasmo-histiocytic. The sympathetic and parasympathetic autonomic nervous systems are always involved. The lesions of random distribution and irregular intensity are always focal, displaying marked differences for each animal. Even when inoculated with the same strains and killed after the same number of days of infection, the animals show lesions of different intensity, some of them sometimes presenting no lesions. Furthermore, morphologically normal ganglia are found beside altered ones. It is also possible that apparently normal ganglia in the vicinity of damaged ganglia cannot function normally. This could explain the disturbances in motility and conductibility that are seen, especially in the chronic stage of infection, and which are largely due to ANS alterations.

Kumar *et al.* (1969) developed an experimental model with mice in order to study the congestive heart failure due to chronic Chagas' myocarditis such as that observed in man. In fact, various mice, having undergone the acute stage and survived for 133 to 218 days, presented pronounced chronic myocarditis, specially in the right heart, with lymphocytic infiltration in intramural ANS. In about half of the cases mural thrombosis was also observed. Cardiac failure was represented by evident cardiomegaly, as well as passive pulmonary and hepatic congestion. According to the authors, these studies, made possible by the availability of the present model of severe decompensated Chagas' disease, yielded some insight into the pathogenesis of the syndrome. The fact that the increase in lesion severity and the appearance of congestive heart failure occurred simultaneously with a change of the parasite virulence in the same inbred strains of mice, constitutes, according to the authors, an argument for the parasite playing the central role in the pathogenesis of the lesion and against the major influence of immune and auto-immune mechanisms. Moreover, according to the authors, the detection of the parasite in the myocardium, the predominance of infiltrative and degenerative lesions, as well as the rarity of perivascular lesions are in agreement with this view.

According to Teixeira *et al.* (1975), the rabbit may be a good experimental animal for the study of the natural history of Chagas' disease. In fact, the authors succeeded in inducing the acute and chronic stages of the disease in rabbits through intraperitoneal inoculation of *T. cruzi*. These stages are very similar to those observed in man, with the appearance, in the chronic stage, of progressive severe cardiopathy with or without megacolon, after a long asymptomatic period. They also showed that it is possible to reproduce the infection chronic stage lesions by successive injections of *T. cruzi* antigenic substances.

In man, from the anatomo-clinical point of view, and according to Bogliolo (1976), Chagas' disease presents the following patterns:

(*a*) Symptomatic or nearly asymptomatic infection in the beginning with no characterization of acute-stage clinical forms; after an intermediary stage of variable duration, there appear one or more of the chronic-stage anatomical forms (Chagas' cardiopathy, megaoesophagus, megacolon). This is believed to be the most common occurrence.

(*b*) Infection with characterization of acute-stage anatomo-clinical forms (septicaemic form, cardiac form, nervous form, etc.); death.

(*c*) Infection with characterization of acute-stage anatomo-clinical forms; intermediary stage of variable duration; appearance of one or more anatomo-clinical forms of chronic stage.

(*d*) Infection with characterization of acute-stage anatomo-clinical forms; clinical cure, even though with persistence of parasitaemia and circulating antibodies.

(*e*) Symptomatic or nearly asymptomatic infection with/or without characterization of acute-stage anatomo-clinical forms; intermediary stage with variable duration; sudden death with apparent characterization of chronic-stage forms.

In Brazil trypanosomiasis usually manifests in the severe anatomo-clinical forms, especially the cardiac and the digestive ones, which are generally incapacitating and responsible for the high death rate of patients "in the prime of life", thus constituting a serious Public Health problem.

1. Human chronic Chagas' cardiopathy

The anatomical characters of chronic chagasic myocarditis are variable and change with every clinical picture. In cases where severe alterations in cardiac rhythm and congestive heart failure develop, optical and electron microscopy show the following lesions:

(*a*) *Chronic inflammation*—The inflammatory infiltrate presents aspects different from those observed in acute chagasic myocarditis, and can be classified into three types:

(*i*) local infiltrate, occasionally with confluent foci (Fig. 25) and when this occurs there is frequently a predominance of lymphocytes which infiltrate the endomysium along each muscle cell;

(*ii*) cellular infiltrate sometimes appearing more polymorphous and displaying a large number of histiocytes, neutrophil granulocytes and eosinophils. Its characters are quite similar to those of acute stage, though more discrete and always focal;

(*iii*) cellular infiltrate occasionally displaying multinuclear giant cells together with histiocytes and other cells which gather and form micronodules, the lesion thus becoming granulomatous and tuberculoid. Such infiltration generally presents a larger number of mast cells in all forms of chronic chagasic myocarditis (Almeida *et al.*, 1974).

(b) *Fibrosis.* The new anatomic character not found in the acute stage is fibrosis. No other type of myocarditis develops it so intensely and acquires such peculiar characters as the chronic chagasic cardiopathy (Bogliolo, 1976). It is represented by the formation of collagenic areas that are irregular in form, distribution and extension, contain a small number of capillaries and have the appearance of granulation tissue. Fibrosis occurs in the endomysium, in substitution for destroyed cells and, to a small extent, plays the role of cicatricial fibrosis of inflammatory origin. The newly formed collagen may dissociate the cardiac cells and surround them until they undergo atrophy and blurring. Fibrosis may also reach the perimysium and then, joining to adjacent fibrosis, give the appearance of interrupted muscle fasciculi fixed to each other by newly formed connective tissue. It must be pointed out that diffuse fibrosis is the sum of all focal fibrosis gradually developed throughout the years, during the continuous progressive cycle of the infection (Bogliolo, 1976).

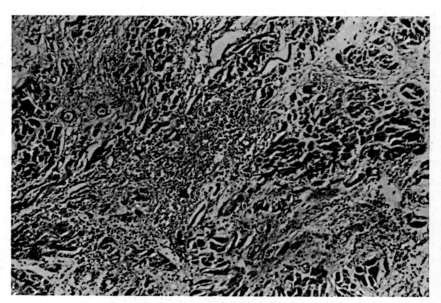

FIG. 25. Chronic phase of *T. cruzi* infection. Human chronic myocarditis. Diffuse lymphocytic infiltrate. Fibrosis, compression and dissociation of muscle cell bundles. Hypotrophic and degenerated muscle cells. × 128.

(c) *The constant degenerative process of muscle cells.* They involve:
(i) mitochondrial alterations (the mitochondria are distributed in a disorderly fashion and show numerical and volumetric changes, crystolysis and lysis of the matrix, vacuolization and increase in the number of mitochondrial granules) (Figs 26 and 27);

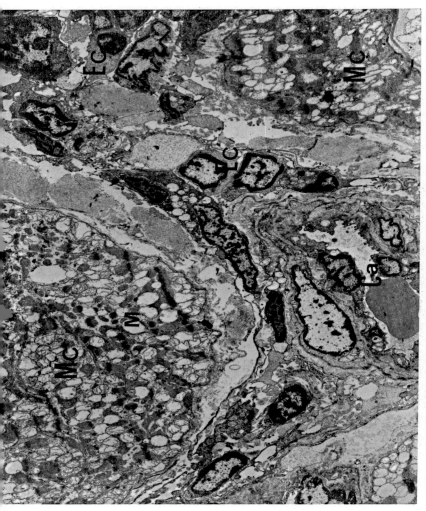

FIG. 26. Chronic phase of *T. cruzi* infection. Human chronic myocarditis. Interstitial fibrosis with infiltrative cells (Ec). Muscle cells (Mc) with swelling and vacuolization of the mitochondria (M). Capillary (Ca). × 18 000.

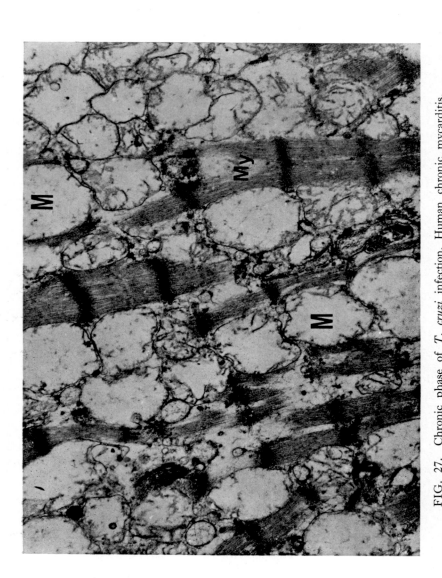

FIG. 27. Chronic phase of *T. cruzi* infection. Human chronic mycarditis. Dissociation of the bundle of myofibrils (My), swelling and vacuolization of the mitochondria (M). × 28 000.

(*ii*) myofibril lesions (widening of the space between myofibrils, with bundle disorganization and dissociation, myocytolysis, torsion and lateral displacement) (Fig. 27);

(*iii*) alterations in the endoplasmic reticulum (cisternae enlarged with probable rupture and blurring of the T system). (Fig. 28);

(*iv*) alterations of the sarcolemma; protrusion, thickening and dehiscence of intercalated disks. All of these degenerative processes are of variable intensity in the different parts of the myocardium. They injure fibres included in the inflammatory foci and fibrotic areas, but also occur in fasciculi not involved in these processes. It is not true that the most intensely injured cells are necessarily related to inflammatory foci (Tafuri *et al.*, 1973a; Tafuri, 1975).

(*d*) *The heart impulse conducting system* was studied by Andrade (1974) in 19 cases. The predominant lesions were found to be fibrosis, atrophy and fragmentation of specific fibres. In most cases, the lower part of AV nodule, the right half of main bundle of Hiss, the proximal portion of the right branch and part of the left branch were injured. In all the cases there was complete blockade of the right branch and demi-blockade of the left. In two cases with right branch blockade, fibrosis was also present in this same branch.

(*e*) *The epicardium and the subepicardial fatty tissue* are constantly injured, usually in an intense way (Raso and Tafuri, 1971). The most frequent lesions are uniform nodular thickening in the ascending portion of the pulmonary artery. These lesions are directly derived from the parasite location in the subepicardial adipose tissue, the probable sequence of the process being as follows:

(*i*) presence of parasites in regions where the fatty tissue occurs most abundantly;

(*ii*) induction of inflammatory reaction, initially of an infiltrative nature;

(*iii*) development into the chronic stage, with replacement of exudate by areolar tissue, at first, and dense tissue, later on. The two main consequences of this development are:

(*iiia*) propagation of the inflammatory process to subepicardial nervous ganglia with partial or total destruction of these structures;

(*iiib*) nodule formation in the epicardium of ventricle and atrium, formation of cicatricial inflammatory patches or plaques which contribute together with other elements such as the vortical lesion (Raso, 1964; Almeida, 1976) to a very peculiar macroscopic appearance of the heart.

(*f*) *Destruction of the intracardiac nervous system* is constant (Köberle, 1960; Lopes, 1965; Lopes *et al.*, 1969) and equally developed both in cases with rhythm alterations and/or irreversible congestive heart failure

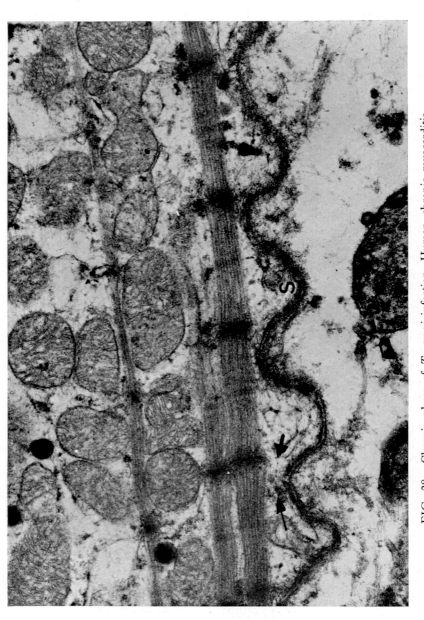

FIG. 28. Chronic phase of *T. cruzi* infection. Human chronic myocarditis. Muscular cell with oedema, protrusion of the sarcolemma (S), with probable rupture and blurring of T system (arrows). × 28 000.

leading to sudden death, and in trypanosomotic myocarditis, no apparent clinical cardiac symptoms in patients who died of other diseases. In fact severe neuronal depopulation could be detected in individuals who did not undergo perceptible heart failure and died of other causes. On the other hand, preservation of a reasonable number of neurons has occurred in cases where death was due to heart failure, accompanied by severe changes in the cardiac rhythm. It seems therefore that subepicardial neuronal depopulation is already present in the acute stage of the disease (Lopes *et al.*, 1976) but that this does not seem to represent the only factor responsible for the appearance of the cardiac rhythmical disturbances and heart failure which characterize the most common cases of chronic chagasic myocarditis.

The investigations on Chagas' disease have not so far allowed a complete tracing of its natural history. Nevertheless, they have thrown some light on the pathogenesis of myocarditis. As regards the different phenomena that characterize it, only some of them seem to be responsible for the peculiar anatomic picture determining the clinical physiognomy of this cardiopathy. According to Bogliolo (1976), they can thus be discriminated:

(*a*) Lack of topographical relationship between parasitized muscle cells, their degeneration, and inflammatory foci, has been emphasized by all researchers since Vianna's first work (1911). Muscle cell destruction and inflammation are not directly related to cell parasitism. In fact, no relationship could be observed between inflammation intensity and number of parasitized myocardium cells. This fact, already evident in the acute stage (Lopes *et al.*, 1976), becomes more pronounced in the chronic phase.

(*b*) Neuronal and cardiac cell destruction directly induced by parasites is minimal. Electron microscopy demonstrates that factors leading to cardiac cell lesions, whether topographically related or not with inflammation, are multiple in number, many of them having already been mentioned when discussing experimental infection.

The phenomena observed in human infections may be summarized as follows:

(*a*) Swelling of the capillary endothelium cytoplasm, lumen reduction and pre-stasis, with consequent disturbance of metabolic exchanges.

(*b*) Alteration of intercellular medium by fibrosis and increase in cell number, disturbing myocell contraction, impulse conduction and nutrition.

(*c*) Disconnection, blurring and probable rupture of transversal tubules (T system) due to sarcoplasmic oedema and/or myocytolysis, interfering with electrolytic exchanges, especially those of Ca^{2+} ion.

(*d*) Intercalated disks dehiscence. Bahr and Jennings (1961) demonstrated that these zones are not under the usual tension; they show zig-zag membranes with a single space, never above 100 Å. In rat experimental chronic myocarditis (Scorza, 1972) and in man (Tafuri, 1975), various cardiac cells undergo membrane widening (larger than 100 Å) at the level of intercalated disks. Bahr and Jennings named these zones "nexus" and interpreted them as electrical synapses, thus suggesting that, electrophysiologically speaking, the myocardium must have a syncytial organization. Due to dehiscence of intercalated disks, the sarcomere contraction mechanism is impaired; the fibrils, not returning to their original size during diastole, are liable to undergo torsion and lateral displacement.

(e) Matrix lysis, mitochondrial crystolysis and swelling may be related to Mg^{2+} ion transport deficiency as well as to Ca^{2+} ion transport impairment. Fibrosis with variable cell population always occurs in myocarditis foci. Lymphocytes, plasmocytes, fibroblasts and mast cells as well as intense collagenic neoformation appear in inflammatory foci. Otherwise diffuse fibrosis unrelated to inflammatory foci can be observed in several areas. The presence of infiltration and connective neoformation contributes to the widening of intercellular spaces (almost double normal width, as compared with control cases). These well-documented fibrosis studies by optical microscopy undoubtedly represent an important step towards the determination of the causes accounting for regressive lesions of cardiac cells.

(f) Lesions of the vagus dorsal nucleus and nerve, as described by Lopes et al. (1969) in chagasic myocarditis patients with congestive cardiac failure and ultrastructural alterations of intracardiac myelinic fibres, probably of vagal nature (Tafuri, 1975), necessarily contribute to alterations of the cardiac cells.

(g) Many of the mechanisms responsible for the progressive destruction of cardiac cells, as well as for the type of inflammation and fibrosis which occurs, are probably a response to an immunological reaction. In fact recent investigations (Santos-Buch and Teixeira, 1974; Teixeira et al. 1975) indicate that rabbit lymphocytes sensitized to T. cruzi exert cytotoxic action on the myocardium muscle cells of this animal in vitro, and also that sub-cellular fractions of both T. cruzi and rabbit myocardium cells have cross antigenic properties. Our electron microscopic study of a human case of acute chagasic myocarditis (Lopes et al., 1976) seemed to show that within 30 days of the onset of the disease the phenomenon described by Santos-Buch and Teixeira (1974) could be observed. In various photomicrographs we verified that lymphocytes were adherent to and/or fused with the cardiac cell plasmalemma or even had penetrated it.

2. Chagasic megaoesophagus and megacolon

The general definition of "mega" (from Greek mega = large, great; as in megaoesophagus, megacolon, megaduodenum, megaureter, megabladder, etc) means the permanent dilatation of hollow and ductal viscera accompanied, or not, by wall thickening and lengthening.

Acquired megaoesophagus and megacolon are rare in Europe (Köberle, 1960) and frequent in South America (Chapadeiro *et al.*, 1964). The high frequency of these pathological conditions led Brazilian authors, especially after the works of Köberle and Nador (1955) and Köberle (1956a, b, 1957, 1961) to admit the existence of a cause–effect relationship; this means that, in Brazil, except for a few cases (congenital megas, toxins, etc), the "megas" are of chagasic aetiology.

The terms chagasic megaoesophagus and megacolon, even though long used, must be criticized, as in most cases clinical symptoms involving disphagy and disturbances of oesophagus peristalsis occur before the development of the macroscopic picture of "mega". That is why new denominations have been suggested for the same entity: aperistalsis (Brasil, 1956), dyskinesia (Habr-Gamma, 1966), achalasia, cardiospasm, etc. In megacolon, the first symptom to appear is constipation and only rarely is it identified before the development of the ectasic stage. Megaoesophagus and megacolon are usually associated and, not infrequently, myocarditis is also present. In 161 megacolon cases (Rezende, 1968), 148 presented oesophagic aperistalsis (91·6%), 117 of them also displaying ectasia.

According to Rezende (1968), megaoesophagus may be precociously developed in chagasic infection, whereas clinical signs of chronic chagasic cardiopathy appear late. However, the exact interval occurring between the onset of infection and the oesophageal symptomatology is still unknown. In 27 cases periodically followed up with radiographs for 7 years, starting from the acute stage, Rezende (1959) observed that only four of them presented clinical digestive signs. Two of these patients presented precocious disphagy, and one of them, megaoesophagus, reaching the ectasic form 5 years after the acute stage.

In congenital Chagas' disease with lesion of the oesophagus, functional changes and dilatation of the organ may occur at a very early stage (Tafuri *et al.*, 1973b).

Except at the initial stage, when only microscopic alterations are found, megaoesophagus and megacolon can be macroscopically characterized by:

(*a*) Variable degree of dilatation, accompanied, or not, by organ lengthening.

(*b*) Wall thickening, mainly due to hypertrophy of the muscularis and to the newly formed connective tissue (fibrosis).

(*c*) Absence of mechanical obstacle.

(*d*) Normal aspect of the terminal portion of the organ, immediately beyond the dilated part.

(*e*) Occurrence or not, of secondary alterations, such as leucoplasia and mucosa ulceration.

By optical microscopy, the following can be observed:

(*a*) Chronic inflammatory infiltration (predominantly lymphocytic) appearing in systematized foci in the *muscularis mucosae*, in the submucosa and, most commonly of all, in the *muscularis propria*.

(*b*) Lesions in the intramural nervous system, especially in Auerbach's plexus (focal or diffuse periganglionitis and ganglionitis, with intense neuronal regressive phenomena, possibly leading to complete destruction of Auerbach's ganglia).

(*c*) Focal or diffuse interstitial intermuscular fibrosis following myositis, periganglionitis and ganglionitis.

(*d*) The presence of the parasite is extremely rare during this stage of the disease (Fig. 29).

Ultrastructural alterations of the myenteric plexus in the megaoesophagus and megacolon are similar, only quantitative differences being observed (Tafuri *et al.*, 1971). In all ganglia lesions were found in the neurons, in the Schwann cells, in the nerve fibres and in the capsule components. Nearly normal neurons were always found by the side of altered ones in the same ganglion. On the other hand, almost completely fibrosed ganglia were also observed.

The submicroscopic alterations of the muscle cells may be summarized as follows:

(*a*) Decrease in cell to cell contact, due to widening of intercellular spaces.

(*b*) Thickening of the plasma membrane, as well as of the electrodense plates and corpuscles.

(*c*) Hypertrophy of a certain number of muscle cells in the neighbourhood of others seen to be normal or even atrophied.

(*d*) Vacuolization of the mitochondria.

(*e*) Presence of amorphous masses and spherical osmiophilic granules next to the degenerated areas.

(*f*) Pyknosis and wrinkling of the nucleus of hypotrophic cells.

The most frequent interstitial alterations observed were:

(*a*) Chronic focal myositis.

(*b*) Focal or diffuse fibrosis.

(*c*) Intense degenerative alteration of the amyelinic and myelinic nervous fibres.

(*d*) Regressive and progressive alterations of the vascular walls (Figs 30, 31).

The data presented above can explain the occurrence of generalized lesions in Chagas' disease in an easily understood way, as the trypanosomes can parasitize any organ or tissue of the body at random. It is difficult, however, to understand why the lesions are more frequent and

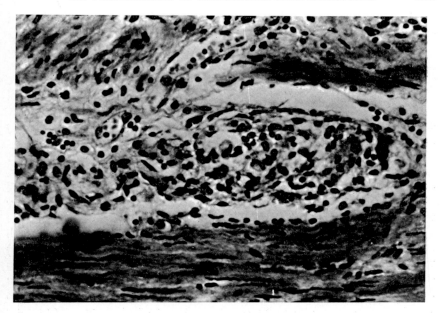

FIG. 29. Chronic phase of *T. cruzi* infection. Human megaoesophagus. Chronic myositis, periganglionitis and ganglionitis with intense inflammatory infiltration of mononuclear cells. Destruction of the neurons. × 200.

more severe in the oesophagus and colon, causing the so-called "megas". It is extremely likely therefore that other factors play important roles in the pathogenesis of the oesophagus and colon lesions. In chagasic megaoesophagus and megacolon, stasis and diskinesia are always observed. Stasis in the megaoesophagus seems to appear when there is alteration in sphincter opening, for diskinesia by itself is unable to induce it (Habr-Gamma, 1966). Supposing stasis to be one of the important factors triggering the mechanism of "mega" formation, we could easily understand the reason why the lesions of the nervous plexus are much more severe in the intestinal tract, where stasis occurs for the following reasons:

(1). Faecal content, accumulating in this part of the intestine, determines its dilatation and compresses the mucosa.

(2). The compressed mucosa undergoes alterations such as ischaemia, and regressive lesions.

(3). Once altered, the mucosa is affected by inflammation.

(4). The inflammation may reach the submucosa and aggravate the already existing lesions of Meissner's plexus caused by *T. cruzi*.

(5). Auerbach's plexus, in turn, is damaged as a consequence of close synaptic relations between the two plexuses.

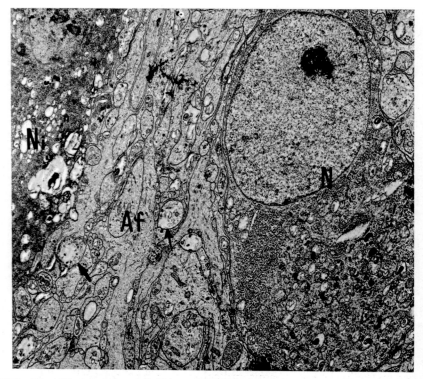

FIG. 30. Chronic phase of *T. cruzi* infection. Human megaoesophagus. Auerbach's ganglion. Normal neuron (N) side by side with another one severely injured (Ni). Normal (Af) and degenerated amyelinic fibres (arrows). × 7200.

(6). The inflammation, secondary to stasis and resulting destruction of plexus and interstitial components, leaves sequelae (interstitial fibrosis), which represent one of the factors responsible for the modification of intermuscular interstitial components.

(7). The muscle cells undergo hypertrophy because of the stronger contraction effort required to overcome the greater resistance of the surroundings (fibrosis) (Fig. 31). On the other hand, interstitial fibrosis altering the structure of the connective tissue around the muscle cells and widening the space between the muscle cells and the capillaries, also leads to decreased metabolic exchanges and, therefore, induces regressive changes of the muscle cells (hypotrophy) or even their death.

(8). Since Auerbach's plexus is closely related with muscle cells, it is easy to understand how myositis and its sequelae, when near the ganglia, may injure them even more.

(9). Finally, it is reasonable to think that the plexus lesions would be aggravated in proportion to the mega duration and intensity.

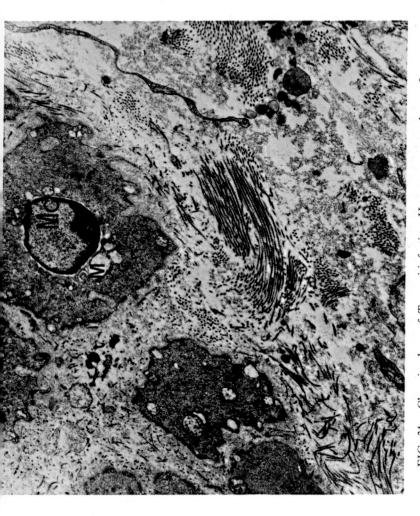

FIG. 31. Chronic phase of *T. cruzi* infection. Human megaoesophagus. Interstitial fibrosis. Muscle cells (Mc) with vacuolization of the mitochondria (M). × 7200.

A comparative study of the injured neurons in Auerbach's plexus with both those remaining healthy in megaoesophagus and those of the control normal oesophagus seemed to show that the non-degenerated neurons in megaoesophagus and megacolon undergo a compensatory hypertrophy (Tafuri and Maria, 1970). The data justifying this hypothesis are:

(a) Volumetric increase of nucleoli.

(b) Increase of ribosomes, resulting in greater electron density of pericarium.

(c) Hypertrophy of Golgi's complex with presence of several dense granular vesicles around it; hypertrophy of neurofilaments and neurotubules.

(d) Volumetric and numerical increase of dense granular vesicles in the nerve fibres.

Based on this fact, we raise the hypothesis that disturbances in megaoesophagus and megacolon peristalsis are caused by hypersecretory activity of parasympathetic neurons with increase in the synthesis and secretion of indolamines, catecholamines and, possibly, other substances. The search for other factors led us to investigate the behaviour of substance P in chagasic mega colon and megaoesophagus (Hial et al., 1973). In mega- and control oesophagus, the levels of substance P were not found to be significantly different. However, since severe denervation occurs in cases of megaoesophagus and megacolon, whereas the plexus is well preserved in the controls, two explanations may be offered for the above findings:

(a) Substance P, found in cases of megaoesophagus and megacolon, does not originate from the nervous plexus.

(b) If the plexus is the source of substance P, then a higher production (or a greater storage) of substance P should be found in "megas" rather than in controls.

The second explanation appears to be the more plausible, as although severe denervation occurs, the amount of substance P found in "megas" is similar to that found in the controls. As in "mega" conditions healthy neurons hypersecrete, it is logical to deduce that the numerical and volumetric increase of granular vesicles must be related to the storage of active substances including substance P (Fig. 32).

Many theories try to explain the dilation and thickness of the oesophagus and colon in cases of "megas". Although the formal genesis of the lesions in the nervous system and muscle cells is only partially known, no satisfactory explanation has so far been offered for the functional alterations observed in chagasic megaoesophagus and megacolon.

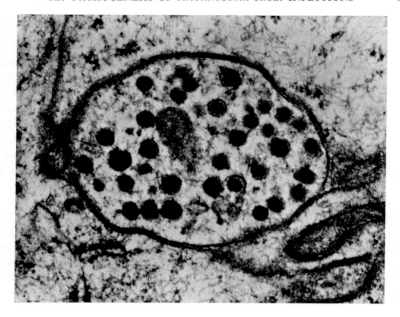

FIG. 32. Chronic phase of *T. cruzi* infection. Human megaoesophagus. Auerbach's plexus. Amyelinic nerve fibre with dense granular vesicles of variable diameter. × 50 000.

III. Lesions of the central nervous system in T. cruzi infections

There have been relatively few studies on the central nervous system (CNS) lesion in Chagas' disease compared with those concerning the cardiac and digestive forms of the infection. However, the detection in Chagas' patients of a decrease in the number of neurons in the cerebellum (Brandão and Zullian, 1966), in the vagus dorsal nucleus (Lopes *et al.*, 1969) and in the hypothalamus (Britto-Costa, 1969; Britto-Costa and Gallins, 1971), as well as the occurrence of minimal disfunction (Jörg and Orlando, 1967) in human cases of chronic encephalomyelitis, probably of chagasic aetiology, show the importance and the need for further research to discover the nature of the injuries by *T. cruzi* to the central nervous system (CNS). The parasitism of CNS cells in *T. cruzi* infection is discrete even in instances of severe systemic infection. However, when *T. cruzi* is directly inoculated into the brain, the parasitism of CNS cells is usually intense and the lesions more severe (Sanabria, 1968). Although the data obtained suggest that the site of inoculation plays an important role in the pathogenesis of CNS injuries, other findings also indicate that the differences in severity of CNS lesions are due to differences in the tropism of *T. cruzi* strains. Amaral *et al.* (1975) observed that, following intraperitoneal inoculation of different *T. cruzi* strains into mice, only PNM strain could induce marked parasitism and severe inflammatory changes in the CNS, although all of the strains were known to cause high parasitaemia. Indeed, *T. cruzi* strains have been reported to present different cellular tropisms, some of them being mainly myotropic, while others are reticulotropic or neurotropic (Brener, 1973). Edgcomb (1970) observed that in 20% of rats naturally infected with *T. cruzi* intense parasitism of CNS cells occurs, which seems to indicate that aside from the route of inoculation and the strain of *T. cruzi*, the susceptibility of the host is also an important factor in the evolution of the infection.

Lesions of the CNS in acute cases of Chagas' disease have been observed in humans (Vianna, 1911; Crowell, 1923; de Coursey, 1935; Johnson and Derivas, 1936; Noetzel *et al.*, 1958; Almeida-Cardoso, 1960; Dominguez and Jaffe, 1962; Borges-Fortes, 1942; Jörg and Orlando, 1967; Alencar, 1964, 1967), and in experimental animals (Vianna, 1911; Mayer and Rocha-Lima, 1914; Villela and Torres, 1925; Alencar and Elejald, 1960; Dominguez and Gavaller, 1962; Jardim, 1967; Menezes, 1964; Menezes and Alcantara, 1965; Britto-Costa, 1969; Britto-Costa and Gallina, 1971; and Amaral *et al.*, 1975). The lesions were described as follows:

(1). Hyperaemia and oedema of the leptomeninges and the brain nervous tissue, frequently associated with focal haemorrhage and focal accumulation of microglial cells.

(2). Presence of parasites in the lumen of blood vessels, in astrocytes and in microglial cells. The neurons were rarely parasitized. In the astrocytes, *T. cruzi* amastigotes multiply, inducing focal lysis in the cytoplasm and the formation of empty vacuoles around them. After rupture of the parasitic nests in the astrocytes and release of the parasites into the interstitium, phagocytosis of the parasites by microglial cells accumulated around the ruptured host cells takes place, giving rise to a granulomatous formation.

(3). The macrophages containing normal or degenerated parasites display irregular contours and many papillary projections, and they contain numerous corpuscles of variable electron density surrounded by a membrane. These corpuscles stain positively for phosphatase and are considered to be lysosomes.

(4). Focal perivascular lymphoplasmocytic infiltrates are usually found, especially around demyelinated areas.

(5). The CNS lesions appearing in the acute stages of Chagas' disease would seem to be reversible, as apart from the decrease in the number of neurons, no further morphological or clinical alterations could be observed in the chronic stage of the disease.

IV. Concluding remarks

The whole sequence of events occurring in the development of *T. cruzi* infection is not yet known, nor are the mechanisms responsible for the changes in local and systemic host response in the various stages of the disease. The events observed in the different phases of the infection point to a change in the host reactivity, and suggest that the mechanisms responsible for such reactivity changes are probably multifold and dependent on various factors. The clinical and anatomopathologic forms observed in Chagas' trypanosomiasis, are possibly related to these changes in host reactivity. Among the various factors likely to interfere in the sequence of events occurring during the evolution of Chagas' disease, and thus determine the clinical–pathological features presented in the chronic stage of the process, are the following:

(1). *T. cruzi* strain infectivity, polymorphism and tropism.
(2). Number of *T. cruzi* inoculated and route of inoculation.
(3). Host's sex, age and genetic constitution.
(4). Repeated infection and acquired resistance.
(5). Nutritional factors.
(6). Local and systemic immunological reactivity.

Researchers engaged in the study of American trypanosomiasis are faced with the following question: What are the factors determining the disruption of the steady state apparently existing between host and parasite during the chronic phase of Chagas' disease, and leading to the appearance of severe evolutive cardiopathy and/or "mega" conditions? As no objective answers to this question have so far been offered, many pathogenetic theories have been developed. Our studies, as well as those of other investigators, show that it is not possible to explain the pathogenesis of lesions found in Chagas' disease through one single factor, such as, for instance, plexular denervation of the hollow organs. More and more evidence shows that the various parasite and host factors playing a role in the appearance and evolution of *T. cruzi*-induced lesions must be well determined and clearly understood before the complete natural history of Chagas' disease can be brought to light.

V. Acknowledgements

The author wishes to express his gratitude to Dr. A. N. Raick for his critical review and translation of the manuscript and to Dr. Lineu Freire-Maia and Dr. E. Chiari for the review of the text.

VI. References

Alencar, A. (1964). Atrofia cortical na cardiopatia crônica chagásica. O Hospital, 66, 807–815.

Alencar, A. (1967). Alterações cerebelares em pacientes com cardiopatia crônica chagásica. Arquivo de Neuropsiquiatria, 25, 191–198.

Alencar, A. and Elejald, P. (1960). Histogenese do granuloma chagásico do S.N.C. de cães jovens. Archivos de Histologia Normal y Patologica, 7, 327–335.

Almeida, H. O. (1976). A "Lesão vorticilar" da cardiopatia chagásica crônica. Thesis, School of Medicine, Federal University, M. Gerais, Belo Horizonte, Brazil.

Almeida, H. O., Lima-Pereira, F. E. and Tafuri, W. L. (1974a). Estudo quantitative dos mastócitos na cardiopatia chagásica crônica. Revista do Instituto de Medicina tropical de São Paulo, 17, 5–9.

Almeida, H. O., Tafuri, W. L., Bogliolo, L. and Cunha, J. C. (1974b). Parasitismo incomum do miocárdio e do esôfago em chagásico crônico, portador da doença de Hodgkin e em uso de imunopressores. Revista da Sociedade Brasileira de Medicina Tropical, 8, 117–121.

Almeida, H. O., Tafuri, W. L., Cunha-Melo, J. R., Freire-Maia, L., Raso, P. and Brener, Z. (1977). Studies on the vesicular component of the Auerbach's Plexus and the substance P content of the Mouse Colon in the Acute Phases of Experimental Trypanosoma Cruzi infection. Virchows Archives Abt. A. Pathological Anatomy and Histology, 376, 353–360.

Almeida-Cardoso, R. A. De (1960). Lesões do sistema nervoso central em 4 casos infantis agudos de doença de Chagas. Boletin do Instituto de Puericultura do Brasil, 17, 101–110.

Almeida-Prado, A. (1959). Aspectos patológicos gerais da doença de Chagas. International Congress on Chagas' disease. July. Rio de Janeiro, Brazil, pg. 32–33.

Amaral, C. F. S., Tafuri, W. L. and Brener, Z. (1975). Frequência do parasitismo encefálico em camundongos experimentalmente inoculados com differentes cepas de T. cruzi. Revista da Sociedade Brasileira de Medicina Tropical, 9, 243–246.

Andrade, S. G. (1973). Caracterização de cepas do Trypanosoma cruzi isoladas do Recôncavo Baiano (contribuição ao estudo da patologia geral da doença de Chagas em nosso meio). Thesis, School of Medicine, Federal University, Bahia, Salvador, Brazil.

Andrade, Z. (1974). Patologia do sistema excito-condutor do coração na mio-cardiopatia chagásica. Revista de Patologia Tropical, Goiânia, 3, 367–428.

Andrade, S. G. and Andrade, S. A. (1966). Estudo histopatológico comparativo das lesões produzidas por cepas do Tripanosoma cruzi. O Hospital, 70, 1267–1278.

Anselmi, A., Gurdiel, O., Suarez, J. A. and Anselmi, G. (1967). Disturbance in the A–V conduction system in Chagas' myocarditis in the dog. Circulation Research, 2, 56–64.

Bahr, G. F. and Jennings, R. B. (1961). Ultrastructure of normal and asphyxic myocardium of the dog. Laboratory Investigation, 10, 548–572.

Barbosa, A. J. A., Pitella, J. E. H. and Rafuri, W. L. (1970). Incidência da cardiopatia chagásica em 15.000 necrópsias consecutivas e sua associação com os megas. Revista da Sociedade Brasileira de Medicina Tropical, 44, 219–223.

Behbehani, M. K. (1971). Multiplication of Trypanosoma (Schisotrypanum) cruzi in mouse peritoneal macrophages. *Transactions of the Royal Society of Tropical Medicine and Hygiene*, **65**, 15–16.

Bogliolo, L. (1976). *In:* "Bogliolo Patologia", pg. 339–352. Guanabara Koogan, Rio de Janeiro, Brazil.

Borges-Fortes, A. (1942). As lesões do sistema nervoso na enfermidade de Chagas. *Jornal dos Clínicos*, **23**, 353–361.

Brandão, H. J. S. and Zullian, R. (1966). Nerve cell depopulation in chronic Chagas' disease. A quantitative study in the cerebellum. *Revista do Instituto de Medicina tropical de São Paulo*, **8**, 281–286.

Brant, T. C. (1966). Matizes regionais da doença de Chagas. *Revista Brasileira de Malariologia e Doencas Tropicais*, **18**, 3–8.

Brasil, A. (1956). Etiopatogenia da "aperistalsis" do esôfago. *Revista Brasileira de Medicina*, **13**, 577–590.

Brener, Z. (1961). Contribuição ao estudo da terapêutica experimental da doença de Chagas. Thesis, Federal University, M. Gerais, Belo Horizonte, Brazil.

Brener, Z. (1973). Biology of *Trypanosoma cruzi*. *Annual Review of Microbiology*, **27**, 347–382.

Brener, Z. and Chiari, E. (1963). Observações sôbre a fase crônica da doença de Chagas experimental no camundongo. *Revista do Instituto de Medicina tropical de Sao Paulo*, **5**, 128–132.

Brener, Z. and Chiari, E. (1965). Aspects of early growth of different *Trypanosoma cruzi* strains in culture medium. *Journal of Parasitology*, **51**, 922–926.

Brener, Z. and Chiari, E. (1971). The effects of some imunosupressive agents in experimental chronic Chagas' disease. *Transactions of the Royal Society of Tropical Medicine and Hygiene*, **65**, 629–636.

Brener, Z., Tafuri, W. L. and Maria, T. A. (1969). An electron microscope study of *Trypanosoma cruzi* intercellular forms in mice treated with an active nitrofuran compound. *Revista do Instituto de Medicina tropical de São Paulo*, **11**, 245–249.

Brener, Z., Chiari, E. and Alvarenga, N. J. (1974). Observations on *Trypanosoma cruzi* strains maintained over an 8-year period in experimentally inoculated mice. *Revista do Instituto de Medicina tropical de São Paulo*, **16**, 39–46.

Britto-Costa, R. (1969). Estudo do hipotálmo anterior na fase crônica da moléstia de Chagas. Thesis, School of Medicine, Ribeirão Preto, São Paulo, Brazil.

Britto-Costa, R. and Gallina, R. A. (1971). Hipotálmo anterior na molestia de Chagas humana. *Revista do Instituto de Medicina tropical de Sao Paulo*, **13**, 92–98.

Burnstock, G. (1972). Purinergic nerves. *Pharmacological Reviews*, **24**, 509–581.

Chagas, C. (1909). Estudos sobre morfologia e o ciclo evolutivo do *Schizotrypanum cruzi*, n. gen. n. sp. agente etiológico de nova entidade morbida do homem. *Memorias do Instituto Oswaldo Cruz*, **1**, 159–219.

Chagas, E. (1935). L'infection experimentale chez l'home par le *Schizotrypanum cruzi*. *Comptes Rendus des Séances de la Société de Biologie et de ses Filiales*, Paris, **118**, 290–292.

Chapadeiro, E., Lopes, E. R., Mesquita, P. M. and Pereira-Lima, F. E. (1964). Incidência de "megas" associados a cardiopatia chagásica. *Revista do Instituto de Medicina tropical de São Paulo*, **6**, 287–291.

Clinton, B. A., Ortiz-Ortiz, L., Garcia, W., Martinez, T. and Capin, R. (1975). *Trypanosoma cruzi*: early immune responses in infected mice. *Experimental Parasitology*, **87**, 417–425.

Costa, J. F. and Costa, A. (1960). Verificações experimentais sobre imunidade humoral na moléstia de Chagas. *Publicacões Médicas de São Paulo*, **31**, 29–37.

Crowell, B. C. (1923). The acute form of American trypanosomiasis: notes on its pathology, with autopsy report and observations on *Trypanosomiasis cruzi* in animals. *American Journal of Tropical Medicine*, **3**, 425–454.

Cunha-Melo, J. R., Freire-Maia, L., Tafuri, W. L. and Maria, T. A. (1970). Mecanismo de ação da toxina purificada de escorpião sôbre o íleo isolado de rato. *Acta Physiologica Latinoamericana*, **20**, 296.

Cunha-Melo, J. R., Freire-Maia, L., Tafuri, W. L. and Maria, T. A. (1973). Mechanism of action of purified Scorpion toxin on the isolated rat intestine. *Toxicon*, **11**, 81–84.

De Coursey, E. (1935). The first fatal case of Chagas' disease observed on the Isthmus of Panama. *American Journal of Tropical Medicine*, **15**, 30–40.

De Robertis, E. D. P. and Bennet, H. S. (1954). Submicroscopic vesicular component in the synapse. *Federation Proceedings*, **13**, 35.

Dias, E. (1932). O *Trypanosoma cruzi* pode evoluir na cavidade geral do *Triatoma megista*. Nota prévia. *Memórias do Instituto Oswaldo Cruz*, **26**, 83–84.

Dias, E. (1933). Immunité naturelle des animaux à froid vis-à-vis de l'infection par le *Trypanosoma cruzi*. *Comptes Rendus des Séances de la Société de Biologie et de ses Filiales, Paris*, **112**, 1474–1475.

Dias, E. (1934). Estudos sôbre o *Schizotrypanum cruzi*. *Memórias do Instituto Oswaldo Cruz*, **28**, 1–110.

Diniz, C. R. and Torres, J. M. (1968). Release of an acetylcholine-like substance from Guinea pig ileum by scorpion venom. *Toxicon*, **5**, 277–281.

Dominguez, A. and Gavallér, B. (1962). Encephalitis chagásica. *Zeitschrift für Tropenmedizin und Parasitologie*, **13**, 308–311.

Dominguez, A. and Jaffé, R. (1962). Beitrage zur Biologie des Entwickungszclus von *Trypanosoma cruzi* in infizierten Organismus. *Zeitschrift für Tropemedizin und Parasitologie*, **13**, 304–307.

Dvorack, J. A. (1976). New *in vitro* approach to quantitation of *Trypanosoma cruzi* vertebrate cell interactions. PAHO International Symposium on New Approaches in American Trypanosomiasis Research. Belo Horizonte, Brazil, 18–21 March 1975. Washington DC. Pan American Health Organization, pg. 109–120.

Dvorack, J. A. and Schmunis, G. A. (1972). *Trypanosoma cruzi*: Interaction with mouse peritoneal macrophages. *Experimental Parasitology*, **32**, 289–300.

Edgcomb, J. (1970). Natural Infection of *Rattus rattus* by *Trypanosoma cruzi* in Panama. *American Journal of Tropical Medicine and Hygiene*, **19**, 767–769.

Freire-Maia, L., Cunha-Melo, J. R., Gomez, M. V., Tafuri, W. L., Maria, T. A., Calixto, S. L. and Futuro-Neto, H. A. (1976a). Studies on the mechanism of action of tityustoxin. *In:* "Animal, Plant and Microbiology Toxins" (K. Hajashi Ohsaka and 4-Sawa, ed.), Vol. 2, pp. 273–285. Plenum Press, New York.

Freire, Maia, L., Cunha-Melo, J. R., Futuro-Neto, H. A., Azevedo, A. D. and Weinberg, J. (1976b). Cholinergic and adrenergic effects of tityustoxin. *General Pharmacology*, **7**, 115–123.

Golgher, R. R., Bertelli, M. S., Peixoto, M. L. and Brener, Z. (1976). Effect of interferon on the development of *Trypanosoma cruzi* in tissue culture "Vero" cells. *Journal of Parasitology*. (Sent for publication).

Gomez de Alcantara, F. (1959). Experimentelle Chagas Kardiomiopathie. *Zeitschrift für Tropenmedizin und Parasitologie, Stuttgart*, **10**, 296–303.

Gonzalez-Cappa, S. M. and Kagan, L. G. (1969). Agar gel immunoelectrophoretic analysis of several strains of *Trypanosoma cruzi*. *Experimental Parasitology*, **25**, 50–57.

Grillo, M. and Pallay, S. L. (1962). "Electromicroscopy" (S. S. Breese, Jr., ed,), Vol. 2. Academic Press, New York and London.

Guimarães, J. P. and Miranda, A. (1959). Megaesôfago em macaco Rhesus com 10 anos de infecção chagásica. International Congress on Chagas' disease, July. Rio de Janeiro, Brazil, pg. 657–671.

Habr-Gamma, A. (1966). Motilidade do colon sigmoide e do reto (contribuição à fisiopatologia do megacolo chagásico). Thesis, School of Medicine, Federal University, São Paulo, Brazil.

Hager, H. and Tafuri, W. L. (1959a). Elektronenoptischer Nachweis sog. neurosekretorischer Elementar granula in marklosen Nervenfasern des Plexus myentericus (Auerbach) des Meerschweischens. *Naturwissenchaften*, **49**, 332–333.

Hager, H. and Tafuri, W. L. (1959b). Elektronenoptische untersuchungen über die Fein-Struktur des Plexus myentericus (Auerbach) in colon des Meerschweinchens (cavia-cobaya). *Archives für Psychiatry und Zeitschrift für Gesund Neurologie*, **199**, 437–471.

Hauschka, T. S. (1947). Sex of host as factor in Chagas' disease. *Journal of Parasitology*, **33**, 399–404.

Hial, W. and Diniz, C. R. (1971). Efeito da escorpiotoxina sôbre o contéudo do substância P do intestino de rato. *Ciência e Cultura de São Paulo*, **33**, 304 (suppl.).

Hial, W., Diniz, C. R., Pittella, J. E. H. and Tafuri, W. L. (1973). Quantitative study of P substance in the megaesophagus megacolon of *Trypanosoma cruzi* infections. *Journal of Tropical Medicine and Hygiene*, **76**, 175–179.

Jardim, E. (1967). Alterações quantitativas das células de Purkinje na moléstia de Chagas experimental no camundongo. *Arquivo de Neuro-Psiquiatria*, **25**, 199–208.

Johnson, C. M. and Derivas, C. T. (1936). Six new cases of Chagas' disease in Panama with review of previous cases. *American Journal of Tropical Medicine*, **16**, 47–57.

Jörg, M. E. and Orlando, A. S. (1967). Neurosíndrome mínino em la tripanosomíasis cruzi crônica. *Memórias do Instituto Oswaldo Cruz*, **65**, 63–80.

Köberle, F. (1956a). Chagaskrankheit: eine Erkrankung der Neurovegetativen Peripherie. *Wiener Klinische Wochenschrift*, **68**, 339–349.

Köberle, F. (1956b). Zur Frage der Enststehung sog. "Idiopathischer Dilatationem" muskularer Hohlorgane. *Virchow's Archiv Abt. A. Pathologische Anatomie*, **329**, 337–362.

Köberle, F. (1957). Patogenia da moléstia de Chagas. Estudo dos órgãos musculares ôcos. *Revista Goiana de Medicina*, **3**, 155–180.

Köberle, F. (1959). Die Chagaskrankheit-ihre Pathogenese und ihre Bedeutung als Vorksseuche. *Zeitschrift für Tropenmedizin und Parasitologie*, **10**, 236–268.

Köberle, F. (1960). Hiperplasia muscular no megaesôfago chagásico. *Revista Goiana de Medicina*, **6**, 147–153.

Köberle, F. (1961). Patología y anatomía patológica de la enfermedad de Chagas. *Boletin de la "Oficina Sanitária Panamericana"*, **51**, 404–428.

Köberle, F. (1967). Zur Pathogenese des Megaösophagus. *Zeitschrift Gastroenterologie*, **5**, 287–290.

Köberle, F. (1968). Chagas' disease and Chagas' syndromes: The pathology of American trypanosomiasis. *Advances in Parasitology*, **6**, 63–116.

Köberle, F. and Nador, E. (1955). Etiologia e patogenia do megaesôfago no Brasil. *Revista Paulista de Medicina*, **47**, 643–661.

Kolodny, M. H. (1939). Seasonal variations in the intensity of experimental infection with *Trypanosoma cruzi*. *American Journal of Hygiene*, **29**, 13–24.

Kolodny, M. H. (1940). The effect of environmental temperature upon experi-

614 W. L. TAFURI

mental trypanosomiasis (*T. cruzi*) of rats. *American Journal of Hygiene*, **32**, 21–23.

Kumar, R., Kline, I. K. and Abelmann, W. H. (1969). Experimental *Trypanosoma cruzi* myocarditis. Relative effects upon the right and left ventricles. *American Journal of Pathology*, **57**, 31–48.

Kumar, R., Kline, I. K. and Abelmann, W. (1970). Imuno-Suppression in experimental acute and subacute chagasic myocarditis. *American Journal of Tropical Medicine and Hygiene*, **19**, 932–939.

Lambrecht, F. L. (1965). Biological variations in trypanosomes and their relation to the epidemiology of Chagas' disease. *Revista do Instituto de Medicina tropical de São Paulo*, **7**, 346–352.

Lima-Pereira, F. E. (1976a). Observações sobre a imunodepressão durante a fase aguda da infecção de camundongos Albinos pelo *Trypanosoma cruzi*. Thesis, School of Medicine, Federal University, M. Gerais, Belo Horizonte, Brazil.

Lima-Pereira, F. E. (1976b). Colloidal carbon uptake by liver and spleen macrophages in *T. cruzi* infection in mice. *Revista Brasileira de Pesquisas Médicas e Biologicas*. (Sent for publication).

Lima-Pereira, F. E. and Sassine, W. A. (1976). Comportamento do macrófagos peritoneais de camundongos com *T. cruzi* (cepa *Y*). *Ciência e Cultura*, **28**, 528.

Lisboa-Bittencourt, A. C. (1960). Sôbre a forma congênita da doença de Chagas. Estudo anátomo-patológico de 6 casos. *Revista do Instituto de Medicina tropical de São Paulo*, **2**, 319–334.

Lopes, E. R. (1965). Contribuição ao estudo dos gânglios cardíacos (sistema nervoso autônomo) em chagásicos crônicos. Thesis, School of Medicine, M. Gerais, Uberaba, Brazil.

Lopes, E. R., Tafuri, W. L. and Chapadeiro, E. (1969). Estudo morfológico e quantitativo dos núcleos dorsal do vago e hipogloso em chagásicos crônicoa com e sem megaesôfago. *Revista do Instituto de Medicina tropical de São Paulo*, 123–129.

Lopes, E. R., Tafuri, W. L., Bogliolo, L., Almeida, H. O., Chapadeiro, E. and Raso, P. (1977). Miocardite chágasica aguda humana (ganglionite subepicárdica; aggressão à fibra Muscular). *Revista do Instituto de Medicina tropical de São Paulo*, **19**, 301–309.

MacClure and Poche, R. (1960). Die experimentelle Chagasmyocarditis der Weiben Maus in elektronmikroskopischen Bild. *Virchows Archives Abt. A. Pathologische Anatomie*, **33**, 405–420.

Macedo, V. O. (1973). Influência da exposição à reinfecção na evoluçao da doença de Chagas (Estudo longitudinal de cinco anos). Thesis, School of Medicine, Federal University, Bahia, Salvador, Brazil.

Machado, A. B. M. and Machado, C. R. S. (1976). Reinervação simpática do coração na doença de Chagas experimental. *Ciência e Cultura*, **27**, 558.

Machado, A. B. M., Machado, C. R. S. and Gomes, C. B. (1975). Depletion of heart norepinephrine in experimental acute myocarditis caused by *Trypanosoma cruzi*. *Experientia*, **31**, 1202–1203.

Martinez-Silva, R., Lopes, V. A. and Chiriboga, J. (1970). Effects of poly I.C. on the course of infection with *Trypanosoma cruzi*. *Proceedings of the Society for Experimental Biology and Medicine*, **134**, 885–888.

Mayer, M., Da Rocha-Lima, H. (1914). Zum verhalten von *Schizotrypanum cruzi* in warm blutern und Arthropoden. *Archives für Tropenmedizin und Hygiene*, **18**, 101–136.

Menezes, H. (1964). Moléstia de Chagas experimental. Lesões do distema nervoso central na fase aguda. *Revista Brasileira de Medicina*, **21**, 21–24.

Menezes, H. and Alcantara, F. G. de (1965). Distribuição dos parasitas (pseudo-

cistos) no sistema nervoso central de ratos infectados experimentalmente pelo
T. cruzi. Revista Goiana de Medicina, **11**, 21–25.

Meyer, H. and Oliveira-Musachio, M. X. (1948). Cultivation of *Trypanosoma cruzi* in tissue cultures: A four-year study. *Parasitology*, **39**, 91–94.

Milder, R. V., Kloetzel, J. and Deane, M. P. (1973). Observation on the inter-action of peritoneal macrophages with *Trypanosoma cruzi*. I. Initial phase of the relationship with blood stream and culture forms *in vitro. Revista do Instituto de Medicina Tropical de São Paulo*, **15**, 386–392.

Nilsson, L., Larsson, I., Hakanson, E., Brodin, B., Pernow, P. and Sundler, F. (1975). Localization of substance P-like immuno-reactivity in mouse gut. *Histochemistry*, **43**, 97–99.

Noetzel, H., Elejalde, P. and Dias, F. (1958). Uber die Gehirnveranderungen bei der Chagaskrankheit. *Zeitschrift für Tropenmedizin und Parasitologie*, **9**, 27–32.

Nogueira, N. (1974). The scope of *T. cruzi* from the vacuolar system of macro-phages. *Journal of Cell Biology*, **63**, 245.

Nogueira, N. and Cohn, Z. (1976). *Trypanosoma cruzi*: Mechanism of entry and intracellular fate in mammalian cells. *Journal of Experimental Medicine*, **143**, 1402–1470.

Nussenzweig, V., Deane, L. M. and Kloetzel, J. (1963). Differences in antigenic constitution strains of *Trypanosoma cruzi. Experimental Parasitology*, **14**, 221–232.

Okumura, M. and Corrêa-Neto, A. (1961). Produção experimental de "megas" em animais inoculados com *Trypanosoma cruzi. Revista do Hospital das Clínicas da Faculdade de Medicina da Universidade de São Paulo*, **16**, 338–341.

Palade, G. E. and Palay, S. L. (1954). Electron microscope observations of inter-neuronal and neuromuscular synapses. *Anatomical Record*, **118**, 335.

Paulino da Costa, C. (1976). Personal communication.

Pizzi, T. (1957). Imunologia de la enfermedad de Chagas. Universidade do Chile, Monografia Biológica no. 71, Santiago (Chile). Stanley.

Pizzi, T. (1961). Immunologia de la enfermedad de Chagas: estado actual del problema. *Bolentin de la Oficina Sanitaria Panamericana*, **51**, 450–464.

Pizzi, T. and Rubio, M. (1955). Aspectos celulares de la inmunidad en la enfer-medad de Chagas. *Boletin Chileno Parasitologia*, **10**, 4–9.

Pizzi, T., Agosin, M., Chriten, R., Holcker, G. and Neghme, A. (1948–1949). Influencia de la constitucion genetica en la resitencia de la laucha en la infeccion experimental por *Trypanosoma cruzi. Biologica* **8/9/10/11**, 43–53.

Pizzi, T., Rubio, M. and Knierim, F. (1953). Contribución al conocimento de los mecanismos inmunitarios en la enfermedad de Chagas experimental de la rata. *Boletin de Informaciones Parasitarias Chilenas*, **8**, 66–72.

Prata, A. (1955). Esquistossomose mansoni—doença de Chagas—megaesôfago—calazar na Bahia. *Arquivo Brasileiro Medicina Naval*, **16**, 4029–4034.

Raso, P. (1964). Contribuição ao estudo da lesão vorticilar (especialmente do vortex esquerdo) na cardite chagásica crônica. Thesis, School of Medicine, Federal University, M. Gerais, Belo Horizonte, Brazil.

Raso, P. and Tafuri, W. L. (1971). Alterações do pericardio na fase crônica da tripanossomíase cruzi humana e nas fases aguda e crônica da moléstia experi-mental. *Revista da Sociedade Brasileira de Medicina Tropical de São Paulo*, **5**, 135–153.

Rezende, J. M. (1959). Forma digestiva da moléstia de Chagas. *Revista Goiana de Medicina*, **5**, 193–227.

Rezende, J. M. (1968). Aspectos clínicos da colopatia chagásica. *Revista Goiana de Medicina*, **14**, 69–72.

Rodrigues da Silva, G. (1966). Doença de Chagas em famílias de duas áreas restritas da cidade de Salvador, Bahia. Thesis, School of Medicine, Federal University, Bahia, Salvador, Brazil.

Romãna, C. and Terracini, E. (1945). Comportamento de las infeciones de lauchas por *S. cruzi*, segun la concentración de parasitos inoculados (infecciones crônicas iniciales). *Anales del Instituto de Medicina Regional, Tucumán*, 1, 141–164.

Rubio, M. D. (1954). Estudio de los factores que intervienen en la virulencia de una cepa de *Trypanosoma cruzi*. Acción de la cortisona en la capacidad de invasión y multiplicación del parasito. *Biologica*, 20, 89–125.

Rubio, M. D. (1956). Estudio de la enfermedad de Chagas experimental del batracio. I. Factores que intervienen en la immunidad natural. *Boletin Chileno de Parasitologia*, 11, 28–32.

Sanabria, A. (1968). Ultrastructure of *Trypanosoma cruzi* in Mouse Brain. *Experimental Parasitology*, 23, 379–391.

Sanabria, A. (1969). Nuevas investigaciones acerca de la ultraestructura e histoquímica del *Trypanosoma cruzi* en el cerebro del raton. *Acta Científica Venezolana*, 20, 32–39.

Santos-Buch, C. A. and Teixeira, A. R. L. (1974). The immunology of experimental Chagas' disease. III. Rejection of Allogeneic heart cells *in vitro*. *Journal of Experimental Medicine*, 140, 38–53.

Scorza, C. (1972). Alterações ultraestruturales de los discos intercalares com *Trypanosoma cruzi* y submetidas a exercício ou reinoculaciones. *Revista Latinoamericana de Microscopia Eletrônica*, 1, 48.

Scorza, C. and Scorza, J. V. (1972a). Acute Myocarditis in rats inoculated with *Trypanosoma cruzi*: Study of animals sacrificed between the fourth and twenty-ninth day after infection. *Revista do Instituto de Medicina tropical, São Paulo*, 14, 171–177.

Scorza, C. and Scorza, J. V. (1972b). The role of inflammatory macrophages in experimental acute chagasic myocarditis. *Journal of Reticulo Entothelial Society*, 11, 601–616.

Scorza, C., Scorza, J. V. and Noorden S. von (1972). Secrecion de fosfatasa acida por formas intracelulares de *Trypanosoma cruzi* en el miocardio de ratas blancas. *Revista Latinoamericana de Microscopia Eletronica*, 1, 26.

Silva, L. H. P. and Nussenzweig, V. (1953). Sobre uma cepa de *Trypanosoma cruzi* altamente virulenta para o camundongo branco. *Folia Clínica et Biologica*, 20, 191–207.

Souza-Campos, E. (1929). Estudo sobre a anatomia patologia do ganglio lynphatico na trypanosomiase americana experimental. Alterações do sistema reticulo endothelial -Corpos intranucleares-Myelopoese. *Anales da Faculdade de Medicina da Universidade de São Paulo*, 4, 75–90.

Streber, F. (1950). Influencia del sexo en infecciones experimentales por *Schiszotrypanum cruzi* Chagas, 1909. *Revista de Paludismo y Medicina Tropical, México*, 2, 73–78.

Tafuri, W. L. (1964). Ultrastructure of vesicular component in the intramural nervous system of the Guinea-pig's intestine. *Zeitschrift für Naturforschung*, 19B, 622–625.

Tafuri, W. L. (1970). Pathogenesis of lesions of the autonomic nervous system of mouse in experimental acute Chagas' disease. Light and electron microscope studies. *American Journal of Tropical Medicine and Hygiene*, 19, 405–417.

Tafuri, W. L. (1971). Light and electron microscope studies of the autonomic nervous system in experimental and human American trypanosomiasis. *Virchows Archives Abt. A. Pathologische Anatomie*, 354, 136–149.

Tafuri, W. L. (1975). Alterações ultra-estruturais dos componentes muscular, intersticial e nervoso do coração, esôfago e intestinos na doença de Chagas experimental e humana. Thesis. School of Medicine, Federal University, Minas Gerais, Belo Horizonte, Brazil.

Tafuri, W. L. and Brener, Z. (1966a). Lesões do sistema nervoso autônomo do camundongo albino na fase crônica da tripanossomiase cruzi experimental. *Revista do Instituto de Medicina tropical de São Paulo*, **8**, 177–183.

Tafuri, W. L. and Brener, Z. (1966b). Lesões do sistema nervoso autônomo do camundongo albino na tripanossomíase cruzi experimental, fase aguda. *O Hospital*, **69**, 371–383.

Tafuri, W. L. and Brener, Z. (1967). Lesões dos plexos de Meissner e de Auerbach do intestino do camundongo albino na fase crônica da tripanossomíase cruzi experimental. *Revista do Instituto de Medicina tropical de São Paulo*, **9**, 149–154.

Tafuri, W. L. and Maria, T. A. (1970). Sobre o comportamento do compomente vesicular neurosecretor no megaesôfago da tripanossomíase cruzi humana. *Revista do Instituto de Medicina tropical de São Paulo*, **12**, 298–309.

Tafuri, W. L. and Raso, P. (1962). Lesões do sistema nervoso autônomo do camundongo albino na tripanosomíase. *O Hospital*, **62**, 1326–1341.

Tafuri, W. L., Maria, T. A. and Lopes, E. R. (1971). Lesões do plexo mientérico do esôfago, do jejuno e do colo de chagásicos crônicos. Estudo ao microscópio electrônico. *Revista do Instituto de Medicina tropical de São Paulo*, **13**, 76–91.

Tafuri, W. L., Lopes, E. R., Chapadeiro, E. and Maria, T. A. (1973a). Microscopia eletrônica do miocárdio na tripanossomíase cruzi humana. *Revista do Instituto de Medicina tropical de São Paulo*, **15**, 347–370.

Tafuri, W. L., Lopes, E. R., Nunan, B. (1973b). Doença de chagas congenita. *Revista do Instituto de Medicina tropical de São Paulo*, **15**, 322–330.

Tafuri, W. L., Maria, T. A., Freire-Maia, L. and Cunha-Melo, J. R. (1974a). Effect of the scorpion toxin on the granular vesicles in the Auerbach's plexus of the rat ileum. *Journal of Neural Transmission*, **35**, 233–240.

Tafuri, W. L., Pittella, J. E. H., Bogliolo, L. and Almeida-Maria, T. (1974b). An electron microscope study of the Auerbach's plexus and determination of substance P of the colon in Hirschsprung's disease. *Virchows Archives Abt. A. Pathological Anatomy and Histology*, **362**, 41–50.

Taliaferro, W. H. and Pizzi, T. (1955). Connective tissue reactions in normal and immunized mice to a reticulotropic strain of *Trypanosoma cruzi*. *Journal of Infectious Disease*, **96**, 199–226.

Teixeira, A. R. L., Teixeira, L. and Santos-Buch, C. A. (1975). The immunology of experimental Chagas' disease. IV. Production of lesions in rabbits similar to those of chronic Chagas disease in man. *American Journal on Pathology*, **80**, 163–180.

Torres, C. B. M. (1941). Sôbre a anatomia patológica da doença de Chagas. *Memórias do Instituto Oswaldo Cruz*, **36**, 391–404.

Torres, C. B. M. and Duarte, E. (1948). Miocardite na forma aguda da doença de Chagas. *Memórias do Instituto Oswaldo Cruz*, **46**, 759–793.

Vianna, G. (1911). Contribuição para o estudo da anatomia patológica da "moléstia de Carlos Chagas". *Memórias do Instituto Oswaldo Cruz*, **3**, 276–294.

Vichi, L. (1964a). Destruição de neurônios motores na medula espinal de ratos na fase aguda da meléstia de Chagas. *Revista do Instituto de Medicina tropical de São Paulo*, **6**, 150–154.

Vichi, L. (1964b). Avaliação quantitativa do parasitismo no coração, vasos da base e coronário do rato, na fase aguda da moléstia de Chagas. *Revista do Instituto de Medicina tropical de São Paulo*, **6**, 292–296.

Villela, E. and Torres, C. B. M. (1925). Lésions histopathologiques dans la paralysie expérimentale à *Schizotrypanum cruzi* chez le chien. Nature des cellulas contenant le parasite dans le système nerveux central. *Comptes Rendus des Seànces de la Société de Biologie et ses Filiales, Paris,* **93,** 133–135.

Warren, L. G. and Borsos, T. (1959). Studies in immune factors occurring in sera of chickens against the crithidia stage of *Trypanosoma cruzi. Journal of Immunology,* **82,** 585–590.

Wood, S. F. (1953). Survival time of metacyclic *Trypanosoma cruzi* in human sweat. *Journal of Parasitology,* **39,** 569–570.

Yaeger, R. G. and Miller, O. N. (1960). Effect of malnutrition on susceptibility of rats to *Trypanosoma cruzi.* III. Pantothenate deficiency. *Experimental Parasitology,* **10,** 232–237.

Yaeger, R. G. and Miller, O. N. (1963). Effect of malnutrition on susceptibility of rats to *Trypanosoma cruzi.* V. Vitamin A deficiency. *Experimental Parasitology,* **14,** 9–14.

13

Biochemical Aspects of the Biology of *Trypanosoma cruzi*

W. E. GUTTERIDGE and G. W. ROGERSON*

*Biological Laboratory, University of Kent,
Canterbury, Kent, England*

I.	Introduction	620
II.	Morphological changes	621
III.	Isolation of the various morphological forms	623
IV.	Energy metabolism	625
	A. Substrates utilized	625
	B. End products of metabolism	626
	C. Pathways of metabolism	627
	D. Oxidation of reduced pyridine nucleotides . . .	629
	E. Synthesis of ATP	633
	F. Conclusions	634
V.	Nucleic acid metabolism	636
	A. Purine metabolism	636
	B. Pyrimidine metabolism	638
	C. Deoxyribonucleotide metabolism	641
	D. Nucleic acid synthesis	642
	E. DNA, especially kinetoplast DNA	643
	F. RNA	644
	G. Nucleic acid catabolism	644
	H. Conclusions	644
VI.	Discussion and Conclusions	645
VII.	Acknowledgements	647
VIII.	References	647

* Present address: Wellcome Research Laboratories, Langley Court, Beckenham, Kent, England.

I. Introduction

Biochemical studies carried out over the last decade have indicated clearly that the morphological changes which occur during the life cycles of many genera of parasitic protozoa, and which are associated with a change from one host to another, are paralleled in many instances by biochemical changes (Trigg and Gutteridge, 1977). Such changes have been related to the adaptation of the parasite to its new host. Undoubtedly the best documented example of such adaptation is in the *Trypanosoma brucei* sub-group of trypanosomes (Bowman *et al.*, 1972; Brown *et al.*, 1973; Newton *et al.*, 1973; Bowman, 1974; Bowman and Flynn, 1976; Trigg and Gutteridge, 1977). Here, there is good evidence that the move from the homeostatically controlled glucose and oxygen rich mammalian bloodstream to the gut of the insect vector (*Glossina* sp.) involves the acquisition of an extensive mitochondrion with numerous plate-like cristae, at least a partially functional tricarboxylic acid (TCA) cycle and a cytochrome-containing respiratory chain. Associated with these acquisitions, there appears to be a metabolic switch in energy metabolism. In the mammalian forms, glucose is catabolized to pyruvate with NADH being reoxidized by the α-glycerophosphate oxidase system (apparent K_m for $O_2 \equiv 2 \cdot 1\ \mu M$). In the culture (insect vector) forms, depending on strain, either a more complete metabolism of glucose or the catabolism of the amino acid proline occurs, the reduced pyridine nucleotides in both cases being reoxidized principally by the respiratory chain (apparent K_m for O_2 by intact organisms $\equiv 0 \cdot 10\ \mu M$). These changes in energy metabolism, which are summarized in Table 1, correlate well with the change of environment, as the contents of the tsetse fly gut are about 20% by weight protein but only 0·1% by weight carbohydrate, and the oxygen concentration of the gut is much lower than that of the mammalian bloodstream. There are also some concomitant changes in lipid content which have been associated with the alternate development and regression of the mitochondrial network.

Trypanosoma cruzi has a complex life cycle which involves development both in a mammal and in an insect vector (various species of triatomine). In fact, the cycle is more complex than that of the *T. brucei* subgroup trypanosomes as in the mammalian host it develops intracellularly. Different morphological forms of the parasite exist and, therefore, there has been much speculation as to how far these environmental and morphological changes are associated with parallel biochemical changes. In this article, we will first discuss in more detail the environments in which *T. cruzi* develops and the morphological forms that it assumes in each of these. We will then consider the studies which have been carried out to date, principally in our own laboratory, in which

Table 1. Comparison of the metabolic status of the different forms of *T. brucei* subgroup trypanosomes.

| Parameter | Blood trypomastigote forms | | Culture procyclic trypomastigote forms |
	Long slender	Short stumpy	
Glycolysis	+	+	+
TCA cycle	$-^a$	Partial	$+^b$
L-a-glycerophosphate oxidase	+	+	Low
Proline oxidase	—	Low	+
Cytochrome chain	—	—	+
Cyanide sensitivity	—	—	Partial
Mitochondria	Very few tubular cristae	Tubular cristae	Plate-like cristae
Growth temperature (°C)	37	37	25

+, Present; —, absent. ^{a} Recent work suggests that some of the enzymes may be present in some strains but *not* the key citrate synthase and succinate dehydrogenase. ^{b} The cycle may only be partial when growing on proline. Based on Table 5.1 of Gutteridge and Coombs (1977).

the biochemistry of the different forms has been compared. So far such studies have encompassed only energy metabolism and nucleic acid metabolism, so no mention will be made of protein and lipid biosynthesis and the metabolism associated with this. Finally, we will assess critically just how far the morphological changes which occur correlate with biochemical changes. No attempt will be made to give a complete review of the biochemistry of *T. cruzi* as most studies have been concerned only with culture epimastigote forms and in any case this information is readily available elsewhere (Brener, 1973; Von Brand, 1973; Bowman and Flynn, 1976; Gutteridge, 1976a; Gutteridge and Coombs, 1977). The chemotherapeutic implications of the differences in metabolism between *T. cruzi* and its mammalian host are also discussed elsewhere (Gutteridge, 1978).

II. Morphological changes

The basic life cycle of *Trypanosoma cruzi* is given in Fig. 1. Note that throughout this article, the classification of trypanosomes given by Hoare (1970, 1972) has been followed. The life cycle of *T. cruzi* has been reviewed by the same author (1972).

Metacyclic trypomastigotes, when inoculated into a mammal, do not multiply in the blood, but rather they penetrate into the cells of various tissues such as the muscle of the heart and intestine. Here they change into the so-called "amastigote" forms which divide repeatedly by binary

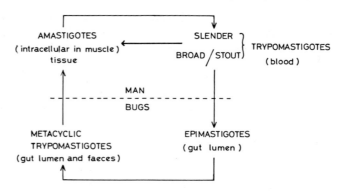

FIG. 1.   Diagram of the basic life cycle of *T. cruzi* (based on Fig. 1.6 of Gutteridge and Coombs, 1977).

fission. It is now clear that the term "amastigote" is a misnomer as the intracellular stages of *T. cruzi* are somewhat pointed and have a short free flagellum (see Lumsden, 1974; Dvorak, 1976; Meyer and de Souza, 1976; Gutteridge, 1976b; Gutteridge *et al.*, 1978). It has been proposed that they should be called "sphaeromastigotes" (Meyer and de Souza, 1976), a term originally suggested by Brack (1968) for the rounded forms found in the insect vector, until a more appropriate name is found. Since there is no evidence that mammalian intracellular forms are indeed the same as Brack's sphaeromastigotes, we will continue in this article to call them "amastigotes".

After a certain number of divisions (Dvorak, 1976), amastigotes give rise to trypomastigote forms which find their way back into the bloodstream. The mechanism of this change has been the subject of some controversy, the centre of which concerns whether there is a direct change by a process of unrolling of the amastigote ("obicular" development) or whether there is an intermediate epimastigote form ("fusiform" development) (see Hoare, 1972). This controversy has not been resolved, possibly because both processes may occur and the phenomenon may be strain related. Our experience with the Sonya strain of *T. cruzi* leads us to support the existence of the fusiform developmental cycle as our preparations of intracellular parasites always contain small numbers of epimastigote forms (see below). This is also the view of Dvorak (1976) from his observations in tissue culture.

It is generally agreed that the blood trypomastigote forms do not divide in the blood, though occasionally organisms with two nuclei and/or two kinetoplasts are seen (see Hoare, 1972). There are two kinds of blood trypomastigote; one is an actively motile slender form with an elongated nucleus, a sub-terminal kinetoplast and a short free flagellum, while the other is a broad form with slow movements, an oval nucleus, an almost terminal kinetoplast and a long free flagellum (Chagas, 1909; Hoare, 1972 for a review of the later literature; Howells and Chiari, 1975). Brener and Chiari (1963) have also described a stout trypomastigote characterized by its bulky aspect, vacuolated cytoplasm and terminal kinetoplast. Which form predominates appears to be a function of both the strain of *T. cruzi* and the age of the infection (Brener and Chiari, 1963; Howells and Chiari, 1975; Cover and Gutteridge, 1978). It has been suggested that it is mainly the slender forms which invade the tissues and thus continue the infection in the mammal, and that it is mainly the broad forms which are infective to the insect vector and thus transmit the infection (Brener, 1969; 1976).

The entire development of *T. cruzi* in the insect vector takes place within the lumen of the gut and again there is controversy as to the exact route followed (see Brack, 1968; Hoare, 1972; Brener and Al-varanga, 1976). Trypomastigotes appear to change initially in the foregut into amastigote and sphaeromastigote forms which multiply by binary fission. By about 24 hours after the blood meal was taken, they have found their way to the mid-gut and most have changed to epimastigotes. This is probably the main form in which division takes place. From about the fourth day onwards, epimastigotes are also present in the rectum. Here, some epimastigotes change, either directly by a gradual migration of the kinetoplast backwards or indirectly through a rounded sphaero-mastigote stage, to form metacyclic trypomastigotes. These are voided in the faeces and can initiate a new infection.

Thus, there are three main environments in which *T. cruzi* occurs: within the cells of the tissues; free in the bloodstream of the mammal; and in the lumen of the gut of the insect vector (Fig. 1). Three different morphological forms predominate in these environments—amastigotes, trypomastigotes and epimastigotes—though numerous transitional forms also occur. The three main morphological forms are readily distinguish-able on the basis of the position of the kinetoplast, the length of the flagellum and the extent of the undulating membrane (see Hoare, 1972). All three forms, however, have mitochondria with plate-like cristae, which has led Brack (1968) to doubt the existence of a mitochondrial cycle in *T. cruzi*. However, the electron microscopic studies of Sanabria (1966) and Maria *et al.* (1972) suggest to Vickerman and Preston (1976) a progressive amplification of mitochondrial substance from intra-cellular amastigote to bloodstream trypomastigote to vector epimastigote.

III. Isolation of the various morphological forms

It is clear from Section II that investigations attempting to correlate environmental, morphological and biochemical changes during the life cycle of *T. cruzi* must include intracellular amastigote, blood trypomastigote and vector epimastigote stages. Ideally, they should also include studies of intracellular epimastigotes and trypomastigotes and insect amastigotes, sphaeromastigotes and metacyclic trypomastigotes, as these are transitional forms which might exhibit partial adaptation. Unfortunately, it has only proved possible so far to isolate intracellular amastigotes and blood trypomastigotes in quantities sufficient for biochemical study. However, the epimastigote forms of *T. cruzi*, which can be grown in culture at 28°C, are morphologically similar to those in the insect vector. It is generally assumed that they are also biochemically similar, but it must be stressed that there is as yet no direct experimental evidence for this assumption. Thus, in this article, we will review comparatively only the biochemistry of the intracellular amastigote, blood trypomastigotes and culture epimastigote forms of *T. cruzi*. Occasional reference will be made to studies with culture trypomastigotes which have been used in a few biochemical studies (Stohlman *et al.*, 1973; Wood, 1975; Wood and Schiller, 1975) but none to culture amastigotes, as, although these can be grown *in vitro* (Pan, 1976), they have yet to be used in biochemical studies. As will be seen below, the data from these studies in fact allow tentative conclusions to be drawn about the other, transitional stages.

In most of the work that will be described, blood trypomastigotes and intracellular amastigotes were isolated mainly from rats (90–110 g weight) which had received 580 R of whole-body γ-irradiation not more than 24 h before subcutaneous inoculation with 10^7 trypomastigotes of the Sonya strain of *T. cruzi* (Gutteridge, 1976b; Gutteridge *et al.*, 1978). Unirradiated chinchillas (250–350 g) were, however, used for some experiments. Blood stages were isolated from rats 8–20 days after infection using a technique involving differential centrifugation to remove most of the erythrocytes and DEAE cellulose chromatography (phosphate–saline–glucose buffer, pH 7·5, I = 0·206) to remove the remaining blood cells. Overall recoveries were usually in the range 30–70%. Parasites were mainly ($\sim$97%) broad forms and were motile and had lost none of their infectivity for mice.

Intracellular stages were isolated from rats 10–15 days after infection or from chinchillas 12–16 days after infection. Hind limb muscle tissue was disrupted in an M.S.E. tissue homogenizer and the homogenate incubated with deoxyribonuclease, collagenase and trypsin. Parasites, contaminated only by a few blood cells, were then obtained by differential centrifugation. For purer preparations ($\sim$0·1% contamination), a terminal sucrose gradient step (0·25–0·70 M linear sucrose gradient, 225 × g for 5 min) was used. Recoveries ranged between 40–70%. About 1–2% of the parasites isolated were epimastigotes and trypomastigotes; the remainder were amastigotes. They were undamaged as judged by light and electron microscopy. However, the infectivity for mice of both these purified preparations and the initial cell homogenates could be accounted for by the epimastigotes and trypomastigotes present in them. In the experiments carried out in this laboratory, culture epimastigote forms of the parasite were harvested by centrifugation from mid-logarithmic phase cultures of organisms grown at 28°C in a modified LIT medium (Gutteridge *et al.*, 1969). Other investigators have used alternative media. Culture trypomastigote forms have been obtained from cultures grown in tissue culture media over a layer of tissue cells (Stohlman *et al.*, 1973).

IV. Energy metabolism

A. SUBSTRATES UTILIZED

Intracellular amastigote, blood trypomastigote and culture epimastigote forms of *T. cruzi* are all able to respire and retain their motility for long periods of time in the absence of exogenous energy sources (Zeledon 1960a; Ryley, 1956; Rogerson and Gutteridge, 1978). This situation contrasts markedly with that of the bloodstream forms of the *T. brucei* subgroup trypanosomes. Such metabolism implies the existence of substantial endogenous reserves of energy (our calculations suggest they should represent about 5% of the dry weight), but so far these have not been characterized. The carbohydrate content of the organism is far too low for this macromolecule to be the endogenous substrate and so it is generally considered that it is either lipid or protein or a mixture of these two macromolecules.

Endogenous reserves, however substantial, must ultimately be replenished from exogenous sources. Studies using manometric, polarographic and amino acid autoanalytical techniques have shown clearly that both monosaccharides such as glucose, fructose, mannose, galactose and xylose and amino acids such as proline, glutamate, leucine and threonine can be taken up and/or oxidized by culture epimastigote forms, though threonine is most likely a source of acetate units for fatty acid synthesis rather than a source of energy (Zeledon, 1960b; Sylvester and Krassner, 1976; Cross *et al.*, 1975; Rogerson and Gutteridge, 1978). The pattern of utilization of monosaccharides and amino acids by intracellular amastigotes and blood trypomastigotes is similar to that of the culture epimastigotes (Rogerson and Gutteridge, 1978).

It has been reported that the fatty acid, palmitate, inhibits the growth of the culture epimastigote forms of *T. cruzi* (Boné and Parent, 1963). However, it has recently been shown that culture trypomastigote forms of *T. cruzi*, in contrast to culture epimastigote forms, can catabolize palmitate and other fatty acids to CO_2, presumably by β-oxidation (Wood, 1975; Wood and Schiller, 1975). We have recently obtained similar results using culture epimastigotes and blood trypomastigotes and have further shown that intracellular amastigotes also catabolize palmitate at an apparently high rate of oxidation (Rogerson and Gutteridge, 1978). Our experiments, unlike those of Wood and Schiller, involved the incubation of organisms in a defined incubation medium containing ^{14}C-palmitate of known specific activity. We have therefore been able to calculate what these apparently high rates of metabolism in the mammalian stages represent in terms of ng atoms of oxygen utilized

Table 2. Rates of respiration of the different forms of *T. cruzi*.

Substrate	ng atoms 0/min/10^8 organisms		
	Culture epimastigote	Blood trypomastigote	Intracellular amastigote
Endogenous[a]	18	27	16
Glucose[a, b]	4·6	3·8	2·9
Palmitate	0·00084	0·0078	0·016

[a] Calculated from polarographic determinations. [b] Assuming glucose-stimulated rate of oxidation is additive to the endogenous rate of respiration. Data of Rogerson and Gutteridge (1978).

(Table 2). We have found that they are 1000 times less than the endogenous rates of metabolism and 180 times less than the glucose-stimulated rates of metabolism. Thus, although there are without doubt marked differences in the rates at which mammalian and culture forms can catabolize fatty acids, it is unlikely that this metabolism has a physiological significance in any stage. Sugars and amino acids should therefore still be regarded as the primary exogenous sources of energy for *T. cruzi*.

B. END PRODUCTS OF METABOLISM

The end products of endogenous metabolism in the blood trypomastigote and culture epimastigote forms are volatile acids and ammonia (Ryley, 1956), suggesting that, at least in part, the endogenous energy reserves are protein in nature. Blood trypomastigotes and culture epimastigotes catabolize glucose to CO_2, succinate and acetate. Lactate is also formed, though probably in most strains only by the blood trypomastigote forms (Ryley, 1956 but see Chang, 1948). Intracellular amastigotes metabolize glucose to products which include CO_2 and succinate; the possible formation of acetate and lactate has not yet been investigated (Rogerson and Gutteridge, 1978). Proline is catabolized in culture epimastigotes to TCA cycle acids and amino acids such as glutamate, aspartate, cysteine and lysine (though not alanine) (Sylvester and Krassner, 1976). The metabolism of this amino acid by other forms of *T. cruzi* has not yet been investigated.

C. PATHWAYS OF METABOLISM

Culture epimastigote forms of *T. cruzi* contain most of the enzymes of the glycolytic pathway (Table 3), form hexose monophosphates and diphosphates from ^{14}C-glucose (Shaw *et al.*, 1964) and show a distribution of radioactivity among the products of ^{14}C-glucose metabolism which infers metabolism through that pathway (Bowman *et al.*, 1963; Mancilla and Naquira, 1964). There is no doubt therefore that the pathway is both present and functional in these forms. Intracellular amastigote and blood trypomastigote forms contain hexokinase, phosphofructokinase and pyruvate kinase (Table 3) and therefore it is likely that the glycolytic pathway functions in these forms also (Rogerson and Gutteridge, 1976 and in preparation).

Table 3. Distribution of the enzymes of energy metabolism in the different forms of *T. cruzi*.

Enzyme	Culture epimastigote	Blood trypomastigote	Intracellular amastigote
Hexokinase	*	+	+
Phosphoglucoisomerase	*		
Phosphofructokinase	*	+	+
Aldolase	*		
Triose phosphate isomerase	*		
Triose phosphate dehydrogenase	*		
Phosphoglycerate kinase			
Phosphoglyceromutase			
Enolase			
Pyruvate kinase	+	+	+
Lactate dehydrogenase	*	+	+
Glucose-6-phosphate dehydrogenase	*	+	+
6-Phosphogluconate dehydrogenase	*	+	+
Pyruvate dehydrogenase	†		
Citrate synthase	+	+	+
Aconitase	*	+	+
Isocitrate dehydrogenase (NADP)	*	+	+
α-Ketoglutarate dehydrogenase			
Succinate thiokinase			
Succinate dehydrogenase	*	+	+
Fumarate hydratase	*	+	+
Malate dehydrogenase	*	+	+
Malic enzyme	+	+	+
Glutamate dehydrogenase	+	+	+

* Enzyme present (see Von Brand, 1973). + Enzyme present (Data of Rogerson and Gutteridge, 1976 and in preparation). † Enzyme present (Data of Miller *et al.* 1976).

Glucose-6-phosphate dehydrogenase and 6-phosphogluconate dehydrogenase are present in all three forms (Table 3), indicating the presence of at least the reductive part of the hexose monophosphate shunt. Bowman *et al.* (1963) have already stressed the importance of this pathway in culture epimastigote forms. Mancilla and Naquira (1964), from experiments in which they incubated these forms in media containing $2\text{-}^{14}\text{C-}$, $6\text{-}^{14}\text{C-}$ and $\text{U-}^{14}\text{C}$-glucose and measured the incorporation into glycerol and CO_2, calculated that the hexose monophosphate shunt contributed 40% towards the catabolism of glucose in the Tulahuean strain and 28% in the Peruvian strain.

The TCA cycle probably functions in all forms. All the enzymes of this cycle have been shown to be present in intracellular amastigote, blood trypomastigote and culture epimastigote forms, with the exception of a-ketoglutarate dehydrogenase and succinate thiokinase (Table 3). Of special interest are the presence of succinate dehydrogenase and citrate synthase which are normally indicative of a fully functional TCA cycle. The TCA cycle intermediates malate, fumarate and a-ketoglutarate have been identified in culture epimastigote forms incubated in the presence of radio-labelled glucose (Shaw *et al.*, 1964). Furthermore, if these forms are incubated in the presence of $3\text{-}^{14}\text{C}$-pyruvate or $2\text{-}^{14}\text{C}$-acetate, radioactivity is found not only in CO_2 but also in succinate, malate, fumarate, aspartate and glutamate (De Boiso and Stoppani, 1973). Thus there is conclusive proof for the presence of a functional TCA cycle in culture epimastigote forms and good evidence that a similar situation exists in the intracellular amastigote and blood trypomastigote stages.

Proline oxidation in culture epimastigote forms probably involves an initial oxidation by proline oxidase to form glutamate which is then metabolized through the complete TCA cycle (Sylvester and Krassner, 1976). In the *T. brucei* subgroup trypanosomes, in contrast, apparent absence of a citrate synthase in organisms growing on proline leads to the formation of alanine as the end product (Evans and Brown, 1972). The presence of proline oxidase has not been demonstrated in intracellular amastigote and blood trypomastigote forms, but a glutamate dehydrogenase is present in all of them (Table 3), no doubt accounting for the ammonia liberated from respiring culture epimastigotes. Since many transaminase activities are present at least in the culture epimastigote forms (Bash-Lewinson and Grossowicz, 1957; Zeledon, 1960c; Cazzulo *et al.*, 1977) other amino acids can be catabolized in conjunction with glutamate dehydrogenase.

The malic enzyme has been identified in all three forms of *T. cruzi* (Table 3). In culture epimastigote forms, there is evidence that it is involved in a pathway for the formation of succinate (Raw, 1959; Bowman *et al.*, 1963). However, other CO_2-fixing enzymes may also occur and the presence of a fumarate reductase activity, which might be coupled to a substrate level phosphorylation, as it is in helminths (Saz, 1972), has not been demonstrated. As Bowman *et al.* (1963) have indicated, succinate formation could equally be due to the low activity of succinate dehydrogenase.

The results of the experiments involving the metabolism of ^{14}C-fatty acids to CO_2 (Wood and Schiller, 1975; Rogerson and Gutteridge, 1978) imply the existence, in intracellular amastigote and blood trypomastigote forms, of a pathway for their degradation such as the β-oxidation pathway found in mammalian cells. No information is available at present, however, about the details of such a pathway.

D. OXIDATION OF REDUCED PYRIDINE NUCLEOTIDES

1. Investigation with whole cells

Lactate dehydrogenase is present in all forms (Table 3) and may account for some of the NADH oxidized. Similarly, if a fumarate reductase activity is indeed present in the organism (see above) the formation of succinate, which occurs in all forms, will lead to the concomitant oxidation of some NADH. However, it seems likely that in all three forms of *T. cruzi* most of the oxidation of reduced pyridine nucleotides involves the respiratory chain or chains.

It has been known for a number of years that blood trypomastigote and culture epimastigote forms of *T. cruzi* have a cyanide-sensitive terminal oxidase (Ryley, 1956; Bowman and Flynn, 1976). It is apparent, however, that in both forms, part of this oxidase activity is insensitive to cyanide, suggesting that more than one terminal oxidase is present. Kallinikova (1968a, b) has demonstrated histochemically in both forms the presence of a cytochrome c oxidase. However, as Bowman and Flynn (1976) have pointed out, this may not necessarily indicate the presence of cytochrome $a + a_3$ since the reaction observed could be linked with the alternative CN^- insensitive oxidase. We have found recently that the oxygen consumption of washed cell suspensions of all three forms of *T. cruzi* was equally and only partially sensitive to inhibition by cyanide and 2-heptyl-4-hydroxyquinoline-N-oxide (HOQNO) (Table 4) (Rogerson and Gutteridge 1977a and in preparation). Salicylhydroxamic acid (SHAM) which specifically inhibits cyanide-insensitive respiration in some plants (Henry and Nyns, 1975) and the α-glycerophosphate oxidase system of the *T. brucei* subgroup trypanosomes, did not however have any detectable (i.e. inhibition was $<5\%$) effect on any form (Table 4). The motility of blood trypomastigotes and culture epimastigotes was also unaffected by it. These results suggest that all three forms of *T. cruzi* have at least two similar respiratory chains and that a dominant, SHAM-sensitive, oxidase similar to the α-glycerophosphate oxidase of the *T. brucei* subgroup trypanosomes is not present in any form.

Table 4. Effects of inhibitors on the oxygen consumption of washed cell suspensions of the different forms of T. cruzi.

Inhibitor	Molarity	Inhibition		
		Culture	Blood	Intracellular
KCN	10^{-3}	69 ± 5	68 ± 4	68 ± 2
HOQNO	10^{-6}	31 ± 8	31 ± 1	34 ± 6
SHAM	3×10^{-3}	<5	<5	<5
Suramin	10^{-5}	<5	<5	<5

Data of Rogerson and Gutteridge (1977).

2. Investigations with mitochondrial preparations

Unpurified and undoubtedly damaged mitochondrial preparations from the three main forms of T. cruzi have succinate, α-glycerophosphate and NADH oxidase activities (Rogerson and Gutteridge, 1977a). In addition, we have shown that culture epimastigote forms have cyanide-sensitive ascorbate + TMPD (N,N,N′,N′-tetramethyl-p-phenylenediamine) cytochrome c oxidase activity.

Succinate oxidase of the culture epimastigote forms is partially sensitive to inhibition by cyanide, antimycin A and HOQNO, confirming the

Table 5. Effects of inhibitors on the oxygen consumption of mitochondrial preparations from culture epimastigote forms of T. cruzi.

Inhibitor	Molarity	% Inhibition		
		Succinate	α-Glycerophosphate	NADH
KCN	10^{-3}	83 ± 7	85 ± 4	<10
HOQNO	10^{-6}	47 ± 11	62 ± 4	<10
Antimycin	3×10^{-6}	$35 \; {}^{+}7$	—	<10
Rotenone	10^{-6}	<10	<10	<30
Amytal	10^{-3}	<10	<10	34 ± 6
Suramin	10^{-3}	<5	100	<10
SHAM	3×10^{-3}	<5	<5	<5

The figures represent the means and, where present, the standard deviations of at least three determinations. Data of Rogerson and Gutteridge, (1977a and in preparation).

presence of two terminal oxidases (Table 5). In contrast NADH oxidase activity is completely insensitive to all of these inhibitors, suggesting either that electrons from exogenously supplied NADH are fed exclusively into the cyanide-insensitive terminal oxidase or that a cytochrome-independent NADH oxidase or peroxidase activity may be present (Table 5). Caution must be exercised when these suggestions are being considered, however, since it must be remembered that the mitochondrial preparations used were damaged. SHAM does not inhibit either succinate- or NADH-stimulated oxidation to any detectable extent (i.e. inhibitions <5%) (Table 5), suggesting that the cyanide-insensitive terminal oxidase is not similar to that present in cyanide-insensitive plants.

The oxidation of α-glycerophosphate is cyanide and antimycin A sensitive, but not SHAM sensitive (Table 5), suggesting that it is a cytochrome-linked oxidation. It is, however, quite sensitive to inhibition by suramin, a known inhibitor of the α-glycerophosphate oxidase of the blood trypomastigote forms of the *T. brucei* subgroup trypanosomes (Bowman and Fairlamb, 1976). In this subgroup, the activity can be separated, using phenazine ethosulphate as an artificial electron acceptor, into dehydrogenase and oxidase components, the former being inhibited by suramin and the latter by SHAM (Bowman and Fairlamb, 1976). The activity in *T. cruzi* can be separated in the same way. We have thus been able to show that in this species, the dehydrogenase component is sensitive to suramin and the oxidase component is sensitive to cyanide (Fig. 2).

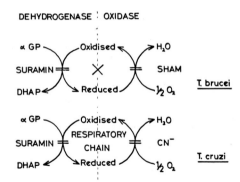

FIG. 2. Comparison between α-glycerophosphate oxidation in *T. brucei* and *T. cruzi*. Data of Rogerson and Gutteridge (1977a and in preparation).

Thus, in two quite separate species of *Trypanosoma* the dehydrogenase components of two distinct α-glycerophosphate oxidase activities are suramin sensitive. It is generally accepted that the *T. brucei* subgroup trypanosomes are more highly evolved than *T. cruzi*. Thus it can be envisaged that the cyanide-insensitive, SHAM-sensitive α-glycerophosphate oxidation of *T. brucei* has evolved from a cytochrome-linked, cyanide-sensitive, SHAM-insensitive oxidase by the retention of the suramin-sensitive dehydrogenase component and the evolution of a new oxidase component. This hypothesis is made more tenable by the recent demonstration that in *T. brucei*, α-glycerophosphate oxidase is a mitochondrial enzyme (Opperdoes and Borst, 1976).

3. Cytochrome studies

Some evidence has been presented for the existence of cytochromes in the culture epimastigote forms, but it is only recently that a systematic and rigorous study has been made of their distribution in the different forms of *T. cruzi*. Thus, in dithionite reduced versus H_2O_2 oxidized difference spectra, a shoulder at 605 nm has been taken as an indication of cytochrome $a + a_3$ and a broad peak at 560 nm as an indication of cytochrome b/c (Ryley, 1956). Cytochrome c_{558} has, however, been purified and characterized from culture epimastigote forms (Hill *et al.*, 1971). A CO-binding pigment, probably cytochrome o, has also been identified in these forms (Hill and Cross, 1973).

There are two basic problems in studying cytochromes in *T. cruzi* by difference spectroscopy. First, any haemin contamination of preparations will obscure the cytochrome peaks, especially those between 600 and 500 nm. Second, some of the absorbance peaks are so close that they cannot be differentiated in spectra run at room temperature. Recently, we have attempted to overcome these problems by culturing epimastigotes for one or two subcultures in the absence of haemin and by running the spectra of broken cell preparations at liquid nitrogen temperatures (Rogerson and Gutteridge, 1977b, and in preparation).

In dithionite reduced versus H_2O_2 oxidized spectra, a peak is then observed at 600 nm and a shoulder at 444 nm which are indicative of cytochrome $a + a_3$. A sharp peak at 558 nm indicates cytochrome b and a shoulder at 554 nm suggests the presence of cytochrome c (note that in low temperature studies, the absorbance peaks at low temperature will have shifted to the ultra-violet compared with those at room temperature). The presence of cytochromes b and c_{558} has been confirmed by the difference spectra of the pyridine haemochromes of the acid acetone extract prepared from broken cell preparations of culture epimastigotes.

In a CO difference spectrum, absorbance peaks at 568, 540 and 417 nm were detected, indicating the presence of a CO-binding pigment similar to cytochrome o. Similar spectra were obtained from active mitochondrial preparations, indicating that we were not simply measuring the spectrum of haemin, though the peaks were reduced by about 70%.

Thus, there is now good evidence for the presence of cytochromes c, b, $a + a_3$ and o in the culture epimastigote forms of *T. cruzi*. Similar studies on particularly well purified preparations of intracellular amastigotes and blood trypomastigotes have shown that the same cytochromes are present in these forms (Rogerson and Gutteridge, 1977b and in preparation) (see Fig. 3 for trypomastigote spectra). Thus, there is now evidence in all three main forms of *T. cruzi* from both spectral and inhibitor studies for a cytochrome-containing respiratory chain which func-

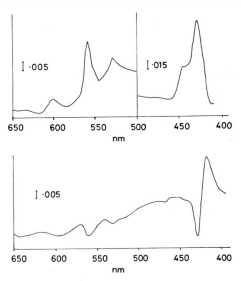

FIG. 3. Low temperature difference spectra of broken cell preparations of the blood trypomastigote forms of *T. cruzi*. Upper trace: dithionite v. H_2O_2; lower trace: dithionite CO v. dithionite. Data of Rogerson and Gutteridge (1977b).

tions in the oxidation of endogenously produced NADH and other electron carriers.

The exact composition of the respiratory chain in *T. cruzi* is not known but it now appears that it is similar to that of the culture forms of other trypanosomatids. It has been proposed by Ray and Cross (1972) that in such chains, cytochromes *b*, *c* and *a* + *a₃* are linked in that order and that there is a branch from this chain before cytochrome *c* involving cytochrome *o*. There is no real evidence for a branched chain rather than two parallel chains but it is clear that there are two terminal oxidases, a cyanide-sensitive cytochrome *a* + *a₃* and a cyanide- and SHAM-insensitive oxidase (possibly cytochrome *o*). Photochemical action spectra have demonstrated the functioning of cytochrome *o* in *Trypanosoma mega*, *Blastocrithidia culicis* and *Leishmania tarentolae* (Kronick and Hill, 1974). There is as yet no equivalent data for *T. cruzi* but all the information available so far suggests that the same situation exists in all three main forms of *T. cruzi*. Its most likely composition is shown in Fig. 4.

E. SYNTHESIS OF ATP

The exact sites of synthesis of ATP in *T. cruzi* are not clear though the evidence described above suggests that the same sites exist in all forms. Some ATP is likely to be generated by substrate level phosphorylations

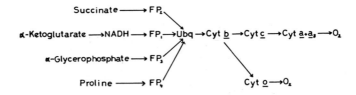

FIG. 4. Possible respiratory chain in *T. cruzi*. Data of Rogerson and Gutteridge (1977a, b).

during glycolysis. Most is likely to be formed during the passage of electrons down the respiratory chain by phosphorylation (De Satre and Stoppani, 1973; Stoppani and De Boiso, 1973). Some may also be formed during the synthesis of acetate and succinate but there is no experimental evidence for this as yet.

F. CONCLUSIONS

The overall picture of energy metabolism in *T. cruzi* which is beginning to emerge is summarized in Fig. 5 and Table 6. Note the similarity of this

Table 6. Comparison of the metabolic status of the different forms of *T. cruzi*.

Parameter	Mammalian forms		Culture epimastigote forms
	Amastigote	Trypomastigote	
Glycolysis	+	+	+
TCA cycle	+	+	+
L-*a*-glycerophosphate oxidation[a]	+	+	+
Proline oxidation	+	+	+
Cytochrome chain	+	+	+
Cyanide sensitivity	Partial	Partial	Partial
Mitochondria	Plate-like cristae	Plate-like cristae	Plate-like cristae
Growth temperature (°C)	37	37	28

[a] Cytochrome linked—see text.

metabolism to that of the culture forms of other trypanosomatids. In contrast to the situation in the *T. brucei* subgroup, no qualitative and few quantitative differences between the intracellular amastigotes, blood trypomastigotes and culture epimastigote forms have emerged (cf Table 1 and Table 6). Thus Brack's (1968) doubts about the absence of a mito-

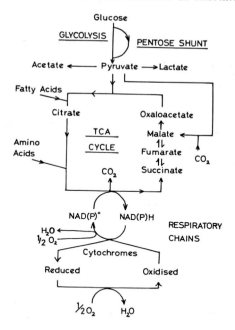

FIG. 5. Likely pathways for energy metabolism in *T. cruzi*. Reproduced from Fig. 3 of Gutteridge (1978).

chondrial cycle in *T. cruzi* appear to have been vindicated.

The only marked quantitative difference which has been found so far concerns the ability of the mammalian forms to catabolize fatty acids at a much greater rate than culture forms. Wood and Schiller (1975) have suggested that such results relate to the environments in which the different forms are found, mammalian forms infecting adipose and muscle tissues which are rich in fatty acids. Since the catabolism of fatty acids appears to be of no great importance in energy metabolism, this view is untenable. The difference, however, does provide us with a ready test to distinguish amastigotes and trypomastigotes from culture epimastigotes and indicates that the flagellated "amastigotes" which we isolate are quite different from the epimastigotes that we culture, even though they are more similar morphologically than we expected. In this connection it would be of interest to measure the rate at which the amastigotes which Pan (1976) can grow *in vitro* are able to catabolize palmitate.

V. Nucleic acid metabolism

A. PURINE METABOLISM

The first study in this area of metabolism was by Fernandes and Castellani (1958) who reported that culture epimastigote forms of *T. cruzi* did not incorporate ^{14}C-glycine into nucleic acid purines and were therefore judged to be unable to synthesize the purine ring *de novo* (see Fig. 6). A comparative study by microautoradiography of the ability of intracellular amastigotes *in situ* in tissue cells and extracellular trypomastigotes in tissue culture to utilize ^{14}C-adenine and ^{14}C-glycine was subsequently carried out by Yoneda (1971). He found substantial incorporation of ^{14}C-glycine by intracellular forms, but not by extracellular forms and therefore concluded that the former synthesized purines *de novo* and the latter salvaged them from preformed purines such as adenine. Some support for these conclusions came later from the studies of Fernandes and Kimura (1973). Thus, it appeared possible that *T. cruzi* is one of two exceptions to the general rule that parasitic protozoa appear unable to synthesize the purine ring *de novo* (Jaffe and Gutteridge, 1974; Gutteridge and Coombs, 1977). The other exception is *Crithidia oncopelti*, which probably contains endosymbiotic bacteria, and therefore is a special case (Gutteridge and Coombs, 1977). Since, in Yoneda's experi-

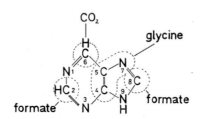

FIG. 6.   Sources of some of the atoms of the purine ring when synthesized *de novo*.

ments, the possibility was not excluded that the ^{14}C-glycine was biosynthesized into purine by the host tissue cell before it was taken up by the parasite, the ability of *T. cruzi* to synthesize purines *de novo* clearly required re-examination.

A detailed study of the ability of washed cell suspensions of isolated intracellular amastigote, blood trypomastigote and culture epimastigote forms to utilize ^{14}C-glycine, ^{14}C-formate and ^{14}C-bicarbonate for nucleic acid synthesis in the absence of added purines has therefore been carried out (Gutteridge and Gaborak, 1979). No radioactivity from any of these precursors has been detected in the nucleic acid purines of intracellular amastigote or culture epimastigote forms. Some radioactivity has, however, been found from ^{14}C-formate but *not* ^{14}C-glycine in the nucleic acid purines of blood trypomastigotes (Fig. 7). It is not clear yet whether

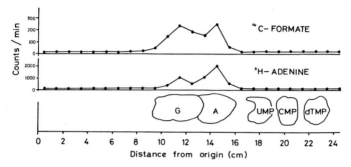

FIG. 7. Distribution along a paper chromatogram (solvent: *iso*propanol/HCl) of radioactivity from the 1*N* HCl hydrolysed nucleic acid fraction of blood trypomastigote forms of *T. cruzi* incubated with either ^{14}C-formate or ^{3}H-adenine.

this incorporation represents more than a minimal amount of synthesis of no great significance, and the possibility that the formate incorporation results from an exchange reaction between formate and the purine ring at carbon 2 (see Fig. 6) has not been excluded. The balance of the evidence at the moment thus favours the view that no form of *T. cruzi* can synthesize *de novo* substantial amounts of nucleic acid purines and that therefore the organism is probably not an exception to the general rule that parasitic protozoa are unable to carry out these reactions.

Absence of purine synthesis *de novo* implies dependence on the host for preformed purine and in keeping with this, there is now evidence for salvage of a range of purine bases and nucleosides by all three major forms of *T. cruzi* (see Fig. 8). There seems to be some preference for free bases rather than nucleosides; there is no direct nucleotide utilization as has been reported to occur in African trypanosomes (Sanchez *et al.*, 1976). Calculations based on the amount of adenine incorporation by culture epimastigote forms in defined media in the presence of radiotracers of known specific activity have indicated that virtually all the purine used in nucleic acid synthesis is derived from the exogenous source (Gutteridge and Gaborak, 1979). The results of these calculations are thus in agreement with conclusions reached in the previous paragraph about the lack of *de novo* purine biosynthesis.

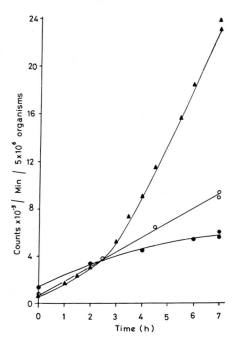

FIG. 8.   Time courses of the incorporation of ^{3}H-adenine (5 μCi/ml and 8 × 10^{-5}M) into the three forms of *T. cruzi*. Key: ▲——▲, culture epimastigote forms; ○——○, blood trypomastigote forms; ●——●, intracellular amastigote forms. Note that no allowance has been made for the greater mass of the culture epimastigote forms. Data of Gutteridge *et al.*, 1978.

The enzymes involved in the utilization of purines and their subsequent interconversion have not been investigated in any form, though the experiments in our own laboratory with ^{14}C-adenine and ^{14}C-guanine have indicated that in all forms, adenine can be converted into guanine and guanine into adenine (Gutteridge and Gaborak, 1979).

B. PYRIMIDINE METABOLISM

A number of investigators have examined the question of the ability of *T. cruzi* to synthesize pyrimidines *de novo* (especially Rey and Fernandes, 1962; Yoneda *et al.*, 1974). All have done this by comparing the utilization of ^{14}C-orotate (as a measure of *de novo* synthesis—see Fig. 9) with that of ^{14}C-uridine. All have reached the conclusion that since ^{14}C-orotate is not well incorporated, pyrimidines in *T. cruzi* are obtained preferentially in all forms by salvage. As with the conclusion about purine synthesis, such an inference is surprising since all the other parasitic protozoa examined to date appear able to synthesize at least some part of their pyrimidine requirement (Jaffe and Gutteridge, 1974; Gutteridge and Coombs, 1977). Since there are clear indications in the literature that malaria parasites, which are unable to salvage pyrimidines, also utilize orotate poorly (Gutteridge and Trigg, 1970), such a conclusion is untenable. Thus the question of the ability of *T. cruzi* to synthesize pyrimidines *de novo* needed re-examination.

It is now clear that whereas orotate is poorly utilized *in vitro* by washed cell suspensions of isolated intracellular amastigotes, blood trypomastigotes and culture epimastigotes even in the absence of added pyrimidines, ^{14}C-bicarbonate is readily incorporated. Calculations based on the amount of the incorporation indicate that it represents a substantial amount of the total pyrimidine being utilized in nucleic acid synthesis and that therefore it is wrong to conclude that *T. cruzi* cannot synthesize the pyrimidine ring (Gutteridge and Gaborak, 1979).

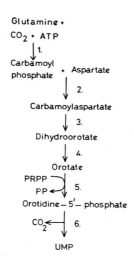

FIG. 9.   Pathway for the synthesis of UMP *de novo*. Enzymes: 1. Carbamoyl phosphate synthetase; 2. aspartate carbamoyl transferase; 3. dihydroorotase; 4. dihydydroorotate dehydrogenase/dihydroorotate hydroxylase (mammal/*T. cruzi* respectively); 5. orotidine-5′-phosphate pyrophosphorylase; 6. orotidine-5′-phosphate decarboxylase. PRPP, phosphoribosylpyrophosphate.

In keeping with this conclusion, dihydroorotate hydroxylase, a key enzyme in the pyrimidine biosynthetic pathway *de novo* (see Fig. 9), has been shown to be present in all forms of *T. cruzi* at similar specific activities (Table 7) (Gutteridge *et al.*, 1979). Calculations based on these

Table 7. Dihydroorotate hydroxylase activity in *T. cruzi*.

Enzyme	n moles orotate/min/mg protein[a]
Culture	0·75 ± 0·17 (4)
Blood	0·67 ± 0·18 (4)
Intracellular	0·47 ± 0·15 (3)
C. fasciculata	0·90 ± 0·17 (4)

[a] Mean, standard deviation and number of determinations. Data of Gutteridge *et al.* (1979).

specific activities have indicated that they are about sufficient to explain the growth rate of the organism, though they are certainly not present in excess. This, however, is not surprising since there is good evidence that the enzyme is a regulatory point of the pathway (it is regulated by orotate, its product) and would therefore not be expected to be present in excess amounts. The mechanism of the reaction appears to be the same in all three forms of *T. cruzi*: it involves the hydroxylation of the 5-position of dihydroorotate to form an unstable intermediate which breaks down to form orotate and water. None of the other enzymes in the *de novo* pyrimidine biosynthetic pathway have yet been investigated.

Ability to synthesize pyrimidines *de novo* does not always imply, as in malaria, a lack of ability to salvage them. Indeed, mention has already been made of the ability of all forms of the parasite to salvage uridine. A quantitative study of the salvage of pyrimidines by all three forms of *T. cruzi* has confirmed these earlier conclusions (Gutteridge and Gaborak, 1979). Thus, of a range of pyrimidines tested, all were utilized to a significant extent (see Fig. 10) and calculations based on the rates of incorporation indicated that a high proportion of the pyrimidines used in nucleic acid synthesis were coming from the exogenous source. One exception to the general result was with ^{3}H-thymidine which was apparently not used by blood trypomastigotes to any great extent, suggesting that these forms do not synthesize much DNA.

Details of the pathways involved in pyrimidine salvage have not been investigated in any form. Pyrimidines have been shown to be interconvertible but the regulation of the balance between synthesis and salvage also remains to be investigated.

C. DEOXYRIBONUCLEOTIDE METABOLISM

The synthesis of deoxyribonucleotides has not been studied so far in

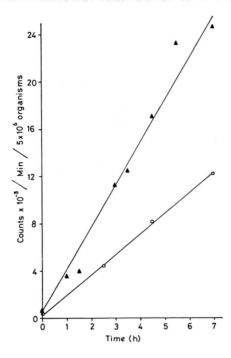

FIG. 10. Time courses of the incorporation of ^{3}H-uracil (5μCi/ml, 8×10^{-5}M) into two forms of *T. cruzi*. Key: ▲——▲, culture epimastigote forms; ○——○, blood trypomastigote forms. Note that no allowance has been made for the greater mass of the culture epimastigote forms.

any form of *T. cruzi*, though it is generally considered likely that it is carried out at the ribonucleoside diphosphate level (Gutteridge and Coombs, 1977). The synthesis of deoxythymidylate (dTMP) has, however, been investigated. In most cells, this methylation is carried out at the nucleoside monophosphate level and involves the conversion of deoxyuridylate (dUMP) to dTMP by the enzyme thymidylate synthase. This enzyme requires N^5, N^{10}-methylenetetrahydrofolate as cofactor, which, in the course of the reaction, is converted to dihydrofolate. It is reformed by the enzyme dihydrofolate reductase and recharged with an active one carbon transfer group by one of a number of possible methyltransferase enzymes.

Two key enzymes of the thymidylate synthase cycle, thymidylate synthase (Al Chalabi, 1975; Al Chalabi and Gutteridge, 1977a) and dihydro-

Table 8. Thymidylate synthase and dihydrofolate reductase activities in *T. cruzi*.

	Specific activities[a]		
Enzyme	Culture	Blood	Intracellular
Thymidylate synthase	1·56 ± 0·16	1·19 ± 0·04	0·35 ± 0·05
Dihydrofolate reductase	150 ± 12	30 ± 10	120 ± 15

[a] ll n moles of product/min/mg protein. Mean and standard deviations of at least 4 determinations. Data of Al Chalabi and Gutteridge (1977a) and Gutteridge *et al.* (1969)·

folate reductase (Gutteridge *et al.*, 1969), have been shown to be present in all three forms of *T. cruzi* (Table 8) and to have similar properties. In addition, experiments on the incorporation of ^{14}C-formate by washed cell suspensions of culture epimastigote forms have shown that radioactivity is incorporated into thymine residues of DNA (Gutteridge and Gaborak, 1979). It seems, therefore, that the thymidylate synthase cycle is present in all three forms of *T. cruzi*, though the natural donor of the active one carbon transfer groups is not known. There is as yet no information as to whether the cofactor tetrahydrofolate is derived from folate or synthesized *de novo* from GTP, *p*-aminobenzoic acid and glutamate.

Besides synthesis *de novo* from dUMP, culture epimastigote forms can also salvage thymidine, but not thymine (Gutteridge and Gaborak, 1979). At low concentrations, it is likely that the salvage of thymidine will be limited since the organism contains a high level of thymidine phosphorylase which will rapidly degrade it to thymine (see Section IV, G). There appears to be relatively little salvage of thymidine by blood trypomastigotes (Gutteridge and Gaborak, 1979). Lack of utilization here probably relates to a lack of DNA synthesis.

D. NUCLEIC ACID SYNTHESIS

The ability of isolated preparations of all forms of *T. cruzi* to incorporate purines and pyrimidines or their precursors into nucleic acids implies that DNA and RNA polymerase activities are present in all forms. However, although some preliminary work has been done on the isolation of the enzymes from culture epimastigote forms (Sims, 1976, Sims and Gutteridge, 1979) they have yet to be characterized and studied in detail.

E. DNA, ESPECIALLY KINETOPLAST DNA

There are about 0·17 pg of DNA per cell in the culture epimastigote forms of *T. cruzi*; culture trypomastigote forms contain slightly higher amounts (Stohlman *et al.*, 1973). Ultracentrifugation in isopycnic CsCl gradients has indicated the presence in intracellular amastigote, blood trypomastigote and culture epimastigote forms of two DNA components, a nuclear component of density 1·710 g/ml ($\sim$ 51% G + C) and a kineto-plast component of 1·689–1·699 g/ml ($\sim$ 40% G + C) (Table 9) (Riou

Table 9. Properties of kinetoplast DNA in *T. cruzi*.

	Nuclear DNA		Kinetoplast DNA	
	Density[a]	Proportion[b]	Density[a]	Proportion[b]
Culture	1·710	80	1·699	20
Blood	1·710	63	1·698	37
Intracellular	1·710	75	1·698	25

[a] g/ml. [b] % of total DNA, derived from densitometer tracings. Data of Riou and Gutteridge (1973) and in preparation.

and Gutteridge, 1978). There appears to be more kinetoplast DNA in the blood trypomastigote forms than in the other stages (Table 9), thus explaining the higher DNA content of these cells. This greater quantity of kinetoplast DNA in the blood trypomastigotes has been related to differences in the appearance in thin section electron micrographs of the kinetoplast of this form compared with the other stages. In intracellular amastigotes and culture epimastigotes, the kinetoplast DNA appears as a double row of regular and well-defined electron dense material, whereas in the blood trypomastigote form, it has a more open, basket-like arrangement and is organized in three or four double-layered rows (Brack, 1968; Meyer, 1968; Rio and Gutteridge, 1978; Vickerman and Preston, 1976).

The kinetoplast DNA in all forms bands rapidly in CsCl gradients, indicating that it is in the form of networks. Each is the equivalent of all the DNA from one kinetoplast (Riou and Gutteridge, 1973). Measurements made of the sedimentation coefficients of the networks from blood trypomastigote and culture epimastigote forms yielded similar values ($\sim$ 5200 S), suggesting that the kinetoplast DNA in the blood trypomastigote forms is composed of an association of two networks rather than of a single large network (Riou and Gutteridge, 1979).

The networks from all forms appear to be composed of a mass of interlocking minicircles of 0·45 μm contour length and what have been described as long linear pieces of DNA, 2–12 μm in length. There is evidence that the minicircles are heterogeneous in both size and base sequence. In intact networks the linear pieces are probably maxicircles and represent the true mitochondrial DNA (Riou and Gutteridge, 1978). The main differences noted between the networks of the different forms were: dimeric and oligomeric circles were present in the kinetoplast DNA of the blood trypomastigote and intracellular amastigote forms in much greater proportion than in the culture epimastigote forms; minicircles in replication were seen only in the blood trypomastigote forms; there were some differences, mainly quantitative, in the gel electrophoretic patterns after endonuclear digestion. No explanation can yet be given for these differences.

No detailed studies have yet been made in any form of *T. cruzi* of either the replication of the kinetoplast DNA networks or the transcription of any genetic information that they might contain.

F. RNA

Ribosomal RNA has been isolated from culture epimastigote forms of *T. cruzi* (Tanowitz *et al.*, 1975) but no comparative study with the other forms of the organism have been carried out. Messenger and transfer RNA species, which are presumably present, have not been investigated in any form.

G. NUCLEIC ACID CATABOLISM

Lysosomes are present in all forms of *T. cruzi* (Vickerman and Preston, 1976) and it is likely that these contain a range of degradative enzymes, including nucleases. Some of these lysosomal enzymes have recently been characterized in culture epimastigote forms, including a very active deoxyribonuclease (Van Hoof *et al.*, 1977). In addition, it has been shown that all forms of *T. cruzi* contain thymidylate phosphatase and thymidine phosphorylase activities (Table 10) and that these two enzymes can function, at least in the culture epimastigote forms, in a catabolic pathway which degrades dTMP to thymine which is then excreted (Al Chalabi, 1975; Al Chalabi and Gutteridge, 1977b).

H. CONCLUSIONS

It is thus apparent that as far as nucleic acid metabolism is concerned, there is a high degree of uniformity in intracellular amastigote, blood trypomastigote and culture epimastigote forms. Of the few differences found, most can be related in the trypomastigotes to a lack of cell

Table 10. Thymidylate phosphatase and thymidine phosphorylase activities in *T. cruzi*.

	Specific activities[a]		
Enzyme	Culture	Blood	Intracellular
Thymidylate phosphatase	29·0 ± 2·2	23·4 ± 1·2	18·2 ± 1·1
Thymidine phosphorylase	29·3 ± 3·3	10·6 ± 0·7	2·3 ± 0·1

[a] All n moles of product/min/mg protein. Mean and standard deviation of at least three determinations. Data of Al Chalabi and Gutteridge (1977b).

division (e.g. lack of utilization of ^{3}H-thymidine and arrangement of kinetoplast DNA).

VI. Discussion and Conclusions

It is clear from this review that although there are marked morphological differences between intracellular amastigote, blood trypomastigote and culture epimastigote forms of *T. cruzi*, no qualitative and a minimal number of quantitative differences appear to be associated with these changes. It must be stressed that at present this conclusion can only be regarded as tentative since there is still much to be done before a complete understanding of energy metabolism and nucleic acid metabolism in the different forms of *T. cruzi* is reached and a start has yet to be made on protein and lipid biosynthesis. However, the major changes seen in the *T. brucei* subgroup trypanosomes relate to energy metabolism and, as Table 6 indicates, enough has now been done in *T. cruzi* to exclude the possible existence of changes of this order of magnitude. There are also changes in lipid content between the different forms of *T. brucei* subgroup trypanosomes. These appear to be less marked than the changes in energy metabolism and in part relate to the alternate development and regression of the mitochondrial network during the life cycle. Since the state of the mitochondrion does not change in *T. cruzi* to this extent, it is unlikely that changes in this species will be so marked. However, since the lipid content of protozoa seems in part to be a function of what is present in its environment (Gutteridge and Coombs, 1977), it is unlikely that there will be no changes.

If it is accepted that there are no major biochemical differences between the three main forms of *T. cruzi*, three important deductions can be made. First, there are unlikely to be biochemical differences between these main forms and intracellular epimastigotes and trypomastigotes and insect amastigotes, sphaeromastigotes and metacyclic trypomastigotes.

Second, pleomorphism in the blood trypomastigote forms is unlikely to be linked with biochemical changes. Third, though caution should still be exercised, the probability is that studies with culture epimastigote forms are pertinent to the situation in intracellular amastigotes and blood trypomastigotes. This last conclusion is particularly important since it means that biochemists need now hesitate less about using culture forms in studies of *T. cruzi* if they do not have facilities available to isolate blood and intracellular stages. It is to be hoped that this will in turn encourage more biochemists to work in this field and produce information required to develop drugs for Chagas' disease on a more rational basis than has been possible hitherto.

The apparent lack of correlation between biochemistry and morphology in *T. cruzi* seems to suggest that, in contrast to the situation in *T. brucei* subgroup trypanosomes, there is also a lack of correlation between biochemistry and the environment. We would argue that this is not so. It is undoubtedly true that *T. cruzi*, in contrast to *T. brucei*, does not adapt to each environment by repressing those parts of its metabolic machinery which are not required in that environment. However, we suggest that instead, it adapts to its different environments by having available at all times the metabolic machinery that it requires in each of them.

The apparent lack of biochemical differences between intracellular and blood stages of *T. cruzi* implies that the evolution to an intracellular form of development in the mammal is not associated with any major loss of autonomy by the parasite as is seen in its extreme form in viruses. It would seem most likely that the move to an intracellular environment should be regarded as a mechanism to escape, at least in part, the immunological reaction of the host.

The apparent lack of correlation between morphology and biochemistry raises the question as to the significance of the morphological changes which occur. These seem to correlate with the physical nature of the environments in which the different stages are found. Thus, the intracellular forms which would gain little advantage from being motile, are found as amastigotes with reduced flagella. The trypomastigote forms must survive in the blood and also seek new host cells. They are presumably adapted for this purpose. The epimastigote forms must retain their position in the gut of the insect vector. They seem to use their long anterior flagella to anchor themselves to the gut wall (Zeledon, 1978).

The marked contrast in the results reported here for *T. cruzi* and those detailed in the literature for the *T. brucei* subgroup trypanosomes raises the question as to the situation in other members of the Kinetoplastida. The blood forms of *Trypanosoma congolense* and *Trypanosoma vivax* have mitochondria with tubular cristae (Vickerman and Preston, 1976) and metabolize glucose beyond pyruvate (Bowman and Flynn, 1976), suggesting that any biochemical changes seen will be less marked than those in *T. brucei* (Trigg and Gutteridge, 1977). In *Trypanosoma lewisi*, both blood trypomastigote and culture epimastigote forms possess mitochondria with plate-like cristae (Vickerman and Preston, 1976) and there is bio-chemical evidence for a functioning TCA cycle and a cyanide-sensitive respiratory chain (Bowman and Flynn, 1976). This suggests that, as in *T. cruzi*, few biochemical changes will occur during its life cycle (Trigg and Gutteridge, 1977). The situation in *Leishmania* is probably similar. Both amastigotes from the mammal and promastigotes in culture have mitochondria with plate-like cristae but it has been suggested that the mitochondrial mass and number of cristae increase with the change from amastigote to promastigote (see Vickerman and Preston, 1976). However, this has been questioned recently by Brun and Krassner (1976) who have reported that the *relative* mass decreases and the relative number of cristae remains constant. Respiration in both forms is at least partially cyanide sensitive. Thus it would seem that the biochemical changes which occur during the life cycles of other members of the Kineto-plastida are much less dramatic than those seen in the *T. brucei* sub-group. It is the situation in *Leishmania* and stercorarian trypanosomes which is the normal; that in salivarian trypanosomes is the unusual.

VII. Acknowledgements

Much of the work discussed in this article was carried out in the Bio-logical Laboratory of the University of Kent. Some of this was done in collaboration with Kausi Al Chalabi, Bryan Cover, Dilip Dave, Maria Gaborak and Paul Sims, all of whom we thank for many helpful dis-cussions. Financial support was provided in part by grants from the Ministry of Overseas Development, London, the World Health Organiza-tion, Geneva and the Wellcome Research Laboratories, Beckenham, Kent. One of us (G.W.R.) was in receipt of a Research Studentship from the Medical Research Council, London.

VIII. References

Al Chalabi, K. (1975). Thymine nucleotide metabolism in the *Trypanosomatidae*. Ph.D. Thesis. University of Kent.

Al Chalabi, K. and Gutteridge, W. E. (1977a). Presence and properties of thymidy-late synthase in trypanosomatids. *Biochimica Biophysica Acta*, **481**, 71–79.

Al Chalabi, K. and Gutteridge, W. E. (1977b). Catabolism of deoxythymidylate in some trypanosomatids. *Parasitology*, **74**, 299–312.

Bash-Lewinson, D. and Grossowicz, N. (1957). Transaminases of *Trypanosoma cruzi*. *Bulletin of the Research Council of Israel*, **6E**, 91–92.

Boné, G. J. and Parent, G. (1963). Stearic acid, an essential growth factor for *Trypanosoma cruzi*. *Journal of General Microbiology*, **31**, 261–266.

Bowman, I. B. R. (1974). Intermediary metabolism of pathogenic flagellates. *In:* "Trypanosomiasis and Leishmaniasis with Special Reference to Chagas'

Disease", pp. 255–271. Ciba Foundation Symposium 20 (New Series). Associated Scientific Publishers, Amsterdam.

Bowman, I. B. R. and Fairlamb, A. H. (1976). L-Glycerol-3-phosphate oxidase in *Trypanosoma brucei* and the effect of suramin. *In:* "Biochemistry of Parasites and Host-Parasite Relationships" (H. van den Bossche, ed.), pp. 501–507. Elsevier North-Holland Biomedical Press, Amsterdam.

Bowman, I. B. R. and Flynn, I. W. (1976). Oxidative metabolism of trypanosomes. *In:* "Biology of the Kinetoplastida" (W. H. R. Lumsden and D. A. Evans, eds), Vol. 1, pp. 435–476. Academic Press, New York.

Bowman, I. B. R., Tobie, E. J. and Von Brand, T. (1963). CO_2 fixation studies with the culture forms of *Trypanosoma cruzi*. *Comparative Biochemistry and Physiology*, 9, 105–114.

Bowman, I. B. R., Srivastava, H. K. and Flynn, I. W. (1972). Adaptations in oxidative metabolism during the transformation of *Trypanosoma rhodesiense* from bloodstream into culture form. *In:* "Comparative Biochemistry of Parasites" (H. Van den Bossche, ed.), pp. 329–342. Academic Press, New York.

Brack, C. (1968). Elektronenmikroskopische untersuchungen zum lebenszyklus von *Trypanosoma cruzi*. Unter besonderer berücksichtigung der entwicklungsformen im veberträger. *Rhodnius prolixus*. *Acta Tropica*, 25, 289–356.

Brener, Z. (1969). The behaviour of slender and stout forms of *Trypanosoma cruzi* in the bloodstream of normal and immune mice. *Annals of Tropical Medicine and Parasitology*, 63, 215–220.

Brener, Z. (1973). Biology of *Trypanosoma cruzi*. *Annual Review of Microbiology*, 27, 347–382.

Brener, Z. (1976). Significance of morphological variation of bloodstream forms. *In:* "American Trypanosomiasis Research", Scientific Publication Number 318, pp. 127–131. Pan American Health Organization, Washington.

Brener, Z. and Alvarenga, N. J. (1976). Life cycle of *T. cruzi* in the vector. *In:* "American Trypanosomiasis Research", Scientific Publication Number 318, pp. 83–86. Pan American Health Organization, Washington.

Brener, Z. and Chiari, E. (1963). Variações morfologicas observadas em differentes amostras de *Trypanosoma cruzi*. *Revista do Instituto de Medicina Tropical de São Paulo*, 5, 220–224.

Brown, R. C., Evans, D. A. and Vickerman, K. (1973). Changes in oxidative metabolism and ultrastructure accompanying differentiation of the mitochondrion in *Trypanosoma brucei*. *International Journal of Parasitology*, 3, 691–704.

Brun, R. and Krassner, S. M. (1976). Quantitative ultrastructural investigations of mitochondrial development in *Leishmania donovani* during transformation. *Journal of Protozoology*, 23, 493–497.

Cazzulo, J. J., Juan, S. M. and Segura, E. L. (1977). Glutamate dehydrogenase and aspartate aminotransferase in *Trypanosoma cruzi*. *Comparative Biochemistry and Physiology*, 56B, 301–303.

Chagas, C. (1909). Nova tripanosomiase human. Estudos sôbre a morphologia eo ciclo evolutivo do *Schizotrypanum cruzi* n. gen. n. sp., ajente etiolojico de nova entidade morbida do homen. *Mem Inst Oswaldo Cruz*, 1, 159–218.

Chang, S. L. (1948). Studies on haemoflagellates. IV. Observations concerning some biochemical activities in culture and respiration of three species of leishmania and *Trypanosoma cruzi*. *Journal of Infectious Diseases*, 82, 109–118.

Cover, B. and Gutteridge, W. E. (1978). The course of infection of *Trypanosoma cruzi* in γ-irradiated rats. *Transactions of the Royal Society of Tropical Medicine and Hygiene*, 72, 596–601.

Cross, G. A., Klein, R. A. and Baker, J. R. (1975). *Trypanosoma cruzi* growth amino acid utilisation and drug action in a defined medium. *Annals of Tropical Medicine and Parasitology*, 69, 513–519.

De Boiso, J. F. and Stoppani, A. O. M. (1973). The mechanism of acetate and pyruvate oxidation by *Trypanosoma cruzi*. *Journal of Protozoology*, **20**, 673–678.

De Satre, M. B. R. and Stoppani, A. O. M. (1973) Demonstration of a Mg^{2+}-activated adenosine triphosphatase in *Trypanosoma cruzi*. *FEBS Letters*, **31**, 137–142.

Dvorak, J. A. (1976). New *in vitro* approach to quantitation of *Trypanosoma cruzi* —vertebrate cell interaction. *In:* "American Trypanosomiosis Research", Scientific Publication Number 318, pp. 109–120. Pan American Health Organization, Washington.

Evans, D. A. and Brown, R. C. (1972). The utilization of glucose and proline by culture forms of *Trypanosoma brucei*. *Journal of Protozoology*, **19**, 686–690.

Fernandes, J. F. and Castellani, O. (1958). Nucleotide and polynucleotide synthesis in *Trypanosoma cruzi*. I. Precursors of purine compounds. *Experimental Parasitology*, **7**, 224–235.

Fernandes, J. F. and Kimura, E. (1973). Biosynthesis of purines and pyrimidines by different forms of *Trypanosoma cruzi*. *In:* "Progress in Protozoology", p. 137. 4th International Congress on Protozoology. Clermont Ferrand.

Gutteridge, W. E. (1976a). Biochemistry of *Trypanosoma cruzi*. *In:* "American Trypanosomiasis Research", Scientific Publication Number 318, pp. 135–140. Pan American Health Organization, Washington.

Gutteridge, W. E. (1976b). Isolation of blood and intracellular forms of *Trypanosoma cruzi* and comparative aspects of nucleic acid metabolism. *In:* "Biochemistry of Parasites and Host-Parasite Relationships" (H. Van den Bossche, ed.), pp. 245–252. Elsevier, North Holland Biomedical Press, Amsterdam.

Gutteridge, W. E. (1978). Biochemical studies of intracellular blood and culture forms of *Trypanosoma cruzi*: possible targets in rational chemotherapy. *In:* "Chagas Disease", Scientific Publication No. 347, pp. 48–58. Pan American Health Organization, Washington.

Gutteridge, W. E. and Coombs, G. H. (1977). Biochemistry of Parasitic Protozoa. The Macmillan Press Ltd., London.

Gutteridge, W. E. and Gaborak, A. M. (1979). A re-examination of purine and pyrimidine synthesis in the three main forms of *Trypanosoma cruzi*. International Journal of Biochemistry. (In press)

Gutteridge, W. E. and Trigg, P. I. (1970). Incorporation of radioactive precursors into DNA and RNA of *Plasmodium knowlesi in vitro*. *Journal of Protozoology*, **17**, 89–96.

Gutteridge, W. E., Knowler, J. and Coombs, J. D. (1969). Growth of *Trypanosoma cruzi* in human heart tissue cells and effects of aminonucleoside of puromycin, trypacidin and aminopterin. *Journal of Protozoology*, **21**, 512–517.

Gutteridge, W. E., Cover, B. and Gaborak, M. (1978). Isolation of blood and intracellular forms of *Trypanosoma cruzi* from rats and other rodents and preliminary studies of their metabolism. *Parasitology*, **76**, 159–176.

Gutteridge, W. E., Dave, O. and Richards, W. H. G. (1979). Conversion of dihydroorotate to orotate in parasitic protozoa. *Biochimica et Biophysica Acta*. (In press)

Henry, M. and Nyns, E. (1975). Cyanide insensitive respiration. An alternative mitochondrial pathway. *Subcellular Biochemistry*, **4**, 1–65.

Hill, G. C. and Cross, G. A. M. (1973). Cyanide-resistant respiration and a branched cytochrome system in *Kinetoplastidae*. *Biochimica et Biophysica Acta*, **305**, 590–596.

Hill, G. C., Gutteridge, W. E. and Mathewson, N. W. (1971). Purification and properties of cytochrome *c* from trypanosomatids. *Biochimica et Biophysica Acta*, **243**, 225–229.

Hoare, C. A. (1970). Systematic description of the mammalian trypanosomes of

Africa. *In:* "The African Trypanosomiases" (H. W. Mulligan, ed,), pp. 25–59. Allen and Unwin, London.

Hoare, C. A. (1972). The Trypanosomes of Mammals. A Zoological Monograph. Blackwell Scientific Publications, Oxford.

Howells, R. E. and Chiari, C. A. (1975). Observations on two strains of *Trypanosoma cruzi* in laboratory mice. *Annals of Tropical Medicine and Parasitology,* **69**, 435–448.

Jaffe, J. J. and Gutteridge, W. E. (1974). Purine and pyrimidine metabolism in protozoa. *Actualités Protozoologiques,* **1**, 23–35.

Kallinikova, V. D. (1968a). Cytochemical study of enzymes of the respiratory chain in the life cycle of *Trypanosoma cruzi* Chagas, 1909. I. Enzymes of the respiratory chain at all stages of the life cycle in vivo and in culture. *Acta Protozoologica,* **5**, 395–403.

Kallinikova, V. D. (1968b). Cytochemical study of enzymes of the respiratory chain in the life cycle of *Trypanosoma cruzi* Chagas, 1909. II. Respiratory enzymes of the crithidial forms in the course of cultivation and some observations on the growth of the culture. *Acta Protozoologica,* **6**, 87–96.

Kronick, P. and Hill, G. C. (1974). Evidence for the functioning of cytochrome *o* in Kinetoplastida. *Biochimica et Biophysica Acta,* **368**, 173–180.

Lumsden, W. H. R. (1974). Leishmaniasis and Trypanosomiasis: the causative agents compared and contrasted. *In:* "Trypanosomiasis and Leishmaniasis with Special Reference to Chagas' Disease", pp. 3–27. Ciba Foundation Symposium Number 20 (New Series), Associated Scientific Publishers, Amsterdam.

Mancilla, R. and Naquira, C. (1964). Comparative metabolism of ^{14}C glucose in two strains of *Trypanosoma cruzi. Journal of Protozoology,* **11**, 509–513.

Maria, T. A., Tafuri, W. and Brener, Z. (1972). The fine structure of different bloodstream forms of *Trypanosoma cruzi. Annals of Tropical Medicine and Parasitology,* **66**, 423–431.

Meyer, H. (1968). The fine structure of the flagellum and kinetoplast chondriome of *Trypanosoma (Schizotrypanum) cruzi* in tissue culture. *Journal of Protozoology,* **15**, 614–621.

Meyer, H. and de Souza, W. (1976). Electron microscopic study of *Trypanosoma cruzi* periplast in tissue cultures. I. Number and arrangement of the peripheral microtubules in the various forms of the parasite's life cycle. *Journal of Protozoology,* **23**, 385–390.

Miller, P. G. G., Linstead, D. J. and Klein, R. A. (1976). Routes for the synthesis and utilization of acetyl CoA in trypanosomatid flagellates. *Parasitology,* **73**, xvi.

Newton, B. A., Cross, G. A. M. and Baker, J. (1973). Differentiation in the Trypanosomatidae. *In:* "Microbial Differentiation" (J. M. Ashworth and J. E. Smith, eds.), pp. 339–374. Cambridge University Press, London.

Opperdoes, F. R. and Borst, P. (1976). The effect of salicylhydroxamic acid on the glycerol-3-phosphate oxidase(GPO) of *Trypanosoma brucei*: Its influence on a *T. brucei* model infection and the intracellular location of GPO. *In* "Biochemistry of Parasites and Host-Parasite relationships" (H. Van den Bossche), ed., pp. 509–517. Elsevier, North-Holland Biomedical Press, Amsterdam.

Pan, S. C. (1976). *In vitro* cultivation of amastigotes of *Trypanosoma cruzi* in cell-free media. *In:* "American Trypanosomiasis Research", Scientific Publications Number 318, pp, 121–126. Pan American Health Organization, Washington.

Raw, I. (1959). Some aspects of carbohydrate metabolism of cultural forms of *Trypanosoma cruzi. Revista do Instituto de Medicina Tropical de São Paulo,* **1**, 192–194.

Ray, S. K. and Cross, G. A. M. (1972). Branched electron transport in *Trypanosoma mega*. *Nature (New Biology)*, London, **237**, 174–175.

Rey, L. and Fernandes, J. F. (1962). Nucleotide and polynucleotide synthesis in *Trypanosoma cruzi*. VII. Precursors of the pyrimidine nucleotide. *Experimental Parasitology*, **12**, 55–60.

Riou, G. and Gutteridge, W. E. (1973). Comparative study of kinetoplast DNA in culture, blood and intracellular forms of *Trypanosoma cruzi*. *Biochemie*, **60**, 365–379.

Rogerson, G. W. and Gutteridge, W. E. (1976). Enzymes of energy metabolism in the culture, blood and intracellular forms of *Trypanosoma cruzi*. *Parasitology*, **73**, xv.

Rogerson, G. W. and Gutteridge, W. E. (1977a). The action of respiratory inhibitors on the culture epimastigote, blood trypomastigote and intracellular amastigotes of *Trypanosoma cruzi*. *Parasitology*, **75**, xxvii.

Rogerson, G. W. and Gutteridge, W. E. (1977b). Cytochromes in the various stages of *Trypanosoma cruzi*. *Journal of Protozoology*, **24**, 42A.

Rogerson, G. W. and Gutteridge, W. E. (1978). Aspects of energy metabolism in *Trypanosoma cruzi*. *Parasitology*, **77**, xi.

Ryley, J. F. (1956). Studies on the metabolism of the protozoa. Comparative carbohydrate metabolism of eleven species of trypanosome. *Biochemical Journal*, **62**, 215–222.

Sanabria, A. (1966). Ultrastructure of *Trypanosome cruzi* in the rectum of *Rhodnius prolixus*. *Experimental Parasitology*, **19**, 276–299.

Sanchez, G., Knight, S. and Strickler, J. (1976). Nucleotide transport in African trypanosomes. *Comparative Biochemistry and Physiology*, **53**, 419–421.

Saz, H. J. (1972). Comparative biochemistry of carbohydrates in nematodes and cestodes. *In:* "Comparative Biochemistry of Parasites" (H. Van den Bossche, ed.), pp. 33–47. Academic Press, New York.

Shaw, J. J., Voller, A. and Bryant, C. (1964). Intermediary carbohydrate metabolism of four species of Trypanosomatidae. *Annals of Tropical Medicine and Parasitology*, **38**, 17–24.

Sims, P. (1976). Mode of action of SQ 18,506 (a 5-nitrofuran drug) against *Trypanosoma cruzi*. Ph.D. thesis. University of Kent.

Sims, P. and Gutteridge, W. E. (1979). Inhibitory action of a nitrofuran (SQ 18506) against nucleic acid synthesis in *Trypanosoma cruzi*. *Biochemical Pharmacology*. (In press)

Stohlman, S. A., Kuwahara, S. S. and Kazan, B. H. (1973). Enzyme, protein and nucleic acid content of two morphological forms of *Trypanosoma (Schizotrypanum) cruzi*. *Archives of Microbiology*, **9**, 301–311.

Stoppani, A. O. M. and De Boiso, J. F. (1973). Oxidative phosphorylation in *Trypanosoma cruzi*. *Experimentia*, **29**, 1494–1496.

Sylvester, D. and Krassner, S. M. (1976). Proline metabolism in *Trypanosoma cruzi* epimastigotes. *Comparative Biochemistry and Physiology*, **55**, 443–449.

Tanowitz, H., Wittner, M., Sueda, M. and Soeira, R. (1975). Studies on ribosomal RNA of *Trypanosoma cruzi*. *Journal of Parasitology*, **61**, 1065–1069.

Trigg, P. I. and Gutteridge, W. E. (1977). Morphological, biochemical and physiological changes occurring during the life cycles of parasitic protozoa. *In:* "Parasite Invasion" (A. E. R. Taylor and R. Muller, eds.), pp. 57–81. Blackwell Scientific Publications, Oxford.

Van Hoof, F., Jadin-Nyssens, M. and Jadin, J. M. (1977). Compared study of digestive enzymes in *Kinetoplastidae*. *In:* "Progress in Protozoology", p. 386. 5th International Congress of Protozoology. New York.

Vickerman, K. and Preston, T. M. (1976). Comparative cell biology of the kinetoplastid flagellates. *In:* "Biology of the Kinetoplastida" (W. H. R. Lumsden and D. A. Evans, eds.), Vol. 1, pp. 35–130. Academic Press, London and New York.

Von Brand, T. (1973). "Biochemistry of Parasites". Second edition. Academic Press, New York and London.

Wood, D. E. (1975). *Trypanosoma cruzi*: fatty acid metabolism *in vitro*. *Experimental Parasitology*, **37**, 60–66.

Wood, D. E. and Schiller, E. L. (1975). *Trypanosoma cruzi*: comparative fatty acid metabolism of the epimastigotes and trypomastigotes *in vitro*. *Experimental Parasitology*, **38**, 202–207.

Yoneda, S. (1971). Some aspects of the purine metabolism of *Trypanosoma cruzi* in tissue culture. *Rev Bras de Pesquisas Med e Biol*, **4**, 205–218.

Yoneda, S., Carvalho, R. P. de S. and Quiroga, M. (1974). Aspects of pyrimidine biosynthesis of *Trypanosoma cruzi*. *Revista do Instituto de Medicina Tropical de São Paulo*, **16**, 324–327.

Zeledon, R. (1960a). Comparative physiological studies on four species of hemoflagellates in culture. I. Endogenous respiration in the presence of glucose. *Journal of Protozoology*, **7**, 146–150.

Zeledon, R. (1960b). Comparative studies on four species of hemoflagellates in culture. II. Effect of carbohydrate and related substances and some amino compounds on the respiration. *Journal of Parasitology*, **46**, 541–551.

Zeledon, R. (1960c). Comparative physiological studies on four species of hemoflagellates in culture. V. Transaminases. *Revista Brasileira de Biologia*, **20**, 409–414.

Zeledon, R. (1978). Ecology of *Trypanosoma cruzi* in the insect vector. *In:* "Chagas' Disease", Scientific Publication Number 347, pp. 59–70. Pan American Health Organization, Washington.

Note added in proof

Since this manuscript was submitted in August 1977, about 50 papers have been published on various aspects of the biochemistry of *T. cruzi*. Most of these have been concerned solely with culture epimastigote forms but some have included data also on the other main forms. Where possible, these have been incorporated into the text. Note, however, that preliminary work has now been carried out on lipid metabolism and some quantitative differences detected (Roitman and Gutteridge, 1978). In addition, De Azevedo and Roitman (1978) have shown that the γ-strain of *T. cruzi* can be grown in a completely defined medium in the absence of added pyrimidine but *not* in the absence of added purine.

References

Roitman, I. and Gutteridge, W. E. (1978). Synthesis of lipids in *Trypanosoma cruzi*. *Pesquisa* Basica em Doença de Chagas. V Reuniao Anual, Caxambu, M.G. Brazil. Resumo A–28.

De Azevedo, H. P. and Roitman, I. (1978). Nutritional requirements of *Trypanosoma cruzi*. Ibid. Resumo A–26.

14

Nutrition of the Kinetoplastida

S. H. HUTNER and C. J. BACCHI

Haskins Laboratories and Department of Biology of Pace University,
New York, USA

and H. BAKER

Departments of Medicine and Preventive Medicine and Community Health,
New Jersey Medical School, East Orange, New Jersey, USA

I.	Introduction	654
II.	Kinetoplastid origins; inferences from nutrition	658
III.	*Crithidia fasciculata* as point of departure for nutritional investigations; substrates for trypanosomatids	660
	A. Basic requirements	660
	B. Haem and protoporphyrin	668
	C. Long-chain fatty acids	670
	D. Amino acids; purines and pyrimidines; vitaminic growth factors	671
	E. Temperature factors	677
IV.	Endosymbionts; detection of external contaminants	677
V.	Lower trypanosomatids, *Leishmania* and *Trypanosoma* compared	678
VI.	A perspective	680
VII.	Acknowledgements	681
VIII.	References	681

. . . all species except the talkative have been allotted the niche and diet that become them.—W. H. Auden: *Ode to Terminus*

I. Introduction

A defined medium—the traditional initial goal of nutritional analysis—serves notice that no additional nutrients have to be sought to ensure sustained growth, however meagre. Such a conclusion is valid for organic factors but not for several trace elements: their essentiality has to be taken on faith that results with other organisms, even if phyletically remote, apply to the Kinetoplastida. As described later, this zone of un-certainty is being narrowed for haemoflagellates (a handy term for Trypanosomatidae)—an effort possibly applicable to the search for new chemotherapy.

Motives for nutritional analysis include: (1) helping to dissect out unique metabolic mechanisms, notably the mitochondrial acrobatics sig-nalling the changes in structure and physiology in African trypanosomes of the subgenus *Trypanozoon* as they adapt from vector to the mammalian bloodstream and back to the invertebrate, with concomitant shifts be-tween predominantly cyanide-sensitive and cyanide-insensitive respira-tion; (2) analysis of factors mediating the intracellularity in the vertebrate characteristic of *Leishmania* and some stercorarian trypanosomes, es-pecially *Trypanosoma cruzi*; (3) the hope that *Leishmania* and *Trypano-soma* are so exquisitely adapted to blood and tissue fluids that some of their as-yet-unidentified growth factors will help elucidate why these milieus sustain leucocytes; (4) that unique growth factors for Trypano-somatidae, absolute or only stimulatory, will inspire synthesis of chemo-therapeutic agents acting as antimetabolites. Also, as media become physiologically realistic, i.e. approximating the makeup of body fluids for those components affecting trypanosomatid metabolism, with excess nutrients pared away, agents acting wholly or partly as antimetabolites will less often be overlooked in screening programmes. Economy is a con-sideration too. Many biochemical and immunological investigations require cells in bulk for extraction of enzymes and antigens; an example is the use of kinetoplast DNA as a diagnostic antigen for lupus ery-thematosus (Slater *et al.*, 1976; Crowe and Kushner, 1977). Identification of limiting nutrients can effect appreciable savings in the use of defined as well as complex media.

Kinetoplastida are unsurpassed among parasites in wealth of accessible forms. One is tempted to regard some as counterparts of extinct stages in evolution of mammalian and avian pathogens from parasites of poikilo-thermic vertebrates. Lower trypanosomatids—gut parasites of inverte-brates—even hark back, via bodonids, to photosynthetic flagellates. As unmatched parasitological evolution appears in unabated course in *Leishmania* and *Trypanosoma* as construed from the rapid emergence in the field of drug-fastness, acquisition of new hosts, and apparent recent abandonment of obligate development in insect vectors ("mechanical" transmission) as in *T. evansi* or complete relinquishment of vector as in *T. equiperdum*.

Nevertheless, Newton (1976) warns: "Determination of the nutritional requirements of kinetoplastid flagellates is proving difficult . . . All we can say at present is that a general pattern of growth requirements is slowly coming to light." Bowman and Flynn (1976) assert: "To correlate the changes in respiratory function at various stages of the life-cycle of trypanosomes, it will be necessary to devise *in vitro* systems to cultivate each stage." We are optimistic that these tall orders can be filled but not by concentrating the main attack on the pathogens; a systematic attack may well first require consolidation of advances with non-pathogens or parasites of negligible economic or medical importance.

Despite these incentives the consensus is that progress in understanding kinetoplastid nutrition is slow (reviews: Taylor and Baker, 1968; Trager, 1974). The milestones document this grudging progress. Novy and McNeal first cultured a trypanosomatid (*Trypanosoma lewisi*) in 1903. A quarter-century ago Cowperthwaite and coworkers (1953) devised the first defined medium for a trypanosomatid (*Crithidia fasciculata*); half a decade ago Cross and Manning (1973) described a virtually defined but far from minimal medium for *T. brucei*, and a preliminary report has followed on suitability of a simplified version of this medium for *T. cruzi* (Azevedo and Roitman, 1977). For purposes of chemotherapy no comprehensively minimal medium has yet been clearly devised for any trypanosomatid.

The genera comprising the Kinetoplastida have been reviewed (Vickerman, 1976; Vickerman and Preston, 1976; lower Trypanosomatidae: Wallace, this volume; *Leishmania*: Zuckerman and Lainson, 1977; Southgate and Wilson, this volume).

It is tempting to arrange the patchy data on nutrition into a gourmet's progress, as kinetoplastids gain access to increasingly richer food from free-living foraging to the richer provender provided by arthropod gut microfloras, with excursions to the haemacoele, as in *T. rangeli*; then to a microflora plied with blood in leeches and haemophagous insects; then breakthrough into the richer internal milieu of vertebrates and adaptation to the steam-tabled smörgåsbord of the homoiotherms. As an additional epicurean adventure, there is the adaptation of some Trypanosomatidae to life in the latex and phloem vessels of some plants, presumably after inoculation by sap-sucking insects (as described later, an axenic phytoflagellate is newly available). These sequences are on occasion drawn upon to buttress evolutionary speculations. Thus Zeledón (1971) posits: lower Trypanosomatidae → *Leishmania* and *Trypanosoma* of poikilotherms → a primitive mammalian trypanosome like *T. cruzi* → other Stercoraria and some of the mammalian species of *Leishmania* and

Endotrypanum → Salivaria "in which some species cannot be cultured, apparently because they cannot revert to the more primitive invertebrate forms."

This scheme reflects the widely (if tacitly) accepted idea of progressive nutritional fastidiousness reflecting a greater utilization of biochemical delicacies marking the escape from invertebrate austerity to vertebrate luxury. This summarizes the prevalent idea of intensified fastidiousness which has enabled the escape from austerity in the invertebrate to luxury in the vertebrate. However plausible it is as a summary description, this scheme may be misleading in particular instances. That fastidiousness, evidenced by failure by competent workers to cultivate some members of groups that are for the most part cultivable, can be inferred from Table 1. Negative results are seldom published except in special circumstances. Thus the present uncultivability of *Blastocrithidia triatomae* would not have emerged were it not that the host insect also harboured *T. cruzi*. *Herpetomonas mariadeanei* had a structural oddity: a flagellum coiled within the cell, hence the effort to cultivate it. The hard-to-cultivate *Leishmania* spp. were peculiarly pathogenic—as are of course all the pathogenic Trypanosomatidae. *Crithidia mellifera* of the honey bee might have remained uncultivated save for trial of an unconventionally acidic (pH 5.2) medium (Langridge and McGhee, 1967). Adherence to Zeledón's theory, and to adornments such as advanced by Baker (1974) that the trypomastigote is an adaptation to life in a bloody, viscous environment, should be in awareness of the skewed samplings of the vast array of species in nature. Progress in nutrition may enable the cultivation of hitherto intractable strains and species, yielding sounder ideas of which mechanisms were inherited by the pathogens from lower Trypanosomatidae and thus armed them to invade vertebrates. Fruitful insights into origin(s) of *Leishmania* and *Trypanosoma* require, then, vastly more knowledge of lower Trypanosomatidae (the paucity of drugs against the pathogens is an argument for this belief). Often the bar to knowledge comes down to poor reproducibility of media or present uncultivability of many important lower and higher Trypanosomatidae.

Some caveats about generalizations should be mentioned:

(1) Kinetoplastida, free-living or parasitic, may have gone in evolutionary directions of their own rather than conforming to orthogenetic nutritional sequences.

(2) Guts of leech and insect may not harbour ancestral-type microfloras; microfloras evolve too.

(3) The leech and arthropod gut may not be a biochemically simpler or less favourable environment than haemocoele or vertebrate interior. It may prove unsafe to assume that nutritional fastidiousness mirrors degree of adaptation of the vertebrate as opposed to a relatively uniform pattern of adaptation to life in invertebrates.

Table 1. Failures to cultivate trypanosomatids belonging to groups having cultivated members.

	Host	Ref.
Blastocrithidia gerridis	*Gerris*	1
B. triatomae	*Triatoma infestans*	2
Herpetomonas mariadeanei	*Muscina stabulans*	3
Leishmania b. braziliensis	Sandflies	4
L. b. guyanensis	Sandflies	4
Trypanosoma		
subgenus *Megatrypanum*	Bats	5
subgenus *Herpetosoma*	Rodents	6

1. Wallace *et al.* (1965); 2. Cerisola *et al.* (1971); F. G. Wallace (pers. commun.); 3. Yoshida *et al.* (1977); no growth in media for 3 other *Herpetomonas* sp.; 4. Bray (1974). Poor growth (if any) on NNN medium; 5. Marinkelle (1976). Three species tried; all negative; 6. Molyneaux (1976). *T. lewisi* cultivable.

(4) Nutritional fastidiousness may not necessarily denote the closeness of adaptation to the homoiothermic as opposed to the poikilothermic vertebrate; nor might capability for intracellular growth denote a greater fastidiousness in *Leishmania* as opposed, say, to the species now included in *Leptomonas*.

Scepticism about nutritional generalizations has a practical side: it may prove imprudent to neglect robust trypanosomatids which, if they prove to have patterns of drug sensitivity paralleling those of particular pathogens, could be useful for initial drug screening. Inasmuch as few practical drugs are at hand—indeed for Chagas' disease there is hardly one (Gutteridge, 1976; Schlemper *et al.*, 1977)—knowledge of the chemotherapeutic patterns for the pathogens is correspondingly sketchy. The formidable cost of developing novel drugs (Hutner, 1977) argues that amenable lower Trypanosomatidae and species of *Leishmania*, e.g. *L. tarentolae* and *L. enriettii*, and of *T. mega* should be scrutinized for metabolic features, detected perhaps most expeditiously as nutritional peculiarities, conceivably exploitable for taxonomy and chemotherapy—which takes into account the long acceptance of patterns of chemotherapy as valid taxonomic characters. There is a need, by this reasoning, for as many transmission lines between easily handled species and the pathogens as there are distinct chemotherapeutic patterns discerned among the pathogens.

Pyrimethamine—a mainstay of malaria chemotherapy—and the antifolic methotrexate—prominent in anti-cancer therapy—were developed with lactobacilli as initial screening organisms. The situation may not be different with Trypanosomatidae: easily reared relatives of the pathogens are available. Lower Trypanosomatidae may, then, be useful stopgaps until culture media for the pathogens (or else for closely allied forms) become easily reproducible and yet incorporate as many as practicable of those metabolites in body fluids which are likely to influence drug trials.

The uncultivability of dyskinetoplastic forms (Vickerman, 1977) portends great difficulties which, when overcome, will yield great rewards: identification of nutrients permitting their cultivation may be tantamount to identifying metabolites originally produced by the parasite's chondriome, now obtained from the host's chondriome. Export of mitochondria-mediated synthetic products seems a neglected aspect of mitochondriology although the list of products is already impressive (Flavell, 1971). Preoccupation with the mitochondrion as power plant has distorted the picture. In trypanosomes, mitochondria atrophy, perhaps furthered by feedback repression tolerated by *petite* mutants of yeast. Yet trypanosomes survive because tissue fluids may be rich in mitochondrial products and, moreover, because trypanosomes may have more transport systems than does yeast to take advantage of this bounty. Optimism about this gambit is nurtured by the amply verified observation that some yeasts can be grown anaerobically (where mitochondrial function is nearly completely suppressed) if given a sterol, e.g. ergosterol, and unsaturated fatty acid, e.g. oleate, to make good suppressed O_2-dependent mitochondrial syntheses (Linnane and Lukens, 1975). That growing trypanosomatids anaerobically has prospects of success is suggested by frequently finding intensely crowded trypanosomatid populations in the gut of invertebrates. One wonders how even super-efficient utilization of carbohydrate and traces of O_2 could sustain such populations; capacities for nutrition under anaerobiosis may be expressed that have been overlooked by emphasis on aerobic metabolism. Recent illustrations of intense crowding include *T. rotatorium* in a leech (Desser, 1976), *T. grayi* in the hindgut of *Glossina* (Molyneux, 1977), and a leptomonad (Gibbs, 1951).

II. Kinetoplastid origins; inferences from nutrition

Before dissecting the nutrients for kinetoplastids, one notes that the Order Kinetoplastida is pretentious in this context, for no member of Suborder Bodonina is in axenic culture—not even the haematozoic *Cryptobia* spp. and the pathogen *Ichthyobodo*, both common in fish hatcheries. The bacteria- and symbiont-bearing *Bodo saltans* (Brooker, 1971) and *Rhynchomonas nasuta* (Swale, 1973) appear highly eligible for axenization since lower trypanosomatids which have been cultured, and which bear bacteria-like symbionts, have simplified exogenous requirements (described later) as compared with the norm for Trypanosomatidae; *B. saltans* and *R. nasuta* are available from the Culture Centre for Algae and Protozoa, Cambridge, England. *R. nasuta* may be better since it is less subject to the constraint on growth observed in flagellates which prefer to glide on surfaces rather than swim freely. Simplifications in maintenance of axenic tetrahymenid ciliates have been effected by taking advantage of commercial availability of dried bacteria beside the usual yeasts, crude lipids, and powdered dehydrated tissues (Keenan *et al.*, 1978). Similar tactics may help in axenizing bodonids.

From morphological resemblances between *Bodo* (and similar genera) and some biflagellated colourless euglenids, e.g. *Anisonema*, one might suppose that resemblances between euglenid and trypanosomatid descriptive biochemistry would be paralleled by nutritional resemblances, as suggested by the *c*-type cytochromes of *Euglena* and *Crithidia*. In respect to amino acid sequences and presence of trimethyllysine, their cytochromes resemble each other more than they do the cytochromes of other eukaryotes (Pettigrew *et al.*, 1975). Yet, although all euglenids examined have a vitamin B_{12} requirement, including the voracious euglenid *Peranema* (Storm and Hutner, 1953), a B_{12} requirement is unreported for Trypanosomatidae. *Peranema* requires sterol; such a requirement has not yet been reported in Kinetoplastida, nor has the trypanosomatid biopterin-folate relationship been reported in euglenids.

Some euglenids, a cryptomonad, volvocines, and a dinoflagellate are "acetate" flagellates, i.e. conspicuously able to utilize acetate as principal or sole substrate. This attribute depends on a glyoxylate cycle. Diagnostic enzymes of the cycle, isocitrate lyase and malate synthase, have been reported from four species of *Leishmania* (Mukkada, 1977) and a *Herpetomonas* (Frugulhetti and Rebello, 1977). This cycle is thought to be primitive because, although found in bacteria, *Tetrahymena*, fungi and metaphytes, it appears absent in metazoa (a report of its occurrence in a nematode remains to be confirmed). But the crucial test—ability of acetate or other 2-carbon substrates to sustain growth—has not been clearly carried out. The likelihood that not exogenous acetate but acetate derived from threonine is the quantitatively importance source of acetate (discussed in the later section on amino acids) argues against acetate being an important substrate in the sense that it is for acetate flagellates.

That haemoflagellates may be particularly ancient parasites (Mattingly, 1965) seems borne out, then, by the nutritional gulf between them and the euglenids if one considers the euglenids as ancestral to bodonids. A haem requirement is not by itself a hallmark of parasitism; haem may be required by the non-pathogenic amoeboflagellate *Naegleria gruberi* (Band and Balamuth, 1974; confirmation is needed however), the slime mould *Physarum polycephalum* (McCullough and Dee, 1976), and the nematode *Caenorhabditis*.

III. *Crithidia fasciculata as point of departure for nutritional investigations; substrates for trypanosomatids*

A. BASIC REQUIREMENTS

Criteria for speciating *Crithidia* are tentative because of their rather uniform structure, uncertainty as to the weight to be accorded to host specificity and to immunological differences, and lack of data on DNA and RNA hybridization. Lumsden (1974) contends that specific distinction in *Leishmania* should be founded on biochemical characters. This applies likewise to *Crithidia* and *Leptomonas*. If nutritional characters are to be drawn on, media must be devised to serve as reference points— nutritional yardsticks—and to discern which biochemical characters are largely independent of variations in media, and which are not. As flexible yardsticks are an absurdity save in relativistic physics, reference media must be reasonably reproducible and not far out of line with ecological realities. Such a medium may be in sight for *C. fasciculata* (Shapiro *et al.*, 1978). How then to minimize subjectivity in formulating a yardstick medium? This has usually been attempted by specifying two cardinal concentrations for each nutrient: for half-maximal and full growth, as employed, for example, for *C. fasciculata* by Kidder and Dutta (1958). We follow the guideline advanced by Ham (1974) for vertebrate-cell culture: the concentration chosen is the middle of the plateau obtained on plots of log concentration of nutrient concentration vs. growth in linear units. Emphasis in the remainder of this review is on reproducibility within each class of nutrient; most information derives from *Crithidia*.

   Crithidia fasciculata is so amenable to manipulation that despite absence of mating behaviour it challenges *Tetrahymena* and yeasts as a biochemical workhorse. Most used is the classical isolate from *Anopheles* (ATCC 11745). Its minimal requirements, aside from haem and the interchangeable biopterin–folic acid duo, are largely conventional, in the pattern familiar for moderately exacting bacteria, notably the common lactic acid bacteria. With lipid factors and the unstable ascorbic acid subtracted, the remaining requirements of insects and vertebrates would be much like *Crithidia*'s, with some variations in purine and pyrimidine requirements. Its intense aerobic fermentation permits a diauxie like that of *Corynebacterium diphtheriae* in media designed for high yield of toxin (Wilson and Miles, 1975): initial rapid glycolysis and, if good aeration is ensured by a high surface:volume ratio and acidification slowed by good buffering and release of NH_4^+, alkalinization then ensues by oxidation of glycolytic products. A clear glycolysis–oxidation diauxie has been detailed for *T. cruzi* (S. L. Chang, 1948; Kallinikova, 1968) which, like other stercorarian trypanosomes, has functional cytochromes throughout its life cycle. The observed pH reversal for *C. fasciculata* has not been rigorously analysed but is elicited under the aforementioned conditions (Tamburro and Hutner, 1971). The main nutritional pattern for *C. fasciculata* has been outlined by Kidder and Dutta (1958); much of what follows here amounts to an updating of that medium. Recent findings with proline, described later, and other amino acids close to the Krebs cycle, add plausibility to the contention of Marr *et al.* (1977), who used shake cultures, that in early log phase *C. fasciculata* depends on amino acids, then shifting to glucose utilization—a pattern shared by *L. donovani* and *L. braziliensis* (Marr and Berens, 1977).

Glucose is especially rapidly utilized by many lower trypanosomatids as is inferred from rapid acidification and growth. It is oxidized faster than sucrose and fructose, but at the same rate as mannose (Cosgrove, 1959). Trehalose, often the most abundant sugar in insect haemolymph (Wyatt, 1975), is not utilized by several species of *Crithidia* and *Leptomonas collosoma* (Cosgrove, 1963). These strains used D-ribose to some extent. Conceivably, under conditions favouring very rapid growth, superiority of the common nucleosides and nucleotides over the free bases (supplied to satisfy the purine requirements) may emerge, attributable to the pentose, for many eukaryotic cells have high-capacity permeases; there is no reason to think that Trypanosomatidae are different. This idea has ecological support. A blood meal is low in carbohydrate (Evans and Brown, 1972). The possibility of nucleic acid-derived pentose as carbon source may have been ignored because of reliance on all-or-nothing trials of substrates. In the Tulahuen strain of *T. cruzi* the pentose pathway accounts for 41% of the glucose catabolized (Mancilla and Naquira, 1964). The abundance of DNA in Stercoraria which, like lower Trypanosomatidae, have an undiminished kinetoplast throughout the life cycle (aside perhaps from intracellular or amastigote stages), might thus be limiting during rapid growth.

Under several conditions the non-reducing sorbitol supports growth almost as well as sucrose for several *Crithidia* isolates (Guttman, 1963). Reducing sugars autoclaved in neutral or alkaline media are subject to decompositions and condensations, some unfavourable, some favourable —some glucose breakdown products are useful Fe transporters (Hutner, 1972). Acidification tends to slow and then terminate growth in traditional media. Good growth of *C. fasciculata* with nonfermentable substrates was obtained with a combination of glycerol, proline, L-malic acid, acetate, excess arginine, and asparagine; the initial pH of 6·9 rose to 7·6 (Tamburro and Hutner, 1971). For alkaline media, as in those at blood pH (7·5), glucose should be added separately after filter-sterilization or, more conveniently, from a slightly acidified concentrated solution which is then autoclaved without damage. Flagellates with a full complement of cytochromes may appreciably oxidize acid substrates if not overwhelmed by glycolysis. Hence it may be feasible to employ initially acidic media, with their advantages of greater stability to autoclaving. Then, if the pH rises during growth, reaching or exeeding blood pH, chemotherapeutic trials with ionizable drugs may be closer to *in vivo* conditions than with media permitting the usual excessive glycolytic acidification. Appreciable pH stabilization without serious slowing of growth was enabled by use of the slowly fermented mannitol in assay of biopterin with *C. fasciculata* (Baker *et al.*, 1974).

The digenetic habit may correlate with a restricted range of usable carbohydrates. Thus *T. lewisi* does not respire sucrose, mannitol or sorbitol; glycerol is oxidized (Ryley, 1951). Slowly utilized sugars may have an advantage beside that of slowing glycolytic acidification; they may be weaker than glucose in suppressing mitochondrial activity while energy from glycolysis is not seriously diminished. Thus Hill and Anderson (1969) employed D-xylose for *C. fasciculata*; such cells had double the O_2 uptake of glucose-grown cells. Glycerol was used similarly by Edwards *et al.* (1975).

Use of D-ribose as all-purpose substrate, i.e., both fuel and synthetic substrate, may be well developed in *Leishmania*, as shown by the life-supportive efficacy, of ribose for *L. tropica* (Dubois,1936); *L. braziliensis* (Medina *et al.*, 1955; Zeledón and Mange, 1967), and the high O_2 consumption of *L. donovani* given ribose (Ghosh and Data, 1971). The rapid catabolism of thymidine to thymine observed in *C. fasciculata* and culture forms of *T. cruzi* (but not in blood forms of *T. lewisi*, *T. congolense*, and culture forms of *T. brucei*) (Chalabi and Gutteridge, 1977) raises the questions: Does the residual deoxyribose share the fate of thymine—excretion? Is a significant proportion assimilated?

An extensive literature indicates that utilization of glycerol as sole substrate correlates nicely in Trypanosomatidae with cytochrome activity (von Brand *et al.*, 1967). Even when not serving as oxidative substrate glycerol can be a valuable carbon source, especially for trypanosomes. Lipids, consisting mainly of phospholipid and neutral fat, are abundant in trypanosomes (Dixon *et al.*, 1970; Godfrey and Taylor, 1972; Oliveira *et al.*, 1977). Suspensions of bloodstream *T. b. rhodesiense* survived with glycerol twice as long as with sugars (Ryley, 1962). Glycerol maintained motility in *T. evansi* in blood after glucose had been metabolically depleted (Balis, 1964). Presumably much of the glycerol enters lipids. Uptake of glycerol is at least in part independent of that for glucose (*Leishmania tropica*: Schaeffer and Mukkada, 1976; *T. b. equiperdum*: Ruff and Read, 1974), which suggests that it may be a useful auxiliary substrate. It seems competitive with glucose for *T. b. gambiense* (Southworth and Read, 1970) which suggests, on the other hand, that glycerol may usefully slow the metabolism of glucose—serving as a glucose buffer, as it were—allowing formation of alkali (NH_4^+ and residues from oxidation of Krebs-cycle acids) to keep pace with glycolytic acidification.

Combinations of glycerol and carbohydrates might well support rapid growth better than either alone; and data on this point would be welcome on another ground: in nature substrates are not present singly.

α- and β-glycerol phosphates are multi-purpose nutrients, the rationale for whose use is largely empirical; biochemical analysis is needed. Commercial mixed α- and β-glycerol phosphates were used as pH buffers for *C. fasciculata* (Bacchi *et al.*, 1969); high concentrations are well tolerated (Ellenbogen *et al.*, 1972). If much of the phospholipid in trypanosomes is metabolically active, trypanosomes might have a higher than usual response to lipid precursors.

A bugbear of defined media is precipitation of $MgNH_4PO_4$ and Fe phosphates. These precipitates may not be inert; they adsorb metal ions and, as mentioned later for small amoebae and *Tetrahymena*, induce phagocytosis. The glycerol phosphates are very soluble. Their phosphate appears to be readily available which is not unexpected given the ubiquity of alkaline phosphatase in animals, for which the β-isomer is a reagent. L-α-glycerol phosphate, a building block of phospholipids, is one of the few substrates oxidized as such by mitochondria, including those of *C. fasciculata* (Kusel and Storey, 1976). It is therefore important to ascertain whether α-glycerophosphate can enter without prior hydrolysis and whether what limits glycerol utilization is glycerol kinase. Do glycerol and glycerol phosphate enter independently of each other, i.e. by different permeases? Several observations bring up the question: *T. evansi* oxidized α-glycerol phosphate appreciably (Harvey, 1949); α-glycerol phosphate maintained the O_2 consumption of suspensions in serum of two normal and two dyskinetoplastic strains of *T. b. gambiense* and *T. evansi* as well as, or better than, glycerol (Fromentin, 1973). Opperdoes *et al.* (1977) wondered whether, in anaerobiosis, glycerol phosphate might yield ATP for African trypanosomes by reversal of the glycerol kinase reaction. The reduction of tetrazolium by washed bloodstream but not culture forms of *T. b. rhodesiense* cells in the presence of α-glycerol phosphate, under aerobic conditions, provides indirect evidence of its activity as substrate for trypanosomes (Ryley, 1966); under anaerobic conditions both blood and culture forms reduced tetrazolium. Should such reduction be coupled to oxidation of NADH, other exogenous electron acceptors may support anaerobic and assist aerobic growth. Unfortunately information on the redox behaviour of intact trypanosomatids and the effects of redox dyes is otherwise scant. There is a high concentration of Na β-glycerol phosphate $5H_2O$—20 g/L—in a defined medium for *T. cruzi* (Azevedo and Roitman, 1977). Glycerol phosphate, because it is hygroscopic, is incompatible with media formulated as dry mixes. Admixture of Na glycerol phosphate with glycerol phosphoric acid provides a simple, wide-range, buffer system. Glycerol exposed to air accumulates peroxides (Bello and Bello, 1976). Perhaps glycerol, a common glycolytic product, may also accumulate in glycerol phosphate-containing media. Antioxidants might therefore improve media, perhaps by shortening the lag phase now observed in the *C. fasciculata* assay of biopterin (Baker *et al.*, 1974; Shapiro *et al.*, 1978). A beginning has been made by inclusion of retinoic and ascorbic acids and tocopherol in the defined medium for *T. brucei* (Cross *et al.*, 1975a).

Some compounds may be nutritionally valuable collectively (if not singly) because they are taken up; they may appear in lipids. Isovaleric acid was preferentially incorporated by *C. fasciculata*, *Blastocrithidia*, and *Leishmania tarentolae* into iso acids and mevalonic acid (Meyer and Holz, 1966). *T. b. rhodesiense*, rich in phosphatidyl inositol, also has choline and ethanolamine phospholipids (Venkatesan and Ormerod, 1976). Choline ethanolamine, serine, and methionine were incorporated into phospholipids by *C. fasciculata* (Palmer, 1974). Information on uptake of inositol is lacking, but since it is a growth factor for many yeasts and, under some conditions, for rodents and the chick (Alam, 1971) it is worth trial; it is included in the medium of Cross *et al.* (1975a). *L. tarentolae* has a puzzling interchangeable requirement for vitamin B_6 or choline (Trager, 1957). Long-chain fatty acids—additional precursors of lipids—are discussed later (Section III, D).

Nonfermentable substrates, aside from glycerol, glycerol phosphate, and proline, have only lately been included routinely in media for *Leishmania* and *Trypanosoma*. The spotlight has been on fermentable substrates, probably because these support rapid growth when sole substrate; and there is the apparent indispensibility of glucose for both haematozoic and culture forms of African trypanosomes. Another reason may seem trivial: the common practice of growing trypanosomatids in tubes. Stationary cultures, to be well aerated, should be in very shallow layers in flat-bottomed vessels. Media in tubes should be sloped and in small volume. Small volumes increase pipetting error and irregularities due to evaporation; sloping increases aeration inhomogeneities. In exploratory work, agitated or aerated cultures are awkward for more than a few vessels. Growth of aerated mass cultures of *T. cruzi*, *L. donovani*, and *Crithidia oncopelti* (symbiont-harbouring strain) exceeded that of stationary cultures 2–2·5 times, reaching 190 million cells of *T. cruzi* per ml of aerated culture (Zilberblatt, 1969). As noted, thinlayer cultures of *C. fasciculata* in defined media have reached comparable densities (Shapiro *et al.*, 1978) in low-form Erlenmeyer flasks, e.g. 5 ml of medium per 25- or 50-ml flask. Another advantage of volumes of 5 ml or more is that fewer serial cultures are needed to rule out effects of nutrients in inocula. This procedure is being used for biopterin assay with *C. fasciculata* (Baker *et al.*, 1978).

Granted that vertebrate blood is better oxygenated than insect gut, surveys of substrates for bloodstream forms of trypanosomes, as an exclusion test for putative substrates for trypanosomatids generally, should be as aerobic as practicable. The aerobiosis of *C. fasciculata* is unmistakable: when growing well, it forms a loose pellicle and even a film on the wall of the culture vessel above the medium. Many trypanosomatids readily grow on blood-agar slopes or plates—another evidence of aerobiosis, likewise the intense O_2 consumption of bloodstream forms of *Trypanozoon*. Growth on blood-agar surfaces by *Leishmania* and *Trypanosoma* may not indicate great tolerance for aerobiosis, for blood catalase destroys growth-inhibiting peroxides. *Crithidia* grows well on defined agar-based media; assistance from exogenous catalase is unnecessary. Support of surface growth by nonfermentable compounds might provide a sensitive test for such substrates and their interactions.

In surveying substrates the basal medium should be devoid of substrate. This ideal was not fully attainable with *C. fasciculata*: arginine, although essential, had substrate activity (Tamburro and Hutner, 1971) —an apparently catabolic suicidal habit. Arginine accumulates in the gut of *Glossina* after a blood meal (Bursell, 1970), which would appear to permit luxury consumption of arginine in vector as well as vertebrate; blood meals in the mosquito may be similarly digested. The catabolic pathway of arginine and its fate in other Trypanosomatidae are unexamined aside from the observation that citrulline, but not ornithine, could replace arginine as essential amino acid (Kidder *et al.*, 1966) for *C. fasciculata*.

High consumption of O_2 by *C. fasciculata* is supported by asparagine (Hunter, 1960) which, as noted, was growth-supportive (Tamburro and Hutner, 1971). Asparagine was not an energy source for blood or culture forms of *T. b. rhodesiense* (Ryley, 1962) and was only slowly oxidized by *T. lewisi* (Moulder, 1948). Nevertheless it may be of value as an alkalinizer, perhaps as substrate as well, assuming that the requisite amidase is present, as likely in *C. fasciculata*.

Proline has emerged as a readily utilized substrate for trypanosomes, *Leishmania*, and *C. fasciculata*, and hence deserves incorporation in defined media. As proline metabolism has been reviewed (Bowman and Flynn, 1976) it will not be discussed except to note that, being a small, lipid-soluble molecule, its permeation is probably insensitive to variations in pH; in *L. tarentolae* it appears to be readily convertible to glutamate—the reverse does not occur (Wagner and Krassner, 1976). In *T. cruzi*, labelled proline yielded labelled Krebs-cycle intermediates, glutamate remaining unlabelled (Sylvester and Krassner, 1976).

Hunter's (1960) survey of respiratory substrates for *C. fasciculata* was at pH 7·4, where acid substrates, being fully ionic, would penetrate comparatively poorly. Glutamine, in which one ionizable group is blocked as compared to glutamate, was second only to glucose. Unfortunately glutamine is instable, which bedevils tissue-cell culture since many cell lines need it. Esters or acyl derivates of Krebs-cycle acids and related amino acids might penetrate better, and hence be utilized better. Such measures, unreported for trypanosomatids, work with some other organisms. Malate is special because its chelation, as in a high-yield pH 6·5 medium for *C. fasciculata* (Shapiro *et al.*, 1978), may promote permeation by enhancing lipid solubility. Uncertainty about the role of lactic dehydrogenase—apparently present in *Leishmania* (Mattock, 1975) and weakly developed in *C. fasciculata* (Bacchi *et al.*, 1970)—is exacerbated by ignorance as to the activity of lactate as a growth substrate. Lactic acid is of course an important constituent of blood; it occurs in some insects adapted to anaerobiosis (Wigglesworth, 1972).

Until recently the absence of defined media for any pathogen compelled recourse to expedients in addition to short-term respirometry so as to detect substrate activity. Thus to identify substrates supporting transformation of *L. donovani* amastigotes to promastigotes, Simpson (1968a) suspended amastigotes from hamster spleen in Medium C devoloped by Trager (1957) for *L. tarentolae* of lizards. Recently transformed promastigotes divided several times but could not be subcultured. The amastigotes, suspended in saline, accompanied by splenic material, transformed only if given glucose or sucrose, with further assistance from aspartic plus glutamic acids, arginine, and histidine, but transformed poorly, surprisingly, with proline and, unsurprisingly, poorly with alanine and glycine.

A largely unexplored group of potential substrates, especially for growth under reduced O_2 tension, are those figuring in the carboxylations and transaminases centering on pyruvate and glutamate. These have been reviewed by Bowman and Flynn (1976) who mention the possibility of promotion of growth by these substrates or their carboxylation products should they act as alternate oxidants of NADH. If effective, the mystery alluded to earlier—what sustains the crowding often seen in the invertebrate gut?—might be solved. An anaplerotic role for these carboxylations, which yield mainly malate in *C. fasciculata* and *T. mega* and succinate in *T. brucei*, both of which may act as oxidants for NADH, thereby yielding ATP, was suggested by Klein *et al.* (1975) and Linstead *et al.* (1975). Have Trypanosomatidae, then, made do with CO_2 as substitute for O_2 under crowding or anaerobiosis? Some helminths, molluscs and other animals (de Zwann *et al.*, 1976; Hochachka, 1976) have exploited CO_2. Compounds eligible to be sources of electron acceptors if not acting directly include glutamate and α-ketoglutarate, aspartic acid and asparagine (viewed as sources of oxaloacetate), pyruvate and malate, fumarate, glycerol, glycerol phosphates, fumarate, and dihydroxyacetone. *T. brucei* often swarms in tissue spaces rather than bloodstream (Goodwin, 1974)—a hint that under some circumstances it prefers low O_2

tension. Even haemolymph may be reducing at some stages in the insect life cycle judged by its content of antioxidants (Atkinson *et al.*, 1973).

Pyruvate may emerge as a special substrate for dense or even anaerobic growth, and growth of *Trypanozoon* generally. Searle and Reiner (1940) noted that, anaerobically, pyruvate activated glucose metabolism of *T. lewisi* with production of lactate. Pyruvate is a glycolytic product of little obvious substrate activity. This may be misleading because, by the time it accumulates, suppression of mitochondrial activity by glucose might be far advanced. Peroxides inhibiting respiration, formed by *T. b. rhodesiense* in the presence of thiols, are removed by pyruvate (Fulton and Spooner, 1956). Media imitating natural materials should include cysteine (cystine is very poorly soluble), but cysteine is poorly tolerated. Pyruvate may form a dissociable condensate with cysteine and so lower its toxicity (Nishiuch *et al.*, 1976). Tissue fluids contain various antioxidants, for example reduced glutathione, tocopherols, and ascorbic acid. Insect haemolymph is rich in phenolic antioxidants, presumably involved in the tanning steps in laying down cuticle (Wyatt, 1975). *T. rangeli* would appear to be a good test organism for media designed to reproduce conditions in haemolymph, given its haemolymph-invading proclivities (D'Alessandro, 1976). The medium employed by Cunningham (1977) for *T. brucei*, *T. b. gambiense*, *T. b. rhodesiense*, *T. congolense*, and *L. donovani* may be hard to reproduce since it is supplemented with 20% (by volume) foetal calf serum.

Sundry observations deal with the activity or non-activity of Krebs-cycle components. Except as noted for *C. fasciculata*, these observations are hard to translate to nutritional terms even where, as in culture forms of *T. b. rhodesiense*, mitochondria may be well developed and significantly respire succinate, α-ketoglutarate, malate but not acetate, pyruvate, lactate, aspartate or alanine (Ryley, 1962). The potential value of these energy sources may not be expressed clearly except after serial transfer when repression of mitochondrial function by glucose or other repressors is shaken off; or they should be tested in company with sources of CO_2— perhaps malate, α-ketoglutarate, or oxalacetate. If acting more as assimilation substrates than energy sources, their entrance may depend on auxiliary energy sources. The distinction between energy and assimilatory substrates is brought out by the observation that in culture forms of *T. cruzi* O_2 consumption was not stimulated by labelled acetate and pyruvate, yet both were oxidized because radioactivity appeared in CO_2, approaching that obtained with glucose; radioactivity appeared in Krebs-cycle intermediates and glycolytic intermediates from pyruvate but not acetate (Boiso and Stoppani, 1973). The conclusion was that *T. cruzi* has a low aerobic metabolism, as evidenced by the mitochondria having few cristae. But the growth media had glucose. A mixed-substrate system, with carbohydrate minimal or even negligible—as may be the predominant condition in the insect gut—may have elicited a different pattern consonant with the growth of *T. cruzi* on glycolytic and oxidation-assimilation substrates. The apparent contradiction with the activity of acetate as a growth stimulant for *T. cruzi* (Little and Oleson, 1951) might thus be resolved.

Acetate has peculiarities in Trypanosomatidae to be reckoned with in designing media. In *C. fasciculata* acetate can originate from pyruvate. In *T. brucei* acetyl-CoA from threonine is a preferred source of lipid carbon even in the presence of high concentrations of exogenous acetate and glucose; the ratio of acetate from pyruvate and from threonine varies from organism to organism (unpublished results of Linstead, Miller and Klein, cited by Linstead *et al.*, 1977). Evidently where threonine is consumed as an acetate source as well as entering into protein, such luxury consumption entails the risk of threonine limiting growth, as strongly implied by its marked diminution in cultures of African trypanosomes (Pittam, 1966) and total disappearance from complex dialysed medium for *T. lewisi* (Dusanic, 1969); hence the remarkably high threonine in the medium of Cross *et al.* (1975a)—357 mg/litre—which stands out from other neutral amino acids which are not as subject to catabolic destruction, e.g. L-isoleucine and L-leucine (each 260 mg/litre). Threonine was completely metabolized.

Rapid assimilation of acetate, to be sustainable, may require maintenance of high levels of threonine and exogenous acetate. The medium of Cross *et al.* had 680 mg/litre of Na acetate, $3H_2O$; glycine—another product of threonine cleavage in haematozoic *T. brucei* (Cross *et al.*, 1975b)—would be present. Another possibility is that, as in *C. fasciculata*, threonine may be synthesized from methionine or even from cysteine in the presence of high levels of folic acid (Kidder and Dewey, 1972).

B. HAEM AND PROTOPORPHYRIN

Haem—prosthetic group of the haemoproteins which are intrinsically required by all Trypanosomatidae—is bothersome. As mentioned, haem catalyses its autoxidative destruction and that of lipids. It tends to become poorly available because of dimerization, polymerization, and aggregation (which is to be expected from its two vinyl groups), and is poorly soluble below neutrality. Most peptones have negligible haem; rich liver infusions may have haem in useful concentrations. We may have largely eliminated haem as a contributor to irreproducibility of media—at least for *C. fasciculata*—by separating the roles of haem as specific growth factor and as Fe carrier (Shapiro *et al.*, 1978). To lessen autoxidation, blood pH for media was abandoned; present media are at pH 6·5. To avoid precipitation, haemin (the usual way to supply haem) had to be used sparingly. The bulk of haem proved to be serving more as iron transporter than as specific growth factor. By resort to multiple Fe-transport agents, the haem concentration was substantially lowered. Another vexation thereby removed was the short shelf-life of defined media for C. fasciculata. The first published defined medium (Cowperthwaite et al., 1953) had specified that haemin be added as a 5 mg/ml solution in 50% aqueous (w/v) triethanolamine. The viscosity of this solution was intended to impede dimerization and slow convection of the oxygenated layer of the solution. Whatever the explanation, the solutions stay usable for months, unlike those prepared in aqueous NaOH. The next published medium replaced the monobasic triethanolamine with the even more viscous dibasic ethylenedinitrilotetra-2-isopropanol ("Quadrol") (Tamburro and Hutner, 1971). Haemin solutions now keep a year or more. Indirect evidence from animal nutrition and model experiments with a bacterium (Shapiro et al., 1977) indicate that haem is an exceedingly efficient Fe source. By supplying Fe^{2+}-chelators (malic and gluconic acids), a nonpermeant Fe^{3+}-chelator (sulphosalicylic acid), together with a permeant Fe^{3+}-chelator (2,3-dihydroxybenzoic acid), and extra Cu and Mo, growth exceeded 10^8 organisms per ml, and the haemin concentration could be lowered to the vitamin level ordinarily attainable only if fresh haemin solution is filter-sterilized and added immediately. These findings may explain the report that ascorbic acid is a growth factor for T. cruzi and Leishmania (Lwoff, 1938, 1951), for ascorbic acid is both antioxidant (as is 2,3-dihydroxybenzoic acid) and a moderately effective Fe^{3+} mobilizer (Hussain et al., 1977). Perhaps such effects account at least partly for the injunction that blood for Leishmania and trypanosome media should be stored for no longer than a week (Taylor and Baker, 1968).

Simpson (1968b) and Gaughan and Krassner (1971) claimed that L. tarentolae cannot satisfy its haem requirement from protoporphyrin (haem without Fe; protoporphyrin IX). This implies that the organism lacks ferrochelatase, the mitochondrial enzyme which mediates the last step of haem synthesis: insertion of Fe into protoporphyrin. In his classical study of the haem requirement, Lwoff (1934) reported that haem was replaceable by protoporphyrin for C. fasciculata, which would indicate that the requirement was essentially for protoporphyrin— that the biosynthetic block preceded it. Chang et al. (1975) showed that the prophyrin requirement could not be satisfied by δ-aminolaevulinic acid or porphobilinogen for symbiont-free Blastocrithidia culicis and C. oncopelti; both lack the enzymes which catalyse the steps immediately preceding protoporphyrin synthesis: uroporphyrin synthase and porphobilinogen ammonia-lyase, i.e. no precursor of porphyrin is active for Trypanosomatidae: urophorphyrin synthesis could not be detected in L. tarentolae or T. conorhini, and haem could be replaced by protoporphyrin but not by δ-aminolaevulinic acid or porphobilinogen (Chang, 1975).

The observation that chromate, selenate, and vanadate accelerated the growth of *L. tarentolae* in a defined medium with taurine as sole sulphur source (Sheets and Krassner, 1974) might be explicable if Fe and Cu were too low for adequate introduction of Fe into protoporphyrin; vanadium and chromate, by displacement of Fe from binding, might increase Fe availability. Further speculation is unwarranted in the absence of knowledge of the relative effects of haem and protoporphyrin on the Fe requirement of, say, *C. fasciculata*, and of the relative efficiency of Fe and Cu transport of *L. tarentolae*.

Accumulation of "pigment" as well as haematin in the gut of *Glossina* after a blood meal (Bursell, 1970) raises the question of whether such pigment, likely to contain free bile pigments, has morphogenetic activity. Nutrient activity might be detectable by haem-sparing, assuming that if bile pigments are metabolically essential, more haem could be channelled towards the respiratory apparatus. Kidder (1967) had briefly asserted that the haem for *C. fasciculata* was spared by bilirubin and biliverdin. Unpublished work by us has not revealed haem-sparing by bilirubin.

As little as 0·1 mM bilirubin completely inhibited growth of *L. tropica* promastigotes; serum albumin was protective (Simon *et al.*, 1976). Haem induced lysis of bloodstream forms of *T. brucei* and *T. congolense*; serum albumin was protective if added before the haem. Lysis was independent of O_2; riboflavin, "a free-radical scavenger", partly protected (Meshnick *et al.*, 1977).

Replacing the haem of digestible haemoproteins, e.g. haemoglobin and cytochrome *c* (Lwoff, 1951), by free haem is therefore not without danger. Haemoproteins must be reservoirs which release haem, presumably by joint action of host and parasite enzymes; sometimes release of haem keeps pace with the parasite's needs, sometimes overtaxing its tolerance. A surge of bile pigments could also be a formidable barrier to gaining a foothold in the haematozoic vector's gut. Eeckhout (1974), to supply *Crithidia luciliae* with ample haem in order to study catalase formation as a function of exogenous haem, used filter-sterilized haemoglobin because haemin was not soluble enough even at pH 7·5.

C. LONG-CHAIN FATTY ACIDS

As these have been reviewed as growth factors and as substrates for trypanosomes (Bowman and Flynn, 1976), this discussion centres on work with lower trypanosomatids. It is unlikely that trials of respiratory activity where the fatty acids are presented as pure compounds can be clear-cut, the margin between metabolic activity and toxicity is very narrow. Dense growth of *C. fasciculata* requires one or another ester of polyoxyethylene sorbitan ("Tween"), notably Tween 40 (palmitate), Tween 40 (stearate), and oleate (Tween 60). The media of Kidder and

Dutta (1958) and Baker *et al.* (1978) have 0·5% Tween 80, that of Shapiro *et al.* (1978) Tween 40 1·0% plus Tween 80 0·1%, and that of Cross *et al.* (1975a) for *T. brucei* Tween 40 0·5 mg%. The Boné and Parent (1963) medium has stearic acid, presumably an essential factor for *T. cruzi*. That the factor is indeed a long-chain fatty acid is supported by the observation that the activity of solvent-extracted serum albumin was restored by oleate (Citri and Grossowicz, 1955). A possibility, perhaps remote, is that the active factors are oxidation products, as suggested by the reports that *C. fasciculata* can carry an α-oxidation of stearate (Avins, 1968). 2-Hydroxypalmitate as well as CO_2 is produced from carboxy-labelled palmitate in a growth medium, with some of the carboxyl C appearing in water-soluble products (Vakirtzi-Lemonias *et al.*, 1972). Wood and Schiller (1975) found that trypomastigotes of *T. cruzi* can convert palmitate to CO_2; some palmitate was incorporated into neutral lipids but at a rate less than that of the epimastigotes.

Some of these perplexities may be lessened by the following observations: (1) long-chain fatty acids inhibited the motility of *L. donovani*, *L. tropica*, and epimastigotes and trypomastigotes of *T. cruzi*; *C. fasciculata* was relatively resistant (Cunningham *et al.*, 1972); (2) African trypanosomes produce free fatty acids from serum lipids and along with lytic lysolecithins which are intensely immunosuppressive (Roberts and Clarkson, 1977; Tizard *et al.*, 1977). Apparently trypanosomes traverse a very narrow path between utilization of long-chain fatty acids and destruction by them; *C. fasciculata* has a much broader margin of safety. Further speculation is unwarranted until more facts are at hand: (1) Can fatty acids be rendered available but non-inhibitory by binding to soluble starch or, perhaps better, Schardinger cyclo-dextrin which forms clathrate complexes with long-chain acids? (2) Is utilization of long-chain acids promoted by carnitine? (3) Can 2-hydroxystearic or 2-hydroxypalmitic acid (both commercially available) spare or replace long-chain acids?

D. AMINO ACIDS; PURINES AND PYRIMIDINES; VITAMINIC GROWTH FACTORS

1. Amino acids

The foregoing account of threonine as acetate source indicates that Trypanosomatidae are not wholly conventional in their amino acid requirements, i.e. they are not like moderately exacting lactic acid bacteria, insects, domestic animals, or man. Allothreonine is an effective precursor of glycine for *C. fasciculata* but cannot replace threonine (Kidder, 1967); glycine stimulates the synthesis of threonine (Kidder and Dutta, 1958). The Kidder–Dutta medium has DL-threonine. It is not known whether

Trypanosomatidae utilize D-threonine. Threonine is probably the only utilizable isomer. Since threonine is apt to be limiting, its presence in initially high concentration incurs the risk of inhibiting uptake of other amino acids, among them tryptophan, whose transport systems may overlap that of threonine. Tryptophan gives rise to 3-indoleacetic acid and tryptophol (which has sleep-inducing activity) in rats infected with *T. b. gambiense* (Stibbs and Seed, 1974). Likewise, phenylalanine gives rise to phenylpyruvate and tyrosine to *p*-hydroxyphenylpyruvate (Stibbs and Seed, 1975). Should these catabolites divert appreciable tryptophan, phenylalanine and tyrosine, so that they have to be provided in higher than ordinary concentration, concentrations of other neutral amino acids might have to be increased to restore transport balances. Such escalation may account for the assertion by Boné *et al.* (1966) that amino acids have to be 5 to 10 times more concentrated for leishmanias and trypanosomes than for *Crithidia*. If tryptophol and indoleacetic acid should significantly spare tryptophan for *C. fasciculata* another distinctive trait of Trypanosomatidae generally might emerge.

Histidine may also be appreciably catabolized. Bash-Lewinson and Grossowicz (1957), working with intact cells and extracts of *T. cruzi*, reported that the transaminase activity of histidine-pyruvate exceeded that with α-ketoglutarate, pyruvate, glutamate, and alanine. Cross *et al.* (1975b) noted that unlike *T. brucei*, in *T. cruzi* serine and histidine also appear to be extensively metabolized judged from their disappearance. The persistence of histidine in media for *T. brucei* was confirmed by Brun and Jenni (1977), as well as that threonine and methionine were used up, methionine and arginine greatly decreased, and glycine, alanine, and aspartic acid increased. In the medium of Shapiro *et al.* (1978), histidine (as free base) was supplied at $1·0$ g/litre, serving as pH buffer, perhaps also as an auxiliary way to transport Fe (and perhaps Cu) into the cell to attain the high concentrations of intracellular Fe required for dense growth, for there is fragmentary evidence that a transport system for histidine may not distinguish between histidine and histidine chelated with Fe (Van Campen, 1972). Haemoglobin is the richest known source of histidine. Histidine forms about 12% by weight of *Glossina* excrement after a blood meal, uric acid and arginine making up about 72 and 7% respectively (Bursell, 1970). A high-arginine, high-histidine medium is then, from the standpoint of life in the gut of a haematophagous vector, ecologically plausible. By similar reasoning, the fact that 19% of the wet weight of vertebrate blood is protein, carbohydrate 0·1%, and lipids 0·6% (Bursell, 1970), renders the search for noncarbohydrate substrates (indeed finding them among amino acids and glycerol) ecologically justifiable.

Excretion of alanine as a glycolytic product, perhaps in all Trypanosomatidae, indicates that it need not be included in media. Isoleucine was stated not to be essential for *L. tarentolae* (Krassner and Flory, 1971). It was essential for *L. donovani* and *L. braziliensis* (Steiger and Steiger, 1977); the contrasts between these leishmanias and *T. brucei* in respect to utilization of amino acids is evident from a tabulation of rates of consumption of amino acids by *L. donovani* and *L. braziliensis* (Steiger and Meshnick, 1977).

Lysine presents another divergence from the metazoan pattern: the L and *meso* isomers of diaminopimelic acid were as active as L-lysine for *C. fasciculata* (Gutteridge, 1969). (Bacteria and plants can use diaminopimelic acid.) Diaminopimelic acid was incorporated into proteins of *C. fasciculata*. Diaminopimelic decarboxylase, which converts the acid to lysine, was absent from acetone-powder preparations of *T. b. rhodesiense* and *T. cruzi*, which opens the possibility that their lysine requirement is of the metazoan type. Since *C. fasciculata* is a possible assay organism of lysine, and since these findings are of obvious taxonomic interest, the comparative biochemistry of lysine in Trypanosomatidae is extraordinarily interesting.

It seems premature to treat here the remarkably diverse patterns for synthesis of lysine and methionine among lower Trypanosomatidae, *T. mega*, and *T. ranarum*, outlined by Guttman (1967). Details were few, and, in the light of present knowledge, better basal media should be applied to elucidate the complicated biosynthetic interrelations among amino acids, growth factors, and inorganic nutrients.

A strain of *Leishmania tarentolae* was reported to grow without organic sulphur; sulphate was utilized in Trager's Medium C (Cruz and Krassner, 1971). Taurine could also serve as sole S source (Sheets and Krassner, 1972); tracer experiments showed assimilation of taurine into methionine. These findings must be received with reserve until verified.

A consequence of the amino acid patterns assuming firm shape is that they may range from lower trypanosomatids, *Leishmania*, and Stercoraria on one side, to Salivaria on the other—a distinction already manifest from gross morphology and from those biochemical fine-structures expressed as differences in patterns of chemotherapy. At the same time, as demonstrated by the metabolism of threonine, the cohesiveness of the family Trypanosomatidae is demonstrated. Perhaps, after this ground is consolidated, amino acid by amino acid, as done for the chick, rat and, foreseeably, for *Tetrahymena thermophila*, it will be in order to investigate whether major groups of Trypanosomatidae differ importantly in utilization of intact proteins. After all, cytochrome *c* (Lwoff, 1938) and haemoglobin (Eeckhout, 1974) do serve as haem sources. *C. fasciculata* may have a well-developed ability to utilize peptides for it can satisfy its leucine requirement from various leucine-containing peptides; *Tetrahymena pyriformis*, on the other hand, tended to be inhibited by those peptides (Kidder and Dewey, 1975).

The remaining essential amino acids for *C. fasciculata*—isoleucine, leucine, and valine—seem conventional. Since both phenylalanine and tyrosine are required, they are not reciprocally sparing as in higher animals, and their biosynthetic blocks are unaffected by biopterin.

2. B vitamins

The vitamins for *C. fasciculata*, aside from haem and folate-biopterin, are commonplace: thiamine, nicotinic acid (alternatively nicotinamide), pantothenate, riboflavin, pyridoxal (alternatively pyridoxamine, not pyridoxine), and biotin. For flexibility and reproducibility in compounding media, it is convenient to have on hand triturates of each nutrient employed at the mg/litre level or below. Pentaerythritol is serviceable for the purpose and seems nutritionally inert. Triturates can be weighed out directly instead of being pipetted from solutions of uncertain stability; vitamins in dilute solution tend to become adsorbed to glass, especially if basic or planar. Thus dilute solutions of choline lost strength rapidly; glass has a negative charge. Plastic bottles are therefore preferable even for temporary solutions, which anyway are best stored frozen. Riboflavin is conveniently dispensed as the monophosphate, which on a molar basis has the same activity as the free vitamin base but is more soluble; its phosphate does not contribute to precipitates. Nicotinamide may be slightly preferable to nicotinic acid, since it may be closer to the coenzyme.

Since biopterin is adequately treated in a standard text (Metzler, 1957), biochemical background here can be reduced to a précis. Ordinary synthesis of biopterin—by bacteria and mammals alike—proceeds by way of a common pteridine precursor with folic acid; this pteridine has a three-carbon side-chain. In folate synthesis the distal two carbons are cleaved; the residual side-chain methylene carbon is then condensed with *p*-aminobenzoic acid and glutamate to form folic acid. In biopterin synthesis the original three-carbon side-chain is retained, and the distal hydroxymethyl group reduced to methyl so that, with some intervening steps, the side-chain becomes 1',2'-dihydroxypropyl. The unique ability of *C. fasciculata*, perhaps of all Trypanosomatidae, shared only with *Paramecium aurelia* (Soldo and Godoy, 1974), is a growth response to biopterin, and which is synergistic with folic acid. The explanation from tracer experiments (Kidder, 1967) is that *Crithidia* cannot synthesize biopterin from the precursor shared with folic acid. Instead, folic acid itself is the precursor. The *p*-aminobenzoylglutamate moiety is removed leaving a hydroxymethyl which is then fused with a two-carbon fragment, thus forming the 1',2'-dihydroxypropyl side-chain of biopterin. The specificity of the biopterin requirement seems an amalgam of the two pathways: in the synthetic pathway via the pre-folate route, biopterin is formed from *L* and *D*-neopterin, where the side chain is 1',2',3'-trihydroxypropyl; L-neopterin and D-neopterin have 56 and 0·22%, respectively, of the activity of biopterin (Leeming and Blair, 1974). The route from folate includes, as postulated, 6-hydroxymethylpterin, which has about 32% of the activity of biopterin (Dewey and Kidder, 1971). This pterin was identified as the growth-promoting factor in spinach chloroplasts (Iwai et al., 1976). The biopterin status of *Phytomonas davidi*, cultivated by McGhee and Postell (1976), thus acquires special interest. L-threo-neopterin is the principal pterin produced by *Serratia indica* (Kobashi and Iwai, 1971) and *Escherichia coli* (Rembold and Heinz, 1971). Like the folates, the coenzyme form of biopterin is the tetrahydro derivative, which is 80% as active as biopterin (Leeming and Blair, 1974). The major material in human urine, as assayed by *Crithidia*, is 7,8-dihydrobiopterin (Leeming and Blair, 1974), likewise in sera, where it is accompanied by another active constituent, probably tetra-hydrobiopterin (Leeming et al., 1976). Evidently, in all the environments mentioned, biopterins–folates are probably seldom if ever limiting—and this without taking into consideration the biopterin-sparing factors to be considered below. Since folates in yeast and plants are predominantly polyglutamates, it will be of interest to quantitate their synergy with biopterin.

Interference by folates in the biopterin assay is easily eliminated. First, biopterin is about 500 times more active than folic acid (as pteroylglutamic acid); 5-methyl-, 10-formyl-, and 5-formyl tetrahydrofolic acid (folinic acid, i.e. citrovorum factor) have less than 0·01% of the activity of biopterin (Leeming and Blair, 1974). Therefore they are diluted out in most samples. Second, autoclaving at pH 4·5 destroys the folates whereas biopterin is unaffected and, if bound, liberated. This procedure, to-gether with the autoclaving of assay flasks at pH 6·5, apparently destroys interference by biopterin-catalysed metabolites.

Since biopterin is a coenzyme for hydroxylations leading from tyrosine to dopa and from tryptophan to serotonin, it is therefore involved in overall synthesis of the neurotransmitters dopamine, norepinephrine, epinephrine, and the pineal hormone melatinin. If these neuro-endo-crines also figure in the metabolism of Trypanosomatidae, then they might spare biopterin—which was indeed observed with *C. fasciculata* with dopa, norepinephrine and epinephrine (Janakidevi et al., 1966a) and 5-hydroxytryptophan and serotonin (Janakidevi et al., 1966b). Un-explored roles for biopterin were revealed by the activity of oleate, linoleic, arachedonic, hexadecanedioate and eicosanedioic acids (Dewey and Kidder, 1966). The activity of crude sphingomyelin was traced to a new methyl-sphingosine subsequently isolated from *Crithidia* cells (Carter et al., 1966).

Given excess thymidine (or thymine) plus biopterin, sparing by folate becomes so vanishingly small as to raise the question of whether *C.*

fasciculata can carry out a limited folic synthesis (Kidder *et al.*, 1967). By serial transfer we (Hutner, Bacchi and Baker, unpublished observations) have demonstrated rigorously that *C. fasciculata* indeed can be grown without folic acid. Kidder and Dewey (1975) advanced two theories to account for growth without folate (which never attains that reached with biopterin plus folate):

(1) Cytoplasmic protein synthesis in *Crithidia* does not require *N*-formylation by a folate coenzyme; the proteins are then exported into the mitochondrion;

(2) *Crithidia* can dispense in this respect with mitochondrial function, like bloodstream trypanosomes.

A third possibility can be advanced: a limited but definite back-synthesis from biopterin to folic acid. Perhaps the best way to settle the issue is to assay biopterin-grown *Crithidia* bodies for total folates with *Tetrahymena* (which respond to polyglutamates), and assays for *p*-aminobenzoic acid. A eukaryotic cell devoid of all folates would indeed be anomalous.

In *C. fasciculata* biopterin has additional functions: it is required for a hydroxylation in its synthesis of orotic acid, the precursor of the common pyrimidines (Kidder and Nolan, 1973), and for synthesis of threonine from methionine (Kidder and Dewey, 1972). The Kidder and Dutta (1958) medium lacks pyrimidines. To secure the most sensitive possible response to biopterin it is obviously necessary to include an assortment of pyrimidines and ample threonine in the assay medium.

Leeming and Blair, for their aforementioned work, independently developed a pH 6·5 medium. This falls into line with the fact that, aside from the better stability of the basal medium, biopterin uptake is optimal at pH 6·0 (Rembold *et al.*, 1974). *C. fasciculata* responds the same on a molar basis to the common purines whether as free bases, nucleosides or nucleotides (Kidder and Dutta, 1958). This may be general, for much the same emerged for "*Leptomonas pessoai*" (now *Herpetomonas samuelpessoai*) grown at 28° and 37°C (Roitman *et al.*, 1972). In older work with biopterin, contamination of nucleosides and nucleotides with biopterin was troublesome, even with "chromatographically pure" products. Pteridines are detected by fluorescence under ultraviolet. On the assumption that in rapid growth interconversions of purines might become limiting, a mixture of purines was recently employed; because of low solubility of guanine, Na_2guanosine-5'-phosphate was used along with hypoxanthine and adenine, and with pyrimidines such as cytosine, uracil and thymine (Shapiro *et al.*, 1978).

Under present conditions the *Culex* isolate of *C. fasciculata* has a somewhat more sensitive response to biopterin (Baker, in press). The fragmentary evidence at hand is that all isolates of *Crithidia* tested so far show the biopterin pattern (Guttman, 1964). *L. tarentolae* also followed the *Crithidia* pattern insofar as *L*-neopterin was approximately one hundredth as active as biopterin (Trager, 1969).

The report by Steinert (1965) that urea favours formation of trypomastigotes of *T. mega* remains unconfirmed. There have been fragmentary reports for *T. mega* and similar phenomena in other trypanosomatids, but it seems unprofitable to review this topic in the absence of detailed work with defined media.

E. TEMPERATURE FACTORS

An intriguing picture has been sketched of a stepwise increase in nutritional fastidiousness of *C. fasciculata* with rising temperature (Guttman, 1963). As experimental details were not given, and the criticality of osmotic pressure with increasing temperature (Ellenbogen *et al.*, 1972) has to be taken into account, discussion is left aside. The temperature adjustments for parasites in passage between vector and warm-blood host might be reflected in differences in nutritional requirements. If special factors for growth at blood heat could be detected, such modified media might support growth of bloodstream forms, and thereby permit benefits such as knowledge bearing on biochemical factors for adjustment to the mammalian host, and also greater validity for *in vitro* tests of putative drugs. There are several reports for *Leishmania* and *Trypanosoma* that *in vitro* growth at 37°C is obtainable, at least for several transfers, after a lesser or greater period of adaptation by growth at intermediate temperatures. Such experiments rest on media still at the witches'-brew stage and therefore outside the scope of this review. The outlook is far from bleak since fairly hardy model organisms are available: among them for trypanosomes, *T. mega*; for *Leishmania*—at least as a start, despite its peculiarly isolated position—*L. enriettii*, notoriously temperature sensitive in the guinea-pig, and having the great virtue of growing well on autoclaved (121°C) blood agar with simple NaCl-glucose overlay (Neal and Miles, 1963).

IV. Endosymbionts; detection of external contaminants

Symbiont-bearing haemoflagellates may be valuable for detecting new growth factors or new approaches to the metabolism of familiar vitamins. Chang (1976) found that asymbiotic strains of *Blastocrithidia culicis* and *Crithidia oncopelti* require a liver factor. The factor for asymbiotic *C. deanei* proved to be nicotinamide; half-maximal growth required 0·02 mg/ml—100 times the equivalent requirement for the *C. fasciculata* control (Mundim and Roitman, 1977).

One value of a common-denominator-defined medium for lower Trypanosomatidae is that it would serve as a sterility-test medium.

Growth with abnormally low or no haem is a time-honoured diagnostic test for endosymbionts. What if the endosymbiont or the external contaminant organisms needed haem? Recourse would then have to be to other indices, the best of all, perhaps, being the lack of response to the B vitamins and biopterin. Charting dose–response curves to these growth factors are also multiple sterility checks. The prevalence of such subtle contaminants as currently uncultivable mycoplasmas should counsel wariness in putting much weight on nutritional conclusions based on the use of unheated natural materials. No mycoplasmas are known which withstand temperatures above 56°C, hence such a treatment might well be a step in establishing a degree of thermolability of postulated growth factors.

V. Lower trypanosomatids, Leishmania and Trypanosoma compared

A picture emerges of the hardiness of *Crithidia fasciculata* and similar species—if species they are. Why so hardy? Is the sampling of *hardy* lower Trypanosomatidae adequate? Is hardiness necessarily proportional to resemblance to the standard strains of *Crithidia*? A good test case is provided by acidophilic strains (species?), i.e. strains whose isolation in the complex maintenance medium of Cowperthwaite *et al.* (1953) only succeeded when the medium was brought to pH 5·0 or so (Langridge and McGhee, 1967; McGhee *et al.*, 1969). We had no difficulty in growing them in defined media for *C. fasciculata* (Hutner, Bacchi and Baker, unpublished observations); indeed some grow so well that should they prove to have a sensitive response to biopterin, they could be practical assay organisms. Evidently the apparent acidophily betokens not so much difference in fundamental requirements or greater fastidiousness, but an unidentified sensitivity to an imbalance or toxicity inherent in certain complex media. As noted, some representatives of other genera of lower Trypanosomatidae conform to the *C. fasciculata* pattern even if able to grow at 37°C (Roitman *et al.*, 1972).

A conspicuous attribute of *C. fasciculata* is wide osmotic tolerance; indeed it behaves like an osmometer, shrinking and slender in hypertonic media, swelling into almost spheroidal shape in hypotonic media (Ellenbogen *et al.*, 1972), with no great loss of viability. It required scrutiny of its contractile vacuole to determine its isosmotic point at 21–28°C to be at 0·12 M NaCl (Cosgrove and Kessel, 1958). Moreover, its membrane tenaciously retains cellular solutes, for dilute suspensions in distilled water remain viable for many hours, which aligns with the observation that *C. fasciculata* swims in ponds from mosquito larva to larva (Clark *et al.*, 1964). Another element in the hardiness of some lower Trypanosomatidae which remains to be explored is their power to create reducing conditions, and their probable concomitant the destruction of noxious peroxides accumulated under aerobic conditions. *C. fasciculata* on glycerol-agar plates reduced nitro-blue tetrazolium—a good measure of respiratory capacity and of colony viability (Cohen and Zahalsky, 1968). *Herpetomonas megaseliae* and *C. harmosa*, both hardy, form colonies on blood agar; outdated human blood is suitable (Keppel and Janovy, 1977).

Another underpinning of nutritional efficiency, perhaps associated with hardiness, is phagotrophy or endocytosis. Much evidence from morphology and uptake of electron-dense or other identifiable materials is that endocytosis occurs in Trypanosomatidae. Perhaps the nearest evidence for endocytosis being nutritionally significant is the demonstration of uptake of ferritin by bloodstream and culture forms of *T. brucei*, with short-stumpy forms developing an enlarged flagellar pocket (Langreth and Balber, 1975). Orias and Rasmussen (1977) showed that a mutant of *Tetrahymena* had normal growth at 28°C; at 37°C, unable to form food vacuoles, growth required extra Fe, Cu, and folinic acid. If these prove to be temperature factors for *C. fasciculata* as well, then variations in endocytosis as a morphogenetic factor can be attacked systematically.

That evolution of Trypanosomatidae was at least partly channelled by the constraint imposed by the composition of haemolymph is suggested by the present picture of their nutrition. As summarized (Jeuniaux, 1971), insect haemolymph has: a reducing power not attributed to fermentable sugars such as glucose, but to ascorbic acid, α-ketonic acids, and unknown substances; extraordinarily high concentrations of organic acids, mainly of the Krebs cycle; glycerol, trehalose, and occasionally sorbitol; a high concentration of acid-soluble organic phosphates, including α-glycerol phosphate and other phospholipid components; and extraordinarily high concentrations of amino acids.

Another method of identifying growth factors—by identifying transport systems for drugs—has scarcely been used. All polar drugs, unless very small, permeate cells by exploiting a pre-existing transport or permease system; a classical example is discovery of *p*-amino benzoic acid as target of sulfanilamide. A counterpart for Trypanosomatidae might be the diamidines. Damper and Patton (1976) found that uptake of pentamidine by *T. brucei* was undiminished by the presence of basic amino acids. Choline and polyamines seem worth trying as antagonists, perhaps in conjunction with natural crudes.

Two extremes of nutritional patterns would meet if *C. fasciculata* becomes an experimental object for studying survival of dyskinetoplastic strains, for its populations are approximately 0·1% dyskinetoplastic (Cosgrove, 1966). To reason by analogy: *Euglena gracilis* Z strain gives rise to 1% white colonies. Given a substrate-rich medium, white strains outgrow green strains. What is the nutritional equivalent for dyskinetoplastic *C. fasciculata*? The principle is the same: in one the damaged organelle is the chloroplast, in the other the mitochondrion–kinetoplast complex. It may be only chance that dyskinetoplasty persists only in haematozoic forms: they have gained natural access to the missing mitochondrial products.

It may be unnecessary to be reminded that even were cultivation of dyskinetoplastic forms solved, other challenges remain. For instance, defined or semi-defined media for *T. brucei* failed for *T. congolense* (Steiger *et al.*, 1977).

VI. A perspective

The remark "the composition of some cultures is so sophisticated that they are more like a 'witches' brew' than a culture medium" (Hoare, 1972) remains apposite. The failure to cultivate any *Cryptobia*, many trypanosomes, difficulties with some leishmanias, and other failures (see Table 1) may denote that such forms, more than others, rely heavily, when in the vector, on soluble substances from microflora and epithelial cells. Those living in leeches and haematophagous insects rely on solutions and a different assortment of cellular debris, and on better oxygenation which entails the intriguing nutritional, as well as the notorious respiratory, gear-changing. Knowledge of haemolymph and blood and tissue-fluid composition should, logically help in understanding the nutritional shifts, even of dyskinetoplastid forms. But the state of culturing the cellular companions of the parasites in the vertebrate milieu, above all of bone-marrow and blood cells, is unedifying. For instance, the phenomena of immunology derive from three main cells—thymus- and bone-marrow-derived lymphocytes and macrophages. None is available as an established cell line (Golub, 1977) except for a few infected with certain oncogenic viruses. These viruses behave like overzealous symbionts; virus-transformed cells need less serum (Fenner *et al.*, 1976). But even for such cells the consequently less needed serum factors or the residual serum factors are unidentified. A case therefore can be made that one escape from that impasse is by elucidating the nutrition of kinetoplastids, especially of the exacting ones. Progress may be plodding but would be systematic and require fewer resources and risks of contamination. Kinetoplastids as probes for tissue-cell nutrition might be an attractive idea to many in affluent countries; workers in third-world countries would probably put chemotherapy and practical immunology ahead.

The most instructive parallel to evolution of parasitism, judged by the wealth of accessible species, ranging from those free-living to an array of parasites living in intimacy with plant or vertebrate cells—some easily cultivable, others hardly or not yet cultivable—may be the mycoplasmas.

Here too progress is slow (Razin, 1973). For instance, urea is an absolute growth factor for one group, but an explanation has not yet been forthcoming. The prevalence of mycoplasmas as contaminants in commercial blood sera and in tissue-cell cultures may account for some of the difficulties in reproducing results derived from serial cultivation of trypanosomatids on media containing unheated blood or blood fractions —a cogent argument for identifying ostensibly thermolabile factors required by Trypanosomatidae. The conclusion (implied in the Introduction) is that investigators of kinetoplastid nutrition, even if drawing efficiently on information from other fields, would still largely be on their own.

The gaps in knowledge of the metabolism of the pathogens are underscored by the scarcity of novel drugs despite barely acceptable toxicities of the few at hand and spread of drug resistance. More flank support may prove to be a necessity, perhaps from a congeries of academic cottage-industries devoted to domesticating kinetoplastids and exploring idiosyncrasies of those in culture. Investigation of *Crithidia* nutrition, with little heed to the pathogens, helped reveal that biopterin is a constituent of blood of tissues of potential chemotherapeutic and fundamental biochemical significance. From that perspective we submit that rearing Kinetoplastida is barely at the end of its theoretical and practical beginnings.

VII. Acknowledgements

Preparation of this article was supported in part by National Science Foundation grant AER-77-02114 to S.H.H.; N.I.H. grant RO1AI 13852 to C.J.B., and U.S. Public Health Service grant FRO5596 to F. S. Cooper (Haskins Laboratories). We are grateful for this aid.

VIII. References

Alam, S. Q. (1971). Inositols. IX. Biochemical systems. *In:* "The Vitamins" W. H. Sebrell, Jr. and R. S. Harris, eds), Second Edition, Vol. 3, pp. 380–394. Academic Press, New York and London.

Atkinson, P. W., Brown, W. V. and Gilby, A. R. (1973). Phenolic compounds from insect cuticle: Identification of some lipid antioxidants. *Insect Biochemistry,* 3, 309–315.

Avins, L. R. (1968). Studies on alpha oxidation of stearic acid by *Tetrahymena pyriformis* and *Crithidia fasciculata*. *Biochemical and Biophysical Research Communications*, 32, 138–142.

Azevedo, H. P. and Roitman, I. (1977). Growth of the Y strain of *Trypanosoma cruzi* in an HX25-modified defined medium. *Journal of Parasitology*, 63, 485.

Bacchi, C. J., Ciaccio, E. I. and Koren, L. E. (1969). Effects of some antitumor agents on growth and glycolytic enzymes of the flagellate *Crithidia*. *Journal of Bacteriology*, 98, 23–28.

Bacchi, C. J., Ciaccio, E. I., O'Connell, K. M. and Hutner, S. H. (1970). Biochemical properties of trypanosomatid lactate dehydrogenases. *Journal of Bacteriology*, **102**, 826–834.

Baker, H., Frank, O., Bacchi, C. J. and Hutner, S. H. (1974). Biopterin content of human and rat fluids and tissues determined protozoologically. *American Journal of Clinical Nutrition*, **27**, 1247–1253.

Baker, H., Frank, O., Shapiro, A. and Hutner, S. H. (1978). Crithidia assay of unconjugated pteridines. *In:* "Methods in Enzymology" (D. B. McCormick and C. D. Wright, eds). Academic Press, New York. In press.

Baker, J. R. (1974). The evolutionary origin and speciation of the genus *Trypanosoma*. *In:* "Evolution in the Microbial World" (M. J. Carlisle and J. J. Skehel, eds), pp. 343–366. 24th Symposium of the Society of General Microbiology. Cambridge University Press, Cambridge.

Balis, J. (1964). Utilisation des glucides et de leurs produits de métabolism par *Trypanosoma evansi* et *Trypanosoma brucei*. *Revue d'Elévage de Medicine Veterinaire des Pays Tropicals*, **17**, 361–368.

Band, R. N. and Balamuth, W. (1974). Hemin replaces serum as a growth requirement of *Naegleria*. *Applied Microbiology*, **24**, 64–65.

Bash-Lewinson, D. and Grossowicz, N. (1957). Transaminases of *Trypanosoma cruzi*. *Bulletin of the Research Council of Israel*, **GE**, 91–92.

Bello, J. and Bello, H. R. (1976). Chemical modification and cross-linking of proteins by impurities in glycerol. *Archives of Biochemistry and Biophysics*, **172**, 608–612.

Berens, R. L. and Marr, J. J. (1977). Phosphofructokinase of *Leishmania donovani* and *Leishmania braziliensis* and its role in glycolysis. *Journal of Protozoology*, **24**, 340–344.

Bishop, A. (1967). Problems in the cultivation of some parasitic protozoa. *Advances in Parasitology*, **5**, 93–138.

Boiso, J. F. and Stoppani, A. O. M. (1973). The mechanism of acetate and pyruvate oxidation by *Trypanosoma cruzi*. *Journal of Protozoology*, **20**, 673–678.

Boné, G. J. and Parent, G. (1963). Stearic acid, an essential growth factor for *Trypanosoma cruzi*. *Journal of General Microbiology*, **31**, 261–266.

Boné, G., Parent, G. and Steinert, M. (1966). Le culture de trypanosoma en milieu défini. 1st International Congress of Parasitology, Rome 1964. Vol. 1, pp. 297–298. Pergamon, Oxford.

Bowman, I. B. R. and Flynn, I. W. (1976). Oxidative metabolism of trypanosomes. *In:* "Biology of the Kinetoplastida" (W. H. R. Lumsden and D. A. Evans, eds), Vol. 1, pp. 436–476. Academic Press, London and New York.

von Brand, T. E. J. and Higgins, H. (1967). Hexose and glycerol absorption by some *Trypanosomatidae*. *Journal of Protozoology*, **13**, 8–14.

Bray, R. S. (1974). *Leishmania*. *Annual Review of Microbiology*, **28**, 189–217.

Brooker, B. (1971). Fine structure of *Bodo saltans* and *Bodo caudatus* (zoomastigophora; Protozoa) and their affinities with the Trypanosomatidae. *Bulletin of British Museum* (Natural History), **22**, 82–102.

Brun, R. and Jenni, L. (1977). A new semi-defined medium for *Trypanosoma brucei* sspp. *Acta Tropica*, **34**, 21–33.

Bursell, E. (1970). Feeding, digestion and excretion. *In:* "The African Trypanosomiases" (H. W. Mulligan, ed.), pp. 305–316. Allen & Unwin, London; Wiley-Interscience, New York.

Carter, H. E., Gaver, R. C. and Yu, R. K. (1966). A novel branched-chain sphingolipid base from *Crithidia fasciculata*. *Biochemical and Biophysical Research Communications*, **22**, 316–320.

Cerisola, J. A., Del Prado, C. E., Rohwedder, R. and Bozzini, J. O. (1971). *Blasto-*

crithidia triatomae n. sp. found in *Triatoma infestans* from Argentina. *Journal of Protozoology*, **18**, 503–506.

Chalabi, K. and Gutteridge, W. E. (1977). Catabolism of deoxythymidylate in some trypanosomatids. *Parasitology*, **74**, 299–312.

Chang, K.-P. (1975). Haematophagous insect and haemoflagellate as hosts for prokaryotic endosymbionts. *In:* "Symbiosis" (D. H. Jennings and D. L. Lee, eds), Vol. 29, pp. 407–428, *Symposia of the Society for Experimental Biology*. Cambridge University Press, Cambridge.

Chang, K.-P. (1976). Symbiote-free hemoflagellates, *Blastocrithidia culicis* and *Crithidia oncopelti*: their liver factor requirement and serologic identity. *Journal of Protozoology*, **23**, 241–244.

Chang, K.-P., Chang, C. S. and Sassa, S. (1975). Heme biosynthesis in bacterium-protozoon symbioses: Enzyme defects in hemoflagellates and complemental role of their intracellular symbiotes. *Proceedings of the National Academy of Sciences, U.S.A.*, **72**, 2979–2983.

Chang, S. L. (1948). Studies on haemoflagellates. IV. Observations concerning some biochemical activities in culture, and respiration of three species of leishmanias and *Trypanosoma cruzi*. *Journal of Infectious Diseases*, **82**, 109–118.

Citri, N. and Grossowicz, N. (1955). A partially defined culture medium for *Trypanosoma cruzi* and some other haemoflagellates. *Journal of Microbiology*, **13**, 273–278.

Clark, T. B., Kellen, W. R., Lindegren, J. E. and Smith, T. A. (1964). The transmission of *Crithidia fasciculata* Léger 1902 in *Culiseta incidens* (*Thomson*). *Journal of Protozoology*, **11**, 400–402.

Cohen, L. and Zahalsky, A. C. (1968). Freezing colonies of *Crithidia* fasciculata on glycerol-agar plates. *Journal of Protozoology*, **15** (supplement), 23.

Cosgrove, W. B. (1959). Utilization of carbohydrate by the mosquito flagellate, *Crithidia fasciculata*. *Canadian Journal of Microbiology*, **5**, 573–578.

Cosgrove, W. B. (1963). Carbohydrate utilization by trypanosomatids from insects. *Experimental Parasitology*, **13**, 173–177.

Cosgrove, W. B. (1966). Acriflavin-induced akinetoplasty in *Crithidia fasciculata*. *Acta Protozoologica*, **4**, 155–160.

Cosgrove, W. B. and Kessell, R. G. (1958). The activity of the contractile vacuole of *Crithidia fasciculata*. *Journal of Protozoology*, **5**, 296–298.

Cowperthwaite, J., Weber, M. M., Packer, L. and Hutner, S. H. (1953). Nutrition of *Herpetomonas* (*Strigomonas*) *cylicidarum*. *Annals of the New York Academy of Sciences*, **56**, 972–981.

Cross, G. A. M. and Manning, J. C. (1973). Cultivation of *Trypanosoma brucei* sspp. in semi-defined media. *Parasitology*, **67**, 315–331.

Cross, G. A. M., Klein, R. A. and Linstead, D. J. (1975a). Utilization of amino acids by *Trypanosoma brucei* in culture: L-threonine as a precursor for acetate. *Parasitology*, **71**, 311–326.

Cross, G. A. M., Klein, R. A. and Baker, J. R. (1975b). *Trypanosoma cruzi*: growth, amino acid utilization and drug action in a defined medium. *Annals of Tropical Medicine and Parasitology*, **69**, 513–514.

Crowe, W. and Kushner, I. G. (1977). An immunofluorescent method using *Crithidia luciliae* to detect antibodies in double-stranded DNA. *Arthritis and Rheumatism*, **20**, 811–814.

Cruz, F. S. da and Krassner, S. M. (1971). Assimilatory sulfate reduction by the hemoflagellate *Leishmania tarentolae*. *Journal of Protozoology*, **18**, 718–722.

Cunningham, I. (1977). New culture medium for maintenance of tsetse tissue and growth of the trypanosomatids. *Journal of Protozoology*, **24**, 325–329.

Cunningham, L. V., Kazan, B. H. and Kuwahara, S. S. (1972). Effect of long-chain fatty acids on some trypanosomatid flagellates. *Journal of General Microbiology*, **70**, 491–496.

D'Alessandro, A. (1976). Biology of *Trypanosoma* (*Herpetosoma*) *rangeli* Tejera, 1920. *In:* "Biology of the Kinetoplastida" (W. H. R. Lumsden and D. A. Evans, eds), Vol. 1, pp. 328–403. Academic Press, London and New York.

Damper, D. and Patton, C. L. (1976). Pentamidine in *Trypanosoma brucei*—kinetics and specificity. *Biochemical Pharmacology*, **25**, 271–276.

Desser, S. S. (1976). The ultrastructure of the epimastigote stage of *Trypanosoma rotatorium* in the leech *Batracobdella picta*. *Canadian Journal of Zoology*, **54**, 1712–1723.

Dewey, V. C. and Kidder, G. W. (1966). Effects of long-chain mono- and decarboxylic acids on the pteridine requirement of *Crithidia*. *Archives of Biochemistry and Biophysics*, **115**, 401–406.

Dewey, V. C. and Kidder, G. W. (1971). Assay of unconjugated pteridines. *In:* "Methods in Enzymology" (D. B. McCormick and L. D. Wright, eds), Vol. 18B, pp. 618–624. Academic Press, New York and London.

de Zwann, A., Kluytmans, J. H. F. and Zandee, D. I. (1976). Facultative anaerobiosis in molluscs. *In:* "Biochemical Adaptation to Environmental Change" (R. M. S. Smellie and J. F. Pennock, eds), pp. 133–168. Biochemical Society Symposium 41. The Biochemical Society, London.

Dixon, H., Ginger, C. D. and Williamson, J. (1970). The lipid composition of blood and culture forms of *Trypanosoma lewisi* and *Trypanosoma rhodesiense* compared with that of their environment. *Comparative Biochemistry and Physiology*, **33**, 111–128.

Dubois, A. (1936). Utilisation des glucides par *Leishmania tropica*. *Compte Rendu des Séances de la Société de Biologie et des ses Filiales*, **70**, 58–59.

Dusanic, D. G. (1969). Cultivation of *Trypanosoma lewisi* in a dialysate medium. I. Amino acid alterations during growth. *Comparative Biochemistry and Physiology*, **30**, 895–901.

Edwards, C., Statham, M. and Lloyd, D. (1975). The preparation of large-scale synchronous cultures of the trypanosomatid, *Crithidia fasciculata*, by cell-size selection; changes in respiration and adenylate charge through the cell-cycle. *Journal of General Microbiology*, **88**, 141–152.

Eeckhout, Y. (1974). Influence of the division rate on catalase activity of the trypanosomatid flagellate *Crithidia luciliae*. *Cytobiologie*, **8**, 247–256.

Ellenbogen, B. R., Hutner, S. H. and Tamburro, K. M. (1972). Temperature-enhanced osmotic growth requirement of *Crithidia*. *Journal of Protozoology*, **19**, 349–354.

Evans, D. A. and Brown, R. C. (1972). The utilization of glucose and proline by culture forms of *Trypanosoma brucei*. *Journal of Protozoology*, **19**, 686–690.

Fenner, F., McAuslan, B. R., Mims, C. A., Sambrook, J. and White, D. O. (1976). "The Biology of Animal Viruses", 2nd ed. Academic Press, New York and London.

Flavell, R. B. (1971). Mitochondrion as a multifunctional organelle. *Nature, London*, **230**, 504–505.

Fromentin, H. (1973). Souches normales et souches dyskinetoplastiques de trypanosomes chez la souris expérimentalement infectée. Consommation comparee d'oxygène. *Protistologica*, **9**, 353–357.

Frugulhetti, I. C. P. and Rebello, M. A. (1977). Atividade de Enzimas do ciclo do glioxalato em *Herpetomonas samuelpessoa*. Abstracts, p. 50, "Pesquisa Básica em Doença da Chagas". IV. Reunãio Anual. Caxambu Dept. of Chemistry, University of São Paulo.

Fulton, J. D. and Spooner, D. F. (1956). Inhibition of the respiration of

Trypanosoma rhodesiense by thiols. *Biochemical Journal*, **63**, 475–481.

Gaughan, P. L. Z. and Krassner, S. M. (1971). Hemin deprivation in culture stages of the hemoflagellate, *Leishmania tarentolae*. *Comparative Biochemistry and Physiology*, **39B**, 5–18.

Ghosh, D. K. and Datta, A. G. (1971). *Leishmania donovani*: assay for a functional pentose phosphate pathway. *Experimental Parasitology*, **29**, 103–109.

Gibbs, A. J. (1951). *Leptomonas capsularis* n. sp. and other flagellates parasitic in *Cletus ochraceus* (Hemiptera). *Parasitology*, **41**, 129–132.

Godfrey, D. G. and Taylor, A. E. R. (1972). *Trypanosoma brucei brucei*: polycations and the release of alanine aminotransferase. *Experimental Parasitology*, **31**, 407–416.

Golub, E. S. (1977). "The Cellular Basis of the Immune Response". Sinauer Associates, Sunderland, Mass.

Goodwin, L. G. (1974). The African scene: mechanisms of pathogenesis in trypanosomiasis. *In:* "Trypanosomiasis and Leishmaniasis", pp. 107–119. Ciba Foundation Symposium 20 (new series). Elsevier, Amsterdam.

Greenblatt, C. L., Jori, L. A. and Cahnmann, H. J. (1969). Chromatographic separation of a rat serum growth factor required by *Trypanosoma lewisi*. *Experimental Parasitology*, **24**, 228–247.

Gutteridge, W. E. (1969). Presence and properties of diaminopimelic acid decarboxylases in the genus *Crithidia*. *Biochemica Biophysica Acta*, **184**, 366–373.

Gutteridge, W. E. (1976). Chemotherapy of Chagas's disease: the present situation. *Tropical Diseases Bulletin*, **73**, 699–705.

Guttman, H. N. (1963). Experimental glimpses at the lower Trypanosomatidae. *Experimental Parasitology*, **14**, 129–142.

Guttman, H. N. (1964). *Crithidia* assay for unconjugated pteridines. *In:* "Pteridine Chemistry" (W. Pfleiderer and E. C. Taylor, eds), pp. 255–266. Pergamon Press, Oxford.

Guttman, H. N. (1967). Patterns of methionine and lysine biosynthesis in the Trypanosomatidae during growth. *Journal of Protozoology*, **14**, 267–271.

Ham, R. (1974). Nutritional requirements of primary cultures. A neglected problem of modern biology. *In Vitro*, **10**, 119–129.

Harvey, S. C. (1949). The carbohydrate metabolism of *Trypanosoma hippicum*. *Journal of Biological Chemistry*, **179**, 435–453.

Hill, G. C. and Anderson, W. A. (1969). Effects of acriflavine on the mitochondria and kinetoplast of *Crithidia fasciculata*. Correlation of fine structure changes with decreased mitochondrial enzyme activity. *Journal of Cell Biology*, **41**, 537–561.

Hoare, C. A. (1972). "The Trypanosomes of Mammals. A Zoological Monograph", p. 53. Blackwell Scientific Publications, Oxford.

Hochachka, P. W. (1976). Design of metabolic and enzymic machinery to fit lifestyle and environment. *In:* "Biochemical Adaptation to Environmental Change" (R. M. S. Smellie and J. F. Pennock, eds), *Biochemical Society Symposium*, **41**, pp. 3–31. The Biochemical Society, London.

Hunter, F. R. (1960). Aerobic metabolism of *Crithidia fasciculata*. *Experimental Parasitology*, **9**, 271–280.

Hussain, M. A. M., Flynn, D. M., Green, N. and Hoffbrand, A. V. (1977). Effect of dose, time and ascorbate on iron excretion after subcutaneous desferrioxamine. *Lancet*, 1977–i, 977–979.

Hutner, S. H. (1972). Inorganic nutrition. *Annual Review of Microbiology*, **26**, 314–348.

Hutner, S. H. (1977). Essay and reviews of recent symptoms on protozoan chemotherapy. *Journal of Protozoology*, **24**, 475–478.

Iwai, K., Bunno, M., Kobashi, M. and Suzuki, T. (1976). Isolation and characterization of 6-hydroxymethylpterin as the *Crithidia* growth-promoting factor from spinach chloroplasts. *Biochimica et Biophysica Acta*, **444**, 613–617.

Janakidevi, K., Dewey, V. C. and Kidder, G. W. (1966a). The biosynthesis of catecholamines in two genera of protozoa. *Journal of Biological Chemistry*, **241**, 2576–2578.

Janakidevi, K., Dewey, W. C. and Kidder, G. W. (1966b). Serotonin in protozoa. *Archives of Biochemistry and Biophysics*, **113**, 758–759.

Jeuniaux, C. (1971). Hemolymph—Arthropoda. *In:* "Chemical Zoology", Arthropoda. Part, B, pp. 63–118 (M. Florkin and B. T. Scheer, eds). Academic Press, New York and London.

Kallinokova, V. D. (1968). Cytochemical studies of enzymes of the respiratory chain in the life cycle of *Trypanosoma cruzi* Chagas, 1909. II. Respiratory enzymes of crithidial forms in the course of cultivation and some observations on the growth of the culture. *Acta Protozoologica*, **6**, 87–96.

Keenan, K., Erlich, E., Donnelly, K. H., Basel, M. B., Hutner, S. H., Kassoff, R. and Crawford, S. A. (1978). Particulate-based axenic media for tetrahymenids. *Journal of Protozoology*, **25**. In press.

Keppel, A. D. and Janovy, J. (1977). *Herpetomonas megaseliae* and *Crithidia harmosa*: growth of blood-agar plates. *Journal of Parasitology*, **63**, 879–882.

Kidder, G. W. (1967). Nitrogen: distribution, nutrition, and metabolism. *In:* "Chemical Zoology. Vol. I. Protozoa" (G. W. Kidder, ed.), pp. 93–159. Academic Press, New York and London.

Kidder, G. W. and Dewey, V. C. (1972). Methionine or folate and phosphoenolpyruvate in the biosynthesis of threonine in *Crithidia fasciculata*. *Journal of Protozoology*, **19**, 93–98.

Kidder, G. W. and Dewey, V. C. (1975). Some aspects of the initiation of protein synthesis in *Crithidia fasciculata* and *Tetrahymena pyriformis*. *Comparative Biochemistry and Physiology*, **52B**, 537–539.

Kidder, G. W. and Dutta, B. N. (1958). The growth and nutrition of *Crithidia fasciculata*. *Journal of General Microbiology*, **18**, 621–638.

Kidder, G. W. and Nolan, L. L. (1973). Pteridine-requiring dihydroorotate hydroxylase from *Crithidia fasciculata*. *Biochemical and Biophysical Research Communications*, **53**, 929–936.

Kidder, G. W., Davis, J. S. and Cousens, K. (1966). Citrulline utilization in *Crithidia*. *Biochemical and Biophysical Research Communications*, **24**, 365–369.

Kidder, G. W., Dewey, V. C. and Rembold, H. (1967). The origin of unconjugated pteridines in *Crithidia fasciculata*. *Archives für Mikrobiologie*, **59**, 180–184.

Killick-Kendrick, R., Molyneux, D. H. and Ashford, R. W. (1974). *Leishmania* in phlebotomid sandflies. I. Modifications of the flagellum associated with attachment to the mid-gut and oesophageal valve of the sandfly. *Proceedings of the Royal Society of London*, **187B**, 409–419.

Klein, A., Linstead, D. J. and Wheeler, M. V. (1975). Carbon dioxide fixation in trypanosomatids. *Parasitology*, **71**, 93–107.

Kobashi, M. and Iwai, K. (1971). Biochemical studies on naturally occurring pteridines. II. Isolation and characterization of *L-threoneopterin*, as the *Crithidia* factor, and of isoxanthopterin produced by *Serratia indica*. *Agricultural and Biological Chemistry*, **35**, 47–50.

Krassner, S. W. and Flory, B. (1971). Essential amino acids in the culture of *Leishmania tarentolae*. *Journal of Parasitology*, **57**, 917–920.

Kusel, J. P. and Storey, B. T. (1976). Midpoint potentials of the mitochondrial cytochromes of *Crithidia fasciculata*. *Journal of Bacteriology*, **127**, 812–816.

Langreth, S. G. and Balber, A. F. (1975). Protein uptake and digestion in blood-stream and culture forms of *Trypanosoma brucei*. *Journal of Protozoology*, **22**, 40–53.

Langridge, D. F. and McGhee, R. B. (1967). *Crithidia mellifera* n. sp. an acidophilic trypanosomatid of the honey bee *Apis mellifera*. *Journal of Protozoology*, **14**, 485–487.

Leeming, R. J. and Blair, J. A. (1974). *Crithidia* factors in human urine. *Biochemical Medicine*, **11**, 122–128.

Leeming, R. J., Blair, J. A., Melikian, V. and O'Gorman, D. J. (1976). Biopterin derivatives in human body fluids and tissues. *Journal of Clinical Pathology*, **29**, 444–451.

Linnane, A. W. and Lukens, H. B. (1975). Isolation of mitochondria and techniques for studying mitochondrial biogenesis in yeasts. *Methods in Cell Biology*, **12**, 285–309.

Linstead, D. J., Klein, R. A. and Eldridge, M. V. (1975). Carboxylation reactions in trypanosomatids. *Transactions of the Royal Society of Tropical Medicine and Hygiene*, **69**, 267–268.

Linstead, D. J., Klein, R. A. and Cross, G. A. M. (1977). Threonine catabolism in *Trypanosoma brucei*. *Journal of General Microbiology*, **101**, 243–251.

Little, P. A. and Oleson, J. J. (1951). The cultivation of *Trypanosoma cruzi*. *Journal of Bacteriology*, **61**, 709–714.

Lumsden, W. H. R. (1974). Biochemical taxonomy of *Leishmania*. *Transactions of the Royal Society of Tropical Medicine and Hygiene*, **68**, 74–75.

Lundberg, W. O. and Järvi, P. (1971). Peroxidation of polyunsaturated fatty compounds. *In:* "Progress in the Chemistry of Fats and Other Lipids" (R. T. Holman, eds), Vol. II, pp. 379–406. Pergamon Press, Oxford.

Lwoff, A. (1934). Die Bedeutung des Blutfarbstoffes für die parasitischen Flagellaten. *Zentralblatt für Bakteriologie, Parasitologie und Infektionskunde. I. Abteilung. Originale*, **130**, 497–518.

Lwoff, M. (1938). L'hématine et l'acide ascorbique, facteurs de croissance pour le flagellé *Schizotrypanum cruzi*. *Comptes Rendus Hebdomadaire des Séances de l'Académie des Sciences, Paris*, **206**, 540–542.

Lwoff, M. (1951). The nutrition of parasite flagellates (Trypanosomidae, Trichomonadinae). *In:* "Biochemistry and Physiology of Protozoa" (A. Lwoff, ed.), Vol. 1, pp. 129–176. Academic Press, New York.

Mancilla, R. and Naquira, C. (1964). Comparative metabolism of C^{14}-glucose in two strains of *Trypanosoma cruzi*. *Journal of Protozoology*, **11**, 509–513.

Marinkelle, C. J. (1976). Biology of the trypanosomes of bats. *In:* "Biology of the Kinetoplastida" (W. H. R. Lumsden and D. A. Evans, eds), Vol. 1, pp. 175–216. Academic Press, London and New York.

Marr, J. J. and Berens, R. L. (1977). Regulation of aerobic fermentation in protozoans. VI. Comparative biochemistry of pathogenic and non-pathogenic protozoans. *Acta Tropica*, **34**, 143–155.

Marr, J. J., Birenbaum, M. E. and Ladenson, J. M. (1977). *Crithidia fasciculata*: Appearance kinetics of intermediates and regulation of aerobic fermentation. *Experimental Parasitology*, **42**, 322–330.

Mattingly, P. F. (1965). The evolution of parasite-arthropod vector systems. *In:* "Evolution of Parasites" (A. E. R. Taylor, ed.), pp. 29–45. Blackwell Scientific Publications, Oxford.

Mattock, N. M. (1975). Electrophoretic investigation of some dehydrogenases in *Leishmania* amastigotes. *Annals of Tropical Medicine and Parasitology*, **69**, 345–348.

McCullough, C. H. R. and Dee, J. (1976). Defined and semi-defined media for the growth of amoebae of *Physarum polycephalum*. *Journal of General Microbiology*, **95**, 151–158.

McGhee, R. B. and Postell, F. J. (1976). Axenic cultivation of *Phytomonas davidi* Lafont (Trypanosomatidae), a symbiote of laticiferous plants (Euphorbiaceae). *Journal of Protozoology*, **23**, 238–241.

McGhee, R. B., Hanson, W. L. and Schmittner, S. M. (1969). Isolation, cloning and determination of biologic characteristics of fine new species of *Crithidia*. *Journal of Protozoology*, **16**, 514–520.

Medina, H., Amaral, D. and Bacila, M. (1955). Estudos sobre o metabolismo de protozoarios do género *Leishmania*. I. Vias de oxidaçao da glucose e do acetato pela *Leishmania braziliensis* Vianna, 1911. *Arquivos de Biologia e Technologia*, **10**, 97–102.

Meshnick, S. R., Chang, K.-P. and Cerami, A. (1977). Heme lysis of the bloodstream forms of *Trypanosoma brucei*. *Biochemical Pharmacology*, **26**, 1923–1928.

Metzler, D. E. (1977). "Biochemistry. The Chemical Reactions of Living Cells". Academic Press, New York and London.

Meyer, H. and Holz, G. G., Jr. (1966). Biosynthesis of lipids by kinetoplastid flagellates. *Journal of Biological Chemistry*, **241**, 5000–5007.

Molyneux, D. H. (1977). The attachment of *Trypanosoma grayi* in the hindgut of *Glossina*. *Protozoology*, **3** (Festschr. C. A. Hoare, F.R.S.) London School of Hygiene and Tropical Medicine.

Moulder, J. W. (1948). The oxidative metabolism of *Trypanosoma lewisi* in a phosphate-saline medium. *Journal of Infectious Diseases*, **83**, 33–41.

Mukkada, A. J. (1977). Tricarboxylic acid and glyoxylate cycles in the *Leishmaniae*. *Acta Tropica*, **34**, 167–175.

Mundim, M. H. and Roitman, I. (1977). Extra nutritional requirements of artificially aposymbiotic *Crithidia deanei*. *Journal of Protozoology*, **24**, 329–331.

Neal, R. A. and Miles, R. A. (1963). Heat blood agar medium for the growth of *Trypanosoma cruzi* and some species of *Leishmania*. *Nature, London*, **198**, 210–211.

Newton, B. A. (1976). Biochemical approaches to the taxonomy of kinetoplastid flagellates. *In:* "Biology of the Kinetoplastida" (W. H. R. Lumsden and D. A. Evans, eds), Vol. 1, pp. 405–434. Academic Press, London and New York.

Nishiuch, Y., Sasaki, M., Nakayasu, M. and Oikawa, A. (1976). Cytotoxicity of cysteine in culture media. *In Vitro*, **12**, 635.

Oliveira, M. M., Timm, S. L. and Costa, S. C. G. (1977). Lipid composition of *Trypanosoma cruzi*. *Comparative and Biochemical Physiology*, **58B**, 195–199.

Orias, E. and Rasmussen, L. (1977). Dual capacity for nutrient uptake in *Tetrahymena*. II. Role of the two systems in vitamin uptake. *Journal of Protozoology*, **24**, 507–511.

Opperdoes, F. R., Borst, P., Bakker, S. and Leene, W. (1977). Localization of glycerol-3-phosphate oxidase in the mitochondrion and particulate NAD-linked glycerol-3-phosphate dehydrogenase in the microbodies of the bloodstream form of *Trypanosoma brucei*. *European Journal of Biochemistry*, **76**, 29–39.

Palmer, F. B. (1974). Biosynthesis of choline and ethanolamine phospholipids in *Crithidia fasciculata*. *Journal of Protozoology*, **21**, 160–163.

Pettigrew, G. W., Leaver, J. L., Meyer, T. E. and Ryle, A. P. (1975). Purification, properties and amino acid sequence of atypical cytochrome *c* from two protozoa, *Euglena gracilis* and *Crithidia oncopelti*. *Biochemical Journal*, **147**, 291–302.

Pittam, M. D. (1966). *In vitro* culture of African trypanosomes in a partially defined medium. *1st International Congress of Parasitology*, Rome, 1964, 1, pp. 330–331. Pergamon Press, Oxford.

Razin, S. (1973). Physiology of mycoplasms. *Advances in Microbial Physiology*, **10**, 1–80.

Rembold, H. and Heinz, G. (1971). L-threo-neopterin, the major pterin in *Escherichia coli* B. *Hoppe-Seyler's Zeitschrift für Physiologische Chemie*, **352**, 1271–1272.

Rembold, H., Vaubel, A. and Rao, P. J. (1974). Effect of sugars, Na^+-, and K^+-ions on biopterin transport in *Crithidia fasciculata*. *Archives of Microbiology*, **97**, 51–62.

Roberts, C. J. and Clarkson, M. J. (1977). Free fatty acids, lysophosphatidyl choline, and pathogenesis of trypanosomiasis. *Lancet*, **1977–i**, 952–953.

Roitman, C., Roitman, I. and Azevedo, H. P. (1972). Growth of an insect trypanosomatid at 37°C in a defined medium. *Journal of Protozoology*, **19**, 346–347.

Ruff, M. D. and Read, C. P. (1974). Specificity of carbohydrate transport in *Trypanosoma equiperdum*. *Parasitology*, **68**, 103–115.

Ryley, J. F. (1951). Studies on the metabolism. *1*. Metabolism of the paracitic flagellate, *Trypanosoma lewisi*. *Biochemical Journal*, **49**, 577–585.

Ryley, J. F. (1962). Studies on the metabolism of the protozoa. 9. Comparative metabolism of blood-stream and culture forms of *Trypanosoma rhodesiense*. *Biochemical Journal*, **85**, 211–223.

Ryley, F. (1966). Histochemical studies on the blood and culture forms of *Trypanosoma rhodesiense*. *In:* "Proceedings of the 1st International Congress of Parasitology, Rome, 1964", Vol. I, pp. 41–42. Pergamon Press, Oxford.

Schaefer, F. W. and Mukkada, A. J. (1976). Specificity of the glucose transport system in *Leishmania tropica* promastigotes. *Journal of Protozoology*, **23**, 446–449.

Schlemper, B. R., Chiari, E. and Brener, Z. (1977). Growth-inhibition drug test with *Trypanosoma cruzi* culture forms. *Journal of Protozoology*, **24**, 544–547.

Searle, D. S. and Reiner, L. (1940). Effect of carbon dioxide on glucose metabolism of trypanosomes. *Proceedings of the Society for Experimental Biology and Medicine*, **43**, 80–82.

Shapiro, A., DiLello, D., Loudis, M. C., Keller, D. and Hutner, S. H. (1977). Minimal requirements in defined media for improved growth of some radioresistant pink tetracocci. *Applied and Environmental Microbiology*, **33**, 1129–1133.

Shapiro, A., Hutner, S. H., Katz, L., Bacchi, C. J., Tamburro, K. O. and Baker, H. (1978). Dense *Crithidia* growth and heme sparing; relation to Fe, Cu, Mo chelation. *Journal of Protozoology*. In press.

Sheets, E. M. and Krassner, S. M. (1972). Taurine utilization in *Leishmania tarentolae*. Abstract of the 47th Meeting of the American Society of Parasitologists, Miami, p. 27.

Sheets, E. G. and Krassner, S. M. (1974). "Trace metabolites"—effect of high concentrations on *Leishmania tarentolae* promastigotes. *Journal of Protozoology*, **21**, 742–744.

Simon, M. W., Rusnak, J. M. and Mukkada, A. J. (1976). Toxicity of bilirubin to *Leishmania tropica* promastigotes. *Experimental Parasitology*, **39**, 51–58.

Simpson, L. (1968a). The leishmania-leptomonad transformation of *Leishmania donovani*: nutritional requirements, respiration changes and antigenic changes. *Journal of Protozoology*, **15**, 201–207.

Simpson, L. (1968b). Effect of acriflavin on the kinetoplast of *Leishmania tarentolae*. Mode of action and physiological correlates of the loss of kinetoplast DNA. *Journal of Cell Biology*, **37**, 660–682.

Slater, N. G. P., Cameron, J. S. and Lessof, M. M. (1976). The *Crithidia luciliae* kinetoplast immunofluorescence test in systemic lupus erythematosus. *Clinical and Experimental Immunology*, **25**, 480–486.

Soldo, A. T. and Godoy, G. A. (1974). A requirement for an unconjugated pteridine for the growth of *Paramecium aurelia*. *Biochimica et Biophysica Acta*, **362**, 521–526.

Southgate, B. A. and Wilson, V. C. L. C. *Leishmania* in lizards. This volume.

Southworth, G. C. and Read, C. P. (1970). Specificity of sugar transport in *Trypanosoma gambiense*. *Journal of Protozoology*, **17**, 396–399.

Steiger, R. F. and Meshnick, S. R. (1977). Amino-acid and glucose utilization of *Leishmania donovani* and *L. braziliensis*. *Transactions of the Royal Society of Tropical Medicine*, **71**, 441–443.

Steiger, R. F. and Steiger, E. (1977). Cultivation of *Leishmania donovani* and *Liehsmania braziliensis* in defined media: nutritional requirements. *Journal of Protozoology*, **24**, 437–441.

Steiger, R. F., Steiger, E., Trager, W. and Schneider, I. (1977). *Trypanosoma congolense*: partial cyclic development in a *Glossina* cell system and oxygen consumption. *Journal of Parasitology*, **63**, 861–867.

Steinert, M. (1965). The morphogenesis of trypanosomes. *In:* "Progress in Protozoology" (abstracts of papers, 2nd International Congress of Protozoology), p. 76. Excerpta Medica, Amsterdam.

Stibbs, H. H. and Seed, J. R. (1974). Short-term metabolism of [^{14}C] tryptophan in rats infected with *Trypanosoma brucei gambiense*. *Journal of Infectious Diseases*, **131**, 459–462.

Stibbs, H. H. and Seed, J. R. (1975). Metabolism of tyrosine and phenylalanine in *Trypanosoma brucei gambiense*. *International Journal of Biochemistry*, **6**, 197–203.

Storm, J. and Hutner, S. H. (1953). Nutrition of *Peranema*. *Annals of the New York Academy of Sciences*, **56**, 901–909.

Swale, E. M. E. (1973). A study of the colourless flagellate *Rhynchomonas nasuta* (Stokes) Klebs. *Biological Journal of the Linnean Society*, **5**, 255–264.

Sylvester, D. and Krassner, S. M. (1976). Proline metabolism in *Trypanosoma cruzi* epimastigotes. *Comparative Biochemistry and Physiology*, **55B**, 443–447.

Tamburro, K. M. and Hutner, S. H. (1971). Carbohydrate-free media for *Crithidia*. *Journal of Protozoology*, **18**, 667–672.

Taylor, A. E. R. and Baker, J. R. (1968). Part 1. Cultivation of protozoa. 1. Trypanosomatidae. *In:* "The Cultivation of Parasites *In Vitro*", pp. 3–52. Blackwell Scientific Publications, Oxford.

Tizard, I. R., Nielsen, K., Mellors, A. and Assoku, R. K. (1977). Free fatty acids and pathogenesis of African trypanosomiasis. *Lancet*, **1977–i**, 750–751.

Trager, W. (1957). Nutrition of a haemoflagellate (*Leishmania tarentolae*) having an interchangeable requirement for choline and pyridoxal. *Journal of Protozoology*, **4**, 269–276.

Trager, W. (1969). Pteridine requirement of the hemoflagellate *Leishmania tarentolae*. *Journal of Protozoology*, **16**, 372–375.

Trager, W. (1974). Nutrition and biosynthetic capabilities of flagellates: problems of *in vitro* cultivaion and differentiation. *In:* "Trypanosomiasis and Leishmaniasis, with Special Reference to Chagas' Disease", pp. 20, 225–245. Ciba Foundation Symposium. Associated Scientific Publishers, Amsterdam.

Vakirtzi-Lemonias, C., Karahalios, C. C. and Levis, G. M. (1972). Fatty acid oxidation in *Crithidia fasciculata*. *Canadian Journal of Biochemistry*, **50**, 501–506.

Van Campen, D. (1972). Effect of histidine and ascorbic acid on the absorption and retention of ^{59}Fe by iron-depleted rats. *Journal of Nutrition*, **102**, 165–170.

Vanfleteren, J. R. (1974). Nematode growth factor. *Nature, London*, **248**, 255–257.

Venkatesan, S. and Ormerod, W. E. (1976). Lipid contents of the slender and stumpy forms of *Trypanosoma brucei rhodesiense*: a comparative study. *Comparative and Biochemical Physiology*, **53B**, 481–487.

Vickerman, K. (1976). The diversity of the kinetoplastid flagellates. *In:* "Biology of the Kinetoplastida" (W. H. R. Lumsden and D. A. Evans, eds), Vol. 1, pp. 1–34. Academic Press, London and New York.

Vickerman, K. (1977). The dyskinetoplasty mutation in *Trypanosoma evansi* and other flagellates. *Protozoology, Vol. III* (Festeschrift in honour of C. A. Hoare), pp. 57–69. London School of Hygiene and Tropical Medicine.

Vickerman, K. and Preston, T. M. (1976). Comparative cell biology of the kinetoplastid flagellates. *In:* "Biology of the Kinetoplastida" (W. H. R. Lumsden, and D. A. Evans, eds), Vol. 1, 35–130.

Wagner, K. P. and Krassner, S. M. (1976). *Leishmania tarentolae*: proline anabolism in promastigotes. *Experimental Parasitology*, **39**, 186–194.

Wallace, F. G., Todd, S. R. and Rogers, W. (1965). Flagellate parasites of water striders with a description of *Leptomonas costoris*, n. sp. *Journal of Protozoology*, **12**, 390–393.

Wigglesworth, V. B. (1972). "The Principles of Insect Physiology", 7th ed., pp. 555–559. Chapman and Hall, London.

Wilson, G. S. and Miles, A. (1975). "Topley and Wilson's Principles of Bacteriology, Virology and Immunity", Vol. 1, pp. 613–645. E. Arnold, London.

Wood, D. E. and Schiller, E. L. (1975). *Trypanosoma cruzi*: fatty acid metabolism *in vitro*. *Experimental Parasitology*, **37**, 60–66.

Wyatt, G. R. (1975). Hemolymph in insects and arachnids—some biochemical features. *In:* "Invertebrate Immunity. Mechanisms of invertebrate vector-parasite relations" (K. Maramorosch and R. E. Shope, eds), pp. 225–240. Academic Press, New York and London.

Yoshida, N., Freymuller, E. and Wallace, F. G. (1977). *Herpetomonas mariadeanei* sp. n. (Protozoa, Trypanosomatidae) from *Muscina stabulans* (Fallen, 1816) (Diptera: Muscidae). Abstract P. 1, "Pesquisa Básica em Doença de Chagas. IV. Reunião Anual. Caxambu". Dept. of Chemistry. University of São Paulo.

Zeledón, R. (1971). Cultivation and transformation of hemoflagellates. *Revista de Biologia Tropical*, **19**, 192–210.

Zeledón, R. and Monge, E. D. (1967). Physiological studies on the culture forms of four strains of *Leishmania braziliensis*. I. Nitrogen content, substrate utilization, and effect of metabolic inhibitors on respiration and its relation to infectivity. *Journal of Parasitology*, **53**, 937–945.

Zilberblat, G. S. (1969). Mass cultivation of pathogenic Trypanosomidae. *In:* "Progress in Protozoology" (abstracts of papers, 3rd International Congress of Protozoology), pp. 21–22. Publishing House "Nauka", Leningrad; Swets and Zeitlinger N. V., Amsterdam.

Zuckerman, A. and Lainson, R. (1977). Leishmania. *In:* "Parasitic Protozoa. Vol. 1. Taxonomy, Kinetoplastids and Flagellates of Fish" (J. P. Kreier, ed.), pp. 57–133. Academic Press, New York and London.

15

Characterization, Nomenclature and Maintenance of Salivarian Trypanosomes

Edited by

W. H. R. LUMSDEN and D. S. KETTERIDGE

Department of Medical Protozoology,
London School of Hygiene and Tropical Medicine,
London, England

I. Introduction 694
   A. Current usages in characterization and taxonomy . . 695
   B. Deficiencies of current usages 695
   C. Requirements of a serviceable system 697
   D. Reviews of practice in allied fields 697

II. Characterization Techniques and their Limitations . . . 699
   A. Intrinsic characters 699
   B. Extrinsic characters 707
   C. Numerical taxonomy 710
   D. Consideration of usefulness of different characters . . 710

III. Definitions and Nomenclature. 711
   A. Terms relating to Linnaean taxa 711
   B. Operational terms without implication of characterization . 711
   C. Terms implying characterization 712
   D. Nomenclature of variable antigen types (VATs). . . 712

IV. Relationship of characterized populations to Linnaean taxa . 713
   A. Genus 713
   B. Section 713
   C. Subgenus 713
   D. Species and subspecies 713

V. Maintenance of reference collections. 714
   A. Living organisms 714
   B. Antigens 714

C. Antisera 714

D. Biochemical products 714

VI. Documentation of reference collections 715

A. Designation of materials 715

VII. References 715

VIII. Appendix A 719

IX. Appendix B 720

X. Appendix C 721

I. Introduction

The Informal Consultation on Antigenic Variation in Trypanosomiasis, held by the World Health Organization in Geneva in December 1975, recognized the need to improve methods of defining, denoting and maintaining salivarian trypanosome materials, and so an international Meeting was arranged—Characterization, Nomenclature and Maintenance of Salivarian Trypanosomes—in the London School of Hygiene and Tropical Medicine in September 1976 to consider these matters. The Meeting brought together twenty-two workers* from the United Kingdom and from the continents of Europe and Africa; it was supported jointly by the Wellcome Trust and the Ministry of Overseas Development of the United Kingdom Government.

The Meeting considered present usages in characterization, taxonomy and laboratory maintenance of the trypanosomes present as pathogens of man (African sleeping sickness) and domestic stock (ngana), and compared these with practices in other fields of microbiology, particularly in other fields of protozoology, in bacteriology and mycology. Methods for the characterization of trypanosomes are developing rapidly at present and are further advanced with these organisms than with any other protozoal pathogen. They may form, therefore, a useful model for the development of similar approaches in other parasitic Protozoa. The recommendations of the Meeting are published in full in the Bulletin of the World Health Organization (Anon. 1978); it has seemed valuable, however, to include in this volume the reports of the discussion on which these recommendations were made, together with a summary of the recommendations. Since most of the contributions were compiled before the recommendations were available to authors, not all of them

---

* *Participants:* J. R. Baker, K. N. Brown, D. G. Godfrey, W. J. Herbert, S. P. Lapage, D. Le Ray, W. H. R. Lumsden, P. Mattern, A. R. Njogu, P. de Raadt, J. Somerville, M. Steinert, N. van Meirvenne, K. Vickerman. *Observers:* D. Barry, E. U. Canning, M. L. Chance, D. S. Ketteridge, M. A. Miles. *Advisers:* L. R. Hill, A. H. S. Onions, A. J. Westlake.

will follow these conventions; but the comparison of usages should be useful and may generate further improvement in practice.

A. CURRENT USAGES IN CHARACTERIZATION AND TAXONOMY

The presently accepted morphological characters used to characterize the salivarian *Trypanosoma* spp. and their taxonomic arrangement are summarized in Table 1. Species names other than those quoted in the Table are in use, but, essentially, uncontroversial morphological differentiation of organisms (based mainly on the characters of the kinetoplast, the flagellum and the undulating membrane) is between the subgenera *Duttonella, Nannomonas* and *Trypanozoon; Pycnomonas* occupies a more dubious position. The morphological differentiation of species within the subgenera is less definite, often involving biometrical operations, separating populations on a statistical basis, rather than individual organisms.

The morphological differentiations described above often correlate with, or are extended by, biological characteristics such as host–parasite relationships. For instance:

The subgeneric classification of *Duttonella, Nannomonas* and *Trypanozoon* correlates with differences in cyclical development in *Glossina* (tsetse fly), i.e. whether cyclical development involves, respectively, the proboscis only, the midgut and the proboscis, or the midgut and the salivary glands.

The clinical picture in man is used to differentiate subspecies of *Trypanosoma* (*Trypanozoon*) *brucei* into "nosodemes", those subspecies which do not infect man (*T.* (*T.*) *b. brucei*) or which cause an acute disease (*T.* (*T.*) *b. rhodesiense*) or a chronic one (*T.* (*T.*) *b. gambiense*).

Beyond these, generally accepted, concepts there are virtually no agreed systems for characterization and taxonomy.

B. DEFICIENCIES OF CURRENT USAGES

In the field, hosts, both mammal and insect, may have undergone several infective episodes, and so the trypanosome populations derived from them, seen in blood films or established in laboratory animals, may be highly heterogeneous. This fact has not always been recognized in the past.

Even for homogeneous trypanosome populations, methods for characterization are in only early stages of development, so that correlations between objectively characterized trypanosome populations and particular pathogenic outcomes are still largely lacking. So also are epidemiological applications, such as the large-scale identification of the animal

Table 1. Main morphological features of some salivarian trypanosomes as seen in blood or tissue fluids of the vertebrate host[a]

Subgenus	Species	Length μm	Breadth μm	Kinetoplast		Posterior end	Free flagellum
				Size	Position		
Duttonella	T. vivax vivax	21–26	1·5–2·0	Large	Terminal	Blunt, rounded	Long
	T. v. viennei	21–26	1·5–2·0				
	T. v. uniforme	14–17	1·5				
Nannomonas	T. congolense	12–18	1·0–2·0	Medium	Sub-terminal, marginal	Usually blunt	Usually absent
	(T. simiae)	17–18	1·0–2·0				
Pycnomonas	T. suis	15	3·5	Small	Sub-terminal	Pointed, very short	Short
Trypanozoon	T. brucei sspp. slender forms	c. 30	1·5	Small	Sub-terminal	Blunt, often truncate	Long
	stumpy forms	c. 18	3·5				
	T. b. evansi	20–28	1·5	Small	Sub-terminal		
	(T. equinum)	20–28	1·5	Absent	—	Blunt or truncate	
	T. b. equiperdum	20–28	1·5	Small	Sub-terminal	Blunt, rounded	Usually absent

[a] Adapted from Baker (1972).

hosts harbouring populations of trypanosomes capable of infecting man, e.g. the reservoirs of *T. (T.) b. rhodesiense* in eastern Africa.

C. REQUIREMENTS OF A SERVICEABLE SYSTEM

Any serviceable system of general taxonomy and description must depend on the development of techniques for the laboratory recognition (i.e., characterization) of homogeneous trypanosome populations. Such a requirement presupposes the purification of the trypanosome populations (by cloning) and the setting-up of systems of identification which are strictly reproducible. There is also a requirement for a standard terminology to allow interlaboratory comparisons.

Initial studies for the development of methods may be on laboratory-adapted stocks in sophisticated situations, but such studies should keep in mind the need to develop as soon as possible simple methods for application in the field to small numbers of organisms.

Such precisely carried-out investigations hold promise of practical application in such spheres as:

pathogenesis; epidemiology in relation to wild and domestic animal hosts; emergence of drug-resistant populations in nature; distribution of specially virulent, and non-virulent, trypanosome populations in nature; immunological studies on pathogenic potential of organisms; recognition of host responses to pathogenic organisms; consideration of the possibility of vaccination procedures or the efficient induction of immunity by controlled husbandry and/or chemotherapy.

D. REVIEWS OF PRACTICE IN ALLIED FIELDS

Such reviews were provided for the consideration of the Meeting for the Sporozoa (E. U. Canning), for the Ciliophora (J. Somerville), for the Procaryotae (S. P. Lapage) and for the fungi (A. H. S. Onions). Short summaries are included here and the more extended treatments are included as Appendices A-C.

1. Sporozoa

Sporozoa are sexually reproducing Protozoa, and the concept of a species is based on sexual compatibility and the production of viable offspring. Subspecies are populations within a species isolated from one another so that distinctive characters are maintained. Terms in use to designate materials include isolate, strain, line and variant (see Appendix A).

2. Ciliophora

At the generic level, the classification of ciliates is based upon morphological and ecological characteristics. Species of ciliates can be accurately defined by their ability to interbreed and produce viable daughter cells. A strain or stock (equivalent usage in different genera) of a ciliate species is a laboratory-maintained culture which is derived from the wild, cloned and given an alphabetical or numerical designation. In certain instances, for example within the genus *Paramecium*, the cloning is a very exacting procedure because the clone is derived from a single cell that has been induced to become genetically homozygous by the process of autogamy. Strains/stocks have been characterized in *Tetrahymena, Paramecium* and other well-studied ciliates with respect to features such as serotype expression, isoenzyme patterns and presence of specific endosymbionts.

3. Bacteria

The Kingdom Procaryotae has been divided into two divisions, the bacteria and the blue-green algae, and several classes of these have been proposed. Lower categories, such as family, tribe, genus and species have been used at such different levels through the Kingdom that they cannot be equated, e.g. some medically-important bacteria have been elevated to disproportionately high rank as compared with other bacteria. Uniform criteria for the levels of taxa in the hierarchy are required. The tendency has been to use the *taxospecies*, based on similarity determined by numerical methods, or *nomenspecies*, based on similarity to a nomenclatural type. Because methods of gene exchange are so various, classification by *genospecies* has not been fruitful. Subspecies is little employed, but other infraspecific terms, e.g. serovar, chemovar, phagovar, *forma specialis*, etc., are in use (see Appendix B).

4. Fungi

The fungi comprise some 250 000 species of widely diverse characteristics which seem to occupy a position separate from both the plant and animal kingdoms. They adopt three distinct methods of nutrition—by photosynthesis, by ingestive nutrition and by absorptive nutrition. Present classification is based on the morphology of the sexual reproductive elements. Sexual reproduction is considered characteristic of fungi, although it has not been observed yet in all fungal taxa.

Classification depends at present on comparison with deposited "type" material. Living cultures are not yet accepted as type material.

Many systems of classification have been proposed but that of Ainsworth (1971) is now fairly generally accepted. Names follow the binominal system. The ranks of taxa follow the International Code of Botanical Nomenclature 1972. However, the Code does not define these ranks. It is generally agreed that all these terms and classification are in general a matter of convenience. However, discussion amongst taxonomists is constant, though each has a fairly definite idea as to what constitutes a species within his area of expertise.

Hawksworth (1974) discusses the concepts of species, subspecies, variety and form.

The terms isolate, strain, line, clone, etc., do not appear in the International Code. However, "An Annotated Glossary of Botanical Nomenclature" by R. McVaugh, R. Ross and F. A. Stafleu (1968) includes them amongst definitions prepared by a committee appointed as a result of the meetings of the Nomenclatural Section at the 10th International Botanical Congress at Edinburgh, 1964. Other sets of definitions are to be found in "A Guide to the Use of Terms in Plant Pathology", prepared in 1973 by the Terminology Sub-committee of the Federation of British Plant Pathologists and issued as Phytopathological Paper No. 17 of the Commonwealth Mycological Institute, Kew. This lists five uses of the word "strain". (See Appendix C.)

II. Characterization Techniques and their Limitations

A. INTRINSIC CHARACTERS (Lumsden, 1974)

1. Morphology

Gross morphological differences between comparable stages of the life-cycles of trypanosomes have been used to distinguish sub-genera and species, e.g. differences in length (*T. vivax* and *T. uniforme*), size and position of kinetoplast (all subgenera), and sustained presence or absence of free flagellum (subgenera *Duttonella* and *Nannomonas*) (Hoare, 1972). Ultrastructural differences also occur at the subgeneric level, e.g. surface coat compact (*Nannomonas*, *Trypanozoon*) or diffuse (*Duttonella*), mitochondrion lying on abflagellar side of nucleus (*Nannomonas*, *Trypanozoon*) instead of adflagellar side (*Duttonella*), tubular mitochondrial cristae present in all bloodstream stages and plate-like cristae in all vector stages (*Duttonella*, *Nannomonas*) or cristae absent in multiplicative bloodstream stage, tubular in non-multiplicative bloodstream stage and vector salivary gland stages, and plate-like cristae present only in vector midgut stages (*Trypanozoon*) (Vickerman, 1974; Vickerman and Preston, 1976).

Structural and ultrastructural characters have not so far proved helpful in distinguishing subspecies of *Trypanozoon*. Dyskinetoplastic stocks* of *T. brucei* and *T. evansi* which are indistinguishable by conventional light microscopy are found at the level of the electron microscope to differ in the distribution of the kinetoplast remnant material. This material may

---

* Terms used in this paper conform to the usages recommended by the Meeting (see p. 711 *et seq.* and Anon. (1978)).

be unitary and central, or fragmented and dispersed within the mito-chondrion (Vickerman and Preston, 1976). New cytochemical staining techniques employing DNA-specific fluorescent stains may enable these differences to be discerned at the level of the light microscope (Hajduk, 1976).

2. Physiological characteristics

(a) *Respiratory mechanism*. Studies on the oxidative metabolism of salivarian trypanosomes again reveal significant differences at the sub-generic level; these differences correlate with the mitochondrial characters and cyclical mitochondrial changes referred to above. This carbohydrate breakdown ranges from aerobic glycolysis in the bloodstream forms of *Trypanozoon* spp. to total oxidation in culture forms of these species (culture forms have hitherto been studied as a convenient analogue of vector midgut forms). *Duttonella* and *Nannomonas* multiplicative blood-stream forms, unlike *Trypanozoon*, produce quantities of carbon dioxide; the stumpy forms of *T. brucei* are capable of limited oxidative decarboxy-lation. A succinoxidase system is present in bloodstream forms of *Duttonella* but not in *Nannomonas* or *Trypanozoon*, though this oxidase develops in culture forms. A cyanide-insensitive glycerophosphate oxi-dase system is reputedly unique to *Trypanozoon* spp. and is the principal pathway for electron transport in the bloodstream forms. However, its presence in *Duttonella* bloodstream forms is strongly suggested by the sensitivity of substrate utilization to m-chlorobenzhydrozamic acid (Vickerman and Evans, 1974), a specific inhibitor of this oxidase in *T. brucei* (Evans and Brown, 1973).

The presence of cytochrome pigments in bloodstream forms of any salivarian trypanosome is at present doubtful, though there is evidence for cyanide sensitivity of culture forms (and presumably vector forms) of *Trypanozoon* and *Nannomonas* spp. The stage at which a functional cyto-chrome oxidase develops during the process of transformation from bloodstream to culture forms has been found to differ from stock to stock (Srivastava and Bowman, 1971; Brown *et al.*, 1973). Whether these differences are actually stock-dependent or reflect differences in tech-niques of handling and cultivation in different laboratories remains to be seen when more stocks have been examined using comparable methods. The same comment applies to differences reported between the various species and subspecies of *Trypanozoon* reviewed in detail by Danforth (1967). Conclusions reached concerning the oxidative metabolism of trypanosomes before the development of methods for minimizing host–cell contamination must be accepted with caution.

(b) *Sensitivity to chemotherapy*. Clinically there is evidence for differences in drug-sensitivity between different subgenera/species and even between different subspecies within the salivarian trypanosomes. Thus, suramin has no pronounced effect on *T. vivax* or *T. congolense* infection in cattle but is curative for *T. brucei* in man and for *T. evansi* in camels. Many of the differences in drug-sensitivity between the *Duttonella*/ *Nannomonas* and *Trypanozoon* subgenera can be explained by the difference in distribution within the host, *Trypanozoon* spp. occurring in extravascular sites while *Duttonella* and *Nannomonas* are confined to the vascular system (Losos and Ikede, 1972; Fink and Dann, 1974; Williamson, 1976).

Quinapyramine B. vet. C. (Antrycide), homidium bromide B. vet. C. (Ethidium) and diminazine aceturate B. vet. C. (Berenil) are all equally lethal *in vitro* against the salivarian trypanosomes, but *in vivo* the first two drugs are much less active against *Trypanozoon*. Berenil, on the other hand, appears to be retained in the tissues so that *Trypanozoon* spp. are also susceptible *in vivo*.

Differences in carbohydrate metabolism may explain the hundred-fold-less sensitivity of *Nannomonas* to aromatic arsenicals *in vitro* as compared with *Trypanozoon* (Williamson, 1976); *Duttonella* is also relatively insensitive. Whether this selectivity reflects differences in enzyme proteins in the region of active thiol groups or differences in membrane permeability barriers is uncertain (Newton, 1974).

The metabolic diversity evident in the salivarian trypanosomes at the subgeneric level may well prove to be extended to subtle quantitative differences at the subspecies level and below; this diversity is particularly evident in the occurrence of drug-resistant stocks (e.g., see Kayembe and Wery, 1972). The biological nature of resistance to a particular drug, i.e. whether it is the result of a genetic mutation, nuclear or cytoplasmic, can seldom be decided, though some stocks retain their drug-resistant property over long periods, the character surviving cyclical transmission and transfer to different mammalian hosts. Drug-resistance markers of proven stability may prove useful not only in characterizing trypanosome stocks but also in experiments to demonstrate genetic recombination in trypanosomes; many of the resistance characters used in such experiments to date have been of doubtful stability or show cross-resistance with other drugs.

3. Macromolecular characteristics

In the absence of known sexual reproduction, the usual zoological criterion for defining a species is unavailable. In some eukaryotes, macromolecular characteristics have been correlated with accepted phylogenetic relationships. A study of macromolecular properties may give insight into the relatedness of many present-day forms. The nucleotide sequence of the genome defines the organism. Macromolecular structures, whether examined at the level of DNA or of gene products, evolve at different rates depending on selection pressure; consequently, the degree of discrimination between taxa can be varied by choosing the appropriate macromolecules. With the analytical techniques now available for the characterization of macromolecules, many of the problems basic to the identification and interrelations of salivarian trypanosomes are being studied. Given sufficient data, a balanced classification, reflecting both evolutionary relationships, and present taxonomic status would be expected.

(a) *DNA. Buoyant density*. The buoyant density of DNA in caesium salt solutions gives a measure of its nucleotide composition. As such, it is only a crude method for the characterization of DNA, giving information on the base composition (G + C : A + T) but insensitive in detecting differences in nucleotide sequences. Certain species of salivarian trypanosomes may be distinguished on the basis of the buoyant densities of nuclear main-band, kinetoplast and other satellite DNAs. However, within the subgenus *Trypanozoon* there is little variation in density values, with the exception of the presence of a (G + C)-rich satellite found in *T. b. gambiense* (Newton and Burnett, 1972). Although crude cell lysates can be analysed, this technique requires the use of sophisticated and expensive instrumentation and is not suitable for field studies. Nevertheless, isolated repetitive genetic sequences, which can be resolved as satellite bands or separated by refinements of buoyant-density analysis, are important sources of material for finer analytical studies (Sections II, A, 3, b and c). For instance, the fraction of fragmented DNA which specifies the sequence of ribosomal RNA (ribosomal DNA) is generally (G + C)-rich and may be isolated by the use of actinomycin D to decrease its density and resolve it from main-band DNA.

High-resolution melting analysis. The effect of increased temperature on double-stranded DNA is to cause a transition to a single-stranded state which can be monitored by an increase in absorption at 260 nm. This transition is represented empirically as a melting profile. Like buoyant density, the melting profile is dependent upon base composition. Regions of DNA rich in A + T melt at a lower temperature than do regions rich in G + C, therefore an analysis of nucleotide distribution can be made. This technique has been successfully applied in giving very sensitive and reproducible results with kinetoplast DNA (kDNA). Substantial differences have been detected between computer-differentiated melting profiles of the kDNA of members of the Kinetoplastida (Steinert and Van Assel, 1974; Steinert *et al.*, 1976), and, within the species *T. mega*, even stocks from different geographical locations have been discriminated (Duys, Van Assel and Steinert, in preparation). However, such analyses require rather large amounts of DNA ($\sim$ 100 μg) and can be performed only in well-equipped laboratories.

Smaller amounts of DNA can be examined with respect to base distribution by the related technique of partial denaturation mapping. This technique requires precise electron microscopic examination of DNA treated with chemical denaturing agents and can be applied only to isolated sequences of limited complexity such as kDNA, other satellite DNAs and ribosomal DNA.

Restriction endonuclease target sequence analysis. Restriction endonucleases are enzymes which recognize and cleave DNA at specific nucleotide sequences. For instance, EcoRI (restriction endonuclease from *Escherichia coli* RTF1), which recognizes a particular sequence of six base pairs, is expected to produce, on average, one scission every 4096 pairs. When applied to DNA consisting of repetitive nucleotide sequences, characteristic banding patterns of the DNA fragments are obtained on gel electrophoresis. This technique is highly sensitive in detecting differences in DNA sequence between organisms and is not influenced by any consideration of the function of that particular sequence. As a result, differences in those sequences which are not under strong selection pressure, and which therefore reflect the most extensive evolutionary divergence, may be examined. Although only small amounts of DNA ($< 1\ \mu g$) are required for this technique, the disadvantage for field application is the necessity to isolate repetitive DNA sequences (e.g., kDNA, rDNA).

Hybridization. Sequence homologies between organisms are currently estimated by molecular hybridization. This reaction is monitored by the extent to which small amounts of radioactively labelled DNA form stable hybrid molecules with unlabelled test DNA. The problems of labelling DNA *in vivo* can be overcome by synthesizing RNA which is complementary to a particular DNA (cRNA) using RNA polymerase.

(a) *Slide hybridization*

This technique is applicable to repetitive DNA sequences only but has the advantage that trace amounts of labelled cRNA can be reacted with preparations of a small number of cells. The reaction, which is monitored autoradiographically, has been performed on denatured kDNA of smears of whole trypanosomes or cell lysates and has discriminated between subspecies of *T. brucei* (Steinert *et al.*, 1976). This technique is relatively simple and could be used in field studies.

(b) *Molecular hybridization in solution*

The hybridization of kDNA with its cRNA has been performed in solution giving quantitative measures of cross-hybridization between some members of the Kinetoplastida (Steinert *et al.*, 1976). This technique could be extended to discern homologies between the nuclear DNAs of salivarian trypanosomes. Because these procedures require high concentrations of DNA and analytical instrumentation they are restricted to well-equipped laboratories. The numerical data obtained from hybridization studies are amenable to analysis which could lead to the establishment of patristic relationships between the salivarian trypanosomes.

(b) *Isoenzymes*. An enzyme is characterized and named by its specific function, and many enzymes of identical function are common to a very wide range of organisms. The molecular structure of each isofunctional enzyme may differ among the various organisms and with many has been shown to be under genetic control. Differences in the molecular structure of these isoenzymes—also called isozymes, multiple forms or enzyme variants—may be associated with differences in electrophoretic mobility, and the positions of equivalent isoenzymes are located after electrophoresis by a highly specific staining reaction to the particular common enzymic activity. The system has several advantages for trypanosomes:

(a) Electrophoresis can be carried out with crude aqueous extracts, containing a complex mixture of enzymes, proteins, etc., because the specificity of the staining reaction picks out just the enzymes required. Even contamination with non-trypanosomal material (e.g., from the host, culture medium) can be tolerated, since controls will demonstrate the position of any foreign isofunctional enzymes.

(b) "Amplification" of the enzyme's presence occurs because it is not the enzyme that is stained but its products, which are formed continuously while the enzyme remains active. Hence only minute amounts of material are required.

(c) The apparatus is relatively inexpensive and many samples can be compared in a short time.

(d) Hitherto most intrinsic characterization has been based on the few morphological variations possible in trypanosomes, but since each enzyme is a separate character and some hundreds are present in any one cell, isoenzyme typing has great potential value for characterization. So far, six isoenzyme systems are providing useful information on trypanosome variation, and others are under development.

Differences between species have been demonstrated by Kilgour and Godfrey (1973) and Bagster and Parr (1973), together with indications of infraspecific differences. Enzyme variants of *T. vivax* showed stability in the field over one year (Kilgour *et al.*, 1975; Kilgour and Godfrey, 1978), and *T. b. gambiense* had a distinctive alanine aminotransferase pattern, while the patterns of its aspartate aminotransferase distinguished between two "serotypes" (Godfrey and Kilgour, 1976).

Isoenzyme characterization methods have the advantage that they are sufficiently simple to allow their use in relatively poorly equipped laboratories.

(c) *Other proteins*. The genetic code determines a protein's molecular structure, which in turn determines its characteristic properties. The differential electrophoresis of isoenzymes, already described, is likely to be indicative of genetic differences between trypanosomes, and the serological reactions, described below, are dependent on the molecular structures of antigens. Current work on the structure of variable antigens of the surface coat (Cross, 1975) should lead to an increased understanding of the characterization of and relationship between different variable antigen types.

4. Immunological characterization

Salivarian trypanosomes possess two clearly differentiated groups of antigens that may be used for classification purposes. These are the variable antigens, and the structural or "common" antigens. Variable antigen, of whatever type, appears completely to coat the trypanosome surface (of the metacyclic and blood-stream forms) including the flagellum, undulating membrane and plasmanemes, so that no common antigen is exposed in living organisms. Immunological techniques applied to intact living organisms therefore detect only variable antigen and give no information above the serodeme level. Such techniques are agglutination and immune lysis tests and some techniques using labelled antibody.

Examination of the common antigens requires that the trypanosome be treated in some way so that these are made available. The organism is usually fixed to a glass slide, or disrupted so as to release the internal components. A whole range of immunological tests can then be applied, from labelled antibody methods (using sera specific for the internal, rather than variable antigens) to analysis by immunoelectrophoresis.

As far as is known, the variable antigens are entirely specific to the trypanosomes. The "common" antigens, however, comprise some that are specific to the Protozoa, and others (heterospecific) that are similar to antigens found in other members of the animal kingdom and bacteria. Both variable and common groups of antigens may be used in classification; the protozoon-specific antigens can differ in a way that parallels the closeness of the evolutionary relationships of the organisms. The mosaic of heterospecific antigens also may differ in closely related organisms such as *T. b. rhodesiense* and *T. b. gambiense* (Parratt and Cobb, 1978; Houba *et al.*, 1969).

Table 2 presents the immunological tests presently found to be the most useful for characterizing salivarian trypanosomes. Immunoelectrophoretic analysis is of special value as it allows a comprehensive characterization of the set of antigens displayed by an organism and affords a test for monitoring the purification of antigens and the production of specific antibodies.

Table 2. Immunological tests applicable to the characterization of salivarian trypanosomes

Tests	Minimum number of organisms required per test	Target	Specificity	Resolution	VAT	Serodeme	Subspecies	Species	Higher taxa
Agglutination	Many (10^6)	Surface	+ to +++[a]	–	+	+	–	–	–
Lysis	Few (10^0–10^1)	Surface	+++	+	+	+	–	–	–
Neutralization	Few (10^0–10^2)	Surface	++	++	+	+	–	–	–
Immuno-fluorescence	One (10^0)	Variable antigen and common antigen	+++	+++	+	+	+	+	+
Immuno-electrophoresis	Many (10^{11})	Variable antigen and common antigen	+++	+++	+	–	+	+	+

[a] Auto-agglutination occurs with *T. congolense* and some *T. brucei* VATs.

B. EXTRINSIC CHARACTERS (Lumsden, 1974)

Extrinsic characters refer to the behaviour of trypanosomes in hosts and in *in vitro* culture. They are used as criteria for the differentiation of salivarian trypanosomes with identical or closely similar morphology within one species whose distinction is desirable for practical purposes. Such criteria are mainly: host ranges, modes of transmission and host–parasite relationships.

1. Relationship to the vertebrate host

(*a*) *Host range.* The subspecies of the species *T. brucei* are classified partly on the basis of the host species which they can infect, e.g., *T. b. brucei* is defined as infective to animals (i.e., considering mainly artiodactyls) but not to man. *T. b. gambiense* and *T. b. rhodesiense* are infective to both animals and man although *T. b. gambiense* in nature may be epidemiologically restricted to man. The infectivity of *T. brucei* sspp. indet. isolations has been tested by the experimental inoculation of trypanosomes, grown in rodents, into human subjects. This procedure is only acceptable in *T. b. rhodesiense* situations in which, if the infection is to establish, it will be of the acute type (see Section II, B, 1, b) and be able to be recognized early by the occurrence of parasitaemia. In recent years promising *in vitro* methods based on DNA characteristics, antigens, isoenzymes and serum sensitivity (see Section II, B, 1, c) have been developed, which may in the future render experiments on man unnecessary.

Another example of a subspecies within the *T. brucei* spp. is *T. b. elephantis*, which has been proposed in the past as a separate subspecies as it is assumed that the elephant is the only vertebrate host. However, whether this is a valid subspecies or identical to *T. b. brucei* still remains controversial.

At various higher levels of classification of the salivarian trypanosomes, the animal host range, though not an essential criterion, can be a convenient aid for identification, for example in the case of *T. b. equiperdum* and *T. suis* (Table 3).

(*b*) *Clinical characters and pathogenicity.* The two *T. brucei* subspecies which infect man are separated on the main criterion of their pathogenicity to man. *T. b. gambiense* is well-adapted to man as a host and causes chronic infections with low parasitaemias. *T. b. rhodesiense* causes acute infections with high parasitaemias. The pathological lesions are identical except that in *T. b. gambiense* infections the course of the disease is spread over several years rather than the weeks or months of the typical *T. b. rhodesiense* infection. There is a clear difference between

Table 3. *Trypanosoma*: designations and general properties of Salivaria

Subgenus	Subspecies	Transmission		Infection rates in tsetse	Natural hosts	Area	Natural hosts: maximal parasitaemia	Infectivity to rodents	Culturability *in vitro*
		Cyclical	Non-cyclical						
Duttonella	T. vivax viennei	—	By biting flies in S. America	—		New World tropics	++	Nil to low	Very difficult
	T. v. vivax	By tsetse in Africa	—	High	Domestic ruminants, game		++	Nil to low	
	T. v. uniforme		—	High	game		++ (?)	Nil	?
Nammomonas	T. congolense		—	Moderate	Domestic animals, game		++	Low to high	Difficult
	(T. simiae)		—	Moderate	Pigs, warthogs		+++	Nil	
Pycnomonas	T. suis		—	Low	Pigs	Africa	+	Nil	?
Trypanozoon	T. brucei brucei		—	Low	Domestic animals, game		++ (rare)	High	Fairly easy
	T. b. rhodesiense		—		Man, cattle, game		++ (in man)	High	
	T. b. gambiense		—		Man, ? animals		±	Low	
	T. b. evansi		By biting flies	—	Camels, horses, cattle, buffalo	Tropics and sub-tropics	++ (rare)	High	Not yet possible
	(T. equinum)		—	—	Horses, cattle	New World tropics	++ (rare)	High	
	T. b. equiperdum		Venereally	—	Horses	Worldwide	±	Low	?

the two infections in that the practically insignificant early signs of *T. b. gambiense* sleeping sickness contrast with the predominantly severe symptoms accompanying parasitaemia in the early stages of the *T. b. rhodesiense* disease.

Results of recent DNA and isoenzyme analyses seem to support the validity of separating *T. b. gambiense* and *T. b. rhodesiense* as distinct subspecies.

As a substitute for the experimental inoculation of human subjects for the differentiation of *T. b. brucei* and *T. b. rhodesiense* (Section II, B, 1, b), the infectivity of *T. brucei* sspp. indet. materials can be tested by incubating trypanosomes in normal human blood, serum or plasma, and subsequently inoculating the mixture into rodents. Retention of infectivity indicates *T. b. rhodesiense*, its loss *T. b. brucei* (Robson and Rickman, 1970; Targett and Wilson, 1973). The agent responsible for this phenomenon is a serum factor which has not yet been clearly defined. There is evidence that different variable antigen types, derived from the same clone, when these are grown in rodents, may differ in their sensitivity to human serum (Van Meirvenne *et al.*, 1976).

2. Relationship to the invertebrate host

(*a*) *Site of development.* The hitherto accepted characteristic that the salivarian metacyclic trypanosomes develop in the anterior station of the tsetse fly is not a definitive criterion for distinguishing the group, since *T. vivax viennei*, *T. brucei evansi* and *T. b. equiperdum* are not cyclically transmissible.

The different developmental sites for each of the subgenera are helpful criteria, but again not definitive because three of the subspecies are not cyclically transmitted.

(*b*) *Infection rates.* The proportion of tsetse flies infected by each of the different subgenera is a useful, but not definitive character, since, although the absence of infection by *T. b. evansi* and *T. b. equiperdum* may be a manifestation of the very low infection-rate typical of other *Trypanozoon*, the absence of infection by *T. v. viennei* differs completely from the high rates typical of its companion subspecies *T. v. vivax*.

3. Behaviour in culture

Until recently (Hirumi, unpublished observations), salivarian trypanosomes have not been maintained in the bloodstream form by serial transfer in culture outside the mammalian host. In blood-containing media, *T. congolense* and *T. brucei* will transform to and can be maintained as flagellates which correspond to vector midgut development stages (reviewed by Bishop, 1967). *T. vivax*, which has no such stage, cannot be maintained in similar media, but some stocks will give rise to vector stages in tsetse cell culture (Trager, 1975). The variable ability of *T. brucei* stocks to develop *in vitro* is to some extent related to the pleomorphism of the trypanosomes in the culture inoculum, i.e., to the physiological state of the flagellates at the time the isolation is made; monomorphic lines rarely give rise to cultures and *T. evansi* sspp. have never been cultivated.

Systematic comparison of the ability of different isolations and stocks to develop in given culture media have been few (Weinman, 1960; Lehmann, 1960, 1961). With the development of more defined media (e.g., Cross and Manning, 1973) to replace the complex blood broths and biphasic media used in these early studies, comparison of different trypanosome lines by their behaviour *in vitro* may become more meaningful.

C. NUMERICAL TAXONOMY

In principle the methods of numerical taxonomy can be applied to any biological groups (Sneath and Sokal, 1973), but their applicability to the salivarian trypanosomes has not yet been established by experiment. The method can utilize data from all quantifiable taxonomic criteria and take them together. For instance, data derived from immunological characterization, isoenzyme patterns, molecular hybridization, determination of size of restriction-endonuclease segments, etc., could be used as characters in a numerical taxonomic study. The experimental results can be subjected to similarity matrix analysis to establish phenetic relationships. Eventually, numerical methods of organism identification should be able to be developed (Pankhurst, 1975).

D. CONSIDERATION OF USEFULNESS OF DIFFERENT CHARACTERS

Intrinsic and extrinsic characters having been reviewed, it was concluded that intrinsic characters were to be preferred to extrinsic ones, as the latter involve factors other than those specifically related to the organism and which are not able to be fully standardized. Of intrinsic characters, macromolecular characteristics, biochemical ones such as organism DNA or isoenzymes, and immunological ones such as determination of the variable antigen type repertoire, appear to be most promising. Such methods may be expected to produce large numbers of analysable characters, so that the possibility of the application of numerical taxonomic identification methods will be able to be investigated.

[The remainder of the Report of the Meeting will be presented here only in summary; for the extended treatment, with explanatory diagrams, reference should be made to WHO (1978).]

III. Definitions and Nomenclature

The terms used to describe organisms or populations of organisms, besides those relating to Linnaean taxa (Section III, A), fall into two classes, those purely operational terms simply descriptive of the laboratory history of the materials (Section III, B) and those related to recognizable characteristics of the organisms (Section III, C).

A. TERMS RELATING TO LINNAEAN TAXA

Salivarian trypanosome species
An assemblage of organisms which can be distinguished from other species by one or more stable discontinuous morphological characters.
Salivarian trypanosome subspecies
Assemblages of organisms within a species which cannot be separated from each other by morphological characters but only by other stable characters.

B. OPERATIONAL TERMS WITHOUT IMPLICATION OF CHARACTERIZATION

Population
The group of trypanosomes present at a given time in a given host or culture.
Sample
That part of a trypanosome population collected on a unique occasion.
Primary isolate
The viable organisms present in a culture or in an experimental animal host following introduction of a sample, or part of a sample, from a naturally infected host.
Stock
Population derived by serial passage *in vivo* and/or *in vitro* from a primary isolation, without any implication of homogeneity or characterization.

Line

A laboratory derivative of a stock maintained in different physical conditions or in a different geographical location.

Stabilate

A sample of organisms viably preserved, usually in replicate, on a unique occasion.

Clone

The trypanosomes derived from a single individual by binary fission.

C. TERMS IMPLYING CHARACTERIZATION

Deme

Trypanosome populations which differ from others of the same species or subspecies in a specified property or set of properties, which may be specified, e.g. serodeme, zymodeme.

Strain

A set of populations originating from a group of trypanosomes of a given species or subspecies present at a given time in a given host or culture and defined by the possession of one or more designated characters.

Variable antigen type (VAT)

The identity of a single trypanosome as determined by the variable antigen expressed at its surface. Certain VATs which tend to arise first, or early, in the course of infections have been termed "basic" or "parent" or "predominant" VATs (Gray, 1965a, b).

Homotype (VA homotype)

VAT expressed by the majority of trypanosomes in a clone and against which monospecific antiserum can be prepared.

Heterotype (VA heterotype)

Heterologous VAT that arises within a clone of assumed homologous VAT.

Reference VAT

The first example of a VAT to be characterized and used as a reference point.

VAT repertoire

All the VATs which can be expressed by a clone.

Serodeme

Populations of trypanosomes each of which can express the same VAT repertoire.

D. NOMENCLATURE OF VARIABLE ANTIGEN TYPES (VATs)

Designation of VATs by the codes proposed by Lumsden *et al.* (1967), which include letters indicating the laboratory and *Trypanosoma* subgenus concerned, with "at" (= antigen type) and a number (e.g., ETat 12 = Edinburgh *Trypanozoon* antigen type 12 or AnTat 10 Antwerp

Trypanozoon antigen type 10) have facilitated interlaboratory exchanges and comparison; but interlaboratory consultation is needed to evolve a more universal system.

IV. Relationship of characterized populations to Linnaean taxa

A. GENUS

As species of only a single genus, *Trypanosoma* Gruby, 1843, were considered, definition at the generic level was not required.

B. SECTION

The terms "Stercoraria" and "Salivaria" were introduced by Hoare (references in Hoare, 1972) as the names of two groups described as "sections" at a level between genus and subgenus, and referring only to trypanosomes of mammals. By the International Code of Zoological Nomenclature no such category is, strictly, permissible; however, the terms have proved very useful and should be retained, although their status may require revision in the future.

C. SUBGENUS

A subgenus of the genus *Trypanosoma* was defined as a group of species defined by common morphological characters; however, other characters are not necessarily excluded. The four subgenera of Salivaria introduced by Hoare (1972) have clarified descriptions and should be retained, although their status may require review in the future.

D. SPECIES AND SUBSPECIES

Taking into account the definition of species proposed in Section III, A, it was recognized that more convincing evidence for the differentiation of many of the commonly accepted taxa at this level (Table 1) was required, e.g. that which might be supplied by macromolecular or immunological characterization (Sections II, A, 3 and 4). Failing such evidence, each salivarian subgenus should be regarded as unispecific.

Subspecies may be distinguished by behavioural differences, by geographical separation, sometimes by mensural differences or by differences in the clinical course of the disease caused. Such differences may, sometimes, correlate with macromolecular or immunological differences.

Where the evidence is insufficient to assign *T. brucei* to a man-infective, or non-man-infective subspecies, it is wise to designate it as *T.*

brucei ssp. indet., so as to draw attention to the need for safety precautions in handling it.

V. Maintenance of reference collections

A. LIVING ORGANISMS

1. Serial passage

Serial passage *in vitro* and *in vivo* has severe limitations for the maintenance of more than a few trypanosome stocks and strains, both logistically and because of the changes in the biological character of the populations following artificial selection under the special conditions of the passage.

2. Stabilation

For the above reasons, reference collections are necessarily of stabilates—in practice, cryopreserved suspensions of trypanosomes in appropriate media.

B. ANTIGENS

The organisms used as reference material for immunological tests should consist of clones available as stabilates. These organisms should be characterized and typed by direct agglutination, lysis, immunofluorescence and/or immunoelectrophoresis, using reference antisera (see Section V, C) before preservation, as well as before actual use.

C. ANTISERA

The optimal procedures to be followed for raising reference antisera against trypanosomes depend on the purpose in view, i.e. whether it be the characterization of whole organisms, in suspension or in films, or of the total antigenic make up of the organisms (see Section II, A, 4) or of particular purified antigens.

D. BIOCHEMICAL PRODUCTS

The requirements for the preservation and storage of trypanosome material for isoenzyme studies are essentially the same as those for antigen preparation: many different techniques are used for the preparation of DNA; it is desirable that organisms should be prepared as far as possible in the same way as for immunological and isoenzyme studies.

VI. Documentation of reference collections

A. DESIGNATION OF MATERIALS

1. Designation of primary isolation

The description of any primary isolation should consist of a list of the following components:

Locality of the primary isolation: one non-hyphenated word of up to ten roman capitals.

The year of isolation: two arabic digits.

Laboratory code: not to exceed five capitals.

Number, which is the specific number of that isolation: in arabic numerals.

In a written description the four elements are separated from each other by a slash character, e.g. SERENGETI/58/EATRO/1716.

2. Designation of derived materials

Any other designation used, e.g. of stock, line, strain or stabilate, should be given in square brackets after the primary isolation designation, quoting a unique coding for the material designated, e.g. [Stabilate TREU 386].

A full, formal designation of a material used would include both designations, e.g. *Trypanosoma brucei* SERENGETI/58/EATRO/1716 [Stabilate TREU 386].

VII. References

Afchain, D., Fruit, J., Petitprez, A., Van Meirvenne, N., Le Ray, D., Bout, D. and Capron, A. (1976). Antigenic analysis of a variant specific component of *Trypanosoma brucei brucei*. Immunochemical purification by affinity chromatography. *Pathologie et Biologie*, **24**, 615–617.

Ainsworth, G. C. (1971). "Ainsworth and Bisby's Dictionary of the Fungi", 6th Edition. Commonwealth Mycological Institute, Kew, Surrey, England.

Anon. (1978). Proposals for the nomenclature of salivarian trypanosomes and for the maintenance of reference collections. *Bulletin of the World Health Organization*, **56**, 467–480. (Edited by W. H. R. Lumsden and D. S. Ketteridge.)

Bagster, I. A. and Parr, C. W. (1973). Trypanosome identification by electrophoresis of soluble enzymes. *Nature, London*, **244**, 364–366.

Baker, J. R. (1972). "Parasitic Protozoa", 2nd Edition. Hutchinson University Library, London.

Bishop, A. (1967). Problems of the cultivation of some parasitic protozoa. *Advances in Parasitology*, **5**, 93–138.

Bowman, I. B. R. and Flynn, I. W. (1976). Oxidative metabolism of trypanosomes. *In:* "Biology of the Kinetoplastida" (W. H. R. Lumsden and D. A. Evans, eds), Volume 1, pp. 435–476. Academic Press, London and New York.

Broom, J. C. and Brown, H. C. (1940). Studies in trypanosomiasis. IV. Notes on the serological characters of *Trypanosoma brucei* after cyclical development in *Glossina morsitans. Transactions of the Royal Society of Tropical Medicine and Hygiene*, **34**, 53–64.

Brown, R. C., Evans, D. A. and Vickerman, K. (1973). Changes in oxidative metabolism and ultrastructure accompanying differentiation of the mitochondrion in *Trypanosoma brucei. International Journal of Parasitology*, **3**, 691–704.

Cross, G. A. M. (1975). Identification, purification and properties of clone-specific glycoprotein antigens constituting the surface coat of *T. brucei. Parasitology*, **71**, 393–417.

Cross, G. A. M. and Manning, J. C. (1973). Cultivation of *Trypanosoma brucei* sspp. in semi-defined and defined media. *Parasitology*, **67**, 315–331.

Damnovic, V., Edwards, S. D. and Thomas, D. (1975). Recovery of haemolytic plaque-forming cells after freeze-drying. *Nature, London*, **235**, 116–119.

Danforth, W. F. (1967). Respiratory Metabolism. *In:* "Research in Protozoology" (T. T. Chen, ed.), Volume 1, pp. 205–306. Pergamon Press, Oxford.

Evans, D. A. and Brown, R. C. (1973). m-Chlorbenzhydroxamic acid—an inhibitor of cyanide insensitive respiration in *Trypanosoma brucei. Journal of Protozoology*, **20**, 157–160.

Fink, E. and Dann, O. (1974). *In:* "Les Moyens de Lutte Contre les Trypanosomes et Leurs Vecteurs". Institut d'Elevage et du Médecine Vétérinaire des Pays Tropicaux, Actes de Colloque, Paris, 12–15 Mars 1974, pp. 297–300. Maisons Alfort, Paris.

Godfrey, D. G. (1975). Biochemical strain characterization of trypanosomes. *International Symposium on New Approaches in American Trypanosomiasis Research, Belo Horizonte, Brazil, 18–21 March 1975.* Pan American Health Organization, Washington DC, USA.

Godfrey, D. G. and Kilgour, V. (1976). Enzyme electrophoresis in characterizing the causative organism of Gambian trypanosomiasis. *Transactions of the Royal Society of Tropical Medicine and Hygiene*, **70**, 219–224.

Gray, A. R. (1965a). Notes on Immunology. Document PD/68.12. World Health Organization, Geneva.

Gray, A. R. (1965b). Antigenic variation in a strain of *Trypanosoma brucei* transmitted by *Glossina morsitans* and *G. palpalis. Journal of General Microbiology*, **41**, 195–214.

Hajduk, S. L. (1976). Demonstration of kinetoplast DNA in dyskinetoplastic strains of *Trypanosoma equiperdum. Science*, **191**, 858–859.

Hawksworth, D. L. (1974). "Mycologist's Handbook". Commonwealth Mycological Institute, Kew, Surrey, England.

Hoare, C. A. (1972). "The Trypanosomes of Mammals". Blackwell Scientific Publications, Oxford.

Houba, V., Brown, K. N. and Allison, A. C. (1969). Heterophile antibodies, M-antiglobulins and immunoglobulins in experimental trypanosomiasis. *Clinical and Experimental Immunology*, **4**, 113–123.

Inoki, S. (1960). Studies on antigenic variation in the Wellcome strain of *Trypanosoma gambiense*. I. Improvements in the technique. *Bikens' Journal*, **3**, 215–222.

International Code of Botanical Nomenclature (1972). See Stafleu (1972).

International Code of Zoological Nomenclature (1964), 2nd Edition. International Trust for Zoological Nomenclature, London.

Kayembe, D. and Wéry, M. (1972). Observations sur la sensibilité aux diamidines de souches de *Trypanosoma gambiense* récemment isolées en République de Zaire. *Annales de la Société belge de Médecine tropicale*, **52**, 1–8.

Kilgour, V. and Godfrey, D. G. (1973). Species-characteristic isoenzymes of two aminotransferases in trypanosomes. *Nature, New Biology*, **244**, 69–70.

Kilgour, V. and Godfrey, D. G. (1978). The persistence in the field of two characteristic isoenzyme patterns in Nigerian *Trypanosoma vivax*. *Annals of Tropical Medicine and Parasitology*. In press.

Kilgour, V., Godfrey, D. G. and Na'isa, B. K. (1975). Isoenzymes of two aminotransferases among *Trypanosoma vivax* in Nigerian cattle. *Annals of Tropical Medicine and Parasitology*, **69**, 329–335.

Lehmann, D. L. (1960). Some culture differences between *Trypanosoma rhodesiense* and *T. brucei* in autoclaved diphasic media. *Annals of Tropical Medicine and Parasitology*, **54**, 419–423.

Lehmann, D. L. (1961). Attempts at the selective cultivation of *Trypanosoma rhodesiense*, *T. brucei* and *T. congolense*. *Annals of Tropical Medicine and Parasitology*, **55**, 440–446.

Le Ray, D. (1975). Structure antigénique de *Trypanosoma brucei* (Protozoa Kinetoplastida). Analyse immunoélectrophorétique et étude comparative. *Annales de la Société belge de Médecine tropicale*, **55**, 129–311.

Le Ray, D., Afchain, D., Jadin, J. B., Capron, A. and Famerée, L. (1971). Interrelations immuno-taxonomiques de *T. brucei*, *T. rhodesiense* et *T. gambiense*. *Annales de Parasitologie humaine et comparée*, **46**, 523–532.

Leupold, F. (1928). Untersuchungen über Rezidivestamme bei Trypanosomen mit hilfe des Reickenberg-Phänomens. *Zeitschrift für Hygiene und Infektioneskrankheit*, **109**, 144–156.

Losos, G. J. and Ikede, B. D. (1972). Review of pathology of diseases in domestic and laboratory animals caused by *Trypanosoma congolense*, *T. vivax*, *T. brucei*, *T. rhodesiense* and *T. gambiense*. *Veterinary Pathology*, **9** (suppl).

Lourie, E. M. and O'Connor, R. J. (1937). A study of *Trypanosoma rhodesiense* relapse strains *in vitro*. *Annals of Tropical Medicine and Parasitology*, **31**, 319–340.

Lumsden, W. H. R. (1974). Biochemical taxonomy of *Leishmania*. *Transactions of the Royal Society of Tropical Medicine and Hygiene*, **68**, 74–75.

Lumsden, W. H. R. and Hardy, G. C. J. (1965). Nomenclature of living parasitic materials. *Nature, London*, **205**, 1032.

Lumsden, W. H. R., Herbert, W. J. and McNeillage, G. J. C. (1967). Nomenclature of antigenic types of trypanosomes. *Veterinary Record*, **81**, 237–238.

Martin, G. W. (1968). The origin and status of fungi. *In:* "The Fungi" (G. C. Ainsworth and A. S. Sussman, eds) Volume 3, pp. 635–648. Academic Press, New York.

Newton, B. A. (1974). The chemotherapy of trypanosomiasis and leishmaniasis: towards a more rational approach. *In:* "Trypanosomiasis and Leishmaniasis", pp. 285–301. Ciba Foundation Symposium 20 (New Series). Elsevier, Amsterdam.

Newton, B. A. (1976). Biochemical approaches to the taxonomy of kinetoplastid flagellates. *In:* "The Biology of the Kinetoplastida" (W. H. R. Lumsden and D. A. Evans, eds), Volume 1, pp. 405–434 and 542. Academic Press, London.

Newton, B. A. and Burnett, J. K. (1972). DNA of Kinetoplastidae: a comparative study. *In:* "Comparative Biochemistry of Parasites" (H. Van den Bossche, ed.), p. 185. Academic Press, New York and London.

Osaki, H. (1959). Studies on the immunological variation in *Trypanosoma gambiense* (serotypes and the mode of relapse). *Biken's Journal*, **2**, 113–127.

Pankhurst, R. J. (1975). "Biological Identification with Computers". Systematics Association Special Volume No. 3. Academic Press, London and New York.

Parratt, D. and Cobb, S. J. (1978). Heterophile antibodies to red cells in human trypanosomiasis. *Clinical and Experimental Immunology*.

Rickman, L. R. and Robson, J. (1970). The testing of proven *Trypanosoma brucei* and *T. rhodesiense* strains by the blood incubation infectivity test. *Bulletin of the World Health Organization*, **42**, 911–916.

Roberts, C. J. (1971). The lack of infectivity to cattle of a strain of *Trypanosoma simiae* transmitted by *Glossina morsitans* and *G. tachinoides*. *Annals of Tropical Medicine and Parasitology*, **65**, 319–326.

Sneath, P. H. A. and Sokal, R. R. (1973). "Numerical Taxonomy". W. H. Freeman, San Francisco.

Srivastava, H. K. and Bowman, I. B. R. (1971). Adaptation in oxidative metabolism of *Trypanosoma rhodesiense* during transformation in culture. *Comparative Biochemistry and Physiology*, **403**, 973–981.

Stafleu, F. A. (1972) (Ed.). International Code of Botanical Nomenclature adopted by the Eleventh International Botanical Congress, Seattle, USA, August 1969. *Regnum Vegetabile*, **82**, 1–426.

Steinert, M. and Van Assel, S. (1974). Base composition heterogeneity in kinetoplast DNA from four species of hemoflagellates. *Biochemical and Biophysical Research Communications*, **61**, 1249–1255.

Steinert, S., Van Assel, S., Borst, P. and Newton, B. A. (1976). Evolution of kinetoplast DNA. *In:* (C. Saccone and A. M. Kroon, eds), *International Conference on the Genetic Function of Mitochondrial DNA*, pp. 71–81. North Holland, Amsterdam.

Targett, G. A. T. and Wilson, V. C. L. C. (1973). The blood incubation infectivity test as a means of distinguishing between *Trypanosoma brucei brucei* and *T. b. rhodesiense*. *International Journal of Parasitology*, **3**, 5–11.

Trager, W. (1975). On the cultivation of *Trypanosoma vivax*. *Journal of Parasitology*, **61**, 3–11.

Van Meirvenne, N., Janssens, P. G. and Magnus, E. (1975a). Antigenic variation in syringe-passaged populations of *Trypanosoma* (*Trypanozoon*) *brucei*. I. Rationalization of the experimental approach. *Annales de la Société belge de Médecine tropicale*, **55**, 1–23.

Van Meirvenne, N., Janssens, P. G., Magnus, E., Lumsden, W. H. R. and Herbert, W. J. (1975b). Antigenic variation in syringe-passaged populations of *Trypanosoma* (*Trypanozoon*) *brucei*. I. Comparative studies of two antigenic type collections. *Annales de la Société belge de Médecine tropicale*, **55**, 25–30.

Van Meirvenne, N., Magnus, E. and Janssens, P. G. (1976). The effect of normal human serum on trypanosomes of distinct antigenic type (ETat 1 to 12) isolated from a strain of *Trypanosoma brucei rhodesiense*. *Annales de la Société belge de Médecine tropicale*, **56**, 55–63.

Vickerman, K. (1965). Polymorphism and mitochondrial activity in sleeping sickness trypanosomes. *Nature, London*, **208**, 762–766.

Vickerman, K. (1974). The ultrastructure of pathogenic flagellates. *In:* "Trypanosomiasis and Leishmaniasis", pp. 171–190. Ciba Foundation Symposium 20 (New Series). Elsevier, Amsterdam.

Vickerman, K. and Evans, D. A. (1974). Studies on the ultrastructure and respiratory physiology of *Trypanosoma vivax* trypomastigote stages. *Transactions of the Royal Society of Tropical Medicine and Hygiene*, **68**, 145.

Vickerman, K. and Preston, T. M. (1976). Comparative cell biology of the kinetoplastid flagellates. *In:* "Biology of the Kinetoplastida" (W. H. R. Lumsden and D. A. Evans, eds), Volume 1, pp. 35–113. Academic Press, London.

Weinman, D. (1960). Cultivation of the African sleeping sickness trypanosomes from blood and cerebrospinal fluids of patients and suspects. *Transactions of the Royal Society of Tropical Medicine and Hygiene*, **54**, 180–190.

Whittaker, R. H. (1969). New concepts of kingdoms of organisms. *Science*, **163**, 150–160.
Williamson, J. (1976). Chemotherapy of African trypanosomiasis. *Tropical Diseases Bulletin*, **73**, 531–542.

VIII. Appendix A

NOMENCLATURAL PRACTICE IN THE SPOROZOA

Sporozoa are sexually reproducing Protozoa which undergo a limited number of asexual generations before gamete production. The concept of species of Sporozoa must include sexual compatibility within the population and production of viable offspring. Subspecies are populations within a species, geographically isolated from one another so that distinctive characters are maintained which would otherwise have been lost by pooling of genes. The limited number of asexual generations and probable recombination of genes during zygotic meiosis suggests that almost every individual in a population will be different. In these respects Sporozoa differ from trypanosomes.

The concepts which should be included are exemplified by the definitions of terms listed below. Their application to Coccidia will be discussed by a working party in an attempt to bring workers in this field into line with other protozoologists and microbiologists.

Isolate

The product of an isolation process (meaning the organisms recovered from a single collection from a naturally infected host); differences from, similarity to, or identity with other isolates are not implicit in this term.

Strain

Descendants of an isolate; a difference from other strains is implicit in this term.

Line

Several parallel populations established from an isolate (strain). These could differ from one another depending on the conditions of passage.

Variant

A population which is not identical with the parent population in all its character; equivalent to a mutant. Not the same as "variety", which is not in use in Zoological Nomenclature, its place being taken by subspecies. It was suggested that consideration be given to replacing the term variant (as in antigenic variant) for trypanosomes by a new term.

IX. Appendix B

NOMENCLATURAL PRACTICE IN THE PROCARYOTES

The Kingdom Procaryotae, comprising the bacteria and the blue-green algae, has been divided into these two Divisions, and several Classes have been proposed, e.g. Mollicutes, red photosynthetic bacteria.

The categories from class to genus have little meaning in modern bacteriology. Family, species, genus and tribe have been used in such different levels among various groups of bacteria that they cannot be equated. The details of some bacteria of medical importance, for example, have been used to elevate them to a disproportionately high rank compared to other bacteria. Many families were grouped arbitrarily on the possession of a character or characters shared by widely disparate groups of bacteria. Some uniform objective criterion of the level of a taxon in the hierarchy of categories is required, though it may not be achieved even with the help of numerical classification or molecular biological techniques.

The tendency has thus been to utilize in bacteriology the *taxospecies*, based on an overall similarity determined by numerical methods, or the nomenspecies, i.e. individuals resembling the nomenclatural type. Methods of gene exchange in bacteria, recombination, transduction, transformation, plasmid transfer and others are so many and varied that the *genospecies* has not proved particularly fruitful, especially as some methods of genetic exchange, e.g., resistance-factor transfer, have been shown to take place between widely different taxa.

Subspecies is little used formally in bacteriology, but infrasubspecific terms are widely used to describe infraspecific taxa, e.g., serovars, chemovars, phagovars, *forma specialis*, etc. The Bacteriological Code does not rule on the naming of infrasubspecific taxa which are not hierarchical and may overlap.

The Bacteriological Code 1976 requires nomination of a type strain for valid publication and recommends deposition in a culture collection, which latter was not made a rule for pragmatic reasons but may be elevated to such at a later date. Reference strains, of no nomenclatural status, may be nominated for infrasubspecific taxa.

A strain of bacteria is derived from a single isolate, usually a colony, and most are not necessarily clones derived from single cells, though such is often assumed. A strain is made up of a series of cultures, those deriving from previous cultures being referred to as subcultures. "Strain" is also used to describe a series of similar strains isolated during given circumstances, for example through an epidemic.

Individual is a term little used in bacteriology, as the determination of the properties of bacteria depend on a study of populations of individual bacteria.

Bacterial species are in general *polythetic*, i.e. possess a number of a set of characteristics possessed by members of the species, rather than *monothetic*, i.e. invariably possessing one or more characteristics specified for membership of the species.

X. Appendix C

NOMENCLATURAL PRACTICE IN THE FUNGI

The fungi are a large cosmopolitan group of greatly varying characteristics and it is estimated that there must be over 250 000 species.

It has been the practice for them to be studied by botanists, possibly because of the structure of the larger species. However, they seem to occupy a position separate from both the plant and the animal kingdoms. Whittaker (1969) suggested that there were three nutritionally distinct groups: (1) those allied to the plant kingdom and characterized by photosynthesis; (2) those allied to the animal kingdom and characterized by ingestive nutrition; and (3) those in which nutrition is absorptive. Other investigations seem to support this, and Martin (1968) concluded that these groups "may reasonably be treated as a discrete major taxonomic unit".

Methods of study are varied as they cover a wide spectrum of structure from the slime moulds (Myxomycetes), or plasmodial forms, to the sporocarps of the higher Basidiomycetes, and can be found as saprobes, symbionts, parasites and hyperparasites. They show sufficient differences of structure for most present classifications to be based on morphology of the sexual reproductive elements. Sexual reproduction is considered characteristic of the fungi though it has not yet been observed in all taxa. Studies using modern techniques such as chemotaxonomy and electronmicroscopy tend to confirm morphological findings but are not used in routine identification.

The basis of classification depends on comparison with deposited "type" material on which the descriptions of the taxa have been based. Living cultures are not accepted as type material, though many species are studied in pure culture.

Subject Index

Ablastin, 468–472
Ablastinogen, 470–471
Acheta domesticus, 230
Aedes aegypti (arthropod), 220
A. albopictus, 220
Agouti paca (Dasyproctidae), 11, 13, 61
Agamidae, 243, 245
Akodon arviculoides (Cricetidae), 16
Alanine aminotransferase (ALAT), 262
Allactaga elater, 198
A. severtzovi, 198
Amblyomma, 125
American visceral leishmaniasis,
  causative agent, 68–75
  control, 87–90
  distribution and incidence in man, 68–69
  epidemiology in Brazil, 75–84
  vector(s), 84–87
Amphibian trypanosomes, 319
  Trypanosoma grylli, 319
  T. mega, 271
  T. rotartorium, 319
Anguidae, 245
Anisonema (euglenid), 659
Anolis sp. 34
Anopheles, 660
  A. gambiae, 216
AnTat 1 antigen type, 497, 498, 499
Antibody types in trypanosomiasis, 534
Anti-F′ antibody, 532
Antigenic identity of clones (*T. brucei* sspp.), 499
Anti-R antibody, 533, 537
Anti-R$_2$ antibody, 538
Anti-SRBC antibody, 536, 537
Anthroponotic cutaneous leishmaniasis in the USSR, 206–208
Anumbius (bird), 134
Aotus trivirgatus (Cebidae), 16, 23, 58

AP antigen type (*T. brucei* sspp.), 499
Apiomerus sp. (arthropod), 235
Apis mellifera (arthropod), 232
Araucaria angustifolia, 65
Arilus cristatus (arthropod), 231
Arthropod Kinetoplastida, biology of, 213–235, 242
  endosymbionts, 219–221
  invertebrate hosts,
    Aedes aegypti, 220
    A. albopictus, 220
    Apiomerus sp., 235
    Apis mellifera, 231
    Arilus cristatus, 231
    Calliphoridae, 226
    Ceratophyllus gallinae, 225
    Chrysomyia chloropyga, 227
    Cimbex americana, 232
    Ctenocephalides canis, 225
    Culex, 221
    Drosophila melanogaster, 219
    D. virilis, 230
    Eurydema ventralis, 234
    Euryophthalmus davisi, 231
    Euschistus servus, 232
    Gerridae, 233
    Hippelates pusio, 218
    Lucilia spp., 231
    Megaselia scalaris, 229
    Mesocercus marginatus, 233
    Musca domestica, 228, 231
    Neodiprion swainei, 229
    Nepa cinerea, 225
    Oncopeltus fasciatus, 232
    Phaenicia sericata, 231
    Phormia regina, 228
    Ranatra linearis, 225
    Triatoma, 221
    T. infestans, 234
    Zelus leucogrammus, 219, 226, 229, 231, 234

Arthropod—*cont.*
life cycles, 216–218
methods of study, 221–224
dried smears, stained, 222
in vitro cultivation, diphasic media
McConnell's, 223
NNN, 223
SNB 9, 223
monophasic medium
Ho Mem, 223–224
morphology, 215–216
pathogenicity, 215
site in host, 219
systematics, 224–235
Blastocrithidia, 233–235
B. apiomerusi, 235
B. culicis, 218, 220, 233, 669, 677
B. euryophthalmi, 218
B. euschisti, 217
B. familiaris, 217
B. galvaoi, 234
B. gerridis, 233, 656, 657
B. leptocoridis, 217
B. ortheae, 217
B. pulicis, 218
B. raabei, 218, 233
B. sandoni, 217
B. triatomae, 122, 214, 217, 234,
657
B. vagoi, 218, 234
Crithidia, 230–232
C. acidophili, 232
C. arili, 231
C. cimbexi, 232
C. deanei, 220, 221, 231, 234, 677
C. epedana, 232
C. fasciculata, 214, 215, 216, 218,
230, 415, 655, 677, 678, 679,
680
C. fasciculata var. *culicis*, 221,
231
C. harmosa, 231, 679
C. luciliae, 218, 227, 228, 231,
234, 670
C. mellificae, 232, 656
C. oncopelti, 144, 214, 215, 220,
221, 231, 644, 669, 677
Herpetomonas, 226–230
H. mariadeanei, 656, 657
H. megaseliae, 218, 229, 679
H. muscarum, 218, 220, 225, 227,
228, 235
H. m. ingenoplastis, 227, 228
H. m. muscarum, 227, 228
H. samuelpessoai (= *L. pessoai*),
215, 225, 229, 234, 676
H. swainei, 215, 229
Leptomonas, 225–226
L. arctocorixae, 216

L. capsularis, 218
L. collosoma, 214, 661
L. craggi, 216
L. ctenocephali, 225
L. ctenocephali var. *chattoni*, 216,
225
L. drosophilae, 216, 219
L. jaculum, 215, 225
L. legerorum, 216, 218
L. lygaei, 217, 218
L. mirabilis, 216, 226, 227, 228
L. mirpiri, 218
L. oestrorum, 216
L. oncopelti, 214, 217
L. oxyuri, 225
L. pattoni, 216
L. pessoai (= *H. samuelpessoai*),
215, 225, 676
L. roubaudi, 216
L. samueli, 226, 234
L. tortum, 218
Rhynchoidomonas, 235
transmission, 218–219
Arthus reaction, 258
Aspartate aminotransferase (ASAT),
262
ATCC 11745 (*Crithidia fasciculata*
isolate), 660
Autophagosome of *T. brucei*, 362–3,
382, 383
Avian trypanosomes, subgenus *Try-
panomorpha*, 319

BA antigen type (*T. brucei* sspp.), 499
Bacteria
in sandflies, 442
nomenclature, 698
Baiomys musculus, 89
Bartonella bacilliformis, 94
Bartonellosis (Carrion's disease), 94, 95
Bassaricyon gabbii, 16, 26
Belyaev's method, for quantitative determination of cutaneous leishmaniasis endemicity, 202
Biochemical characterization
of lizard *Leishmania*, 262
of *T. cruzi*, 144–153
of unidentified Neotropical Suprapylaria (*Leishmania*), 90, 91
Biology of *Leishmania* in phlebotomine
sandflies, 395–449
factors affecting development, 429–
442
attachment to chitin, 441
concomitant infections, 442
digestion of blood meal, 437–438
insusceptibility of sandfly, 430–433
number of ingested parasites, 433–
435

Biology—*cont.*
  sugars, 438–440
  time, temperature and humidity, 435–437
  mammalian *Leishmania*, 400–422
  pathogenicity to sandfly, 428–429
  saurian *Leishmania*, 423–428
Blastocrithidia, 214, 218, 219, 233–235
  infections of Triatominae, 185
  (for species, see Arthropod Kinetoplastida, systematics)
B-lymphocyte mitogen(s), 534, 541
Bodo, 213, 277, 659
B. caudatus, 277
B. saltans, 658
Bodo-Cryptobia lineage, 275
Borrelinavirus swainei, 215
Bradypus griseus (Bradypodidae), 17
B. infuscatus, 16, 23
Brucella, 534

Caenorhabditis (nematode), 659
Calliphoridae (arthropods), 226
Callithrix jacchus (Callithricidae), 82
Caluromys philander (Didelphidae), 18
Candida albicans antigen, immunoassay of, 510
Canis aureus (Canidae), 208
C. familiaris, 13, 16, 18, 19
Cardiopathy (Chagas' disease), 551, 593–600
Carnoy's fluid, 28
Carrion's disease (Bartonellosis), 94, 95
Cavia aperea (Caviidae), 65, 66
C. porcellus, 18, 65
Cebus (monkey), 58
Ceratophyllus canis (arthropod), 87
C. gallinae, 225
C. felix, 87
Cercoplasma, 225
Cerdocyon thous (Canidae), 18, 19, 25, 78, 80, 82, 84, 88
Chagasic megacolon and megaeosophagus, 600–606
Chagoma, 550, 552
Chemovar, 698
Choleopus didactylus (Bradypodidae), 13, 17, 23, 25, 78
C. hoffmani, 16, 17, 23, 40
Chondriome (of *T. brucei*), 360–361
Chrysomyia chloropyga, 227
Ciliophora, 697–698
Cimbex americana (arthropod), 232
Cimex lectularis, 125
Classification of leishmanias, revised, 8–11
Classification of neotropical leishmanias, past, 3–8
Clone, 712

Coccidiascus legeri (fungus), 215
Coendou n.sp. (Erithizontidae), 67
Coendou sp., 11, 18, 24, 26
Coendou prehensilis, 18, 24, 67
C. p. prehensilis, 24, 67
C. rothschildi, 4, 18, 66
Complement-fixation test (CFT)
  for *T. cruzi* infections, 122
  for visceral leishmaniasis, 89
Control of American visceral leishmaniasis, 87–90
Control of Chagas' disease, future research, 153–155
Corynebacterium diphtheriae, 660
Cowperthwaite's medium, 230
  use of, 231, 232, 678
Cricetus auratus auratus, 439
C. griseus, 250
Crithidia, 214, 215, 216, 217, 221, 230–232, 659, 678, 681
  (for species, see Arthropod Kinetoplastida, systematics)
Cryptobia, 658, 680
C. congeri, 300
C. helicis, 275, 277, 321
C. intestinalis, 277
C. vaginalis, 275, 277
Ctenocephalides canis (arthropod), 225
Culex (arthropod), 221

Dasyprocta sp. (Dasyproctidae), 17, 24
D. azurae, 13
D. punctata, 18
DAT (direct agglutination test), 123
DEAE cellulose column, 326
Deme, 712
Diagnosis of *T. cruzi*, 121–124
Didelphis marsupialis (Didelphidae), 17, 23, 24, 31, 45, 46, 80
D. paraguayensis, 82
Difco agar base medium for *Leishmania*, 29
Diphasic media for lower trypanosomatids, 223
Diplomys labilis, 19, 44
Dipus sagitta, 198
Direct agglutination test (DAT) for *T. cruzi*, 123
DNA analysis of trypanosomes, 490, 702–704
DNA buoyant density, application
  differentiation of lizard and mammalian *Leishmania*, 262
  techniques, 535, 702–704
Dried smears, staining for arthropod Kinetoplastida, 222
Drosophila (arthropod), 231
D. melanogaster, 215, 219
D. virilis, 230

Dyskinetoplasty in fish trypanosomes, 273

Eagle's MEM medium, 304, 305, 306
Echimys spp., 82
Eliomys sp., 359
ELISA (enzyme-linked immunosorbent assay), 123
Endosymbionts, 219–221, 667–668
Endotrypanum, 20, 32, 46, 47, 321, 375, 656
E. schaudinni, 39, 40, 78
Enzyme electrophoresis, application, 145, 151, 186, 262
Enzyme-linked immunosorbent assay (ELISA), 123
Epidemiology of leishmaniasis, in USSR, 197–209
   of visceral leishmaniasis in Brazil, 75–84
Epstein-Barr virus (EBV), 524, 540
Equus asinus (Equidae), 13
E. caballus, 13
Erythrocyte antigens (heterophile), 524
Escherichia coli, 675
ETat serodeme, 497, 505
   ETat 1, 2, 3 and 5 antigen types, 497, 499
Euglena, 659
E. gracilis, 679
Eurydema ventralis (arthropod) 234
Euryophthalmus davisi (arthropod), 231
Euschistus servus (arthropod), 232

F (Forssman-like) antigen, 532, 533, 536, 538
Felis catus (Felidae), 13, 19
Fish haemoflagellates, biology of, 270–327
   cell structure, 271–279
      Trypanoplasma, 275–279
      Trypanosoma, 271–275
   in vitro cultivation, 303–306
      Trypanoplasma, 306
      Trypanosoma, 303–306
   life cycle, 279–303
      natural infections, 301–303
      transmission, 279
      vector phase, 280–285
         Trypanoplasma, 283–285
         Trypanosoma, 281–283
      vertebrate phase, 285–300
      chemotherapy, 296
      development, 285–287
      effect of temperature, 287–288
      host specificity, 294–296
      immune response, 288–290
      pathogenicity, 290–293
         Trypanoplasma, 290–292

Trypanosoma, 292–293
      pleomorphism, 296–300, 315–316
         Trypanoplasma, 299–300
         Trypanosoma, 297–299
      stress factors, 288
      virulence, 293–294
   taxonomic considerations
      (including species list of parasites and hosts), 307–325
      Trypanoplasma, 320–325
      Trypanosoma, 307–320
         monomorphic, 316–318
         pleomorphic, 315–316
   vectors (leeches)
      Bactrochobdella tricarinata, 279
      Branchellion torpedinus, 279
      Calobdella punctata, 279, 281
      C. vivida, 279
      Cystobranchus virginicus, 279
      Hemiclepsis sp., 301
      H. marginata, 279, 280, 281, 282, 286
      Hirudo nipponica, 279
      H. tractina, 279
      Johanssonia sp., 279, 280, 282
      Piscicola sp., 279, 280, 301
      P. funduli, 279
      P. geometra, 279, 280, 283, 285, 286
      P. salmostica, 279, 280, 286, 302
      Platybdella muricata, 279
      P. scorpii, 279
      P. soleae, 279
      Pontobdella sp., 279
      P. muricata, 281
      Trachelobdella lubricata, 279
   vertebrate hosts
      Acerina cernus, 295
      Acipenser ruthenus, 290
      Barbus conchonius, 297
      Carassius auratus auratus, 327
      Carassius carassius, 327
      Catostomus commersonii, 296
      Cattus rhotheus, 302
      Clarius batrachus, 314
      C. clarias, 314
      Gobio albipinnatus, 314
      G. gobio, 314
      Lebistes reticulatus, 296
      Lota lota, 292
      Misgurnus anguillicaudatus, 303
      Oncorhynchus kisutch, 291, 302
      O. tschawytscha, 295
      Ophiocephalus striatus, 303, 304
      Parasilurus asotus, 314
      Perca fluviatilis, 304
      Phoxinus phoxinus, 290
      Puntius conchonius, 295, 296
      Raja sp., 314

Fish haemoflagellates, vertebrate hosts
—cont.
  R. punctata, 292
  Rhinichthys catratulus, 327
  R. cataractae, 295
  Siniperca chua-tsi, 314
  (for other hosts, see under alpha-
    betical list of parasites: Try-
    panoplasma, 321–323, and Try-
    panosoma, 307–313)
Forcipomyia spp. (arthropod), 94
Forssman antibody, 532
Forssman antigen(s), 525
  negative, 532
  positive, 532, 538
Fungi, 215, 698–699
  infections in sandflies, 442
  nomenclatural practice, 721

Galea spixii, 82
Gallus domesticus, 489, 538
Gekkonidae, 243, 245
Genome (of trypanosome stock), 502
  operons, 502
Genospecies, 698
Gerridae (arthropods), 233
Giemsa-colophonium method for Leish-
  mania, 28
Giemsa's stain, use of, 222, 407, 411
Glossina (arthropod), 219, 658, 672, 695
  G. fuscipes, 496
  G. morsitans, 503
  G. pallidipes, 496, 503
  G. palpalis, 489
Glucose-6-phosphate dehydrogenase
  (G-6-PDH), 262
Guinea pig kidney (GPK) cells, 532

Haematomonas carassii, 319
Heated bovine erythrocyte (HBE) sus-
  pension, 532
Hemidesmosomes, 400, 401
Hemiechinus auritus, 198
Herpetomonas, 214, 215, 216, 217, 219,
  220, 226–230, 401, 403, 659
  (for species, see Arthropod
    Kinetoplastida, systematics)
  H. hemidactyli (= L. hemidactyli), 246
Herpetosoma complex, 314
Hertig's apparatus, 421
Heteromys, 61
  H. anomalus, 18
  H. desmarestianus, 17, 49
Heterophile antigen-antibody systems,
  525–528
Heterophile antibodies in Trypanosoma
  infections, 524–542
  application for diagnosis, 535–537
  biological significance, 541–542

detection of, 544–545
  diagnostic significance, 539–540
  in human trypanosomiasis, 530–537
  in Trypanosoma spp. other than
    T. b. gambiense and rhodesiense,
    537–539
  nature of, 528–530
Heterophile antibody tests for disease
  diagnosis, 528, 530
Heterophile antigens in Trypanosoma
  infections, 524–528
Heterotype, 712
Hippelates pusio (arthropod), 218
HoMem medium (modification), use of,
  223–224
Homotype, 712
Hoplomys gymnuras (Echimyidae), 13
Hypopylaria, neotropical, 9, 34
Hystryx leucura, 198

Icthyobodo, 658
Identification of sandfly blood meals, 33
IgA antibody, 528
IgG antibody, 528, 538
  in T. cruzi infections, 153
Iguanidae, 243
Immune-complex hypersensitivity, 511
Indirect fluorescent antibody test
  (IFAT) for T. cruzi, 123
Indirect haemagglutination test (IHAT)
  for T. cruzi, 123
Isocitrate dehydrogenase (IDH), 262
Isoenzyme techniques, 490, 535, 704
Isoenzymes of trypanosomatids, 399

Johnston's medium, 304

Kala-azar, Indian, 87
Kannabateomys amblyonx (Echimyidae),
  13
K-DNA, 407
Karatomorpha, 213
Kerodon rupestris, 82
Kinetoplastida, nutrition, 654–681
  Crithidia fasciculata, 660–677
    amino acids, purines, pyrimidines,
      671–677
    basic requirements, 660–668
    haem and protoporphyrin, 668–
      671
    long-chain fatty acids, 670–671
    temperature factors, 677
    vitamin growth factors, 674–677
  comparison of lower Trypanosoma-
    tidae, Leishmania and Trypano-
    soma, 658–659
  endosymbionts, 677–678
  origins of kinetoplastids, nutritional
    evidence, 658–659

Klossiella, 371
Köberle's theory, 552–553

Laboratory transmission of *Leishmania* species, by bite of experimentally infected sandfly, 397
Lacertidae, 243, 245
Leishmania, 214, 654, 655, 656, 657, 659, 660, 662, 664, 665, 666, 679, 673, 677
Leishmania spp., 656
trinomial classification, 253
L. adleri, 7, 9, 243, 244, 246, 247, 250, 255 256, 257, 258, 260, 262, 425, 426
L. aethiopica (see *L. tropica* complex)
L. agamae, 9, 244, 246, 247, 262, 426
L. braziliensis complex, 4, 7, 9, 27, 29, 31, 78, 116, 398, 404, 405, 408, 410, 433, 441, 444, 447, 448
L. braziliensis, 6, 8, 14, 26, 30, 33, 80, 91, 255, 257, 258, 403, 405, 407, 417, 433, 441, 661, 662, 673
L. b. braziliensis, 6, 9, 14, 29, 32, 36–38, 398, 401, 403, 408, 410, 411, 413, 417, 422, 429, 433, 657
L. b. guyanensis, 9, 15, 30, 33, 38–39, 71, 90, 97, 398, 401, 417, 422, 657
L. b. panamensis, 9, 23, 29, 30, 39–43, 408, 417, 433, 437
L. braziliensis unidentified subspecies, 44–48
L. ceramodactyli, 7, 9, 244, 247, 427
L. chagasi (see *L. donovani* complex)
"*L. chagasi*" (= *L. donovani*), 411 413
L. chameleonis, 242–244, 423
L. davidi, 423
L. donovani complex, 10
L. chagasi, 22, 23, 26, 27, 68–90
distribution and incidence in man, 68–69
identification, 69–75
vector(s), 84–87
L. donovani, 26, 27, 69, 70, 71, 75, 143, 249, 255, 256, 257, 258, 261, 396, 397, 403, 404, 416, 417, 418, 419, 421, 422, 426, 432, 434, 435, 436, 438, 441, 445, 661, 662, 664, 666, 667, 671, 673
L. infantum, 22, 26, 27, 255, 396, 398, 401, 403, 407, 411, 416, 417, 418, 420, 430, 432, 434, 436, 437, 445
L. enriettii, 65–66, 68, 257, 258, 657, 677
L. gymnodactyli, 243, 244, 256, 428
L. hemidactyli, 243, 244

L. henrici, 34, 242, 243, 244, 423
L. hertigi complex, 10, 11, 23, 26, 81
L. h. deanei, 24, 67–68
L. h. hertigi, 66–67, 68
L. infantum (see *L. donovani* complex)
L. mexicana complex, 4, 10, 27, 29, 30, 90, 432
L. mexicana, 6, 8, 11, 14, 26, 33, 398, 403
L. m. amazonensis, 6, 11, 14, 15, 23, 24, 55–60, 63, 64, 71, 79, 80, 301, 396, 397, 398, 400, 403, 404, 405, 410, 411, 415, 418, 429, 433, 436
L. m. aristedesi nov. subspecies, 61–63, 64
L. m. mexicana, 6, 26, 49–53, 63, 64, 71, 90, 246, 250, 255, 397, 404, 417, 432
L. m. pifanoi, 60–61, 63, 250
L. mexicana unidentified subspecies, 63–64
L. peruviana, 91–97, 116
epidemiology, 93–97
experimental infection of animals, 92–93
history of 'uta', 91–92
L. tarentolae, 7, 9, 243, 244, 247, 250, 255, 257, 258, 260, 262, 423, 424, 425
life-cycle in sandfly, 423–425
nutrition, 657, 664, 665, 666, 669, 670, 673, 676
physiology and biochemistry, 261–262
L. tropica complex, 10
L. aethiopica, 10, 428
L. major, 90, 198, 199, 201
L. tropica, 26, 70, 91, 96, 116, 403, 408, 410, 411
L. zmeevi, 244
Leishmaniasis in the USSR, epidemiology, 197–209
anthroponotic cutaneous leishmaniasis, 206–208
vectors, 206
differences between anthroponotic and zoonotic types, 207
visceral leishmaniasis, 208–209
vectors, 209
zoonotic cutaneous leishmaniasis, 198–206
artificial immunization, 206
vectors, 199
vertebrate hosts, 198
Leishmanin skin test, 250–260
leishmanin positivity rates, 260–261
Leishman's stain, 257
Leptomonas, 214, 216, 218, 219, 225–226, 242, 425, 435, 657, 660

Leptomonas—*cont.*
(for species, see Arthropod Kinetoplastida, systematics)
Leptospira, 78
Line, definition, 711–712
Liomys irroratus, 89
Lipid metabolism of *T. brucei*, 361–
362
Liverpool antigen type (*T. brucei* sspp.),
499
Lizard (Saurian) *Leishmania*, 241–262
historical aspects and evolutionary
trends, 242–243
morphology and life-cycle, 245–248
parasite, 245–247
transmission and vector, 247–248
relationship of lizard and mammalian
Leishmania species, 248–253
parasites, 243, 244
reptilian hosts, 243, 244, 245
(see also *Leishmania* and lizard
species)
physiology and biochemistry, 261–262
relationship to human leishmaniasis,
253–261
cross-immunity, 256–260
influence on epidemiology, 260–261
serology, 253–256
Lizard species (natural and experimental hosts of lizard *Leish-
mania*),
Acanthodactylus bosbianus asper, 249
Agama caucasica, 245, 248, 249
A. mutabilis, 249
A. sanguinolenta, 244, 245, 248, 249,
251
A. stellio, 244, 247
Alsophylax pipiens, 244
Ameiva ameiva, 250
Anolis sp., 34, 242, 244, 423
Basilicus vittatus, 250
Ceramodactylus doriae, 244, 427
Chamaeleon pumilus, 244
Cnemidophorus lemniscatus, 250, 423
Crossobamon eversamani, 245
Dipsosaurus dorsalis, 250
Eremias grammica, 245, 249
E. guttulata guttulata, 245, 249, 251
E. intermedia, 245, 249, 251
E. i. grammica, 244
E. lineolata, 245, 249
E. scripta scripta, 245
E. velox, 245, 249, 251
Eumeces schneideri, 249
E. s. principes, 245
E. taeniolatus, 245
Gonatodes vittatus, 250
Gymnodactylus caspius, 244, 245, 247,
248, 249, 251

G. russowi, 248
Hemidactylus sp., 250
Hemidactylus brooki, 244
H. turcicus, 244, 428
Iguana iguana, 250
Lacerta viridis, 249
Latastia longicaudata, 244, 247, 425
Mabuya aurata, 245, 249
M. mabouya, 250
M. striata, 249
Opisaurus apodus, 245
Phyrynocephalus helioscopus, 245
P. interscapularis, 245, 249, 251
P. mystaceus, 245, 249
P. raddei raddei, 245
Polychrus marmoratus, 250
Tarentola mauritanica, 243, 244, 250,
423
Lower Trypanosomatidae, 213–235,
657
Lutzomyia (see Psychodidae)
Lycalopex vetulus (Canidae), 19, 82, 83

Macaca mulatta, 530
Macacus rhesus, 94
Macrophage cultures for lizard *Leish-
mania* cultivation, 250–253
Malate dehydrogenase (MDH), 262
Mammalian *Leishmania* within sandfly,
400–422
development in bloodmeal, 403–405
establishment of infection, 405–410
invasion of head, 413–415
migration, 410–411
morphology, 400–403
proboscis forms, 416–418
transmission by bite, 418–422
Marmosa sp. (Didelphidae), 17, 24
M. fuscata, 18
M. mitis, 18
M. murina, 17
M. robinsoni, 11, 18, 61
Marmota sp., 359
McConnell's medium, use of, 223
Medium 199, 306
Megatrypanum, 215, 657
Meriones libycus, 198
M. meridianus, 198
M. persicus, 198
M. tamariscinus, 198
Metachirus (Didelphidae), 62
M. nudicaudatus, 17, 23, 24
Morphological forms of *Leishmania*
within sandfly, 400–418
amastigote, 400
in the proboscis, 416–418
paramastigotes, 400, 401
in ileum, pylorus, 408–410
in pharynx, 413–418

Morphological—*cont.*
　promastigotes, 400–401, 416–418
　　haptomonad, 400, 401, 407, 415
　　hemidesmosomes, 400, 401, 408,
　　　410, 411, 413, 415
　　nectomonad, 400, 401, 407
Mus musculus, 89, 126, 132, 198, 462
Mustela nivalis, 198

Naegleria gruberi, 659
Nasua nasua (Procyonidae), 16, 23
Neacomys spinosus (Cricetidae), 17
Nectomys squamipes (Cricetidae), 17, 49
Neotoma mexicana, 89
Neotropical Hypopylaria, 9, 34
Neotropical leishmanias of uncertain
　status, 91–97
Neotropical Peripylaria, 9, 35–48
Neotropical Suprapylaria, 9–11, 48–91,
　116
　L. chagasi, 68–90
　L. enriettii, 65–66
　L. hertigi deanei, 67–68
　L. h. hertigi, 66–67
　Leishmania mexicana amazonensis, 55–
　　60
　L. m. aristedesi nov. subspecies, 61–63
　L. m. mexicana, unidentified subsp.,
　　63–64
　L. m. pifanoi, 60–61
　L. mexicana, 49–53
　unidentified parasites, 90–91
Nesokia indica, 198
4N diphasic medium, 306
NNN medium, use of, 29, 93, 223, 306
　for *L. chagasi*, 79
　for lizard *Leishmania*, 243, 250, 257
Nomenspecies, 698
Nosodeme(s), 341
Nutrition of Kinetoplastida, 654–681
Nyctomys sumichrasti (Cricetidae), 17, 49

Oncopeltus (arthropod), 221, 231
Oncopeltus fasciatus, 214, 220, 230
Operons, 502
Opisthomastigote (*Herpetomonas*), 401,
　403
Oryzomys spp. (Cricetidae), 24, 59, 62,
　63, 64, 82, 94, 96
O. capito, 11, 16, 17, 18, 23, 55, 56, 61
O. concolor, 16, 17, 38
O. eliurus, 13
O. macconnelli, 17
O. nigripes, 16
Ototylomys (Cricetidae), 64
O. phyllotis, 17, 49
Oxoid agar base for *Leishmania* cultiva-
　tion, 29

Pacui virus, 59
Paul–Bunnell test, 540
Paramecium aurelia, 674, 678
Peranema (euglenid), 659
Peripylaria, neotropical, 9, 35–48, 116
Phacellodomus, 134
Phagovar, 698
Phlebotomine sandflies,
　laboratory-bred species, 446–467
　physiology and behaviour, 443–447
　species (see under Psychodidae)
Phyllostomus hastatus (Phyllostomidae),
　13
Phyllotis spp., 94, 95
Physiology and behaviour of sandflies,
　443–447
Physorum polycephalum (slime mould),
　659
Phytohaemagglutinin, 541
Phytomonas, 242, 321
P. davidi, 675
P. elmassiani, 214, 216
Plasmaneme, 353
Plasmodium berghei, 189
P. falciparum, 364
Pleomorphism of *Trypanosoma brucei*,
　342–354
Pneumocystis carinii, 119, 371
Pokeweed mitogen, 541
Polygyra albolabria, 321
Polymorphism in *T. cruzi*, 548
Ponselle's blood agar medium, 306
Ponselle's fixative, 222
Population, 711
Potos flavus (Procyonidae), 16, 26
Primary isolate, 711
Procaryotes, 698
　nomenclature practice, 720–721
Procyon cancrivorus (Procyonidae), 82
Proechimys (Echimyidae), 61, 62, 64
　transmission of *Pacui* virus, 59
P. guyannensis, 13, 17, 18, 23, 24, 36,
　45, 46, 55
P. oris, 77
P. semispinosus, 11, 13, 18, 19, 23, 61
Pulex irritans, 87
Psammomys obesus, 198
Psychodidae Phlebotominae species
　Lutzomyia spp., 441
　Lu. anduzei, 12, 86
　Lu. antunesi, 12
　Lu. atroclavata (= *Lu. guadeloupensis*),
　　86
　Lu. barretoi, 89
　Lu. battistinii, 95
　Lu. carpenteri, 42
　Lu. cavernicola, 74
　Lu. cayennensis, 89
　Lu. chiapanensis, 89

Psychodidae—*cont.*
Lu. *coelhoi*, 73
Lu. *cortelezzii*, 48, 86, 96
Lu. *cruciata*, 12, 49, 50, 53, 73, 89, 397, 433
Lu. *deleoni*, 89
Lu. *dendrophila*, 12
Lu. *evansi*, 89
Lu. *fischeri*, 72
Lu. *flaviscutellata*, 17, 18, 42, 55, 58, 59, 60, 61, 62, 63, 64, 71, 73, 397, 433, 466
Lu. *flaviscutellata-olmeca* complex, 52, 61, 64, 432
Lu. *furcata*, 12
Lu. *gomezi*, 12, 16, 40, 42, 43, 68, 72, 73, 74, 429, 433, 437, 446
Lu. *imperatrix*, 95
Lu. *intermedia*, 12, 16, 36, 37, 72, 73, 85, 86, 433
Lu. *longipalpis*, 3, 12, 20, 47, 68, 71, 72, 73, 74, 75, 77, 78, 80, 81, 83, 88, 89, 90, 96, 116, 247, 253, 397, 398, 405, 408, 411, 413, 415, 417, 418, 419, 420, 428, 429, 432, 433, 434, 436, 446, 447
vector of *L. chagasi*, 84, 87
Lu. *micropyga*, 34
Lu. *migonei*, 12, 47, 48, 96
Lu. *monticola*, 65, 66, 73, 74
Lu. *noguchi*, 94, 95
Lu. *olmeca*, 43, 64, 433
Lu. *o. bicolor*, 43, 62
Lu. *o. olmeca*, 17, 42, 49, 50, 52, 53, 71
Lu. *ovallesi*, 12, 49, 50, 73
Lu. *panamensis*, 432, 433
Lu. *permira*, 12, 50, 53
Lu. *peruensis*, 94, 95, 96
Lu. *pescei*, 95
Lu. *pessoai*, 12, 16, 36, 397, 433
Lu. *renei*, 47, 72, 73, 74, 397, 417, 432, 433
Lu. *rorotaensis*, 34
Lu. *sallesi*, 73
Lu. *sanguinaria*, 12, 68, 72, 73, 74, 417, 429, 437, 446
Lu. *shannoni*, 12, 49, 50, 73, 86
Lu. *steatopyga*, 50
Lu. *trapidoi*, 12, 16, 39, 40, 42, 43, 72, 433, 437, 439, 446
Lu. *trinidadensis*, 34, 50, 446
Lu. *tuberculata*, 12
Lu. *umbratilis*, 15, 16, 33, 38, 39, 47, 71, 398, 417
Lu. *verrucarum*, 94, 95, 96
Lu. *vespertilionis*, 446
Lu. *whitmani*, 12, 47, 72, 73, 86
Lu. *ylephiletor*, 12, 16, 17, 40, 42, 43, 44, 72, 73, 417, 432, 433
Lu. *yuilli*, 12, 46, 47
Phlebotomus *andrejevi*, 199, 201
P. *ariasi*, 398, 411, 417, 420, 421, 422, 430, 434, 435, 436, 437, 438, 439, 441, 444, 445, 446, 447
P. *argentipes*, 396, 397, 404, 416, 417, 421, 422, 432
P. *chinensis*, 208, 403, 417, 421, 432
P. *caucasicus*, 39, 199, 201, 208, 244, 248, 249
P. *kandelaki*, 208
P. *longipes*, 428, 439, 443, 447
P. *major*, 71, 417, 431, 435, 437
P. *mongolensis*, 199, 201, 208, 403
P. *orientalis*, 434, 439, 444
P. *papatasi*, 39, 199, 201, 203, 206, 207, 244, 247, 248, 397, 403, 408, 410, 416, 420, 421, 424, 425, 426, 427, 428, 429, 431, 432, 434, 437, 439, 443, 444, 445, 447
P. *perfiliewi*, 432
P. *perniciosus*, 84, 396, 416, 418, 420, 432, 434, 436, 446
P. *sergenti*, 206, 207, 417, 429, 431, 436, 437
Psychodopygus *amazonensis*, 13
Ps. *arthuri*, 74
Ps. *bispinosa*, 73
Ps. *complexus*, 46, 47
Ps. *davisi*, 13, 47, 86
Ps. *geniculata*, 72
Ps. *panamensis*, 13, 16, 39, 40, 42, 43, 49, 50, 53, 72
Ps. *paraensis*, 13, 46
Ps. *pessoana*, 40, 43, 72
Ps. *squamiventris*, 46
Ps. *tintinnabulus*, 46
Ps. *wellcomei*, 13, 16, 32, 37, 398, 408, 411, 417, 429, 433
Sergentomyia *antennata*, 423, 425
S. *arpaklensis*, 248
S. *bedfordi*, 439
S. *clydei*, 243, 244, 248
S. *minuta*, 244, 247, 248, 423, 424, 425, 428
S. *minuta minuta*, 244, 247
S. *murgabiensis* (= S. *sintoni*, = S. *arpaklensis*), 428, 429
S. *schwetzi*, 248
S. *sintoni*, 244, 248

R (rat and rabbit) antigen, 532, 533, 536
Rattus sp. (Muridae), 462
R. *rattus*, 13, 17, 23, 45, 46, 82
Reference VAT, 712
Rhipicephalus, 125
Rhipidomys *cearanus*, 82
Rhombomys *opimus*, 39, 198

Rhyncoidomonas, 214, 219, 235
(for species, see Arthropod Kinetoplastida, systematics)
Rhyncomonas, 277
R. nasuta, 658

Saimiri (monkey), 58
Salivaria, 8, 713
Salivarian trypanosomes
characterization techniques, 699–610
extrinsic characters, 707–710
intrinsic characters, 699–710
numerical taxonomy, 710
definitions and nomenclature, 711–
713
operational terms, 711–712
terms implying characterization,
712
relating to Linnean taxa, 711
nomenclature and maintenance, 694–
715
reference collection, documentation,
715
maintenance, 714
Salivarian trypanosome species, definition, 711
Salivarian trypanosome subspecies,
definition, 711
Salmonella, 534
Sample, definition, 711
Sanguinus geoffroyi (Callithricidae), 16,
23
Saurian (lizard) cell cultures, for cultivation of lizard *Leishmania*, 250
Saurian hosts of *Leishmania* (see Lizard
species)
Saurian *Leishmania*, 241–262, 398, 423–
428, 442, 444
attachment of parasite in sandfly,
446
sites of development in sandfly, 441
species, 244
(see also *Leishmania* species)
Scinciidae, 243, 245
Section, definition, 713
Hypopylaria, 9, 34
Peripylaria, 9, 35–48, 116
Suprapylaria, 9–11, 48–91, 116
Sergentomyia, 244, 423
(see also Psychodidae)
Serodeme, 712
Serological tests for *T. cruzi*, 122–123
Serovar, 698
Serratia indica, 675
Sheep erythrocytes (SRBC), 534
Shortt's modification of NNN medium,
223, 305
SNB9 diphasic medium, 223, 305
Sigmodon hispidus (Cricetidae), 17, 49

South American leishmaniasis,
epidemiology, rôle of animals
as reservoirs of human leishmaniasis, 14–33
detection by isolation of *Leishmania*, 27–33
detection by identification of
sandfly bloodmeals, 33
human population, 14–15
mammalian hosts (other than
man), 22–27
phlebotomine sandfly population, 15–22
in Neotropical Hypopylaria, 34
in Neotropical Peripylaria, 35–38
L. braziliensis braziliensis, 36–38
L. b. guyanensis, 39–43
L. b. panamensis, 39–43
L. b. unidentified subspecies, 44–
48
in Argentina, 47–48
Brazil, 45–47
Colombia, 44–45
Costa Rica, 44
El Salvador, 44
Honduras, 44
Nicaragua, 44
Panama, 44
other countries, 48
in Neotropical Suprapylaria, 48–91
L. mexicana mexicana, 49–53
L. m. amazonensis, 55–60
L. m. pifanoi, 60–61
L. m. aristedesi, 61–63
L. mexicana subspecies from
Trinidad, 63–64
L. enriettii, 65–66
L. hertigi hertigi, 66–67
L. hertigi deanei, 67–68
L. chagasi, 68–90
unidentified parasites, 90–91
in Neotropical leishmanias of un-
certain status, 91–97
L. peruviana, 91–97
past classification of neotropical leish-
manias, 3–8
revised classification of leishmanias,
8–11
Section Hypopylaria, 9
Section Peripylaria, 9
Section Suprapylaria, 9–11
Species, 713
Spermophilopsis leptodactilus, 198
Sporozoa, 697
nomenclatural practice, 719
SRBC (sheep erythrocytes), 534
Stabilate, 712
Stercoraria, 8, 713
Stock, 143, 711

Strain, 342, 712
Streptococcus pneumoniae, 524
Strigomonas, 216
S. oncopelti, 257, 258
Subgenus, 713
Subspecies, 713
Sugars, nutrition of sandflies, 438–440
Suprapylaria, neotropical, 9–11, 48–91
Sylvilagos sp., 88
Systematics of arthropod Kinetoplastida, 224–235
Szidat's law, 214

Tamandua tetradactyla (Edentata), 82
Taxospecies, 698
Tetrahymena, 659, 660, 663, 676, 679, 698
T. pyriformis, 673
T. thermophila, 673
"Tinde" experiment (*Trypanosoma brucei rhodesiense*), 502–503
Tobie's medium, 304
Thecadactylus rapicaudus (Gekkonidae), 34
Transovarial transmission, 247
Triatominae, vectors of *T. cruzi*
  Cavernicola pilosa, 128, 133, 134
  Eratyrus mucronatus, 128
  Linshcosteus confumus, 186
  L. costalis, 186
  Microtriamota sp. indet., 128
  Panstrongylus geniculatus, 128, 135
  P. herreri, 142
  P. lignarius, 128
  P. megistus, 118, 131, 132, 133, 135, 148, 186
  P. rufotuberculatus, 128, 136
  Parabelminus sp. n., 133
  Paratriatoma spp., 134
  Psammolestes sp., 134
  P. tertius, 132, 133
  Rhodnius sp., 122
  Rhodnius sp.n., 128
  R. amazonensis, 128
  R. brethesi, 128, 131
  R. domesticus, 133
  R. pallescens, 130, 131, 142
  R. paraensis, 186
  R. pictipes, 128, 135
  R. prolixus, 128, 130, 131, 132, 135, 142, 185, 187, 190
  R. robustus, 128
  Triatoma arthurneivai, 135
  T. barberi, 127
  T. brasiliensis, 131, 132
  T. cavernicola, 186
  T. dimidiata, 130, 131, 142
  T. gerstaeckeri, 129, 135
  T. infestans, 127, 234
  T. lectularis, 129

T. maculata, 128
T. protracta, 127, 129, 135
T. recurva, 129
T. rubida, 129
T. rubrofasciata, 122, 128, 185
T. rubrovaria, 127, 128
T. sanguisuga, 129
T. sordida, 135, 137, 185
T. tibiamaculata, 133, 145
Trichinella spiralis, 474
Trinomial classification of *Leishmania* species, 253
Trypanomorpha (avian trypanosome), 319
Trypanoplasma from freshwater fishes
  T. abramidis, 280, 321
  T. acipenseris, 322
  T. barbi, 280, 322
  T. borelli, 276, 277, 278, 280, 285, 286, 287, 289, 290, 291, 292, 294, 295, 296, 300, 302, 303, 306, 322, 323, 324, 325, 326
  T. capoetobramae, 322
  T. carassii, 314, 320, 322
  T. cataractae, 295, 301, 306, 322, 325, 326
  T. catastomi, 296, 299, 300, 322
  T. clariae, 322
  T. commersoni, 294
  T. cyprini, 291, 322, 324
  T. cyprini (= *T. borelli*), 296, 306
  T. erythroculteri, 322
  T. gandei, 322
  T. guernei, 279, 280, 322
  T. guerneyorum, 284, 295, 299, 322, 325
  T. keysselitzi, 322, 324
  T. lomakini, 322
  T. makeevi, 322, 325
  T. markewitschi, 322
  T. megalobrami, 322
  T. mirabilis, 322
  T. misgurni, 322
  T. ninae kohl-yakimovi, 322
  T. pseudocaphirhynchi, 322
  T. rutili, 322
  T. salmositica, 279, 280, 286, 291, 295, 302, 303, 322, 325, 327
  T. sarcocheilichthys, 310
  T. tincae, 322, 324
  T. truttae, 322, 325
  T. valentini, 279, 322, 325
  T. varium, 288, 306, 323
  T. willoughbii, 306, 323
Trypanoplasma sp. from *Misgurnus anguillicaudatus*, 303, 306
Trypanoplasma spp., unnamed, 323
Trypanoplasma from marine fish
  T. bullocki, 295, 323

Trypanoplasma from marine fish—*cont.*
    T. parmae, 323
Trypanoplasma spp., unnamed, 323
Trypanosoma in freshwater fish,
    T. abramis, 307
    T. acanthobramae, 307
    T. albopunctatus, 307
    T. acerinae, 295, 307
    T. amurensis, 307
    T. andrade-silvae, 307
    T. anguillae, 295
    T. anguillicola, 307
    T. anura, 307
    T. aristichthysi, 307
    T. armeti, 307
    T. ataevi, 307
    T. bancrofti, 307
    T. barbatulae, 298, 307
    T. barbi, 307
    T. batrachi, 307
    T. batrachocephali, 307
    T. bliccae, 308
    T. bourouli, 308
    T. caressi, 308
    T. catostomi, 308
    T. chagasi, 308
    T. cheni, 308
    T. chetostomi, 308
    T. choudhuryi, 308
    T. clariae, 308
    T. clariae var. *batrachi,* 308
    T. cobitis, 308, 319
    T. ctenopharyngodoni, 308
    T. danilewskyi, 271, 273, 281, 282,
        283, 285, 286, 287, 288, 289, 290,
        293, 294, 295, 296, 297, 301, 303,
        304, 305, 306, 308, 314
        strain Ma, 304
        strain Ms, 305
    T. danilewskyi var. *saccobranchi,* 308
    T. dogieli, 308
    T. dorbygnii, 308
    T. elegans, 295, 303, 308
    T. elongatus, 308
    T. ezenami, 313
    T. ferreirae, 308
    T. francirochai, 308
    T. gachuii, 308
    T. gandhei, 308
    T. gasimagomedovi, 308
    T. gerraroi, 308
    T. granulosum, 273, 280, 281, 296,
        303, 308, 326
    T. hypostomi, 308
    T. iheringi, 308
    T. langeroni, 308
    T. larsi, 308
    T. latinucleata, 308
    T. laverani, 309

    T. leucisci, 309
    T. liocassis, 309
    T. loricariae, 309
    T. lotai, 292, 309
    T. luciopercae, 309
    T. macrodonis, 309
    T. maguri, 292, 309
    T. malopteruri, 309
    T. margaritiferi, 309
    T. markewitschi, 309
    T. marplatensis, 309
    T. minuta, 309
    T. mukasai, 309
    T. mukundi, 309
    T. mylopharyngodoni, 309
    T. napolesi, 309
    T. nikitini, 309
    T. occidentalis, 309
    T. ophiocephali, 309
    T. orientalis, 309
    T. pancali, 309
    T. parasiluri, 309
    T. pellegrini, 309
    T. percae, 280, 295, 297, 303, 304,
        309, 326
    T. percae canadensis, 309
    T. phoxini, 281, 309
    T. piavae, 309
    T. pingi, 309, 314
    T. piracicahoe, 309
    T. piscium, 315
    T. plecostomi, 309
    T. pseudobagri, 310
    T. punctati, 310, 315
    T. rebeloi, 310
    T. regani, 310
    T. remaki, 295, 297, 310, 326
    T. rhamdiae, 310
    T. roulei, 310
    T. saccobranchi, 310
    T. sarcochilichthys, 310
    T. scardinii, 303, 310
    T. scerinae, 280
    T. schulmani, 310
    T. serranoi, 310
    T. siluri, 310
    T. simondi, 310
    T. siniperca, 310
    T. squalii, 280, 310
    T. striata, 303, 304, 306, 310
    T. strigaticeps, 310
    T. synodontis, 310
    T. tchangi, 310
    T. tincae, 301, 310
    T. tobeyi, 310
    T. toddi, 310
    T. trigogasterae, 310
    T. vittati, 292, 310
    T. wangi, 310

Trypanosoma—cont.
T. wincheniense, 310, 314
  (= *T.? danilewskyi*), 303, 305
T. zillii, 310
T. zungaroi, 310
Trypanosoma sp. from *Misgurnus anguillicaudatus*, 303
Trypanosoma spp., unnamed, 310–311
Trypanosoma from marine fishes
T. aegefini, 313
T. aulopi, 311
T. balistes, 312
T. bleniclini, 312
T. boissoni, 271, 304, 305, 312, 326
T. bothi, 312
T. callionymi, 312
T. capigobii, 312
T. carchariasi, 312
T. cataphracti, 312
T. caulopsettae, 312
T. cephalacanthi, 304, 312
T. coelorhynchi, 312
T. congiopodi, 312
T. cotti, 281, 312
T. delagei, 312
T. dohrni, 312
T. flesi, 312, 323
T. froesi, 312
T. gargantua, 270, 297, 312
T. giganteum, 270, 282, 297, 312
T. gobii, 312
T. heptatreti, 312
T. laternae, 312
T. limandae, 312
T. murmanensis, 280, 282, 292, 294, 298, 299, 312
T. myoxocephali, 312
T. nudigobii, 312
T. pacifica, 303, 313
T. parapercis, 313
T. platessae, 289, 292, 294, 302, 303, 313, 326
T. pulchra, 313
T. rajae, 271, 273, 281, 297, 303, 313, 314
T. scorpaenae, 313
T. scyllii, 281, 303, 313
T. soleae, 281, 313
T. sphaeroidis, 304, 313
T. torpedinis, 313
T. triglae, 313, 326
T. t. senegalensis, 304, 305, 313
T. tripterygium, 313
T. variabile, 282, 292, 298, 313, 314
T. yakimovi, 313
T. zeugopteri, 313
Trypanosoma spp., unnamed, 313
Trypanosoma diasi, 122
Trypanosoma (*Duttonella*), 695, 699,

700, 701
T. vivax, 149, 340, 342, 492, 496, 501, 503, 539, 544, 704, 709
T. vivax uniforme, 696, 699, 708
T. vivax viennei, 696, 708, 709
T. vivax vivax, 696, 699, 701, 708, 709
T. freitasi, 122
T. grayi, 658
T. grylli, 319
Trypanosoma (*Herpetosoma*), 657
infections in rodents, immunity to, 461–476
antigen and antigenic variation, 472–473
cell surface, nature of, 464, 473
immunization, 473–474
persistence of infection, 474–475
course of infection, 462–463
determinants of infection,
immunological, 464–472
ablastin, 468–472
immunodepression, 465–466, 474
passive transfer, 466–467
non-immunological, 463–464
persistence of infection, 474–475
T. (*H.*) *blanchardi*, 415
T. (*H.*) *lewisi*, 122, 138, 356, 374, 462–476, 655, 662, 665, 668
T. (*H.*) *musculi*, 462–476
T. (*H.*) *rangeli*, 122, 131, 138, 462, 491, 667
T. (*H.*) *rangeli*-like parasites, 128
"*T. majus*", 345
T. mega, 151, 271, 657, 666, 673, 677
T. (*Megatrypanum*), 657
T. (*M.*) *conorhini*, 122, 125, 128, 138, 271, 669
T. (*M.*) *legeri*, 122
T. (*M.*) *theileri*, 493
T. minasense, 118, 122
"*T. minus*", 345
T. (*Nannomonas*), 695, 699, 700, 701
T. congolense, 290, 340, 342, 492, 495, 500, 539, 544, 696, 701, 708, 709
nutrition, 662, 667, 670, 680
T. simiae, 487, 492, 696, 708
T. (*Pycnomonas*), 695
T. suis, 492, 696, 707, 708
T. ranarum, 673
T. rhodesiense (see also *T.* (*Trypanozoon*)), 290, 341
T. rotartorium, 319, 658
T. saimirii, 122
T. (*Schizotrypanum*) *cruzi*, 123, 188–190, 214, 215, 234, 326, 360, 364, 371, 487, 491, 537, 538, 548–609, 620–647, 654, 655, 656, 660, 662, 663, 664, 665, 667, 669, 671, 672

T. (*Schizotrypanum*) *cruzi—cont.*
  biochemical aspects of biology, 620–647
  energy metabolism, 625–635
    end products, 626
    oxidation of reduced pyridine nucleotides, 629–633
    pathways, 627–629
    substrates utilized, 625–626
    synthesis of ATP, 633–634
  isolation of different morphological forms, 623–625
  nucleic acid metabolism, 636–645
    deoxyribonucleotide metabolism, 641–642
    DNA (kinetoplastic), 643–644
    nucleic acid catabolism, 644
    nucleic acid synthesis, 642
    purine metabolism, 636–638
    pyrimidine, metabolism, 638–641
  biochemical characterization, 144–153
    DNA buoyant density, 150–153
    enzyme electrophoresis, 145–150
  distribution, 124–125
    mammalian hosts, 124, 125
      Artiodactyla, 124
      Carnivora
        Bassariscus, 129
        Mephitis, 124, 129
        Nasua, 124
        Procyon, 124, 129
        Urocyon, 124
      Chiroptera, 124
      Edentata
        Dasypus, 124, 129
        D. novemcinctus, 118, 128
        Tamandua tetradactyla, 128
      Lagomorpha, 124
      Marsupialia
        Didelphis, 123, 124, 129, 130, 133, 139, 145
        Didelphis spp., 131
        D. azarae, 132, 133
        D. marsupialis, 128, 186
        Lutreolina, 124
        Marmosa, 124
        M. cinerea, 128
        Philander opossum, 128
      Primates
        Alouatta, 124
        Callithrix, 124
        C. penicillata, 118
        Leontocebus, 124
        Macaca mulatta, 186
        M. philippensis, 185
        Saimiri, 124
        S. sciurius, 128
      Rodentia
        Ammospermophilus, 129

Coendou, 124
      Echimys chrysurus, 128, 186
      Nectomys squamipes, 128
      Neotoma, 124, 129, 134
      Peromyscus, 129
      Rattus, 124
      Rattus spp., 131
      R. rattus, 122, 128
      R. r. frugivorus, 132
  triatomid vector, 124, 172–178
    (see also Triatominae)
  diagnosis, 121–124
  heterogeneity, evidence for, 137–144
    biometric, 137–138
    drug sensitivity, 141–142
    enteromegaly, 140–141
    histotropism, 139
    immunological, 143–144
    infectivity to vectors, 142–143
    ultrastructural, 138
    virulence, 139
  identification of parasite,
    behavioural characteristics, 121
    biochemical characterization, 144–153
    morphology, 120–121, 621–623
  pathogenesis of infections, 548–609
    host-dependent factors, 550–552
    lesions of the central nervous system (CNS), 607–608
    natural history of Chagas' disease, 552–606
      acute phase, 553–591
        cardiopathy, 581–584
        lesions of ANS, 558
      chronic phase, 591–606
        human cardiopathy, 593–600
        megacolon and megaoesophagus, 600–606
    parasite-dependent factors, 548–549
  transmission cycles, 126–137
    enzootic *T. cruzi,*
      Amazon basin, 127–129
      U.S.A., 129–130
    sylvatic and domestic, 130–134
      continuous, 130–131
      discontinuous, 131–134
      detection of continuity between cycles, 136–137
      detection of sylvatic Triatominae, 134–136
      their significance, 126–127
  transmission, secondary modes of,
    blood transfusion, 125
    congenital, 125
    contamination with urine and faeces, 125

T. (Schizotrypanium) cruzi—cont.
  fly-borne contamination, 125
  laboratory accident, 125
  oral, 125
  via infected maternal milk, 125
  vector(s)
    bibliography, 178–184
    control, 156
    detection of sylvatic species, 134–136
    distribution, habitat and species (Appendix), 172–178
T. (S.) dionisii, 152, 154, 189
T. simiae (see also *T. (Nannomonas)*), 487, 492, 696, 708
T. suis (see also *T. (Pycnomonas)*), 492
T. thecadactyli, 34
T. theileri (see also *T. (Megatrypanum)*), 493
Trypanosoma (Trypanozoon), 408, 472, 654, 666, 667, 695, 699, 700, 701, 702
  T. brucei, 143, 145, 149, 340–384, 399, 491, 662, 664, 665, 666, 668, 670, 671, 672, 673, 679, 680, 706, 709, 710, 714
    culture forms, their significance, 357–358
    development in the mammalian host, 340–384
    life-cycle(s) in vertebrate host,
      "aberrant' forms in the blood, their significance, 354–357
    hypothetical life-cycles, 375–383
    parasitaemia, its relationship to pathological lesions, 358–359
    pleomorphism, in chicken embryos, 358
    pleomorphism, its significance, 353–354
    pleomorphism, stages in the blood, 342, 343
    filaments, 352–353
    hypothesis to account for variability, 345, 352
    methods of examination, 342–344
    tissue stages, 363–375
    ultrastructural differences, 360–363
    taxonomy, 341–342, 710
  T. brucei sspp., 151, 492, 495, 497, 505, 538, 695, 696, 699, 700, 701, 703, 707, 709
    antigenic identity of clone(s), 499
  T. b. brucei, 121, 490, 493, 494, 495, 500, 501, 504, 507, 532, 539, 544, 695, 697, 705, 707, 708, 709
    host range, 487
    pedigree of variable antigen type WiTat 1, 488
T. b. elephantis, 707
T. b. equiperdum, 662, 696, 707, 708, 709
T. b. evansi, 696, 699, 701, 708, 709
T. b. gambiense, 151, 494, 495, 496, 500, 501, 530, 532, 533, 536, 537, 544, 662, 663, 667, 672, 673, 695, 702, 704, 705, 707, 708, 709
  antigenic pattern, 539
T. b. rhodesiense, 485, 489, 494, 496, 500, 502, 508, 530, 532, 533, 536, 537, 544, 662, 663, 664, 665, 667
  antigenic pattern, 539
  "Tinde" experiment, 502–503
  variable antigen type ETat 2, 494, 495
T. equinum, 399, 696, 708
T. evansi, 342, 354, 356, 357, 360, 365, 375, 492, 496, 504, 539, 655, 663
  dyskinetoplastic stock, 504
T. evansi sspp., 399, 710
Trypanosomatidae, 242
  conjugation, 399
  evolution, 679
T. vespertilionis, 121, 148
T. vivax (see *T. (Duttonella)*)
Trypanosome-associated heterophile antibodies, methodology, 544–545
Trypanosome infections, virulence in vertebrate hosts, 482–514
  heterophile antibodies, 524–542

Varanidae, 245
VAT (variable antigen type), nomenclature, 712–713
VAT repertoire, 712
Vectors (leeches) of fish haemoflagellates, 279–286
Vectors of leishmaniasis in the USSR, 206, 209
Vector of *Leishmania chagasi,* 84–87
Vector(s) of *T. cruzi,*
  bibliography, 178–184
  control, 156
  detection of sylvatic species, 134–136
  distribution, habitat and species, 172–178
  experimental, other than Triatominae, 125
Vertebrate hosts of zoonotic cutaneous leishmaniasis,
  in Afghanistan, 198
  in Africa, 198
  in Iran, 198
  in Israel, 198
  in South America, 22–27
  see also *L. braziliensis, L. hertigi* and *L. mexicana* complex)

Virulence of trypanosomes, in the
    vertebrate host, 482–514
  changes in virulence, 500–505
    following exposure to high tem-
      perature, 504–505
    following passage,
      in laboratory animals or un-
        natural hosts, 500–502
      in natural hosts, 502–504
    induced by drugs, 504
  definition, 482, 506
  evaluation, 482–485
  evolutionary aspects, 486–490
    adaptation, 486–487
    identification of natural host, 487–
      490
  influence of host body-size, 493–494
  pathological basis, 485–486, 506–511
  range in different hosts, 491–493
    T. brucei ssp., 492
    T. congolense, 492
    T. evansi, 492
    T. equiperdum, 492
    T. simiae, 492
    T. suis, 492
    T. vivax, 492
  relationship to mechanisms of try-
    panosome, pathogenicity, 511–
    514
  virulence of different stocks of a
    single species, 494–496

Visceral leishmaniasis
  in Brazil, epidemiology, 75–84
  in South America, 68–90
  in USSR, 208–209
Vitamin B_{12}, 659
Vormela peregusna, 198
Vulpes corsak (Canidae), 208
V. vulpes, 208

WITat 1 variable antigen type, 499,
    538, 539, 544
  antigenic pattern, 539
WITat 2, 3 and 4 variable antigen types,
    499

Xenodiagnosis, 121–122

Yaeger liver-infusion-tryptose medium,
    29

Zeledon's theory of evolution, 655–656
Zelus leucogrammus (arthropod), 219,
    226, 229, 231, 234
Zoonotic cutaneous leishmaniasis in
    USSR, 198–206
Zooprophylaxis, natural, 260
Zygodontomys (Cricetidae), 61
Z. microtinus, 13
Z. pixuna, 82